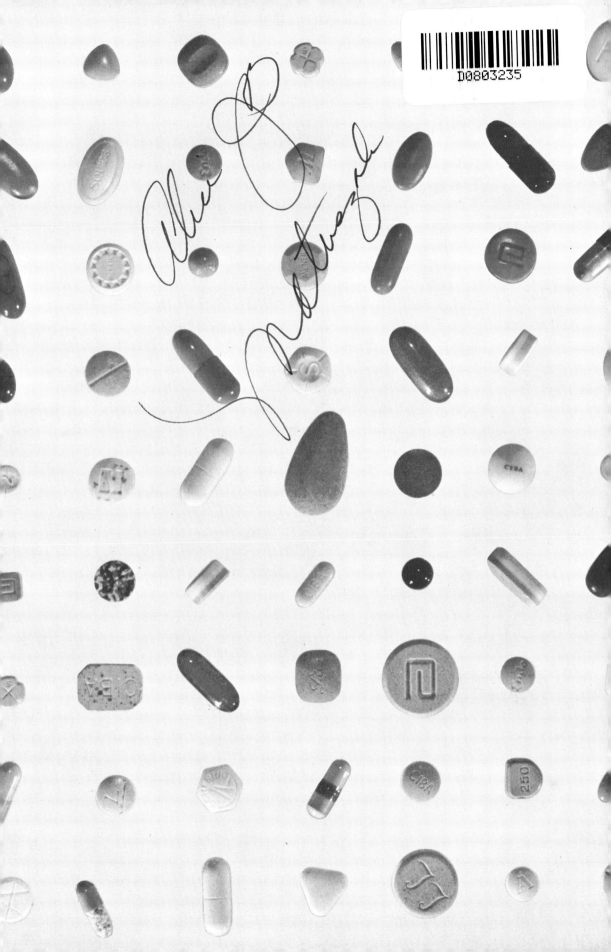

Introduction
to
Pharmaceutical
Dosage Forms

I am a Pharmacist

I am a specialist in medications

I supply medicines and pharmaceuticals to those who need them.
I prepare and compound special dosage forms.
I control the storage and preservation of all medications in my care.

I am a custodian of medical information

My library is a ready source of drug knowledge.
My files contain thousands of specific drug names and tens of thousands of
     facts about them.
My records include the medication and health history of entire families.
My journals and meetings report advances in pharmacy from around the
     world.

I am a companion of the physician

I am a partner in the case of every patient who takes any kind of medication.
I am a consultant on the merits of different therapeutic agents.
I am the connecting link between physician and patient and the final check on
     the safety of medicines.

I am a counselor to the patient

I help the patient understand the proper use of prescription medication.
I assist in the patient's choice of nonprescription drugs or in the decision to
     consult a physician.
I advise the patient on matters of prescription storage and potency.

I am a guardian of the public health

My pharmacy is a center for health-care information.
I encourage and promote sound personal health practices.
My services are available to all at all times.

This is my calling · This is my pride

Author Unknown

SECOND EDITION

Introduction
to
Pharmaceutical
Dosage Forms

Howard C. Ansel, Ph.D.
Head, Department of Pharmacy and Professor
of Pharmacy, School of Pharmacy,
University of Georgia

LEA & FEBIGER · PHILADELPHIA · 1976

Library of Congress Cataloging in Publication Data

Ansel, Howard C 1933–
  Introduction to pharmaceutical dosage forms.

  1. Drugs.   2. Pharmacology.   I. Title.
[DNLM: 1. Dosage forms. QV748 A618i]
RM300.A57   1976   615'.4   76-2487
ISBN 0-8121-0561-3

1st Edition, 1969
 Reprinted, 1972
2nd Edition, 1976

Published in Great Britain by Henry Kimpton Publishers, London
Printed in the United States of America

Preface

The SECOND edition of *Introduction to Pharmaceutical Dosage Forms* represents a major revision of the first edition, both in content and organization, although the purpose of the text remains the same—to present to the beginning pharmacy student introductory concepts of dosage form design, manufacture, and utilization.

In contrast to the traditional organization of the first edition, based solely on the physical characteristics of the various dosage forms, the second edition is arranged according to routes of administration. For instance, the various dosage forms applied topically to the skin, including those which are solutions, suspensions, powders, or semisolids, are all discussed in the chapter covering dermatological preparations.

It is felt that this new organizational approach will enable the student to better relate the basic information on drugs and dosage forms to their actual use in drug therapy. It also provides the student with the concept of dosage form alternatives in patient care. It is intended that the new structure and content of the text will contribute to the beginning pharmacy student's understanding of the role of the pharmacist as both the provider of medication and the source of information to other health professionals on the selection and use of pharmaceuticals.

As in the first edition, appropriate consideration is given in the beginning chapters to such topics as drug action, drug dosage, drug standards, dosage form design, bioavailability and good manufacturing practice. The official compendia again serve as the foundation for the drugs and dosage forms discussed in the text, although a number of nonofficial preparations are also included, as rectal and vaginal foams, ophthalmic inserts, and otic preparations. Continued from the first edition is the practice of identifying commercial counterpart products for the official preparations discussed.

An appendix chapter dealing with pharmaceutical measurement has been added and includes discussion of the systems of weight and measure, and the equipment and techniques used to measure liquids and to weigh on the pharmaceutical balance.

My sincere appreciation is extended to a number of my colleagues who have shared their thoughts with me pertaining to the revision of this text. I would particularly like to thank H. Douglas Johnson, Ph.D. for preparing the definitions of the official drug categories as they appear in the Appendix; to Larry A. Sternson, Ph.D. for his contributions to the discussion of drug solubility; to William F. Pillow, Jr. of Eli Lilly and Company and to John S. Ruggiero, Ph.D. of the Pharmaceutical Manufacturers Association, for their generous contributions to the text. I would also like to thank my secretary, Mrs. Kay Oliver, for her patience and help in the preparation of the manuscript, and to Mr. Martin C. Dallago and Mr. John F. Spahr of Lea & Febiger for their editorial assistance.

HOWARD C. ANSEL

Athens, Georgia

Contents

Chapter 1

Introduction to Drugs and Pharmacy

A DRUG may be defined as an agent intended for use in the diagnosis, mitigation, treatment, cure, or prevention of disease in man or in other animals. One of the most astounding qualities of drugs is the diversity of their actions and effects on the body. Drugs categorized as ecbolics or oxytocics stimulate the activity of the uterine muscle, but other drugs act as uterine muscle relaxants. Some drugs selectively stimulate the cardiac muscle, the smooth muscles, or the skeletal muscles; other drugs have the opposite effect. Mydriatic drugs dilate the pupil of the eye; miotics constrict or diminish pupillary size. Drugs can render blood more coagulable or less coagulable; they can increase the hemoglobin content of the erythrocytes or expand blood volume.

Drugs termed emetics induce vomiting, whereas antiemetic drugs have the opposite effect. Diuretic drugs increase the flow of urine, sudorific drugs promote sweating, expectorant drugs increase respiratory tract fluid, and cathartics or laxatives promote the evacuation of the bowel. Other drugs may decrease the flow of urine, diminish body secretions, or induce constipation.

Drugs can be employed to reduce headache, pain, fever, thyroid activity, sneezing, rhinitis, insomnia, gastric acidity, motion sickness, and mental depression. Drugs can elevate the mood, the blood pressure, or the activity of the endocrine glands. Drugs can combat infectious disease, destroy intestinal worms, or act as antidotes against the poisoning effects of still other drugs. Antineoplastic drugs provide one means of attacking the cancerous process; radioactive pharmaceuticals provide another.

Drugs may be used to diagnose diabetes, liver malfunction, tuberculosis, or pregnancy, or they may be employed to replenish a body deficient in antibodies, vitamins, hormones, electrolytes, protein, enzymes, or blood. Drugs may be used to prevent measles, poliomyelitis, or pregnancy or to assist the maintenance of pregnancy or to extend life itself.

Certainly the vast array of effective medicinal agents available today represents one of man's greatest scientific accomplishments. It would be frightening to perceive of our civilization devoid of these remarkable and beneficial agents. Through their use, many of the diseases which have plagued mankind throughout history, as smallpox and poliomyelitis, are now facing extinction. Illnesses such as diabetes, hypertension, and mental depression are now effectively controlled with modern drugs. Today's surgical procedures would be virtually impossible without the benefit of general anesthetics, analgesics, antibiotics, blood transfusions, and intravenous fluids and nutrients.

The process of drug discovery and development is no simple task. It involves the collective contributions of many scientific specialists including organic, physical, and analytical chemists, biochemists, bacteriologists, physiologists, pharmacologists, toxicologists, hematologists, immunologists, endocrinologists, pathologists, biostatisticians, pharmaceutical scientists, clinical physicians and many others.

After a potential new drug substance is discovered and has undergone definitive chemical and physical characterization, a great deal of biological information must be gathered. The basic *pharmacology* or the nature and mechanism of action of the drug on the biological system must be determined including toxicologic features. A study must be made of the drug's site and rate of absorption, its pattern of distribution and concentration within the body, its duration of action, and the method and rate of its elimination or excretion. Information must be obtained on the drug's metabolic degradation and the activity of any of its metabolites.

A comprehensive study must be made of the drug's short term and long term effects on various body cells, tissues, and organs. Highly specific information may be obtained, as the effect of the drug on the fetus of a pregnant animal or its ability to pass to a nursing baby through the breast milk of its mother. Many a promising new drug has been abandoned because of its potential to cause excessive or hazardous adverse effects.

A new drug's most effective routes of administration (e.g., oral, rectal, parenteral) must be determined and guidelines established concerning the dosage recommended for persons of varying ages, weights, and states of illness. To facilitate administration of the drug by the selected routes, appropriate *dosage forms* as tablets, capsules, injections, suppositories, ointments, aerosols, and others are formulated and prepared. These dosage forms are highly sophisticated pharmaceutical drug delivery systems. Their design, development, production, and use are a prime example of the application of the pharmaceutical sciences—the blending of the basic, applied, and clinical sciences with pharmaceutical technology.

Each particular pharmaceutical product is a formulation unique unto itself. In addition to the active therapeutic ingredients, a pharmaceutical formulation also contains a number of nontherapeutic agents. These agents are generally referred to as *pharmaceutical adjuncts*, *excipients* or *necessities*, and it is through their use that a formulation achieves its unique composition and characteristic physical appearance. Included are such things as fillers, thickeners, vehicles, suspending agents, tablet disintegrants, stabilizing agents, preservatives, flavors, colorants, and sweeteners. *Dosage units*, as capsules, tablets, or "unit-dose" packages of liquid medications, are designed to contain a specified quantity of medication for ease and accuracy of dosage administration.

In order to assure the stability of a drug in a formulation and the continued effectiveness of the drug product throughout its usual shelf life,[1] the principles of chemistry, physical phar-

macy, microbiology, and pharmaceutical technology must be applied. The formulation must be such that all components are physically and chemically compatible, including the active therapeutic agents, the pharmaceutical necessities, and the packaging materials. The formulation must be preserved against decomposition due to chemical degradation and protected from microbial contamination and the destructive influences of excessive heat, light, and moisture. The therapeutic ingredients must be released from the dosage form in the proper amount and in such a manner that the onset and duration of the drug's action is that which is desired. The pharmaceutical product must lend itself to efficient administration and must possess attractive features of flavor, odor, color, and texture that enhance patient acceptance. Finally, the product must be effectively packaged and clearly and completely labeled according to existing legal regulations.

Once prepared, the pharmaceutical product must be properly administered if the patient is to receive maximum benefit. The medication must be taken in sufficient quantity, at specified intervals, and for an indicated duration of time. The effectiveness of the medication in achieving the prescriber's objectives should be reevaluated at regular intervals and necessary adjustments made in the dosage, *dosage regimen* or dosage schedule, dosage form, or indeed, in the choice of the drug administered. Patient expressions of disappointment in his rate of progress or complaints of side effects to the prescribed drug should be evaluated upon report and decisions made as to the continuance, minor adjustment, or major change in drug therapy. Prior to initially taking a medication, a patient should be warned of any expected minor side effects, and of foods, beverages, and/or other drugs which may interfere with the effectiveness of the medication or with the course of therapy.

Through professional interaction and communication with other health professionals the pharmacist is able to contribute greatly to patient care. His intimate knowledge of drug ac-

---

[1]The term "shelf life" refers to the length of time a drug product may remain on the (pharmacist's) shelf, in the original package and under usual environmental conditions, and retain an acceptable level of its original potency and overall quality. In most instances solid dosage forms, as tablets and capsules, have a shelf life of 5 years from the date of manufacture. Usually

liquid dosage forms, disperse systems as aerosols and emulsions, and semisolid forms as ointments and suppositories have shorter shelf lives. However, a great deal depends upon the individual chemical and physical characteristics of the active ingredients, the formulative materials, and the packaging employed. Poor storage conditions, with extremes of temperature, humidity, and light can adversely affect the stability of pharmaceutical products.

tions, drug therapy, dosage form design and utilization, available pharmaceutical products, and drug information sources makes him a vital member of the health care team. He is entrusted with the legal responsibility for the procurement, storage, control and distribution of effective pharmaceutical products and for the compounding and filling of prescription orders. Utilizing his extensive training and knowledge, the pharmacist serves the patient as an advisor on drugs and encourages their safe and proper utilization. The pharmacist delivers pharmaceutical services in a variety of community and institutional health care environments and effectively utilizes record-keeping and monitoring techniques in safeguarding the public health.

To appreciate the progress that has been made in drug discovery and development in recent years and to provide some background for the study of modern drugs and pharmaceutical dosage forms, it is important to examine pharmacy's heritage.

The Heritage of Pharmacy

Drugs, in the form of vegetation and minerals, have existed longer than man himself. Human disease and man's instinct to survive have, through the ages, led to their discovery. The use of drugs, crude though they may have been, undoubtedly dates back long prior to recorded history, for the instinct of primitive man to relieve the pain of a wound by bathing it in cool water or by soothing it with a fresh leaf or protecting it with mud is within the realm of belief. From experience primitive man would learn that certain therapy was more effective than others, and from these beginnings the practice of drug therapy began.

Among many early races, disease was believed to be caused by the entrance of demons or evil spirits into the body. The treatment quite naturally involved ridding the body of the supernatural intruders. From the earliest records of history it is evident that the primary methods of doing so were through the use of spiritual incantations, the application of noisome materials, and the administration of specific herbs or plants.

The First Apothecary

Before the days of the priestcraft, the wise man or woman of the tribe, whose knowledge of the healing qualities of plants had been gathered through experience or handed down by word of mouth, was called upon to attend to the sick or wounded and prepare the remedy. It was in the preparation of the medicinal materials that the art of the apothecary originated.

The art of the apothecary has always been associated with the mysterious, and its practitioners were believed to have connection with the world of spirits and thus performed as intermediaries between the seen and the unseen. The belief that a drug had magical associations meant that its action, for good or for evil, did not depend upon its natural qualities alone. The compassion of a god, the observance of ceremonies, the absence of evil spirits, and the healing intent of the dispenser were individually and collectively needed to make the drug therapeutically effective. Because of this, the tribal apothecary was one to be feared, respected, trusted, sometimes mistrusted, worshipped, and revered, for it was through his potions that spiritual contact was made and upon which the cures or failures depended. Throughout history the knowledge of drugs and their application to disease has always meant power. In the Homeric epics, the term *pharmakon* (Gr.) from which our word *pharmacy* was derived connotes a charm or a drug that can be used for good or for evil purposes. Many of the tribal apothecary's failures were doubtless due to impotent medicines, inappropriate medicines, underdosage, overdosage, and even poisoning. His successes may be attributed to an appropriate drug based on his experience, coincidence of proper therapy, inconsequential effect of the therapy for an individual with a nonfatal illness, or *placebo effects*, that is, successful treatment due to psychologic rather than therapeutic effects. Even today, placebo therapy with nonpotent or inconsequential chemicals is successfully employed in the treatment of individual patients and is a routine practice in the clinical evaluation of new drugs where group response to the effects of the actual drug and the placebo are compared and evaluated.

As time passed, the art of the apothecary became combined with priestly functions, and among the early civilizations the priest-magician or priest-physician became the healer of the body as well as of the soul. Pharmacy and medicine are indistinguishable in their early history, since their practice was generally the function of the tribal religious leaders.

Early Drugs

Due to the patience and intellect of the archeologist, the types and the specific drugs employed in the early history of drug therapy are not as indefinable as one might suspect. Numerous ancient tablets, scrolls, and other relics dating as far back as 3000 B.C. have been uncovered and deciphered by archeological scholars to the delight of historians of both medicine and pharmacy, for contained in these ancient documents are specific associations with our common heritage.

Perhaps the most famous of these surviving memorials is the *Papyrus Ebers*, a continuous scroll some 60 feet long and a foot wide dating back to the sixteenth century before Christ. This document, which is now preserved at the University of Leipzig, is named for the noted German Egyptologist, Georg Ebers, who discovered it in the tomb of a mummy and partly translated it during the last half of the nineteenth century. Since that time, many scholars have participated in the translation of the document's challenging hieroglyphics, and although they are not unanimous in their interpretations there is little doubt that by 1550 B.C. the Egyptians were using many of the same drugs and dosage forms still employed today.

The text of the Ebers Papyrus is dominated by drug formulas, with more than 800 formulas or prescriptions being described and over 700 different drugs being mentioned. The drugs referred to are chiefly botanic, although mineral and animal drugs are also noted. Such currently used botanic drugs as acacia, castor bean (from which we express castor oil), and fennel are mentioned along with apparent references to such minerals as iron oxide, sodium carbonate, sodium chloride, and sulfur. Animal excrements were also employed in drug therapy.

The formulative vehicles of the day were beer, wine, milk, and honey. Many of the pharmaceutical formulas employed two dozen or more different medicinal agents, a type of preparation later referred to as a "polypharmacal." Mortars, hand mills, sieves, and balances were commonly used by the Egyptians in their compounding of suppositories, gargles, pills, inhalations, troches, lotions, ointments, plasters, and enemas.

Introduction of the Scientific Viewpoint

Throughout history many individuals have contributed to the advancement of the health sciences. Notable among those whose genius and creativeness had a revolutionary influence on the development of pharmacy and medicine were Hippocrates (ca. 460–377 B.C.), Dioscorides (1st century A.D.), Galen (ca. 130–200 A.D.), and Paracelsus (1493–1541 A.D.).

Hippocrates was a Greek physician who is credited with the introduction of scientific pharmacy and medicine. He rationalized medicine, systematized medical knowledge, and put the practice of medicine on a high ethical plane. His thinking on the ethics and science of medicine dominated the medical writings of his and successive generations, and his concepts and precepts are embodied into the now renowned Hippocratic oath of ethical behavior for the healing professions. His works included the descriptions of hundreds of drugs, and it was during this period that the term *pharmakon* came to mean a purifying remedy for good only, transcending the previous connotation of a charm or drug for good or for evil purposes. Because of his pioneering work in medical science and his inspirational teachings and advanced philosophies that have become a part of modern medicine, Hippocrates is honored by being called the "Father of Medicine."

Dioscorides, a Greek physician and botanist, was the first to deal with botany as an applied science of pharmacy. His work, *De Materia Medica*, is considered a milestone in the development of pharmaceutical botany and in the studies of naturally occurring medicinal materials. This area of study is today known as pharmacognosy, a term formed from two Greek words, *pharmakon*, drug, and *gnōsis*, knowledge. Many of the drugs described by Dioscorides, as aspidium, opium, ergot, hyoscyamus, and cinnamon, are also used in medicine today. His descriptions of the art of identifying and collecting natural drug products, the methods of their proper storage, and the means of detecting adulterants or contaminants were the standards of the period and established the need for additional work and the guidelines for future investigations.

Claudius Galen, a Greek pharmacist-physician who attained Roman citizenship, aimed to create a perfect system of physiology, pathology, and treatment and formulated doctrines that were followed for 1500 years. He was one of the most prolific authors of his or any other era, having been credited with 500 treatises on medicine and some 250 others on subjects of philosophy, law, and grammar. His medical writings include descriptions of numerous drugs of natural origin with a profusion of drug formulas and methods of compounding. He originated so many preparations of vegetable drugs by mixing or melting the individual ingredients that the area of pharmaceutical preparations has been commonly referred to as "Galenic pharmacy." Perhaps the most famous of his formulas is one for a cold cream, called Galen's Cerate, which is remarkably similar in formulation to some in use today.

Pharmacy remained a function of medicine until the increasing variety of drugs and the growing complexity of compounding demanded specialists who could devote full attention to the art. Pharmacy was officially separated from medicine for the first time in 1240 when a decree of the German Emperor Frederick II regulated the practice of pharmacy within that part of his kingdom called the Two Sicilies. His edict separating the two professions acknowledged that pharmacy required special knowledge, skill, initiative, and responsibility if adequate care to the medical needs of the people was to be guaranteed. Pharmacists were obligated by oath to prepare reliable drugs of uniform quality according to their art. Any exploitation of the patient through business relations between the pharmacist and the physician was strictly forbidden. Between that time and the evolution of chemistry as an exact science, pharmacy and chemistry became united somewhat as pharmacy and medicine had been.

Perhaps no man in history exercised such a revolutionary influence on pharmacy and medicine as did Aureolus Philippus Theophrastus Bombastus von Hohenheim, a Swiss physician and chemist who called himself Paracelsus. He influenced tremendously the transformation of pharmacy from a profession based primarily on botanic science to one based on chemical science. Some of his chemical observations were astounding for his time and for their anticipation of later discoveries. He believed that it was possible to prepare a specific medicinal agent for use in combating each specific disease and introduced a host of chemical substances to internal therapy. Some of the formulas he devised, some of the names he coined, and some of the theories he advanced have become a part of our daily practice of pharmacy.

Early Research

As the knowledge of the basic sciences increased, so did their application to pharmacy. The opportunity was presented for the investiga-

tion of medicinal materials on a firm scientific basis, and the challenge was accepted by numerous pharmacists who conducted their research in the backrooms and basements of their pharmacies. Noteworthy among them was Karl Wilhelm Scheele (1742–1786), a Swedish pharmacist who is perhaps the most famous of all pharmacists because of his scientific genius and dramatic discoveries. Among his discoveries were the chemicals lactic acid, citric acid, oxalic acid, tartaric acid, and arsenic acid. He identified glycerin, invented new methods of preparing calomel and benzoic acid, and discovered oxygen a year prior to Priestley.

The isolation of morphine from opium by the German pharmacist Friedrich Sertürner (1783–1841) in 1805 prompted a series of isolations of other active materials from medicinal plants by a score of French pharmacists. Joseph Caventou (1795–1877) and Joseph Pelletier (1788–1842) combined their talents and isolated quinine and cinchonine from cinchona, and strychnine and brucine from nux vomica. Pelletier together with Pierre Robiquet (1780–1840) isolated caffeine, and Robiquet independently separated codeine from opium. Methodically one chemical after another was isolated from plant drugs and identified as an agent responsible for the plants' medicinal activity. Today we are still engaged in this fascinating activity as we probe nature for more useful and more specific therapeutic agents.

Throughout Europe during the late 18th century and the beginning of the 19th century, pharmacists like Pelletier and Sertürner were held in great esteem by their communities because of their intellect and technical abilities. They applied the art and the science of pharmacy to the preparation of drug products that were of the highest standards of purity, uniformity, and efficacy possible at that time. The extraction and isolation of various active constituents from crude or unprocessed drugs were a major breakthrough in the development of concentrated dosage forms of uniform strength containing singly effective therapeutic agents of natural origin. Many pharmacists of the period began to manufacture quality pharmaceutical products on a small but steadily increasing scale to meet the growing drug needs of their communities. Some of today's gigantic pharmaceutical manufacturing companies developed from these progressive prescription laboratories of over a century and a half ago.

Although many of the drugs indigenous to America and first used by the American Indian were adopted by the settlers, the vast majority of drugs needed in this country before the 19th century were imported from Europe, either as the raw materials or as finished pharmaceutical products. With the Revolutionary War, however, it became more difficult to import drugs, and the American pharmacist was stimulated to acquire the scientific and technologic expertise of his European contemporary. From this period until the Civil War, pharmaceutical manufacture as we know it today was in its infancy in this country, but some of the pharmaceutical firms established during that period are still preparing drugs. Three firms are known to have been established before 1826, with 22 additional ones having their origin in the subsequent half century. In 1821, the first American school of pharmacy was established in Philadelphia.

The United States Pharmacopeia

The term *pharmacopeia* comes from the Greek, *pharmakon*, meaning "drug," and *poiein*, meaning "make," and the combination indicates any recipe or formula or other standards required to make or prepare a drug. The term was first used in 1580 in connection with a local book of drug standards in Bergamo, Italy. From that time on there were countless city, state, and national pharmacopeias published by various European pharmaceutical societies. As time passed, the value of a uniform set of drug standards within a nation became apparent. In England, for example, three city pharmacopeias— the London, the Edinburgh, and the Dublin— were official throughout the kingdom until 1864, when they were replaced by the British Pharmacopoeia (BP).

In the United States drug standards were first provided on a national basis in 1820, when the first *United States Pharmacopeia* (USP) was published. The need for drug standards was recognized, however, in this country long before the first USP was published. For convenience and because of their familiarity with them, colonial physicians and apothecaries used the pharmacopeias and other references of their various homelands. The first American pharmacopeia was the so-called "Lititz Pharmacopeia," published in 1778 at Lititz, Pennsylvania, for use by the Military Hospital of the United States Army. It was a 32-page booklet containing information on 84 internal and 16 external drugs and preparations.

During the last decade of the 18th century, several attempts were made by various local medical societies to collate drug information, set appropriate standards, and prepare an extensive American pharmacopeia of the drugs in use at that time. In 1808 the Massachusetts Medical Society published a 272-page pharmacopeia containing information or monographs on 536 drugs and pharmaceutical preparations. Included were monographs on many drugs indigenous to America, which were not described in the European pharmacopeias of the day.

On January 6, 1817, Dr. Lyman Spalding, a physician from New York City, submitted a plan to the Medical Society of the County of New York for the creation of a national pharmacopeia. Dr. Spalding's efforts were later to result in his being recognized as the "Father of the United States Pharmacopeia." He proposed dividing the United States as then known into four geographical districts—the Northern, Middle, Southern, and Western. The plan provided for calling a convention in each of these districts, to be composed of delegates from all medical societies and medical schools within them. Where there was as yet no incorporated medical society or medical school, voluntary associations of physicians and surgeons were invited to assist in the undertaking. Each district's convention was to draft a pharmacopeia and appoint delegates to a general convention to be held later in Washington, D.C. At the general convention, the four district pharmacopeias were to be compiled into a single national pharmacopeia.

Draft pharmacopeias were submitted to the convention by only the Northern and Middle districts. These were reviewed, consolidated, and adopted by the first United States Pharmacopeial Convention assembled in Washington, D.C., on January 1, 1820. The first *United States Pharmacopeia* was published on December 15, 1820, in English and also in Latin, then the international language of medicine, to render the book more intelligible to physicians and pharmacists of any nationality. Within its 272 pages were listed 217 drugs considered worthy of recognition, many of them taken from the Massachusetts Pharmacopeia, which is considered by some to be the precursor to the USP. The objective of the first USP was clearly stated in its preface and still serves as the guideline for drug admissions. It reads in part:

"It is the objective of a Pharmacopeia to select from among substances which possess medicinal power, those, the utility of which is most fully established and best understood; and to form from them preparations and compositions, in which their powers may be exerted to the greatest advantage. It should likewise distinguish those articles by convenient and definite names, such as may prevent trouble or uncertainty in the intercourse of physicians and apothecaries."

Before adjourning, the Convention adopted a Constitution and Bylaws, with provisions for subsequent meetings of the Convention leading to a revised *United States Pharmacopeia* every 10 years. As many new drugs entered into drug therapy, the need for more frequent issuance of standards became increasingly apparent. In 1900, the Pharmacopeial Convention granted authority to issue supplements to the currently official USP whenever necessary to maintain satisfactory standards. At the 1940 meeting of the Convention, it was decided to revise the Pharmacopeia every 5 years while maintaining the use of periodic supplements. The *United States Pharmacopeia* was last revised on September 1, 1975, with the issuance of the USP XIX, the 19th revision of the compendium.

The first United States Pharmacopeial Convention was composed exclusively of physicians. In 1830, and again in 1840, prominent pharmacists were invited to assist in the revision, and in recognition of their contributions pharmacists were awarded full membership in the Convention of 1850 and have participated regularly ever since. Indeed, by 1870 the *Pharmacopeia* was so nearly in the hands of pharmacists that vigorous efforts were required to revive interest in it among physicians. The present Bylaws provide that a minimum of one-third of the members of the Board of Trustees and of the Committee of Revision shall represent the medical profession.

After the appearance of the first USP, the art and science of both pharmacy and medicine changed remarkably. Prior to 1820, the drugs employed in the treatment of disease had been much the same for centuries. The *Pharmacopeia* of 1820 reflected the fact that the apothecary of that day was competent at collecting and identifying botanic drugs and preparing from them the mixtures and preparations required by the physician. The individual pharmacist

seemed quite fulfilled as he applied his total art to the creation of elegant pharmaceutical preparations from crude botanic materials. It was a time that would never be seen again because of the impending upsurge in technologic capabilities and the steady development of the basic sciences, particularly synthetic organic chemistry.

The second half of the 19th century brought great and far-reaching changes. The United States was now under the full impact of the industrial revolution. The steam engine, which used water power to turn mills that powdered crude botanic drugs, was replaced by the gas, diesel, or electric motor. New machinery was substituted for the old whenever and wherever possible, and often machinery from other industries was adapted to the special needs of pharmaceutical manufacturing. Mixers from the baking industry, centrifugal machines from the laundry industry, and sugarcoating pans from the candy industry were a few examples of the type of improvisations made. Production increased rapidly, but the new industry had to wait for the scientific revolution before it could claim newer and better drugs for mankind. A symbiosis was needed between science and the advancing technology.

Chemotherapy

By 1880, the industrial manufacture of chemicals and pharmaceutical products had become well established in this country, and the pharmacist was relying heavily upon commercial sources for his drug supply. Synthetic organic chemistry began to have its influence on drug therapy. The isolations of some active constituents of plant drugs had led to knowledge of their chemical structure. From this arose methods of synthetically duplicating the same structures, as well as manipulating molecular structure to produce organic chemicals yet undiscovered in nature. In 1872 the synthesis of salicylic acid from phenol inaugurated the synthesis of a group of analgesic compounds. Other new chemicals synthesized for the first time were phenolphthalein, a laxative, and sleep-producing derivatives of barbituric acid called "barbiturates." A new source of drugs, synthetic organic chemistry, welcomed the turn into the 20th century.

Until this time, drugs created through the genius of the synthetic organic chemist relieved a host of maladies, but none had been found to be curative—none, that is, until 1910, when arsphenamine, a specific agent against syphilis, was introduced to medical science. This was the start of an era of chemotherapy, an era in which the diseases of mankind became curable through the use of specific chemical agents. The concepts, discoveries, and inspirational work that led mankind to this glorious period are credited to Paul Ehrlich, the German bacteriologist who together with a Japanese colleague, Sahachiro Hata, discovered arsphenamine. Today most of our new drugs, whether they be curative or palliative, originate in the flask of the synthetic organic chemist.

Federal Regulation

The advancement of science, both basic and applied, led to drugs of a more complex nature and to more of them. The drug standards advanced by the USP were more than ever needed to protect the public by insuring the purity and uniformity of the drugs administered. The authority of the *United States Pharmacopeia* in setting these standards was recognized fairly early in the statutes of some states, but federal recognition did not come about until June 30, 1906, when President Theodore Roosevelt signed into law the first federal Pure Food and Drug Act. This law designated the USP as establishing the standard of strength, quality, and purity of medicinal agents recognized within it, when sold in interstate commerce for medicinal use. The *National Formulary* (NF), a publication of the American Pharmaceutical Association, was given the same legal standing by the law. Thus, the USP and the NF of current revision are called "official compendia." Among other things, the law of 1906 requires that whenever the designations "USP" or "NF" are used or implied on drug labeling with respect to official drugs or preparations, the products must conform to the physical and chemical standards as set forth for the drug in the compendium monograph. With the passage of the law of 1906, the USP and the NF became indispensable to the entire American drug trade.

The National Formulary

When the American Pharmaceutical Association was organized in 1852, the only authoritative and generally recognized book of drug standards available was the third revision of the *United States Pharmacopeia*. In order to serve as a therapeutic guide to the medical profession, its scope, then as now, was restricted to drugs of established therapeutic merit. Because of this policy of strict selectivity, many drugs and formulas that were widely accepted and used by the medical profession were not granted admission to early revisions of the *Pharmacopeia*. As a type of a protest, and in keeping with the original objectives of the American Pharmaceutical Association to establish standardization of drugs and formulas, certain pharmacists, with the sanction of their national organization, prepared a formulary containing many of the popular drugs and formulas denied admission to the *Pharmacopeia*. The first edition was published in 1888 under the title *National Formulary of Unofficial Preparations*. The designation *Unofficial Preparations* reflected the protest mood of the authors, since the *Pharmacopeia* had earlier adopted the term "official" as applying to the drugs for which it provided standards. The title was changed to *National Formulary* when the Pure Food and Drug Act of 1906 made it an *official* compendium. The early editions of the *National Formulary* served mainly as a convenience to practicing pharmacists by providing uniform names of drugs and preparations and working directions for the small-scale manufacture of popular pharmaceutical preparations prescribed by physicians. Today the drugs and formulas included in each new edition of the *National Formulary* are selected on the basis of therapeutic or pharmaceutic merit, not because of popularity or extent of use. However, they are still selected from among those drugs and preparations not voted admission to the concurrent revision of the *Pharmacopeia*. The determination of the drugs and preparations to be admitted, along with their chemical and physical standards, is entrusted to the chairman and ten members of the National Formulary Board, appointed by the Board of Trustees of the American Pharmaceutical Association. Like the *Pharmacopeia*, the *National Formulary* was originally revised every 10 years, but since 1940 a new edition has appeared every 5 years. Between editions, revision announcements or supplements are issued as required. The currently official *National Formulary*, the 14th edition (NF XIV), replaced the previous edition on September 1, 1975.

On January 2, 1975, the United States

Pharmacopeial Convention, Inc. purchased the National Formulary, unifying the official compendia and thereby provided the mechanism for a single, national compendium.

The progress made in the science and technology of pharmacy, in drug therapy, and in the practice of pharmacy and medicine is reflected in each new edition or revision of the official compendia. The deletion of Latin titles for drugs, the elimination of many synonyms for drugs, and the demise of the apothecaries' system of weights and measures in favor of the metric system are compendia changes that are of historic significance. The steadily diminishing number of official galenicals and polypharmacal preparations and their replacement by synthetic organic medicinals, biologic products, and radioactive pharmaceuticals reflect the progress of drug therapy and our improved technologic capabilities. Our increased development of and dependence upon new analytical techniques can be demonstrated by the steady incorporation of new methods of analysis into the text of the compendia. Such recommended methods as ultraviolet, infrared, and atomic absorption spectrophotometry, nonaqueous titrimetry, fluorometry, polarography, turbidimetry, gas-liquid chromatography, and complexometry are testimony of increased scientific competence, the diversity and complexity of drugs and pharmaceutical products, and the increased investment of pharmaceutical research and manufacturing firms in drug production and quality control.

The standards advanced by the *United States Pharmacopeia* and the *National Formulary* are put to active use by all members of the health care industry who share the responsibility and enjoy the public's trust for assuring the availability of quality drugs and pharmaceutical products. Included in this group are pharmacists, physicians, dentists, veterinarians, nurses, producers and suppliers of bulk chemicals for use in drug production, large and small manufacturers of pharmaceutical products, drugs procurement officers of various private and public health agencies and institutions, drug regulatory and enforcement agencies, and many others.

To provide direct laboratory assistance to the *National Formulary* and the *United States Pharmacopeia*, the Drug Standards Laboratory of the American Pharmaceutical Association Foundation was established in 1961. This analytical laboratory was jointly sponsored by the American Pharmaceutical Association, the American Medical Association, and the United States Pharmacopeial Convention, until its purchase in 1975 by the latter organization. The Laboratory's main functions are to develop specifications for new drugs, check new drug specifications proposed by others, assist in the development of official monographs, improve existing compendia monographs through the incorporation of more sophisticated analytical procedures, develop and evaluate new analytical methods which may be employed in the analysis of drugs in their basic state or in dosage forms, participate in collaborative studies with other laboratories with regard to drug standards, and to provide laboratory services regarding special problems relating to drugs and dosage forms.

Other Pharmacopeias and Drug Standards

In addition to the USP and the NF, other references of drug standards such as the *Homeopathic Pharmacopeia of the United States* and the *International Pharmacopoeia* (IP) provide additional guidelines for drug quality required by certain practitioners and agencies. The *Homeopathic Pharmacopeia* is employed by a dwindling number of pharmacists and homeopathists and by law enforcement agencies which must insure the quality of homeopathic drugs. The term *homeopathy* was coined by Samuel Hahnemann (1755–1843) from the Greek *homoios*, meaning similar, and *pathos*, meaning disease. In essence, the philosophy of homeopathy is that like cures like: that is, a drug that produces in healthy persons the effects or set of symptoms of the illness present will cure the disease. Embodied in the homeopathic approach are (1) the testing of a drug on healthy persons to find the drug's effects so that it may be employed against the same symptoms manifesting a disease in an ill person, (2) the use of only minute doses of drugs in therapy, (3) the administration of not more than one drug at a time, and (4) the treatment of the entire symptom complex of the patient, not just one symptom. The *Homeopathic Pharmacopeia* is essential for pharmacists who prepare drugs to be used in the practice of homeopathy.

The *Pharmacopeia Internationalis*, or *International Pharmacopoeia*, is published by the World Health Organization (WHO) of the United Nations with the cooperation of member countries. It is intended as a recommendation to national pharmacopeial revision committees to modify their respective pharmacopeias according to the international standards adopted. It has no legal authority, only the mutual respect and recognition accorded it by the participating countries in their joint effort to provide acceptable drug standards on an international basis. The first volume of the *Pharmacopoeia Internationalis* was published in 1951. It has been revised periodically since that time.

A number of countries publish their own pharmacopeias, including Great Britain, France, Italy, Japan, India, East Germany, Norway, and the Union of Soviet Socialist Republics. Many of these pharmacopeias are utilized by multinational companies who develop and market products on an international basis. Countries not having a national pharmacopeia frequently adopt one of another country for their use in setting and regulating drug standards. The pharmacopeia selected is usually one based on geographic proximity, a common heritage or language, or a similarity of drugs and pharmaceutical products used.

In the United States, in addition to the official compendia, important drug standards are provided by means of the specifications set forth in individual New Drug and Antibiotic Applications approved by the Food and Drug Administration. The approved standards for individually marketed drugs must be rigidly adhered to by the manufacturer thereby maintaining the established quality of the product.

The Development
of New Drugs

The drug or pharmaceutical industry is a complex blend of interdependent persons, professions, trades, companies, and organizations, each engaged in activities directed toward providing for the drug requirements of the nation. In the broad sense, the pharmaceutical industry encompasses all persons involved or required between the time a drug is first envisioned in the mind of a scientist to the time it is consumed by the patient. In the narrow sense, it is frequently used synonymously with the term "industrial pharmacy," which refers to the

pharmaceutical research and manufacturing companies providing pharmacists with medicines in prefabricated or ready-to-take form. Some firms specialize in manufacturing *proprietary* drug products, or those sold over-the-counter and advertised and promoted directly to the public. Other firms limit their activities to the production of *ethical* pharmaceuticals, or those products that may be prescription drugs or over-the-counter drugs but are promoted directly to the medical and pharmaceutical practitioner and not to the general public. Many of the large companies manufacture both categories of pharmaceutical with some having subsidiary companies to specialize in either of the two functions.

The pharmaceutical industry in the United States grew phenomenally during World War II and in the years immediately following. The upsurge in the domestic production of drugs and pharmaceutical products stemmed in part from the wartime hazards and consequent undependability of overseas shipping, the unavailability of drugs from former sources in the enemy camp or control, and the increased need for drugs of all kinds, especially those of lifesaving capabilities. One such drug is penicillin, which became commercially available in 1944, some 15 years after serendipitous discovery in England by Sir Alexander Fleming. The delay in the development of penicillin was in part due to a poor appreciation for its potential, and thus for many years it was not investigated with the required vigor.

After the war, other antibiotics were developed and today there is a host of them, some effective against limited types of microorganisms with others having a broad range of activity against pathogens. The postwar boom in drug discovery continued and has provided many drugs important to the conquest of disease. Vaccines, such as those effective in preventing poliomyelitis, measles, and influenza, have been as beneficial to mankind in preventing disease as have the antibiotic drugs in curing disease. New pharmacological categories of drugs were developed in this period, including oral hypoglycemic drugs effective against certain types of diabetes mellitus, antineoplastic drugs active against the cancerous process, immunosuppressive agents which assist the body's acceptance of organ transplants, oral contraceptives, which prevent pregnancy, and a host of tranquilizers and antidepressant drugs that provide assistance to the emotionally distraught or distressed.

Most of the basic and applied research leading to the development of new drugs and ethical pharmaceuticals is performed by the major drug companies, which comprise approximately 15% of the nation's drug manufacturing firms but account for over 95% of the nation's total sales of ethical drugs. These companies by and large comprise the membership of the Pharmaceutical Manufacturers Association (the PMA), an organization founded in 1958 as the successor to the American Pharmaceutical Manufacturers Association and the American Drug Manufacturers Association. It is generally regarded as the spokesman for the prescription-drug manufacturers in matters of medical and pharmaceutical science, technologic advancements in drug manufacturing methods, and drug marketing matters. Its member companies have been largely responsible for establishing the United States as a world leader in the creation and development of new drugs and pharmaceutical products. New drugs are also being created in the laboratories of research scientists employed by academic and nonprofit research institutions; however, they too are ultimately supplied as finished drug products to the community pharmacist by the industrial pharmaceutical manufacturing firms.

Sources of New Drugs

New drugs may be discovered from a variety of natural sources or created synthetically in the laboratory. They may be found quite by accident or as the result of many years of tireless pursuit.

Throughout history, plant materials have served as a reservoir of potential new drugs. It has been estimated that only 8% of the plant species thus far identified have been investigated for medicinal agents. Certain major contributions to modern drug therapy may be attributed to the successful conversion of botanic folklore remedies into modern wonder drugs. The chemical reserpine, a tranquilizer and hypotensive agent, is an example of a medicinal chemical isolated by design from the folklore remedy *Rauwolfia serpentina*. Another plant drug, periwinkle or *Vinca rosea*, was scientifically investigated as a result of its reputation in folklore as an agent useful in the treatment of diabetes mellitus. Plant extractives yielded two potent drugs, which when screened for pharmacologic activity surprisingly exhibited anti-

tumor capabilities. These two materials, vinblastine and vincristine, since have been used successfully in prolonging life and reducing the suffering of patients afflicted with certain types of cancer. After the isolation and structural identification of active plant constituents, organic chemists may recreate them by total synthesis in the laboratory or more importantly use the natural chemical as the starting material in the creation of slightly different chemical structures through molecule manipulation procedures. The new structures, termed semisynthetic drugs, may have a slightly or vastly different pharmacologic activity than the starting substance, depending upon the nature and extent of chemical alteration. Other plant constituents which in themselves may be inactive or rather unimportant therapeutically may be employed in the semisynthetic process to yield important drugs with profound pharmacologic activity. For example, the various species of *Dioscorea*, popularly known as Mexican yams, are rich in a chemical nucleus called the "steroid" structure from which hormonal chemicals like cortisone and estrogens, the female sex hormones, are semisynthetically produced.

Animals have served man in his search for drugs in a number of ways. They not only have yielded to drug testing and biologic assay procedures but also have provided drugs fashioned from their own tissues or through their biologic processes. Hormonal substances such as thyroid extract, insulin, and pituitary hormone obtained from the endocrine glands of cattle, sheep, and swine are lifesaving drugs employed daily as replacement therapy in the human body. The urine of pregnant mares is a rich source of estrogens. Knowledge of the structural architecture of the individual hormonal substances has led to the production of a variety of synthetic and semisynthetic compounds with hormone-like activity. The synthetic chemicals in oral contraceptive agents are a notable example. The use of animals in the production of various biologic products, including serums, antitoxins, and vaccines, has been of lifesaving significance ever since the pioneering work of Dr. Edward Jenner on the smallpox vaccine in England in 1796. Today, the poliomyelitis vaccine is prepared in cultures of minced monkey tissue, the mumps and influenza vaccines in fluids of the chick embryo, the rubella (German measles) vaccine in duck embryo or rabbit kidney cell cultures, and the smallpox vaccine in chick embryonic fluid or from the lymph of calves inoculated with vaccinia virus. Tomorrow, vaccines for syphilis, leprosy, and cancer may be developed through the utilization of cell and tissue cultures.

The production of antibiotics through the induced proliferative growth of specific microorganisms has resulted in such lifesaving drugs as penicillin, streptomycin, and chloramphenicol. In addition, a host of semisynthetic antibiotics have resulted through the knowledge of the chemical structure and activity of these compounds. Undoubtedly new and more effective antibiotic substances will be discovered in soil samples, and from these, additional congeners will be prepared in future years. An important by-product of antibiotic production has been cyanocobalamin or vitamin B_{12}, a metabolic product of *Streptomyces griseus* used in the production of the antibiotic streptomycin.

Certainly the richest source of potential drugs is the flask of the synthetic organic chemist. Through his art he creates not only chemical modifications of known structures but also totally new synthetic organic compounds. These new chemical entities may resemble older drugs in both chemical structure and pharmacologic activity and, indeed, may be synthesized for that very reason. Frequently, however, a new drug elicits an effect that was neither sought nor expected. For example, advances in the area of antidepressant agents were made possible by the chance observation that the antitubercular agent, iproniazid, produced marked elevation in mood when administered to tubercular patients. On another occasion, the clinical observation that a new sulfa drug produced symptoms resembling those produced in diabetics after an overdose of insulin was the key to the development of oral hypoglycemic agents or antidiabetic drugs. The fortuitous discovery that a new antihistaminic agent, chlorpromazine, has tranquilizing effects represented the breakthrough in efforts to produce drugs useful in treating emotional distress. Each year new chemical entities demonstrate both safety and efficacy and win approval of the Food and Drug Administration for marketing. As they demonstrate sufficient merit they are incorporated into the official compendia, and if they prove superior to the older drugs, they may displace them in medical practice.

A drug need not be a new chemical entity to be considered a "new drug" by the Food and Drug Administration and therefore subject to the aforementioned requirements for proof of safety and efficacy. A well-known chemical formulated in a new manner with different excipients, coatings, solvents, vehicles, or other formulative materials results in a pharmaceutical product that has not been examined for safety and efficacy and therefore is a "new drug" under the law. It is well recognized that different methods of manufacture or different formulative additives can considerably alter the therapeutic efficacy of a product through chemical or physical interference with the therapeutic agents. A new combination of two or more old drugs or a change in the usual proportions of drugs in an established combination product can be considered "new" if a question of safety or efficacy is introduced by the alteration. A proposed new use for an old drug, a new dosage schedule or regimen, a proposed new route of administration, or a new dosage form can cause an old drug to be reconsidered for safety and efficacy. An old drug also may be considered "new" if the proposed manufacturer of it has never before received FDA approval for marketing the product even though his competitors have.

Drug Product Development and Marketing

As depicted in Figure 1-1, drug product development activities begin during the early stages of the investigation of a new drug and continue through the actual manufacturing or production of the product.

The new drug substance, which may be produced by organic synthesis, fermentation, or extraction, must be prepared in sufficient quantity to meet the projected large scale production of the dosage form. This scale-up work is generally performed by the organic chemists and chemical engineers of the process research and development group. Similarly, the product development scientists who developed the initial drug formulation in pilot plant work, collaborate with the technical people in the production area, engineers, machinists, and quality control specialists in developing the capability for the large scale production of the dosage form. Once in actual production, the mechanics, electricians, plumbers, and other maintenance personnel insure continued function of the complex machinery. In-plant information

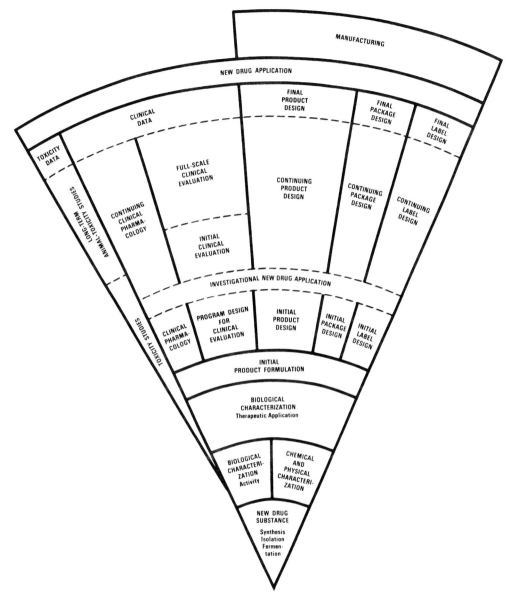

Fig. 1-1. *Schematic representation of development of a new drug. Five years or more may elapse after the isolation or synthesis of a new drug substance before it becomes available as a pharmaceutical product. During this period each new substance is subjected to intensive testing and study, first to characterize its activity and then to determine its safety and effectiveness. (Courtesy of Eli Lilly and Company)*

systems and control procedures are developed to conform with established good manufacturing practice. Double check systems and methods of electronic data processing are integrated into the quality control procedures.

Throughout the developmental stages, extensive testing must be undertaken to insure the chemical and physical stability of the product.

Drug stability in proposed packaging materials must be tested as well as stability under various conditions of storage.

The legal department is active in the development of patent protection for the new drug and for the assignment of a trademark name. Together with the medical department, they work to develop product literature, labeling, and promotion materials. This work involves interaction with literature scientists, the art and printing departments, and the plastics, glass, paper, or other container and packaging suppliers. Marketing analysts, the financial department, and sales personnel become involved in the upcoming promotion of the product to the prescribing practitioner.

As the drug is first advertised and promoted to the medical profession through professional journals, direct mailing, and personal visits by the manufacturer's professional representatives, the drug products are being shipped to the wholesale drug firms, hospitals, and community pharmacies throughout the nation. With the writing of the first prescription for the product by the physician, the filling of the order by the community or institutional pharmacist, and the taking of the drug by the patient, the product joins the armamentarium of drug therapy.

The Need for Standards

The importance of drug standards, even among the nontherapeutic pharmaceutical necessities employed in product formulations, was tragically demonstrated in 1938. The then-new wonder drug, sulfanilamide, which was not soluble in the most commonly used pharmaceutical solvents of the day, was prepared and distributed by a reputable manufacturer as an elixir, solubilized with diethylene glycol. Before the product could be removed from the market, over 100 persons had lost their lives due to the toxic effects of the formulation's solvent, diethylene glycol. The necessity for proper product formulation and for thorough pharmacologic testing of the therapeutic agent and of the completed pharmaceutical product was painfully recognized. Congress responded with the Federal Food, Drug, and Cosmetic Act of 1938 and the creation of the Food and Drug Administration (FDA) to administer and enforce it. Included in the Act is a provision that prohibits the use of any new drug without the prior filing of a New Drug Application (NDA) with the Food and Drug Administration. The medical officers of the FDA grant or deny permission to distribute a new product after reviewing the applicant's filed data on the product's ingredients, manufacturing processes, toxicologic studies on animals, therapeutic claims, and clinical trails on human beings. Although the Act of 1938

required pharmaceutical products to be safe for human use, it should be noted that it did not require them to be efficacious.

By its nature, medical progress involves risk, for no drug is guaranteed completely safe and no drug is completely understood. This lack of understanding resulted in the drug tragedy of the century, if not of all time, in 1960. A new synthetic drug, called thalidomide, recommended as a sedative and tranquilizer, was being sold in Europe without the requirement of a physician's prescription. It was a drug of especial interest due to its apparent lack of toxicity even at extreme dosage levels. It was hoped that it would replace the barbiturates in popularity as a sedative and therefore prevent the frequent deaths caused from accidental and intentional overdosage with barbiturates. An American firm was awaiting FDA approval for marketing in this country when reports of a strange effect of the drug's use began to filter in from Europe. Thalidomide given to women during pregnancy produced phocomelia or an arrested development of the limbs of the newborn infant. Thousands of children were affected to various extents. Some were born with neither arms nor legs; others, with partially formed limbs. The more fortunate were born with only disfigurations of the nose, eyes, and ears. Those more severely afflicted died, the result of internal malformation of the heart or gastrointestinal tract. This drug catastrophe, which for the most part did not affect American citizens, spurred Congress to strengthen the existing laws regarding new drugs. Without dissent, on October 10, 1962, the Kefauver-Harris Drug Amendments to the Food, Drug, and Cosmetic Act of 1938 were passed by both houses of Congress. The purpose of the enactment was to insure a greater amount of safety in the drugs made available to our citizens, and for the first time the manufacturer was required to prove the drug efficacious before it would be granted FDA approval for marketing.

Clinical Testing of New Drugs

Under the Food, Drug and Cosmetic Act as amended, the sponsor of a new drug (usually a drug manufacturer, but occasionally a research institution, an individual or a group of medical researchers) is required to file with the FDA a "Notice of Claimed Investigational Exemption for a New Drug'' (IND) before the drug can be clinically tested on human beings. After submission of such a notice, the investigator must delay use of the drug in human subjects for a period of not less than 30 days from the date the FDA acknowledges receipt of the IND. This 30-day period may be waived or extended by the FDA upon a showing of good cause.

Among the items included in the IND are the following: the name and address of the sponsor of the drug; the name and chemical description of the drug substance to be investigated; a quantitative list of the active and inactive components of the dosage form to be administered; the source or supplier and method of preparation of the drug to be administered; a statement relating to the methods, facilities, and controls employed in the manufacture, processing, packaging and labeling of the new drug to assure appropriate standards of identity, strength, quality, and purity; a thorough presentation of all preclinical (animal) studies of the drug including the names and qualifications of the investigators and the names and locations of the laboratories in which the work was performed; the relation between the preclinical studies and the proposed clinical studies; information on any clinical studies performed in other countries and any related bibliography of publications on the new drug; if the new drug is a combination of previously investigated components, a complete preclinical and clinical summary of these components when administered singly and any data or expectations relating to the effect when combined; copies of labeling and other pertinent information to be distributed to the proposed clinical investigators of the drug; the names and summaries of the training and experience of the proposed clinical investigators; the name of the persons following the progress of the study and collating and evaluating the data received from the investigators; a description of the facilities in which the drug will be investigated; and a complete protocol on the methodology to be employed in the clinical investigation, including the method of selection of subjects for the investigation, the method and route of drug administration, the studies to be performed in the evaluation of the safety and effectiveness of the new drug, and the assurance of the safety and protection of the human subjects participating in the investigation.

The human subjects participating in these clinical investigations do so at their own choosing. The sponsor of the investigation must certify that each person who will receive the drug during the investigational period will give his *informed consent;* that is, he will be informed of the purpose and nature of the investigation and the potential risks involved, and will give his written consent to participate. Appropriate consent forms are used for this purpose.

The Investigational Drug Branch of the FDA is charged with the responsibility of reviewing and evaluating the applications for clinical testing. A sponsor of a new drug will usually be permitted to proceed with his clinical investigation if the IND submitted is complete and the Agency is satisfied with the preclinical data and the entire protocol of the planned investigation. There are generally four "phases" to the clinical investigation of a drug, with each one entered into only after the successful completion of the preceding phase.

Phase I of clinical testing involves a few, carefully chosen, *healthy volunteers.* The initial dose of the drug administered is usually quite low, based on the prior experience with animal studies. If the first dose is well tolerated, the investigation is continued with the administration of additional and carefully scheduled doses. Throughout the investigation, the subjects are closely observed and examined by expert clinicians. Among the basic data collected during this phase include the rate of the drug's absorption; the rate and level of its concentration in the blood; its rate and method of elimination from the body, and toxicological effect, if any, in body tissues and major organs; and changes in the blood forming organs or in the normal physiologic processes of the body. The subjects' ability to tolerate the drug are observed and any unpleasant effects of the drug are recorded. If Phase I is successful in demonstrating sufficient tolerance to the drug and if the order of toxicity remains low, Phase II of clinical testing is begun.

Actual patients suffering from a malady against which the new drug indicated promise through its pharmacological activity are treated in limited numbers and under close observation during Phase II of clinical testing. The main purpose of Phase II is to determine the efficacy of the new drug in treating the disease against which it is being tested and to detect side effects or toxicity symptoms not manifest in the animal studies or in studies with healthy volunteers.

Clinicians familiar with the disease being

treated with the investigational drug are utilized during Phase II studies. During this phase, additional data are collected relating to the drug's patterns of absorption, distribution, and excretion, and drug metabolites which may be formed are identified. Each patient is monitored for the appearance of side effects while the dose of the drug is carefully increased to determine the minimal effective dose. Following this determination, the dose is extended beyond the minimally effective dose to ascertain the dosage level at which a patient reveals extremely undesirable or intolerable toxic or adverse effects from the drug. The greater the range between the amount of drug determined to be minimally effective and that determined to cause severe side effects, the greater is the safety margin of the drug and the greater the promise for effective use in drug therapy.

If the clinical results of Phase II indicate continued promise for the new drug and if the margin of safety appears to be good, Phase III may be embarked upon. In this phase, private practitioners of varying backgrounds and experiences are brought into the investigations by the more experienced clinicians. The objective is to determine the usefulness of the new drug in the hands of the community practitioner. Depending upon the nature of the drug and the disease for which it is recommended, this phase may involve a thousand or more patients. During this phase, the participating practitioners report on their findings to the principal investigator of the new drug and he relays the information and his evaluation to the Food and Drug Administration. Information about possible adverse effects due to the drug are evaluated upon receipt and the information disseminated to all participating practitioners. Should the data warrant it, a clinical investigation may be terminated at any point during the clinical trials.

If during these three phases of clinical testing the drug demonstrates sufficient safety and significant therapeutic effect, the sponsor of the drug may file a New Drug Application (NDA) with the Food and Drug Administration. The application contains a highly organized and complete presentation of all of the preclinical and clinical data that the sponsor has obtained during his investigation of the drug. In addition, the sponsor presents drug stability data and precise information regarding dosage form composition, method of manufacture, documentation of product uniformity as obtained from pilot plant studies,[1] and proposed product labeling. This application is studied by the Medical Evaluation Branch of the Food and Drug Administration, which decides whether to allow the sponsor to market the drug, to disallow marketing, or to require additional data before rendering a judgment. Should the sponsor of the drug be accorded a favorable decision, the FDA continues to require good manufacturing procedures, adequate scientific control over these procedures, continued receipt of information pertinent to the drug's side effects and toxicity, fairness in promotion and advertising, and above all the right to remove the drug from the market, temporarily or permanently, should further study later be justified.

The receipt of marketing status for a new drug product does not terminate a company's investigation of the activity of the drug. Continued clinical investigations, often referred to as Phase IV studies, add to the understanding of the mechanism of the drug's actions and frequently reveal new therapeutic applications or indications for the drug. Should the drug demonstrate usefulness in treating patients with diseases or illnesses other than that for which the drug was originally approved, the drug's sponsor can apply to the FDA for permission to promote and market the drug for the "new indication." The FDA would once again evaluate the new clinical data and make a determination. Phase IV studies may continue as long as useful information is gathered on the safety and effectiveness of the product. As additional experience is gained with the drug, newly revealed adverse effects may also be generated and new cautions or restrictions to the use of the drug imposed.

Additional Standards for Safety and Effectiveness

Once into the full implementation of the procedures required for the evaluation of new drugs, the FDA turned its attention to the examination of products which had entered the marketplace between 1938 and 1962 and thus were never reviewed and "approved" under the same

---

[1] Pilot plant studies refer to the product developmental work that must precede large scale production. The pilot plant work includes all aspects of product formulation, manufacture, stability testing, and dosage form efficacy studies.

criteria for safety and efficacy as were the drugs marketed after 1962. The FDA initiated this Drug Efficacy Study in 1966 through an agreement reached with the National Academy of Sciences-National Research Council (NAS/NRC) for the review for safety and efficacy of some 4000 drug products then on the market. The NAS/NRC review was conducted by 30 panels of physicians, all experts in their fields. The drug products reviewed were primarily prescription drugs; however, over 400 nonprescription drugs were included in the study. In 1969, upon receipt of the NAS/NRC findings, a special task force of the FDA's Bureau of Drugs, called the Drug Efficacy Study Implementation (DESI) Project Office, began reviewing the NAS/NRC recommendations, preparing FDA findings, and setting up the necessary procedures for implementation through regulation. The products that were found to comply with the statutory requirements for safety and efficacy and bore correct labeling were allowed to remain on the market. Those that did not comply were either removed from the market by regulatory action or required to make the necessary changes in labeling, formulation, or submission of suitable additional data as was considered necessary to conform to the regulatory requirements.

An outgrowth of the NAS/NRC Drug Efficacy Study was the review by the FDA of "combination" prescription products; that is, products containing two or more medicinal agents in a fixed dosage unit as a tablet, capsule or teaspoonful. Among the disadvantages cited in the use of fixed combination products include the lack of flexibility in adjusting the dosage of each therapeutic component to meet an individual patient's needs, the exposure of patients to additional and unnecessary drugs when perhaps a single drug would meet the therapeutic requirements, and the increased possibility of adverse drug reactions through the administration of multiple drugs, perhaps without increasing efficacy. The advantages cited for the use of fixed combination products include the likelihood of greater adherence to a therapeutic regimen by the patient, and greater patient convenience and economy than if each of the therapeutic ingredients was given separately but concurrently.

The essence of the Agency regulations, issued in October, 1971, held that combination products must offer to the patient a therapeutic advantage over any of the components administered separately.[1] Thus, when two or more medicinal agents are combined into a single dosage unit, each must effectively contribute to the therapeutic claims for the product. Further, the dosage of each component must be at a level which is both safe and effective for a significant number of patients who require concurrent therapy with the drugs in the combination product. It is also permitted to add a second drug to a first if the added drug enhances the safety or effectiveness of the principal ingredient or minimizes the potential for abuse of the principal ingredient.

Another major effort of the Food and Drug Administration in achieving the goals of the 1962 Drug Amendments involved the massive review of nonprescription drug products. This effort which began in 1972 involved the use of expert scientific panels to review the safety, effectiveness, and labeling of the various categories of nonprescription drugs. As was the case with prescription drugs, products not conforming to the established standards were to be removed from the market unless they were reformulated, relabeled or otherwise changed to meet the prevailing standards.

In another development related to drug product effectiveness, the Food and Drug Administration, the American Pharmaceutical Association, the Academy of Pharmaceutical Sciences, the USP, the NF, and other scientific and professional bodies, organizations, and agencies have become increasingly interested in drug *bioavailability* studies. Bioavailability is defined by the FDA as:[2]

> "The degree to which a drug is absorbed from the drug product into the body or to the site of action."

It has become well established that the rate and extent to which a drug in a dosage form becomes available for biologic absorption or utilization may depend to a great extent upon the materials utilized in the formulation or the method of manufacture. Thus, the same drug when formulated in *different* dosage forms may be found to possess different bioavailability characteristics and thus exhibit different clinical effectiveness. Further, two seemingly "identical" or "equivalent" products, of the same

---

[1] Federal Register, 36, No 200, October 15, 1971.
[2] Federal Register, 38, #3, 885–887, Jan. 5, 1973.

drug, in the same dosage strength and in the *same* dosage form type, but differing in formulative materials or method of manufacture, may vary widely in bioavailability and thus in clinical effectiveness. The following terms are used to define the type or level of "equivalency" between drug products.[1]

Chemical equivalents—Drug products that contain the same amounts of the same therapeutically active ingredients in the same dosage forms and that meet present compendial standards.

Biological equivalents—Chemical equivalents which, when administered to the same individuals in the same dosage regimen, will result in comparable bioavailability.

Therapeutic equivalents—Chemical equivalents which, when administered to the same individuals in the same dosage regimen, will provide essentially the same efficacy and/or toxicity.

Drug bioavailability is an important measure of the efficacy of dosage forms in acting as drug delivery systems. The various criteria for the design and development of effective dosage forms will be discussed more thoroughly in Chapter 3.

The Drug Listing Act of 1972 was enacted to provide the Food and Drug Administration with the legislative authority to compile a list of currently marketed drugs in order to assist the Agency in the enforcement of Federal laws requiring that drugs be safe and effective and not adulterated or misbranded.[2] Under the regulations of the Act, each firm which manufactures or repackages drugs for ultimate sale or distribution to patients or consumers must register with the FDA and submit appropriate information for listing. All foreign drug manufacturing and distributing firms whose products are imported into the United States are also included in this regulation. Exempt from the registration and listing requirement are hospitals, clinics, and the various health practitioners who prepare pharmaceutical products for use in their respective institutions and practices. Also exempt

are research and teaching institutions in which drug products are prepared for purposes other than sale. Each registrant is assigned a permanent registration number, following the format of the National Drug Code (NDC) numbering system. Under this system, the first 5 numeric characters of 10-character code identify the manufacturer or distributor and are referred to as the "Labeler Code." The last 5 numeric characters of the 10-character code identify the drug formulation and the trade package size and type. The segment which identifies the drug formulation is known as the "Product Code," and the segment which identifies the trade package size and type is called the "Package Code." The manufacturer or distributor determines the ratio of use of the last 5 digits for the two codes, as a 3-to-2 digit Product Code-Package Code configuration (e.g. 542-12) or a 4-to-1 digit configuration (e.g. 5421-2). Only one such type of configuration may be selected for use by a manufacturer or distributor who then assigns a code number to each of his products to be included in the drug listing. A final code number is presented as the example: "NCD 15643-542-12."

The FDA requests, but does not require, that the National Drug Code number appear on all drug labeling, including the label of any prescription drug container furnished to a consumer. In some instances, manufacturers imprint the NDC number directly on the dosage units, as capsules and tablets, for rapid and positive identification when the number is matched in the *National Drug Code Directory* or against a decoding list provided by the manufacturer. Once a number is assigned to a drug product it is a permanent assignment. Even in instances in which a drug manufacturer discontinues the manufacture and distribution of a product, the number may not be used again. If a drug product is substantially changed, as through an alteration in the active ingredients, dosage form, or product name, a new NDC number is assigned to the product by the registrant and the FDA advised accordingly.

The product information received by the FDA is processed and stored by computer to provide easy access to the following types of information:

1. A list of all drug products.
2. A list of all drug products broken down by labeled indications or pharmacologic category.

[1] "Drug Bioequivalence," A Report of the Office of Technology Assessment, Drug Bioequivalence Study Panel, Congress of the United States, Washington, D.C. 1974.
[2] Federal Register, 38, No. 44, March 7, 1973.

3. A list of all drug products, broken down by manufacturer.
4. A list of drug product's active ingredients.
5. A list of a drug product's inactive ingredients.
6. A list of drug products containing a particular ingredient.
7. A list of drug products newly marketed or remarketed.
8. A list of drug products discontinued.
9. All labeling of drug products.
10. All advertising of drug products.

Once in full operation, the drug listing program will enable the FDA to monitor the quality of all drugs on the market in this country.

In a continuing effort to assure the standards for drug quality control, the Food and Drug Administration's regulations provide not only for the inspection and certification of pharmaceutical manufacturing procedures and facilities, but also for the field surveillance and assay of products obtained from the shelves of retail distributors.[1]

In instances in which it is found that a manufacturer is not meeting the established standards for drug product quality, that manufacturer will be denied permission to continue to produce products for distribution until he does comply with the standards. In instances in which it is found by the FDA or by a manufacturer that a marketed product presents a threat or a potential threat to consumer safety, that product may be "recalled" or sought for return to the manufacturer from its depth of distribution.

A drug product recall may be initiated by the FDA or by the manufacturer, the latter case being termed a "voluntary recall." A numerical

classification, as follows, indicates the degree of consumer hazards associated with the product being recalled:[2]

Class I Recalls—This is an emergency situation involving the removal from the market of a product in which the *consequences are immediate or long-range, life threatening,* and involve a direct cause-effect relationship. (Examples: label mix-up of a potent drug; botulism toxin in foods; defective heart valves distributed for use in surgery.)

Class II Recalls—This is a priority situation in which the consequences may be immediate or long-range but only *possibly* or *potentially* life threatening or hazardous to health. (Examples: sub- or superpotent drug that is *not* life saving in nature; improperly calibrated thermometers.)

Class III Recalls—This is a routine situation in which the consequences to life (if any) are *remote or nonexistent.* Products recalled because of adulteration (contamination) or misbranding not involving a health hazard. (Examples: Ordinary labeling violations of FDA regulations; defects in food relating to esthetic qualities.)

The "depth of recall," or the level of market removal or correction (as wholesaler, retailer, consumer), depends upon the nature of the product, the urgency of the situation, and depth to which the product has been distributed. The lot numbers of packaging control numbers on the containers or labels of the manufactured products help in identifying the specific lot or batch of product to be recalled.

Classification of Drugs

Drugs approved for marketing by the Food and Drug Administration are categorized according to the manner in which they may be legally obtained by the patient. Drugs deemed safe enough for use by the layman in the self-treatment of simple conditions for which competent medical care is not generally sought are classified as "over-the-counter" (O.T.C.) drugs and may be sold without the requirement of a physician's prescription. This status assigned to a drug product by the FDA may be changed

---

[1] In the fiscal year ended June 30, 1973 the FDA made some 7,000 inspections in some 2,700 drug plants to assure compliance with the Agency's "Good Manufacturing Practices," (see Chapter 2). This covered some 97% of the country's "major manufacturers," of drugs for human use who are responsible for some 95% of the prescription drugs marketed in this country. In addition, some 9,000 samples of drugs for human use were analyzed by the FDA in its laboratories. During the fiscal year ended June 30, 1974 some 19,000 drug samples were collected and analyzed, the sharp increase attributed to the highly automated testing methods developed by the FDA during that period, largely in its National Center for Drug Analysis (NCDA) at St. Louis. Quality Control Reports, "The Gold Sheet," 8, No. 2, February, 1974; 8, No. 5, May, 1974.

[2] Quality Control Reports, "The Gold Sheet," October, 1973.

should more stringent control over the drug's distribution and use later be warranted. Other drugs that are considered useful only after expert diagnosis or too dangerous for use in self-medication are made available only on the prescription of a licensed practitioner. These drugs are referred to as "Legend" drugs, since it is a requirement of their labeling to bear the legend: "Caution: Federal Law Prohibits Dispensing Without Prescription," under the provisions of the Durham-Humphrey Amendment of 1952 to the Federal Food, Drug, and Cosmetic Act. Drugs so designated may also change legal status from time to time according to the judgments of the Food and Drug Administration and the firm that distributes the product. New drugs that have not been shown to be safe in self-medication are generally limited to prescription dispensing until such time that they are considered useful and safe enough for the layman to use at his discretion.

According to the Durham-Humphrey Amendment, prescriptions for Legend drugs may not be refilled (dispensed again after the initial filling of the prescription) without the express consent of the prescriber. The refill status of prescriptions for certain Legend drugs known to be subject to public abuse was further regulated with the passage of the Drug Abuse Control Amendments of 1965 and then by the Comprehensive Drug Abuse Prevention and Control Act of 1970.

The Comprehensive Drug Abuse Prevention and Control Act of 1970 served to consolidate and codify drug control authority into a single statute. Under its provisions, the Drug Abuse Control Amendments of 1965, the Harrison Narcotic Act of 1914, and other related laws governing stimulants, depressants, narcotics and hallucinogenics were repealed and replaced by regulatory framework administered by the Bureau of Narcotics and Dangerous Drugs (BNDD) of the Department of Justice. In 1973, under another reorganization plan, the Drug Enforcement Administration (DEA) was established in the Department of Justice and took over the functions of the Bureau of Narcotics and Dangerous Drugs, which was abolished, and also the drug intelligence, investigation, and enforcement roles of several other governmental agencies.

The Comprehensive Drug Abuse Prevention and Control Act of 1970 established five "Schedules" for the classification and control of drug substances which are subject to public abuse. These schedules, which continue in effect under the jurisdiction of the DEA, provide for decreasing levels of control from Schedule I drugs to those classified as Schedule V drugs. The drugs in the five Schedules may be described as follows:

Schedule I—Drugs with no accepted medical use, or other substances, with a high potential for abuse. In this category are heroin, LSD, and similar items, but virtually any non-medical substance that is being abused can be placed in this category.
Schedule II—Drugs with accepted medical uses and a high potential for abuse which, if abused, may lead to severe psychological or physical dependence.
Schedule III—Drugs with accepted medical uses and a potential for abuse less than those listed in Schedules I and II which, if abused, may lead to moderate or low psychological dependence or high physical dependence.
Schedule IV—Drugs with accepted medical uses and low potential for abuse relative to those in Schedule III which, if abused, may lead to limited physical dependence or psychological dependence relative to drugs in Schedule III.
Schedule V—Drugs with accepted medical uses and low potential for abuse relative to those in Schedule IV and which, if abused, may lead to limited physical dependence or psychological dependence relative to drugs in Schedule IV.

It should be noted that in all instances, local and state laws may enhance the Federal drug laws but may not be used to weaken them. All drug laws are intended to protect the health and welfare of the public and serve as guidelines to members of the health professions to be used by them along with their professional judgment. Working together, the physician, the pharmacist, the drug manufacturers, the drug regulatory agencies, and others involved in the health of our citizens can insure the availability and proper use of the finest drugs for the diagnosis, treatment, cure, or prevention of disease.

The Practice of Pharmacy

Graduate pharmacists perform capably in the many and varied areas in which the pharmaceutical sciences and the professional aspects of pharmacy are applied. Pharmacists working for pharmaceutical research, manufacturing, and distributing firms become involved in virtually every phase of drug product development, production, marketing, and management functions. In government service, pharmacists play active roles in drug regulation, procurement, distribution, and utilization. Teaching institutions utilize pharmacists in the education and training of not only pharmacy students, but students in the allied health professions. Pharmacists who practice in the nation's community pharmacies and in health care institutions do so in virtually every type of facility and environment in which pharmaceuticals are stored, dispensed, or administered.

Pharmacists in industry contribute greatly to the areas of product development and production. Their knowledge of the basic and pharmaceutical sciences, dosage form design, and the technical aspects of production fits well with this major function of industrial pharmacy firms.

Nowadays a number of pharmacy graduates have additional undergraduate degrees in such areas as organic or analytical chemistry or in microbiology or biochemistry, and with their interest and background are able to work effectively in pharmaceutical research. Pharmacists with advanced degrees in the basic or pharmaceutical sciences, or in other areas as health care administration, marketing, law, or medicine contribute to their industrial employers in their respective areas of expertise.

In addition to the areas of drug research, product development, and production, many pharmacists in industry may be found working in such varied areas as in drug materials procurement; in public, trade, or professional relations; as scientific, technical, or professional information specialists; in liaison work with governmental agencies, educational or research institutions, or professional organizations; or in marketing, advertising, promotion, or pharmaceutical sales work. Pharmacists in industry also become involved in management and in the various administrative functions of the industrial firm.

In government service, pharmacists may become involved in administrative functions, as in the development and implementation of health care programs in the design and enforcement of regulations involving drug quality standards, good manufacturing practices, and drug distribution and utilization practices. Pharmacists also practice their profession in government supported hospitals, clinics, and specialized health care institutions.

Career opportunities for pharmacists in government service at the Federal level include positions in the military service, in the Public Health Service, and in such Civil Service agencies as the Food and Drug Administration, Veterans Administration, Department of Health, Education, and Welfare, Drug Enforcement Administration of the Department of Justice, National Institutes of Health, and others. At the State and local level, many pharmacists find rewarding careers in developing programs for drug procurement, distribution and utilization in the various health departments, welfare departments or agencies, drug investigation and regulatory agencies, clinics and health-care institutions, and also with state boards of pharmacy.

A number of pharmacists serve their profession in positions with various professional organizations, as state and national pharmaceutical associations.

Schools of pharmacy utilize pharmacists, some with and some without advanced degrees, to teach in the professional curriculum, to conduct pharmaceutical research, and to participate in the service and continuing education functions of the school. Although most of the educators working full time for the school do so within the classrooms and laboratories of the academic institution, many others provide professional instruction in the practice or clinical setting. A good number of part-time pharmacist-educators also are employed by schools of pharmacy to provide professional instruction within the academic institution or in affiliated teaching hospitals, medical specialty clinics, hospital pharmacies, drug information centers, nursing homes and extended care facilities, drug abuse clinics, health departments, mental health hospitals or clinics, community pharmacies, and other places in which pharmaceutical services are delivered. Many community and institutional pharmacy practitioners are serving educational institutions as "preceptors," and provide pharmacy students with educational experiences within their own daily practice of pharmacy.

In 1971, the National Center for Health Services Research and Development issued a Report of the "Task Force on the Pharmacist's

Clinical Role."[1] The Report was based on professional "functions" of the pharmacist as they were required then and as they were expected to be required in the years immediately ahead. Although a few of these functions were recognized as requiring a change in the law for their legal implementation (as the pharmacist's treatment of minor illness), they were included in the report to reflect reasonable future functions of the pharmacist in terms of his training and in relation to the health care needs of the patient. The Report classified the clinical functions of the pharmacist into seven main categories and described each one as follows:

A. Dispensing and Administering Drugs

The responsibility for dispensing medication upon an order from a physician rests with the pharmacist and his staff. The physician has a legal right to dispense, although in general he does not do so. Exceptions are found in rural communities where a pharmacist is not available and in those few cases there the physician chooses to dispense. When the pharmacist performs the dispensing function, it is assumed that he has drugs available by both brand and established (generic) names in products which are of known and acceptable quality. Furthermore, it is assumed that he has the knowledge to exert a discriminating judgment in selecting a drug product when several products of the same therapeutic class are available that meet the needs of the patient. When generic-name drugs are dispensed, it is assumed that if there is a potential savings the patient will benefit.

1. The pharmacist receives and interprets the drug order and either supervises the dispensing function or performs it himself.
2. The pharmacist should consult with the physician when the latter prescribes products of suspected or known low quality, or when a question arises as to the appropriateness of a drug or drug product in light of the patient's condition.

[1] "Report of Task Force on the Pharmacist's Clinical Role," National Center for Health Services Research and Development, Department of Health, Education, and Welfare, Public Health, Service, Health Services and Mental Health Administration, *HSRD Briefs*, No. 4, 1971.

3. The pharmacist has a responsibility for personally dispensing or supervising the filling of orders that require technical knowledge and skill, such as preparing and dispensing intravenous fluids, radiopharmaceuticals, and compounded prescriptions, etc.
4. The pharmacist's dispensing function in the hospital overlaps with the administration of drugs, an act performed traditionally by the nurse. This is manifest today or will be in the future through (a) administration of medicines by the pharmacist, (b) administration by a technician who works under the supervision of the pharmacist, or (c) administration by a nurse who is responsible for this act. In addition to the pharmacist's potential responsibility for administration of bedside medication, his responsibilities could include the starting of as well as sharing in the assessment of intravenous therapy, and administering drugs in special programs, i.e., cancer chemotherapy.
5. The pharmacist, wherever he practices, may administer biological products for immunizations, i.e., polio (oral or injectable) and smallpox vaccines.
6. The pharmacist's function in preparing the dispensing medication extends logically to inclusion of the function of administering drugs.

Combining these functions provides for improved drug-use control. The nurse realizes that her traditional role in administering drugs is one delegated by the physician, but she appears amenable to the transfer of this role to the pharmacist. If this transfer takes place, the pharmacist's function would include responsibility for administering drugs; and his decision may determine who performs individual tasks. There are ethical, legal and economic problems today that provide barriers to this transfer of function, but model state health legislation may eliminate some of them. In addition, the pharmacist will require special training if he is to serve such an expanded role.

B. Prescribing Drugs

The physician determines if drug therapy is indicated and usually chooses the drug to be used as part of his overall therapy. Under certain circumstances the pharmacist does assist in planning drug therapy, and at times may prescribe medications at the request of the physician.

1. Pharmacists, in reissuing prescriptions designated to be refilled at the request of the patient (p.r.n.), may be regarded as performing a prescribing function.
2. Pharmacists, in complying with "standing orders" of the physician, may be performing an independent prescribing function. "Standing orders" refers to a prearranged plan or understanding between the physician and the pharmacist which permits the latter to dispense medications under certain circumstances without the immediate concurrence of the physician.
3. Pharmacists and pharmacy residents often help medical students to plan drug regimens.
4. Physicians may share responsibility for prescribing with the pharmacist when the latter has demonstrated competence. This may include the selection of drugs, the dosage forms and frequency of use, based upon the physician's diagnosis.
5. Pharmacists prescribe over-the-counter (OTC) drugs. Also, by recommending against the purchase and/or use of OTC drugs, they enter into the prescribing function.
6. Pharmacists prescribe medications in emergency situations when it appears to be in the best interest of the patient.
7. Pharmacists, after consultation with the prescriber, may select and dispense a drug other than the one prescribed by the physician, when they practice under the authority of the drug formulary system.
8. Pharmacists may be considered to be performing a prescribing function when they reply to inquiries from patients about continued use of medications previously prescribed.

C. Documenting Professional Activities

The pharmacist is required to keep certain records of his activities in order to meet legal requirements. These are largely operational in nature and pertain to the acquisition and dispensing of narcotics, dangerous drugs, and appliances. In addition to keeping legally-required records, the pharmacist should keep records to document his activities related to patient care. The following are reasonable functions for the pharmacist to perform:

1. The pharmacist should obtain a drug history by recording medications currently used (prescription and OTC) and idiosyncrasies to specific drugs. He notes the past history of drug and/or chemical intoxication and present exposure to industrial, domestic and/or environmental chemicals, etc. The pharmacist may be able to obtain a detailed drug history by using check off forms. This history becomes the medication part of the patient profile record developed by the health care team. In the community the pharmacist may use a system designed to meet the limitations of both his and the patient's time. This may include the use of a self-administered questionnaire and of automated equipment to provide record linkage with other health care providers used by the patient.
2. The pharmacist should have a meeting with the patient for purposes of reviewing instructions and counseling for home use of medications (a) at time of discharge from the hospital or (b) at time of delivery of medication to him at his community pharmacy. These instructions include mode of administration, conditions of storage, time of renewal, and signs of untoward reactions. The patient is advised in the event of an unanticipated drug reaction to contact the physician or, if the physician is unavailable, the pharmacist.
3. The pharmacist in the hospital or other health care facility has access to the patient's chart and has the obligation to notify the physician when real or potential drug problems arise, such as development of an adverse drug reaction. He also checks charts to determine if changes in drug therapy are properly recorded. In outpatient clinics, the pharmacist may dispense or administer medication directly from instructions in the chart order.
4. The pharmacist, among others, makes proper reporting of adverse drug reactions (ADR) to those collecting ADR data.
5. The pharmacist's records in the community indicate when patients should renew their prescriptions; and if they fail to do so, the pharmacist should contact them in order to assure continuity of care. This is a follow-up function, primarily applicable to, but not limited to, the chronically ill patient.
6. The pharmacist prepares adequate records to assure himself of a documented source of expanding clinical experience which en-

hances his services as a drug specialist and consultant. The pharmacist in the hospital should make rounds with the physician and others on the health care team, or independently as appropriate. In the community setting, his direct contact with patients and physicians permits him to acquire a body of experience through which he becomes a useful clinician in the total care of patients.

7. The pharmacist's function in reviewing chart orders and other documents is to focus on four questions: (a) Is use of these drugs or this drug necessary? (b) Are they the drugs of choice (best drugs for need)? (c) Is the monitoring effort directed to the desired effects? (d) Is the monitoring effort designed to identify adverse drug reactions?

8. The pharmacist in the community setting does not have, in all cases, the equivalent of the patient's hospital chart. He may have no data on the patient's diagnosis or condition; in fact, he may not know whether the physician is treating symptoms or a specifically diagnosed disease. The pharmacist's record, therefore, becomes the historical record of drug utilization, which in time defines the pattern of prescribing of the physician and the pattern (rate, cost, etc.) of utilization by the patient. This permits a periodic review and control function by the pharmacist. The record permits him to monitor therapy for both under- and over-utilization and to identify patients procuring drugs from multiple sources unknown to the physician(s). It also provides an opportunity to acquire information upon which rates of clinical response to individual drugs can be determined by epidemiologic techniques. These data, in correlation with other health records, provide a basis for judgments in which a benefit/risk ratio can be established or, expressed otherwise, an index for predicting likely drug effectiveness.

D. Direct Patient Involvement

The pharmacist should have a direct contact with the patient when he enters or leaves either the hospital system or the community (non-hospital) system. The objective of this contact in either case is the same, but implementation is adapted to fulfill local needs. The pharmacist should be capable of performing the following functions:

1. Conduct an admission interview, or equivalent, to obtain the drug history.

2. Conduct a discharge interview, or equivalent, to review instructions and provide counsel for home use of medications.

3. Provide patient education in personal health matters, i.e., smoking, drug abuse, need for annual health checkup and other preventive measures.

4. Provide patient education and referral when patients are continually using laxatives, antacids, analgesics, etc., or when patients describe symptoms such as one of the cardinal signs of cancer.

5. Screen patients and direct them to sources of appropriate services—a triage function based on the pharmacist's knowledge of community resources, services and means for obtaining access to them.

6. Provide instructions for home use of medications; how and when to take, how to store, cautions in use, when to reorder, expiration date, when to see the physician.

7. Provide instructions in the use of appliances such as inhalers, colostomy bags, trusses, etc. Anatomical models and other demonstration equipment are useful. Special facilities to insure privacy are desirable.

8. Interpret physician's instructions as they relate to drug therapy as well as the total treatment regimen.

9. Conduct rounds in the hospital and develop a system in the community for following a patient's progress when under drug treatment. The monitoring of patients should determine if patients are taking their medicines.

10. Acquaint patients with the name of their pharmacist and how he can be reached. A pharmacist should make arrangements with other pharmacists to provide for the special needs of his patients when he is not available.

E. Reviewing Drug Utilization

Some functions in this section have been noted, in part, previously.

1. Demonstrating concern for the need for organized programs to review and control drug utilization.

2. Developing and/or promoting planned drug utilization review programs.
3. Developing techniques that will lead to identification of drug prescribing patterns by physicians and drug use patterns by patients.
4. Disseminating accurate information concerning the use of drugs to physicians, other members of the health care team, and the public.
5. Implementing a local formulary system of drug-use control in the hospital and in the community.

F. Education

Education refers to those ongoing activities that are designed to influence the prescribing, the dispensing and the use of drugs. The pharmacist's goal as a member of the health care team is to improve patient care by improving the use of drugs and lessening the degree of misuse. Specific functions include:

1. Participation in continuing education through self-directed study and other methods.
2. Organization of inservice and continuing education programs—seminars, lectures, etc., for hospital staffs, group medical practices and professional societies.
3. Participation in the health education of the patient.
4. Participation in public information programs to promote respect for drugs as agents of good health.
5. Participation in the activity of the Pharmacy and Therapeutics Committee or its equivalent organization.
6. Organization of drug information service for physicians and other clinicians.
7. Participation in special programs in the hospital, such as grand rounds, teaching rounds, nursing conferences, medical staff meetings, etc.

G. Consultation

The pharmacist should exert a consultative function by being available to the physician and other clinicians and to the patient for advice and guidance. Although his role as consultant is based primarily on his role as a drug specialist, it is based also on his knowledge of personal and public health matters, community health re-

sources, the treatment of minor illnesses, etc. The pharmacist exerts an *active* role when performing as a consultant. Particular consultations are carried out with the physician and patient concerning:

1. The screening process. For example, the pharmacist might perform certain screening procedures, i.e., determine blood pressure, and in consultation with a physician at some remote point decide what measures should be taken. This is part of the triage function.
2. The selection of drugs and monitoring of drug therapy.
3. The refusal to furnish medication when the best evidence supports this position.
4. The referral of patients to sources of competent medical care.

This Report captures the various aspects of professional practice and the aspirations of today's pharmacist. By definition, a profession is founded upon an art, built upon specialized intellectual training, and has as its primary objective the performing of a service to the betterment of mankind. The principles upon which the professional practice of pharmacy is based are embodied in the Code of Ethics of the American Pharmaceutical Association.

American Pharmaceutical Association Code of Ethics*

preamble

These principles of professional conduct for pharmacists are established to guide the pharmacist in his relationship with patients, fellow practitioners, other health professionals and the public.

section 1

A pharmacist should hold the health and safety of patients to be of first consideration; he should render to each patient the full measure of his ability as an essential health practitioner.

section 2

A pharmacist should never knowingly condone the dispensing, promoting or distributing of drugs or medical devices, or assist therein, which are not of good quality, which do not meet standards required by law or which lack therapeutic value for the patient.

section 3

A pharmacist should always strive to perfect and enlarge his professional knowledge. He should utilize and make available this knowledge as may be required in accordance with his best professional judgment.

section 4

A pharmacist has the duty to observe the law, to uphold the dignity and honor of the profession, and to accept its ethical principles. He should not engage in any activity that will bring discredit to the profession and should expose, without fear or favor, illegal or unethical conduct in the profession.

section 5

A pharmacist should seek at all times only fair and reasonable remuneration for his services. He should never agree to, or participate in, transactions with practitioners of other health professions or any other person under which fees are divided or which may cause financial or other exploitation in connection with the rendering of his professional services.

section 6

A pharmacist should respect the confidential and personal nature of his professional records; except where the best interest of the patient requires or the law demands, he should not disclose such information to anyone without proper patient authorization.

section 7

A pharmacist should not agree to practice under terms or conditions which tend to interfere with or impair the proper exercise of his professional judgment and skill, which tend to cause a deterioration of the quality of his service or which require him to consent to unethical conduct.

section 8

A pharmacist should strive to provide information to patients regarding professional services truthfully, accurately and fully, and should avoid misleading patients regarding the nature, cost, or value of the pharmacist's professional services.

section 9

A pharmacist should associate with organizations having for their objective the betterment of the profession of pharmacy; he should contribute of his time and funds to carry on the work of these organizations.

Selected Reading

Edwards, C. C.: Closing the Gap: OTC Drugs. FDA Papers, February, 1972.

History of National Formulary in *National Formulary*, 14th Edition, Washington, D.C., American Pharmaceutical Association, 1975.

History of the Pharmacopeia of the United States in *United States Pharmacopeia*, 19th revision, New York, The United States Pharmacopeial Convention, Inc., 1975.

Simmons, H. E.: Assuring Total Drug Quality. *J. Amer. Pharm. Assoc. NS13*:96–98, 1973.

Slavin, M.: The National Drug Code. *J. Amer. Pharm. Assoc., NS9*:460–490, 1969.

Sonnedecker, G.: *Kremer's and Urdang's History of Pharmacy*, 3rd Ed. Philadelphia, J. B. Lippincott Co., 1963.

Soos, D. E.: Development and Significance of Modern Pharmacopeias. *Cosmo Pharma., 3*:7–15, 1966.

Special Meeting of the House of Delegates, Proceedings, American Pharmaceutical Association, *J. Amer. Pharm. Assoc., NS13*:21–44, 1973.

The Pharmacist's Role in Product Selection, *J. Am. Pharm. Assoc., NS11*:181–199, 1971.

Allan, F. M.: Standardization of Drug Names. *J.A.M.A., 299*:541–543, 1974.

Jerome, J. B.: The USAN Nomenclature System. *J.A.M.A., 232*:294–299, 1975.

CHAPTER 2

Drug Standards and Good Manufacturing Practice

T HE *United States Pharmacopeia* and the *National Formulary* adopt drugs and drug standards reflecting the best in the current practices of medicine and pharmacy and provide suitable tests and assay procedures for demonstrating compliance with these standards. In fulfilling this function, the compendia become legal documents, every statement of which must be of a high degree of clarity and specificity.

The raw materials employed in the preparation of dosage forms or pharmaceutical preparations must meet rigorous standards of quality, purity, and potency in order that these attributes may be imparted to the resulting drug products. The individual components of each official preparation generally include both therapeutic and pharmaceutic materials, the latter employed for the purpose of enhancing the stability and pharmaceutical elegance of the product. Each agent, therapeutic or pharmaceutic, is represented in an individual compendium monograph and also in the monograph of the preparation in which it is a component. For example, in the official formula for Pentobarbital Sodium Elixir, USP (Fig. 2-1), the chemical

pentobarbital sodium is the therapeutic or medicinally active agent present, and therefore its name appears in the official title. In addition to the pentobarbital sodium, the formula calls for specific amounts of alcohol, glycerin, diluted hydrochloric acid, syrup, and purified water to dissolve the drug and maintain it in solution and provide a sweet liquid vehicle, orange oil to impart a pleasant odor and flavor, and caramel to provide the characteristic color to the preparation. In order that the elixir might be of the same strength, alcoholic content, sweetness, odor, taste, and color each and every time the official preparation is made, it is essential that each starting material, the pentobarbital sodium as well as the supportive pharmaceutical adjuncts, be of uniform quality and present in the same proportions.

It should be noted that many pharmaceutical products on the market, especially those which are combinations of therapeutic ingredients, are not represented by formulation or dosage form monographs in the official compendia. However, the individual components in these products are either represented by monographs in the compendia or are otherwise approved as a part of the manufacturer's drug applications and listings with the Food and Drug Administration and thus together with the approved product meet the designated standards.

An example of a typical drug monograph appearing in the *United States Pharmacopeia* is that for the therapeutic agent chlorambucil. The official monograph for chlorambucil is reproduced in Figure 2-2. A glance at the monograph reveals the type of information generally appearing for organic medicinal agents.

Following the official title or name of the chemical, its graphic or structural formula is presented along with empirical formula, molecular weight, established chemical names and the drug's Chemical Abstracts Service (CAS) Registry Number. The CAS Registry Number identifies each compound uniquely in the CAS computer-oriented information retrieval system. Appearing next in the monograph is reference to the drug's therapeutic category, the physical description and solubility characteristics of the drug, its definition, which states its standard of chemical purity, a cautionary statement which reflects the toxic nature of the agent, packaging and storage recommendations, and chemical and physical tests and the prescribed method of assay to substantiate the identification and

Pentobarbital Sodium Elixir

Category: Hypnotic; sedative.
Usual dose:
Hypnotic—100 mg at bedtime.
Sedative—20 mg three or four times a day.
Usual dose range: 50 to 200 mg daily.
Usual pediatric dose:
Sedative—2 mg per kg of body weight or 60 mg
per square meter of body surface, three times
a day.
Elixir available—Elixir usually available contains the following amount of pentobarbital
sodium: 20 mg per 5 ml.
Dispensing information—
Advice: Drowsiness may occur which may impair ability to drive or perform other tasks
requiring alertness. Avoid alcoholic beverages.
▶ Pentobarbital Sodium Elixir contains, in each
100 ml, not less than 375 mg and not more
than 425 mg of $C_{11}H_{17}N_2NaO_3$.
Pentobarbital Sodium Elixir may be prepared as
follows.

PENTOBARBITAL SODIUM	4	g
GLYCERIN	450	ml
ALCOHOL	150	ml
ORANGE OIL	0.75	ml
CARAMEL	2	g
SYRUP	150	ml
DILUTED HYDROCHLORIC ACID . .	6	ml
PURIFIED WATER, a sufficient quantity, to make	1000	ml

Dissolve the pentobarbital sodium in 200 ml
of purified water, then add the glycerin, alcohol,
orange oil, caramel, and syrup. Mix, and add the
diluted hydrochloric acid and sufficient purified
water to make the product measure 1000 ml.
Mix, and filter, if necessary.

Packaging and storage—Preserve in tight containers.
Identification—The pentobarbital obtained in the
Assay, when recrystallized from hot alcohol and dried
at 105° for 30 minutes, responds to *Identification test
A* under *Pentobarbital Sodium,* page 368, beginning
with "melts between 127° and 133°."
Assay—Transfer 25 ml of Pentobarbital Sodium
Elixir, accurately measured, to a separator, acidify
with diluted hydrochloric acid, and saturate with sodium chloride. Completely extract the pentobarbital
with successive 25-ml portions of chloroform. Wash
the combined chloroform extracts with 10 ml of water,
then extract the water with 10 ml of chloroform, adding the latter to the main chloroform solution. Filter
through a pledget of cotton or small filter paper, moistened with chloroform, into a tared beaker, evaporate
the chloroform on a steam bath, with the aid of a
current of air, add 10 ml of ether, and again evaporate.
Dry the residue at 105° for 2 hours, cool in a desiccator, and weigh: the weight of the residue, multiplied by
1.097, represents the weight of $C_{11}H_{17}N_2NaO_3$ in the
portion of the Elixir taken.
Alcohol content, page 634: between 12 and 18% of
C_2H_5OH.

Fig. 2-1.

purity of the chemical. The monograph for
Chlorambucil Tablets (Fig. 2-3) presents information on the pharmacologic category, dose,
strength of tablets commercially available, dispensing information for use by the pharmacist
and prescribing physician, recommendations for
packaging and storage, and the appropriate
tests, standards, and assay procedures to assure
the overall quality and uniformity of the dosage
form.

In each monograph, the standards set forth
are specific for the individual therapeutic agent,
pharmaceutical necessity, or dosage form and
vary with the particular requirements to insure
purity, potency, and overall quality.

Nomenclature

The initial part of each drug monograph
consists of the official title or name of the drug,
pharmaceutic agent or preparation. The official
titles for preparations contain the name of the

primary or most distinguishing component(s)
and the type of dosage form, as: *Pentobarbital
Sodium Elixir* and *Chlorambucil Tablets.*

Drugs or agents of zoological or botanic origin are named according to the rules set forth by
the International Botanical Congress and the
International Zoological Congress. The inorganic salts are named according to the established precedent of a cation-anion order, as
sodium chloride. It is in the area of naming pure
organic chemicals of synthetic or natural origin
that most of the current efforts in drug nomenclature are directed, since this group represents
today's most prolific source of new drugs.

The official title for a drug substance is referred to as the drug's *nonproprietary* or *public*
name, in contrast to the *proprietary* or brand or
trademark names given the chemical substance
by specific manufacturers or distributors of the
drug. The term *generic name,* although erroneously applied, has been used extensively in referring to the nonproprietary names of drugs.

Chlorambucil*

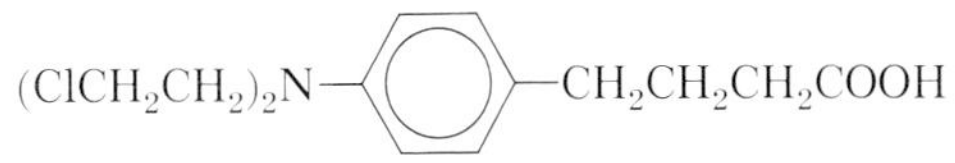

$(ClCH_2CH_2)_2N$—⬡—$CH_2CH_2CH_2COOH$

$C_{14}H_{19}Cl_2NO_2$ 304.22 Benzenebutanoic acid, 4-[bis(2-chloroethyl)amino]-4-[*p*-[Bis (2-chloroethyl)amino]phenyl]butyric acid [305-03-3].

Category: See *Chlorambucil Tablets.*

Description: Off-white, slightly granular powder.

Solubility: Very slightly soluble in water; freely soluble in acetone; soluble in dilute alkali.

▶ Chlorambucil contains not less than 98.0% and not more than 101.0% of $C_{14}H_{19}Cl_2NO_2$, calculated on the anhydrous basis.

Caution—Great care should be taken to prevent inhaling particles of Chlorambucil and exposing the skin to it.

Packaging and storage—Preserve in tight, light-resistant containers.

Identification—

A: The infrared absorption spectrum of a 1 in 125 solution in carbon disulfide, in a 1-mm cell, exhibits maxima only at the same wavelengths as that of a similar solution of USP Chlorambucil Reference Standard.

B: Dissolve 50 mg in 5 ml of acetone, and dilute with water to 10 ml. Add 1 drop of diluted sulfuric acid, then add 4 drops of silver nitrate TS: no opalescence is observed immediately (*absence of chloride ion*). Warm the solution on a steam bath: opalescence develops (*presence of ionizable chlorine*).

Melting range, page 651: between 65° and 69°.

Water, *Method 1*, page 668: not more than 0.5%.

Assay—Dissolve about 200 mg of Chlorambucil, accurately weighed, in 10 ml of acetone, add 10 ml of water, and titrate with 0.1 N sodium hydroxide, using phenolphthalein TS as the indicator. Each ml of 0.1 N sodium hydroxide is equivalent to 30.42 mg of $C_{14}H_{19}Cl_2NO_2$.

*Patented.

Fig. 2-2.

The value of designating each drug by a single nonproprietary name is obvious in terms of achieving simplicity and uniformity in drug nomenclature. The nonproprietary name of a drug serves numerous and varied purposes. Its principal function is to identify the substance to which it applies through its designated name, which may be used without restriction by the professional and lay public, in contrast to the brand name, which may be registered as a trademark with the United States Patent Office for the exclusive use of the registrant. If the drug is protected by a patent, indicated with an asterisk in the monograph, generally only one such manufacturer's trademark exists. When a chemical agent is not protected with a patent, any drug manufacturer may coin a brand name, obtain a trademark, and manufacture and distribute the drug under the exclusive use of the name. Many manufacturers may engage in this activity for a single chemical compound, each promoting his product under a different name. Through the use of a single nonproprietary name for a drug, the nature of drug products of different manufacturers and of different dosage forms is more exactly identified, for it is required by law to use the nonproprietary name whenever the brand name is used in drug advertising, promotion, and labeling. The common designation for a drug facilitates communication among scientists, teachers, and the practitioners in the health fields.

Naming a Drug

The selection of a single nonproprietary name for older organic chemicals has been mostly a matter of accepting the name most widely accepted scientifically through the years. The early selection of a single nonproprietary name for a newly synthesized or discovered chemical is important to reduce the likelihood of its being referred to by several different names in the chemical, drug, and medical literature. Even so, a newly found organic chemical is normally referred to by a minimum of three and often four different names on its way to a recognized place in therapeutics.

When first synthesized, or identified from a natural source, an organic compound is represented by an *empirical formula*, as $C_{14}H_{19}Cl_2NO_2$ for chlorambucil, which indicates the number and the relationship of the atoms comprising the molecule. As knowledge of the relative locations of these atoms is gained, the compound receives a *systematic chemical name,* as 4-{*p*-[Bis(2-chloroethyl)-amino]phenyl} butyric acid for chlorambucil. To be adequate and fully specific, the name must reveal every part of the compound's molecular structure, so that it describes only the compound concerned and no other. The systematic name is generally so formidable that it soon is replaced in scientific communication by a condensed name, which, although less descriptive chemically, is understood to refer only to that chemical compound. This new name may be the first attempt

Chlorambucil Tablets

Category: Antineoplastic.

Usual dose: Initial, 100 to 200 µg per kg of body weight once a day.

Maintenance, 30 to 100 µg per kg of body weight daily.

Usual dose range: 30 to 200 µg per kg of body weight daily.

Usual pediatric dose: 100 to 200 µg per kg of body weight or 4.5 mg per square meter of body surface, once a day.

Tablets available—Tablets usually available contain 2 mg of chlorambucil.

Dispensing information—

Note: This drug should be taken only under strict medical supervision.

Advice: Notify physician if fever, sore throat, or unusual bleeding or bruising occurs.

▶ Chlorambucil Tablets contain not less than 93.0% and not more than 107.0% of the labeled amount of $C_{14}H_{19}Cl_2NO_2$.

Packaging and storage—Preserve coated Tablets in well-closed containers; preserve uncoated Tablets in well-closed, light-resistant containers.

Identification—Shake a quantity of finely powdered Tablets, equivalent to about 16 mg of chlorambucil, with 20 ml of carbon disulfide. Filter, evaporate to dryness, and dissolve the residue in 2 ml of carbon disulfide: the resulting solution responds to *Identification test A* under *Chlorambucil*, page 76.

Disintegration, page 650: 30 minutes.

Content uniformity, page 648: meet the requirements for *Tablets.*

Assay—[*Caution—Exercise great care in the storage and use of isopropyl ether, since it is highly flammable and it tends to form explosive peroxides on standing.*] Wash 100 ml of isopropyl ether by shaking with four 25-ml portions of water, and discard the water washings. Weigh and finely powder not less than 20 Chlorambucil Tablets. Weigh accurately a portion of the powder, equivalent to about 4 mg of chlorambucil, and transfer to a separator containing 5 ml of monobasic potassium phosphate solution (1 in 10). Immediately shake with 15 ml of washed isopropyl ether for about 30 seconds. Draw off the lower, aqueous layer into a second separator, and pour the isopropyl ether layer into a 50-ml volumetric flask. Extract the aqueous layer with three 10-ml portions of washed isopropyl ether, each time drawing off the aqueous layer into the alternate separator, and transfer the ether layer to the volumetric flask. Dilute with the washed isopropyl ether to volume. Dissolve an accurately weighed quantity of USP Chlorambucil Reference Standard in washed isopropyl ether, and dilute quantitatively and stepwise with washed isopropyl ether to obtain a Standard solution having a known concentration of about 80 µg per ml. Concomitantly determine the absorbances of both solutions in 1-cm cells at the wavelength of maximum absorbance at about 301 nm, with a suitable spectrophotometer, using washed isopropyl ether as the blank. Calculate the quantity, in mg, of $C_{14}H_{19}Cl_2NO_2$ in the portion of the Tablets taken by the formula $0.05C(A_U/A_S)$, in which C is the concentration, in µg per ml, of USP Chlorambucil Reference Standard in the Standard solution, and A_U and A_S are the absorbances of the solution from Chlorambucil Tablets and the Standard solution, respectively.

Fig. 2-3.

at assigning the nonproprietary name, or it may be an intermediate designation as a *code number,* which generally stays with the compound through its initial laboratory investigation for pharmacologic activity and through the human clinical trials. The practice of using code numbers for test substances is not new; Paul Ehrlich made it famous a half century ago when he numbered the compounds employed in his search for the "magic bullet" to cure syphilis. His compound "606" became more famous than the chemical's other names of arsphenamine and Salvarsan. Today many companies give their new compounds code numbers for their intralaboratory use prior to the assignment of a nonproprietary name. These code numbers generally take the form of an identifying prefix letter or letters that identify the drug's sponsor, followed by a number that further identifies the test compound.

When the results of clinical testing indicate that a compound has sufficient merit to warrant marketing, a *nonproprietary* and usually a *proprietary name* are assigned to the drug. Should the drug receive recognition in an official compendium, the nonproprietary name established during the period of the drug's early usage is generally adopted. It should be pointed out that nonproprietary names are issued only for single agents whereas proprietary or trademark names may be associated with a single chemical entity or with a mixture of chemicals comprising a specific proprietary product.

The USAN Council

Today the task of designating appropriate nonproprietary names for newly found chemical agents rests primarily with the United States Adopted Names Council (USAN Council). This organized effort at coining nonproprietary names for drugs was inaugurated in 1961 as a joint project of the American Medical Association and the United States Pharmacopeial Convention. They were joined in 1964 by the American Pharmaceutical Association to form the USAN Council; in 1967, the Food and Drug Administration was invited to take part in the work of the Council and to place a representative on it. Financial support for the Council programs is contributed by the three nongovernmental organizations, with the American Medical Association maintaining the secretariat and the USP Convention publishing the United States Adopted Names (USAN) in cumulative form each year.

A proposal for a USAN usually originates from a firm or an individual who has developed a substance of potential therapeutic usefulness to the point where there is a distinct possibility of its being marketed in the United States. Occasionally, the initiative is taken by the USAN Council in the form of a request to parties interested in a substance for which a nonproprietary name appears to be lacking. Proposals are expected to conform to the Council's guidelines for coining nonproprietary names. In general, the name should (1) be short and distinctive in sound and spelling and not be such that it is easily confused with existing names, (2) indicate the general pharmacologic or therapeutic class into which the substance falls or the general chemical nature of the substance if the latter is associated with the specific pharmacologic activity, (3) embody the syllable or syllables characteristic of a related group of compounds. It is recommended that drugs of the following categories bear the appropriate syllable in their nonproprietary names (Table 2-1).

When general agreement on a name has been reached between the Council and the drug's sponsor, it is circulated in the Trademark Bulletin of the Pharmaceutical Manufacturers Association as a "Proposed USAN." This indicates the Council's intention to adopt the name and serves notice on those who wish to protest the selection within 30 days of its appearance. The tentatively adopted USAN is then submitted for consideration by various American and foreign drug regulatory agencies, including the World Health Organization, the British Pharmacopoeia Commission, the French Codex, the Nordic Pharmacopeia, the United States Pharmacopeia, the National Formulary, and the U.S. Food and

Drug Administration. If no objections are raised, adoption is considered final, and the USAN is published in the various literature of the medical and pharmaceutical professions. Disputes are settled by a six-member, appointed board, known as the USAN Review Board. The findings of this Board are regarded as final and beyond appeal.

Under the 1962 Drug Amendments, the Secretary of the Department of Health, Education, and Welfare has authority to designate the nonproprietary name for any drug in the interest of usefulness or simplicity. The authority is generally delegated to the Commissioner of the Food and Drug Administration within the Department. As of 1973, a total of 450 names had been selected under this authority, all of which are identical to or derived from the corresponding USAN. With the creation of the USAN Council and the cooperation of the interested parties on a worldwide basis, the problem of nonproprietary drug nomenclature has been greatly reduced in recent years.

Drug Category

A statement of drug category is provided in each monograph to indicate the therapeutic or pharmaceutic basis for each drug's recognition in the compendium. The statements, which are intentionally brief, represent the best known or most widely recognized use of each drug. The category statement is intended to serve as general information and not to limit the use of the agent or to imply that it has no application other than that which is listed.

In pharmacy, the main systems for classifying or categorizing drugs are as follows:

(1) Classification according to the anatomical site of action.
(2) Classification according to therapeutic activity or application.
(3) Classification according to the pharmacological mechanism of action.
(4) Classification according to the source of origin or the chemical and pharmacological properties of the drug.

Under these schemes, for example, pentobarbital sodium could be classified respectively as: (1) a drug acting on the central nervous system, (2) a sedative and hypnotic, (3) a central nervous system depressant, and (4) a derivative of barbi-

Table 2-1. SOME USAN RECOMMENDED PREFIXES AND SUFFIXES
FOR THE CONSTRUCTION OF NONPROPRIETARY NAMES OF DRUGS

anabolic steroids	bol-; or -bol-
analgesics (meperidine series)	-eridine
androgens	-andr-; or
	-stan-; or
	-ster-
anesthetics, local	-caine
anorexics	-orex
anti-adrenergics (beta receptor)	-olol
antibiotics (cephalosporanic acid derivatives)	cef-
antibiotics (polyene derivatives)	-tricin
antibiotics produced by *Streptomyces* strains	-mycin
antibiotics (rifamycin derivatives)	-rifin
antibiotics (tetracycline derivatives)	-cycline
anticoagulants (coumarin type)	-arol
anticonvulsants, hydantoin	-toin
antimicrobial sulfonamides	sulfa-
barbituric acid derivatives	-barb
bronchodilators (phenethylamine derivatives)	-terol
corticotropins, synthetic	-actide
cortisone derivatives	-cort-
dibenzazepine compounds (imipramine type-straight side chain)	-pramine
diuretics (sulfamoylbenzoic acid derivatives)	-pamide
diuretics (thiazide derivatives)	-thiazide
estrogens	-estr-
hypoglycemics, oral { guanidine	-formin
sulfonamide	gli-
iodine-containing contrast media	io-
mercurials	-mer-
morphinan derivatives that are narcotic antagonists or agonists	-orphan
5-nitrofuran derivatives	nifur-
normorphone derivatives that are narcotic antagonists	nal-
penicillins (6-aminopenicillanic acid derivatives)	-cillin
progestins	-gest-
prostaglandin derivatives	-prost-
steroids that are acetonide derivatives	-onide
tranquilizers (benzodiazepine derivatives)	-azepam
tranquilizers (propanediol and pentanediol series)	-bamate

turic acid. In the official compendia, there is an overlapping of the methods used in categorizing drugs. For the most part, however, the second method is most frequently used and functions as a therapeutic guide to physicians and others.

Mechanism of Drug Action

In general, drugs exert their effects by one of three means: (1) by exerting a physical action, such as the protective effects of ointments and lotions upon topical application; (2) by reacting chemically outside of the body's cells—for example, antacids to counteract excess acidity in the

stomach or antibiotics to act against invading pathogenic microorganisms; or (3) by modifying the metabolic activity of the body's cells. The majority of drugs in use today act in the third manner by affecting the specialized cells of the brain, liver, heart, blood vessels, kidneys, nerve ganglia or endings, and other tissues. The processes of life and metabolism within the body's cells involve intricate enzymatic reactions. Each component of these complex enzyme systems is vital to the normal functioning of the cell. The vitamins, for example, are indispensable to life because they are necessary components of essential enzyme systems. On the other hand, many poisons, including drugs in overdosage, exert their toxic effects by inactivating life-sustaining enzyme systems. Drugs modify the metabolism of cells by (1) adsorption on the cell membrane or surface, (2) penetration of the cell membrane, or (3) chemical combination with cellular components. Any of these actions alters the function of the cell and initiates a series of biochemical and physiological changes that result in the drug's effects and provide the basis for its categorization. The initial drug-cell interaction is appropriately termed the drug's "action"; the resulting events are properly referred to as its "effects."

For established therapeutic agents, most of the drug effects are predictable and desirable. However, no drug is so specific not to possess the potential for the production of accompanying undesirable effects. Some of these undesirable effects, termed *adverse drug reactions*, may be quite minor and easily tolerated by the patient. However, others may be quite disturbing and intolerable and may be so severe to be life-threatening. An adverse drug reaction may be expected or unexpected and may be related to the dose administered or may be a function of the drug in relation to the patient's biochemical or pathological state, the presence of other medication given concomitantly, the patient's psychologic disposition, the diet, or an idiosyncrasy or allergy to the drug substance. In each instance in which an adverse drug reaction is expected or occurs, the drug's benefit to the patient must be weighed against the risk and appropriate decisions and measures taken.

The action of most drugs takes place at the molecular level with the drug molecules interacting with the molecules of the cell structure or its contents (Fig. 2-4).

The selectivity and specificity of drugs for a certain body tissue—for example, drugs that act primarily on the nerves, heart, or kidney—are related to specific sites on or within the cells, receptive only to chemicals of a particular chemical structure and configuration. The cellular component directly involved in the action of a drug is termed its *receptor*. The chemical groups that participate in the drug-receptor combination and the adjacent portions of the receptor that favor or hinder access of the drug to these active groups are known as *receptor groups* or *receptor sites*. Although receptors for most drugs have yet to be identified, they, like the active centers of enzymes, are thought to be carboxyl, amino, sulfhydryl, phosphate, and similar reactive groups oriented on or in the cell in a pattern complementary to that of the drugs with which they react. The binding of a drug to the receptor is thought to be accomplished mainly by ionic and other relatively weak reversible bonds. Occasionally, firm covalent bonding is involved, and the drug effect is then very slowly reversible. Because receptor sites bind chemicals with specific chemical groupings and orientation,

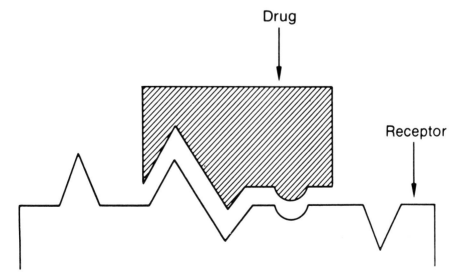

Fig. 2-4. *Schematic drawing of receptor site and substrate (drug) (From "How Modern Medicines are Discovered," Frank H. Clark, Ed., Courtesy of Futura Publishing Company, Inc.)*

many chemicals that are but slight modifications of an initial or parent compound possess the same pharmacologic effect. Basically, the structure of a chemical compound affects two properties that are closely interrelated to its biological activity—its physical characteristics and its chemical reactivity. Such properties determine, for example, whether the molecule can permeate the various barriers between the external medium and the site of biochemical action within the cell and arrive at that site in adequate concentration. Modifications in a chemical's structure can alter the speed of drug action, the duration of the effects, and toxic or undesirable side effects. There are numerous derivatives of barbituric acid, including pentobarbital; each is a sedative, but each differs in its degree of activity and its onset and duration of action. Certain cells within the body are capable of receiving drug substances without eliciting a drug effect. These cells are important in the transport of drugs throughout the body, in their detoxification by metabolism or chemical breakdown, and in their ultimate elimination from the body.

Drugs may act by influencing any of the steps involved in the maintenance of normal cell function. Thus they may individually act to enhance or prevent cell metabolism. The effects of drug action may be described as either stimulation, depression, or irritation. An increased activity of specialized cells due to the presence of drugs is referred to as "stimulation." A decrease in cellular activity is called "depression." Pentobarbital is a depressant to the cells of the central nervous system. The degree of activity of depressants can usually be governed by the size of the dose; thus pentobarbital in greater than sedative doses may be employed as a hypnotic, or a drug that induces sleep. Stimulant drugs may stimulate cells to a point of inactivity resembling the effects of depressant drugs but comparable to physiological fatigue. This type of overstimulation is reversible and is only temporary, with the cells returning to normal activity as the drug is removed from the body through the metabolic process. Irritant drugs are useful in provoking idle cells to normal activity, but if used for extended periods of time or in excessive concentration, they may result in the destruction of tissue. Mercury salts, for example, are irritant to the tubules of the kidney and may cause death of cells with loss of kidney function. In proper dosage regimen, the irritant

action of mercury compounds is used to increase the flow of urine or promote diuresis. Many laxative and cathartic drugs exert their action by the irritation of the lining of the intestinal wall with resultant peristalsis and consequent laxation. Brief definitions of some of the categories used in the compendia are presented in the Appendix.

The physical and chemical aspects of the drug substance and factors of dosage form design which can affect the action of a drug will be discussed in the next chapter.

Dosage Statements

Monographs for therapeutic agents generally contain two or more statements concerning dosage. Normally given are the *usual dose* of the drug and the *usual dosage range.* The usual dose of a drug may be defined as that amount which may be expected ordinarily to produce, in adults, the medicinal effect for which it was officially recognized. It serves as a guide to physicians who then may vary the dose depending upon the particular requirements of the patient. The usual dosage range for a drug indicates the quantitative range or amounts of the drug that may be prescribed within the framework of usual medical practice. Doses falling outside of the usual dosage range may be questioned by the pharmacist as being either underdosage or overdosage, as the case may be, and subject to further scrutiny and consultation with the prescribing medical practitioner. For drugs which may be administered to children, a *usual pediatric dose* may be included in the monograph. Whenever a drug is administered by a route other than oral—as by injection, inhalation, or rectally—the officially stated dose is for that designated means of administration.

The schedule of dosage, or the *dosage regimen,* is indicated for those drugs that are best taken at specific intervals (e.g., every 8 hours) or at specific times (e.g., at bedtime, before meals, or on arising in the morning). Single doses are given for some drugs and daily doses for others, depending upon the type of material and the therapeutic purpose of the medication. When a drug like thyroid is generally taken for extended periods of time, a daily dose is appropriate. When a drug like aspirin is taken occasionally and whenever needed for an acute condition, a single dose is more appropriate. For certain drugs, an *initial, priming,* or *loading* dose may be required to attain a certain desired concentration of the drug in the blood or tissues, which may then be maintained through the subsequent administration of regularly scheduled *maintenance doses*. Digoxin, a cardiotonic agent, is a good example of a drug which is administered in this way. The initial goal of digoxin therapy is to achieve the desired *level of digoxin* in the patient through the administration of the drug four or more times a day at first. This is then usually followed by a single daily dose to maintain the desired blood level of the drug.

For drugs like pentobarbital that produce more than one effect, depending upon the dose administered, the dose for each of the effects is given. Thus in doses of 20 mg, pentobarbital will usually produce sedation in the adult patient, whereas in doses of 100 mg, the same drug will likely have a hypnotic effect. Pharmaceutical preparations are generally formulated so that the usual dose is provided in a convenient unit of the dosage form—as in one tablet, capsule, or suppository or in one teaspoonful (5 ml) or tablespoonful (15 ml) of a liquid preparation. In the case of pentobarbital sodium elixir, there are 4 mg of pentobarbital sodium present in each milliliter of elixir; thus if one wanted to issue a sedative dose of the preparation, one or two teaspoonfuls would generally suffice. For hypnotic doses, a tablespoonful or more of the elixir might be required.

Certain biological products, as Tetanus Human Immune Globulin, may have two different usual doses, one the *prophylactic dose*, or that amount administered to protect the patient from contracting the illness, and the second, the *therapeutic dose* which is administered to a patient after exposure or contraction of the illness. The recommended doses of vaccines and other biological products including antibiotics and endocrine products are sometimes expressed in *units of activity* rather than in specific quantitative amounts of the drug substance. Units of activity derived from biological assay methods reflect a drug's potency and become necessary when suitable chemical assay methods are unavailable for a particular drug. Drugs from natural sources, with unknown or varying complex chemical composition, may vary in potency, one batch to another, even though the same quantitative amount of material is present. Biological assays are useful in determining relative potencies of different

batches of the same drug and in their standardization. The potency of a given drug is based on the comparison with an international reference standard of that drug. Insulin injection, for example, is prepared to contain 40, 80, 100, or 500 Insulin units of activity in each milliliter of injection in order to meet all dosage requirements in a convenient amount of injection. These units of activity reflect the relative potency of the different preparations in terms of biological activity and are uniform on an international basis. Since the biological activities of different products, such as penicillin, poliomyelitis vaccine, and insulin, are so varied, the units of activity for each is specific for one drug only and has no relation between the units of activity for another drug.

All doses in the USP and the NF, with the exception of those expressed in units of activity, are stated in terms of the metric system. Also, all weights, volumes, and linear dimensions of materials present in the official formulas, monographs, and in assay and test methods are indicated with metric units of measurement. The metric and other systems of pharmaceutical measurement are presented in the Appendix.

Factors Affecting Drug Dosage

The dose of a drug has been appropriately described as an amount which is "enough but not too much," the idea being to produce the drug's optimum therapeutic effect in a particular patient with the lowest possible dose. The dose of a given drug is an individual thing, with many factors contributing to its size and effectiveness. The correct dose of aspirin in relieving the pain of a headache would be the smallest effective amount and likely would vary from individual to individual and, indeed, within the same individual from one occasion to another. The familiar bell-shaped curve, presented in Figure 2-5 shows that in a normal distribution of patients, a drug's usual dose will provide what might be called an average effect in the majority of individuals. In a portion of the patients, however, the drug will produce little effect, whereas in another group of similar size, the drug will produce an effect greater than the average effect. The amount of drug that will generally produce the desired effect in the majority of patients is considered the drug's usual dose and would likely be the starter dose for an individual taking the drug for the first time.

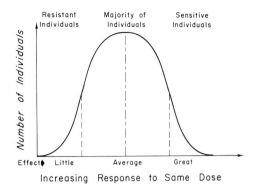

Fig. 2-5. *Drug effect in a population sample.*

From this initial dose the physician may, if necessary, increase or decrease subsequent doses to meet the particular requirements of his patient.

In order for a drug to provide systemic effects, it must be absorbed from its route of administration at a suitable rate, be distributed in adequate concentration to the receptor sites, and remain there for a sufficient duration of time. One measure of a drug's absorption characteristics is the determination of its blood serum concentration at various time intervals following administration. For each drug, a correlation can be made between its blood serum concentration and the presentation of drug effects. An average blood serum concentration of a drug can be determined that represents the minimum concentration that can be expected to produce the drug's desired effects in a patient. This concentration is referred to as the *Minimum Effective Concentration* (MEC). As shown in Figure 2-6, for a hypothetical drug, the serum concentration of the drug reaches the MEC 2 hours following its administration, achieves a

peak concentration in 4 hours and decreases below the MEC in 10 hours. If it would be desired to maintain the drug serum concentration above the MEC for a longer period of time, a second dose of the drug would be required at approximately the 8-hour time frame. The time-blood level figures stated in Figure 2-6 are examples. In practice, the figures would vary, depending on the drug itself, its chemical and physical characteristics, the dosage form type as well as pathological state of the patient, his diet, concomitant drug therapy, and other considerations. Factors of dosage form design affecting the biological availability of a drug for absorption will be considered more extensively in the following chapter. The second level of blood serum concentration of drug labeled MTC in Figure 2-6 refers to the *Minimum Toxic Concentration*. Drug serum concentrations above this level would produce dose-related toxic effects in the average individual and would negate the desirable effects of the drug while challenging the safety of the patient. Ideally, the serum drug concentration in a well-dosed patient would be maintained between the MEC and the MTC for the period that drug effects are desired.

The *median effective dose* of a drug is that amount which will produce the desired intensity of effect in 50% of the individuals tested and the *median toxic dose* is that amount which will produce a defined toxic effect in 50% of the individuals tested. The relationship between the desired and undesired effects of a drug is commonly expressed as the *therapeutic index* and is defined as the ratio between a drug's median toxic dose and its median effective dose, TD50/ED50. Thus, a drug with a therapeutic index of 15 would be expected to have a greater margin of safety in its use than a drug with a

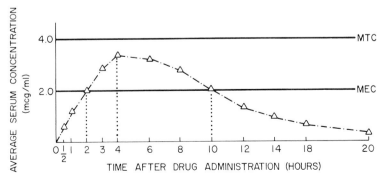

Fig. 2-6. *Example of a blood level curve for a hypothetical drug as a function of time following oral administration. MEC stands for* minimum effective concentration *and MTC for* minimum toxic concentration.

therapeutic index of 5. For certain drugs, like digoxin and digitoxin, the therapeutic index may be as low as 2 and extreme caution must be exercised in the administration of agents such as these.

The therapeutic index has to be viewed as a general guide to the margin of safety of a drug, with each patient and his response to a drug considered separately. The therapeutic index does not take into account individual patient idiosyncrasy by which some patients react differently to a drug than do most persons. Further, since the criteria for determining the therapeutic index involve the use of median figures and intentionally narrow definitions of "effectiveness" and "toxicity," the index does not reflect extremes of the population sample and, depending upon the definitions of effectiveness and toxicity used, a number of therapeutic indexes may be determined for a single drug. For instance, the median effective dose for aspirin can be determined for simple headache, migraine headache, arthritic pain, fever, or other conditions and a different ED50 and therapeutic index calculated. Factors that can influence the proper dose of a drug for a given patient include the patient's age, weight, sex, pathological state, his tolerance to the drug, the time of the drug's administration, the route of administration, the concurrent administration of other drugs, and a variety of physiologic and psychologic factors. Some of these factors will be considered briefly here.

1. AGE. The age of the individual being treated is a usual consideration in the determination of drug dosage, especially in the young or very old. Newborn infants, particularly those born prematurely, are abnormally sensitive to certain drugs because of the immature state of their hepatic and renal function by which drugs are normally inactivated and eliminated from the body. Failure to detoxify and eliminate drugs results in their accumulation in the tissues to a toxic level. Aged individuals may also respond abnormally to a usual amount of a drug due to impaired ability to inactivate or excrete drugs or because of other concurrent pathology.

Before there was an understanding of the physiologic differences between adult and pediatric patients, the latter were treated with drugs as if they were merely miniature adults. Various rules of dosage in which the pediatric dose was a fraction of the adult dose, based on relative age, were created for youngsters. Today these rules are not in general use since age alone is no longer considered to be a singularly valid criterion for use in the determination of children's dosage, especially when calculated from a *usual* adult dose which itself provides wide clinical variations in response. Instead, the *usual pediatric dose*, determined for specific drugs and dosage forms by clinical evaluation, is utilized. These pediatric doses are included in drug literature and in pharmaceutical product labeling and are used as guidelines to be considered with other factors in the dosage determination for a specific pediatric patient.

2. BODY WEIGHT. The official usual doses for drugs are considered generally suitable for 70 kg (150 pound) individuals. The ratio between the amount of drug administered and the size of the body influences the drug concentration at its site of action. Therefore, drug dosage may require adjustment from the usual adult dose for abnormally lean or obese patients. The determination of drug dosage for youngsters on the basis of body weight is considered more dependable than that based strictly on age. However, the consideration of the individual drug and patient's pathological and physiological state still reigns supreme and limits the clinical utility of any *general* rule of pediatric dosage.

Many monographs and commercial pharmaceutical products present adult and pediatric doses in terms of body weight, as shown in Figure 2-3 for Chlorambucil Tablets.

3. BODY SURFACE AREA. Other methods of determining drug dosage have been proposed in preference to those based solely on age or weight. One such method has as its basis the recognition that a close correlation exists between a large number of physiological processes and body surface area (BSA). A formula for the determination of a child's dose based on relative body surface area and the adult dose is:

$$\frac{\text{Surface area of child's body}}{\text{Surface area of adult's body}} \times \text{Adult Usual Dose}$$
$$= \text{Approximate Child's Dose}$$

The surface area of individuals may be determined from a nomogram composed of scales of height, weight, and surface area. Two such nomograms are presented in the Appendix. Surface area is indicated where a straight line drawn to connect the height and weight of an individual intersects the surface area column. The administration of a total adult dose is considered appropriate when the body surface area reaches 1.7 square meters; thus this figure may be employed in the denominator of the above formula.

Referring to Figure 2-3 once again, the usual pediatric dose of chlorambucil based on BSA is 4.5 mg per square meter. Using the nomogram for calculating the BSA of children and using the example of a child weighing 15 kg and measuring 100 cm in height, the surface area would be 0.64 square meter. Thus, the dose of chlorambucil for this child would be: 4.5 mg $\times$ 0.64 = 2.88 mg once a day.

4. SEX. Women are thought to be more susceptible to the effects of certain drugs than are men, and in some instances this difference is considered sufficient to necessitate reduction in dosage. During pregnancy, caution is necessary in the administration of drugs that might affect the uterus or fetus. A number of drugs have been shown to be readily transported from the maternal to the fetal circulation including such agents as: alcohol, anesthetic gases, barbiturates, narcotic and non-narcotic analgesics, anticoagulants, anti-infective agents, and many others.[1] Fetal exposure to agents such as these has resulted in adverse effects to the fetus, sometimes resulting in death *in utero* or in congenital damage to the neonate. The fetus is apparently more sensitive to the effects of certain drugs than is the mother. For instance, respiration in the fetus may be halted at a level of general anesthesia that does not impair maternal respiration. Also, because of the undeveloped and thus ineffective drug detoxication and excretion mechanisms present in the fetus, concentrations of drugs may actually reach a higher level in the fetus than in the maternal circulation. The addiction of newborn infants to narcotic drugs as heroin and morphine due to the maternal use of these agents during pregnancy is not an uncommon occurrence. The same result occurs when an infant is breast-fed by a narcotic dependent mother. The transfer of drugs from the mother to the nursing infant through human milk may occur with a wide variety of drugs with the drug effects becoming manifest in the infant.[2] Thus, pregnant women and nursing mothers should use medications only with the advice and under the guidance of their physician.

5. PATHOLOGICAL STATE. The effects of certain drugs may be modified by the pathological condition of the patient and must be considered in determining the drug to use as well as its proper dose. The terms *warning* and *precautions* are used in the drug literature and labeling to alert the physician to certain restrictions or cautions in the use of a particular drug. A "precaution" to the use of a drug is less restrictive than is a "warning" and is intended to advise the prescriber of some possible problems attendant with the use of the drug and to alert him to take the necessary precautions or countermeasures. For instance, associated with the use of tetracycline antibiotic drugs is the possibility of resultant overgrowth of nonsusceptible organisms including fungi. If such a superinfection occurs, the physician may wish to prescribe an alternate drug. A "warning" is used in instances in which the potential for patient harm is greater than in instances in which the "precaution" is used. For example, if tetracycline is used in the presence of renal impairment, it may lead to the excessive systemic accumulation of the drug and possible liver toxicity. Under such conditions, lower than usual doses are indicated, and if therapy is prolonged, blood serum levels of the drug should be taken and the patient monitored at regular intervals to assure the maintenance of non-toxic levels of the drug. Also, liver function tests may be performed to detect possible liver damage. Drugs having a high danger potential in a given therapeutic situation should be used only when the possible benefit to the patient exceeds the possible risk and when no other suitable drug with a lesser toxicity is available. The term *contraindication* is used in drug literature and labeling to indicate an *absolute prohibition* to the use of a drug in the presence of certain stated conditions. It is the most restrictive of the warnings which limit the use of drugs. Contraindications exist to the use of most drugs, and the physician and pharmacist should be knowledgeable of them to protect the patient from harm. Generally, any drug is contraindicated in a patient with a known allergy or hypersensitivity to the particular agent. Specifically, many drugs have contraindications to their use which are unique or associated with the specific drug or with its general pharmacologic category. For example, since an increased risk of thromboembolic disease associated with

[1]"Hazards of Medication," by Eric W. Martin, Philadelphia, J. B. Lippincott Co., 1972, pp. 274–280.
[2]O'Brien, T. E.: Excretion of Drugs in Human Milk, *Am. J. Hosp. Pharm.*, 31:844, 1974.

the use of hormonal contraceptives has been shown, the use of these drugs in persons with a history of thrombophlebitis or thromboembolic disorders is considered dangerous and is contraindicated. Estrogen-containing contraceptives are also contraindicated in the presence of a known or suspected carcinoma of the breast or other estrogen-dependent neoplasia.

6. TOLERANCE. The ability to endure the influence of a drug, particularly when acquired by a continued use of the substance, is referred to as drug *tolerance*. It is usually developed to a specific drug or to its chemical congeners; in the latter instance it is referred to as *cross-tolerance*. The effect of drug tolerance is that the drug dosage must be increased to maintain a given therapeutic response. Tolerance occurs commonly to the use of such drugs as antihistaminics, narcotic analgesics, and barbiturates. After the development of tolerance to a certain drug or type of drug, normal sensitivity may be regained only by suspending the drug's administration for a period of time. For most drugs, the development of tolerance can be minimized by initiating therapy with the lowest effective dose and by avoiding prolonged administration.

7. CONCOMITANT DRUG THERAPY. The effects of a drug may be modified by the prior or concurrent administration of another drug. Such interferences between drugs are referred to as *drug-drug interactions* and are due to the chemical or physical interaction between the drugs or to an alteration of the absorption, distribution, metabolism, or excretion patterns of one of the drugs. The effects of drug-drug interactions may be desirable and beneficial to the patient or they may be detrimental. An example of a beneficial interaction involves the drugs probenecid and penicillin or its derivatives. Given concomitantly, probenecid causes the prolongation of penicillin serum levels, enabling a reduction in the total dose of penicillin required as well as in the frequency of its administration. This has the effect of reducing the incidence of missed dosage administration by patients.

A detrimental interaction between drugs may be exemplified by that between certain metal ions and the antibiotic tetracycline or its derivatives. Tetracyclines can combine with the metal ions calcium, magnesium, aluminum, and iron in the gastrointestinal tract to form complexes that are poorly absorbed. Many antacid drugs are particularly rich in calcium, magnesium, and aluminum and should be avoided during tetracycline administration. If offending antacids and tetracycline are both required in a patient, they should be given alternately according to a strict schedule which avoids their simultaneous presence during the period allowed for tetracycline absorption. Certain calcium containing foods, as milk, cheese, and other dairy products must similarly be restricted during tetracycline administration.

Another example of drug-drug interaction which can alter the effectiveness of a given dose of a drug involves the drug phenobarbital and the anticoagulant drug warfarin. Phenobarbital stimulates liver microsomal enzymes which can result in the increased rate of metabolism of a number of drugs including warfarin. Thus, a person stabilized on a specific dose of warfarin may require an increased dosage level of that drug if phenobarbital is subsequently added to the therapeutic regimen. Conversely, if a patient is stabilized on a level of warfarin while also being administered phenobarbital, the dosage of warfarin would likely need to be decreased if the phenobarbital therapy is discontinued.

The study of drug interactions with other drugs, with foods, and with clinical laboratory tests is becoming an important facet of drug therapy and pharmacy practice. A number of excellent reference sources are now available in this area for student and practitioner use.

8. TIME OF ADMINISTRATION. The time at which a drug is administered sometimes influences dosage. This is especially true for oral therapy in relation to meals. Absorption proceeds more rapidly if the stomach and upper portions of the intestinal tract are free of food, and an amount of a drug that is effective when taken before a meal may be ineffective if administered during or after eating. On the other hand, irritating drugs are better tolerated by the patient if food is present in the stomach to dilute the drug's concentration.

The proper schedule of a drug's dosage (as "four times a day," or "every 8 hours") is a factor of the illness and the body drug level desired, the physicochemical nature of the drug itself, the dosage form design, and the degree and rate of the drug's absorption, distribution, metabolism and elimination from the body. These factors which play a part in drug dosage and in dosage form design will be discussed in the next chapter.

9. ROUTE OF ADMINISTRATION. The dosage of a

given drug may vary, depending upon the dosage form employed and the route of administration utilized. This is due to the different rates and extents of absorption resulting from the various means of administering drugs. Drugs administered intravenously enter the blood stream directly and thus the full amount administered is present in the blood. In contrast, drugs administered orally are rarely, if ever, fully absorbed due to the various physical, chemical, and biologic barriers to their absorption, including interactions with the gastric and intestinal contents. Thus in many instances, a lesser parenteral (injectable) dose of a drug is required than the oral dose to achieve the same blood levels of drug or clinical effects. This is not to say that adequate absorption cannot take place from the various body sites. Excellent absorption of certain drugs can be achieved from the rectum, gastrointestinal tract, under the tongue, and from other sites. However, each drug has to be studied individually to determine the best routes of its administration and then suitable dosage forms designed to carry the necessary amount of drug to meet the desired clinical requirements.

Commercially prepared dosage forms contain fixed amounts of drugs designed to meet the *usual dosage* requirements of patients. The liquid dosage forms, as injections, syrups and elixirs, are flexible in that they permit the dosage administered to be easily adjusted simply by altering the volume of product used. Some tablets are *scored* or grooved to permit even breaking to facilitate the accurate administration of partial dosage units. However, some dosage forms as capsules and unscored tablets do not permit easy and accurate partial dosage unit administration. Thus, to provide greater flexibility in the selection and use of commercially prepared dosage forms, manufacturers generally prepare more than a single strength of a given drug product. For instance, phenobarbital tablets are commercially available containing 15, 30, 60, and 100 mg of phenobarbital. Information as to the available strengths of drug products is provided to the pharmacist by means of drug package inserts, drug literature, reference books, and also through the official compendia monographs.

Dispensing Information

Included in certain official monographs is information pertinent to the effective use of the drug or dosage form. The information relates to such things as the drug's minor or major adverse effects, proper drug storage and stability considerations, possible drug-drug or drug-food interactions, proper methods or times for the administration of the medication, important contraindications to the use of the medication, important signs of drug overdosage, and others. This type of information is used by the pharmacist at his professional discretion to insure the safety and welfare of his patients. The information itself is not unique to the official compendia. It is typical of the kind of information that the pharmacist accumulates through his professional education, professional literature, and experience and which he applies in his practice. Examples of the types of information presented in the official monographs are as follows:

Bisacodyl Tablets:

Do not use when abdominal pain, nausea, or vomiting is present.

Do not chew or break tablet coating. Do not take within 1 hour after ingestion of antacids or milk. Usually effective overnight or within 6 hours.

Castor Oil:

Should not be taken during pregnancy or menstruation. Do not use when abdominal pain, nausea, or vomiting is present.

Usually effective within 2 hours. Preferably taken on an empty stomach. May be taken with juices to mask the taste.

Dicumarol Capsules:

The dosage schedule prescribed by the physician must be strictly followed. Do not take or discontinue any other medication without the consent of the physician. Notify physician at the earliest signs of unusual bleeding or bruising, blood in the urine, or red or tarry black stools. Changes in alcoholic intake may alter response to the medication.

Diphenhydramine Hydrochloride Capsules:

Drowsiness impairing ability to drive or perform other tasks requiring alertness may occur. Avoid alcoholic beverages.

Doxycycline Hyclate Capsules:

Possible interference with absorption by divalent and trivalent cations.

Possible enamel damage and discoloration of teeth of infants and children may occur.

Epinephrine Injection:

Protect the solution from light and do not use if it is brown or contains a precipitate.

Ergotamine Tartrate Tablets:

Initiate therapy at onset of (migraine) attack. Lie down in a quiet and darkened room for 2 hours after taking the medication.

Penicillin G Potassium Tablets:

Inquire whether patient is allergic to penicillin.

Thyroid Tablets:

Notify physician if signs of overdose (sweating, diarrhea, headache, heart palpitations) occur.

Physical and Chemical Standards

In order to assure the identity and consistent high quality of drugs and drug preparations, each monograph contains the appropriate standards, tests, and assay procedures which must be met. Drugs and drug products which are not represented by official monographs must meet similar standards to comply with FDA requirements.

The Chemical Entity

Appearing in the monograph for each inorganic and organic chemical is information identifying the chemical nature of the substance. For inorganic chemicals like sodium chloride the data include the chemical formula, $NaCl$, and the respective molecular weight. For organic substances, as chlorambucil, included are the chemical's structural formula, its complete chemical name, empirical formula, and molecular weight. Some official drugs like thyroid are not pure chemicals but mixtures of chemicals

and therefore no structural formula can accurately describe their chemical nature. Quality standards, tests, and assays for these drugs as well as for the pure chemical substances are included in the monograph for each article.

Official Definitions

For most official chemicals or drugs, a definition of drug identity is provided in the monograph. Official definitions of inorganic and organic chemicals include a statement of composition giving the established minimum or both minimum and maximum percentage of the chemical required as determined by the official assay provided or referred to in the monograph. Chlorambucil, for example, to be of official quality, must contain not less than 98.0% and not more than 101.0% of the pure agent, $C_{14}H_{19}Cl_2NO_2$, calculated on an anhydrous basis.

The official definition of vegetable drugs indicates as far as possible the part or parts of the plant constituting the drug substance and the botanical name or names of the plant or plants yielding the drug. Orange oil, for example, is a volatile oil obtained by expression from the fresh peel of the ripe fruit of *Citrus sinensis*. The name *Linné* following the drug's botanic origin refers to the Swedish botanist, Carl von Linné (1707–1778), who established a system of scientifically classifying and naming botanicals. The established minimum and maximum percentages of the active or important drug constituents are also stated in the definition, and assay methods are provided to determine them. Official orange oil, for instance, must contain between 1.2 and 2.5% aldehydes determined by the assay provided. Although there is a mixture of aldehydes present, their separate isolation and identification is not only difficult but of little consequence to the quality of the oil: therefore the total aldehyde content is calculated as if it were the single chemical, decanal, itself an aldehyde present in the oil.

The official definition for animal drugs is much the same as for botanic drugs. The source of the drug is given, sometimes as a general source, as thyroid from thyroid glands of domesticated animals used for food by man, and sometimes as a specific zoological source, as for chymotrypsin, a proteolytic enzyme crystallized from an extract of the pancreas gland of the ox, *Bos taurus*. When applicable, the active constituents of animal drugs are indicated, the standards defined, and the appropriate assays provided.

Vegetable and animal drugs should be free of such extraneous material as dirt, animal excreta, nonrequired animal or plant parts, and other adulterants oftentimes found in commercial lots of crude natural drugs. This requirement is particularly important if the crude drug is to be employed as such in the preparation of dosage forms. Digitalis leaves, for instance, are finely powdered and compressed directly into tablets. On the other hand, belladonna leaves are subjected to total extraction by alcohol and water and the extract used in preparing belladonna tincture with the drug-exhausted leaves discarded. If the drugs employed in this manner are contaminated, so would be the resultant pharmaceutical preparations. On the other hand, if natural products are used as the source of specific chemical agents that are removed from the crude drug and chemically purified, the gross contaminants are of considerably less consequence to the desired products. Naturally occurring drugs should also be free of mold or insect infestation. It is permissible to employ suitable fumigants (chloroform, carbon tetrachloride, methyl bromide) to prevent contamination by insects. Crude drugs should be properly dried after collection to prevent enzymatic deterioration and mold formation.

Physical Descriptions

Each drug substance in the official compendia is characterized in its monograph by a description of its physical nature. In general, the descriptions include pertinent distinguishing features of the material—for example, its physical state in nature (solid, liquid, or gas), and if a solid, its crystalline or amorphous character, if a liquid, its relative fluidity, and for all materials, usual color, odor, or taste features. The physical descriptions of drugs are not intended to serve as a means of positive identification, but rather as a pharmaceutic guide to enable the detection of mislabeled drugs, deteriorated drugs, or drugs contaminated with foreign matter.

Tests for Quality Assurance

Depending on the nature of a particular therapeutic or pharmaceutic substance, various physical, chemical, and biological tests are spec-

ified in the monograph to assure purity, stability, and potency of the starting materials employed in the preparation of pharmaceutical products. In this manner, the final preparations inherit the qualities of the standardized starting materials. To emphasize the scope of quality control extended over materials employed in formulations, Table 2-2 presents the physical, chemical, and biological tests and limits required of the materials used in the preparation of pentobarbital sodium elixir.

The tests and limits for impurities established by these monographs are selected for those chemicals most likely to be present as contaminants. The impurities generally are due to processes of chemical manufacture of the drug or to the drug's deterioration. Glycerin, for example, may be prepared in a number of different ways, each utilizing a different starting material and different reagents and resulting in different impurities. These processes include the use of lead oxide, chlorine gas, animal fats and oils, and beet sugar molasses; the respective contaminants resulting from these processes are heavy metals, chlorinated compounds, fatty acids and esters, and glucose. The limits to which each of these may be present in official glycerin is provided in the monograph. The monograph also prescribes a test for acrolein, an intensely pungent material resulting from the deterioration of glycerin.

Pentobarbital sodium elixir, once prepared, is assayed for pentobarbital sodium and alcohol content. Similarly, each official chemical and finished pharmaceutical product has its own designated physical, chemical, and biological requirements that must be met before it can be referred to as being official. In addition to the usual tests required, some dosage forms have special requirements. For example, capsules and tablets must meet requirements for weight variation to insure batch-to-batch uniformity in their weight. Tablets must also meet disintegration tests to guarantee the release of the medication once the tablet is swallowed. Suppositories must melt, soften, or dissolve at body temperature to release the medication they carry. Injectable and ophthalmic preparations must be sterile to protect the patient against infection. These and other characteristics of the various dosage forms will be discussed in succeeding chapters. The monographs for pharmaceutical preparations include working directions for the manufacture of small batches of product, gener-

Table 2-2. THE QUALITY CONTROL PROFILE OF THE INGREDIENTS IN PENTOBARBITAL SODIUM ELIXIR USP XIX

Pentobarbital Sodium:	Appearance
	Solubility
	Identification
	pH
	Loss of drying
	Isomer content
	Readily carbonizable sub-
	    stances
	Free pentobarbital
	Heavy metals
	Assay
		Alcohol:
		(*Cont.*)
			Nonvolatile residue
			Water-insoluble substances
			Aldehydes and other foreign organic
			    substances
			Amyl alcohol and nonvolatile,
			    carbonizable substances, etc.
			Fusel oil constituents
			Methyl ketones, isopropyl alcohol,
			    and tertiary butyl alcohol, metha-
			    nol

Orange Oil:	Appearance, odor, and taste Solubility Specific gravity Angular rotation Refractive index Ultraviolet absorbance Heavy metals Residue on evaporation Foreign oils	Glycerin:	Appearance and odor Neutral solutions Solubility Identification Specific gravity Color Residue on ignition Chloride Sulfate Arsenic Heavy metals Readily carbonizable substances
Caramel:	Appearance Specific gravity Purity Ash		Chlorinated compounds Acrolein, glucose, and ammonium compounds Fatty acids and esters
Purified Water:	Appearance Neutral pH Chloride Sulfate Ammonia Calcium Carbon dioxide Heavy metals Oxidizable substances Total solids Bacteriological purity	Sucrose: (in Syrup)	Appearance Solutions neutral to litmus Solubility Specific rotation Residue on ignition Chloride Sulfate Calcium Heavy metals Invert sugar
Alcohol:	Appearance Boiling point Flammability Solubility Specific gravity Acidity	Diluted Hydrochloric Acid:	Specific gravity Residue on ignition Free bromide or chlorine Sulfate Sulfite Arsenic Heavy metals Assay

ally 1000 ml if a liquid, and 1000 g if a solid. These formulas may be enlarged or reduced to prepare greater or lesser amounts; however, the final products should be uniform and of the same potency.

In addition to the basic tests provided in the monographs for controlling the quality of medicinal agents, most pharmaceutical manufacturers employ supportive measures to insure the safety and efficacy of their products. One such measure is the in-process control of drug quality (Figs. 2-7 and 2-8). By this is meant the control

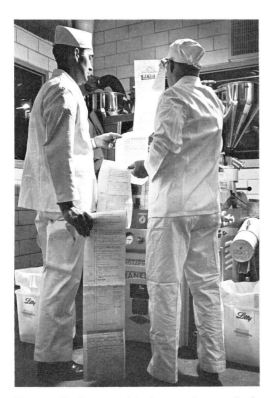

Fig. 2-7. *Quality control in the manufacture of tablets. The manufacturing ticket lists the ingredients of a given item, describes how they are to be combined, and specifies the checks and tests necessary for safety and purity. (Courtesy of Eli Lilly and Company)*

over the pharmaceutical product during the entire course of its manufacture, from the raw materials through the packaging, labeling, and

storage of the finished product. The purpose of the in-process control is to insure against detectable and significant human errors, those of equipment failure, abnormal raw material, or other such influences. The procedures may be elaborate or simple. They may involve complex instruments, or they may depend on employees' observations of drug odor, color, or consistency. The human and instrumental controls in pharmaceutical manufacturing help to assure dose-to-dose uniformity within as well as between drug batches.

Packaging, Labeling, and Storage

Most monographs contain a statement dealing with the proper method of packaging and storing individual drugs or pharmaceutical preparations. Most frequently, drugs have to be protected against conditions of excessive heat, light, and moisture to maintain the original quality and potency throughout storage periods.

Containers

The official compendia terms applying to conditions of storage and types of containers have definite meaning and must not be loosely interpreted. According to the USP and the NF, a *container* is the device that holds a drug and is, or may be, in direct contact with the drug. The *immediate container* is that which is in direct

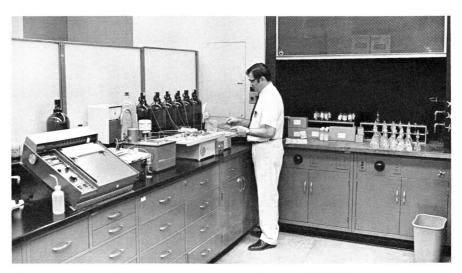

Fig. 2-8. *Scene of a portion of a quality control laboratory (Courtesy of Eli Lilly and Company)*

contact with the drug at all times. The *closure* is part of the container. The container, including the closure, should be clean and dry prior to its being filled with the drug. The container must not interact physically or chemically with the drug placed in it so as to alter to any significant degree the strength, quality, or purity beyond the official requirements for that particular drug.

Containers may be classified according to their ability to protect their contents from external conditions. The minimally acceptable container is termed a *well-closed container*. It protects the contents from extraneous solids and from loss of the drug under ordinary conditions of handling, shipment, storage, and distribution. A *tight container* protects the contents from contamination by extraneous liquids, solids, or vapors, from loss of the drug, and from efflorescence, deliquescence, or evaporation under the usual conditions of handling, shipment, storage, and distribution. A tight container is capable of reclosure to its original capability after being opened. A *hermetic container* is impervious to air or any other gas under the ordinary or customary conditions of handling, shipment, storage, and distribution. Hermetic containers which are sterile are generally used to hold pharmaceutical preparations intended for injection or parenteral administration. These containers may be *single-dose containers* in which the quantity of sterile drug contained is intended as a single dose and which once opened cannot be resealed with assurance that sterility has been maintained. These containers are commonly referred to as ampuls. A *multiple-dose container* is a hermetic container which permits withdrawal of successive portions of the contents without changing the strength or endangering the quality or purity of the remaining portion. These containers are commonly referred to as vials. Examples of ampuls and vials are shown in Figure 2-9.

Other dosage forms, as tablets, capsules, and oral liquids, are also packaged in *multiple-unit* and in *single-unit* containers. Examples of single-unit and multiple-unit packages are shown in Figure 2-10. A single-use package is termed a *unit-dose* package at the time a prescribing physician orders that particular amount of the drug for a specific patient. The single-unit packaging of drugs may be performed on a large scale by the industrial manufacturer or distributor or on a smaller in-house

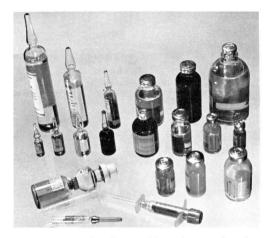

Fig. 2-9. *Examples of injectable products packaged in single-dose (ampuls) and multiple-dose (vials) containers and in unit-dose syringes.*

scale by the pharmacy actually dispensing the medication. In each instance, the single-unit package is appropriately labeled with information on the drug contents to insure the positive identification of the medication. Although single-unit packaging has particular usefulness in institutional settings as hospitals and extended care facilities it is not limited to such. Many outpatients find single-unit packages a convenient and sanitary means of maintaining and utilizing their medication. Among the advantages cited for single-unit packaging and unit-dose dispensing are the following: positive identification of each dosage unit after it leaves the pharmacy or nursing station and the consequent reduction of medication errors, reduced contamination of the drug by virtue of its protective wrapping, reduced preparation and dispensing time, greater ease of inventory control in the pharmacy or nursing station, and elimination of waste through better medication management with less discarded medication.

Most hospitals with unit-dose systems use strip packaging equipment for the packaging of oral solids (Fig. 2-11). Such equipment hermetically seals solid dosage forms into four-sided pouches and imprints dose identification on each package at the same time. The equipment can be adjusted to produce individual single-cut packages or perforated strips or rolls of singly packaged dosage units. The packaging materials may be paper, foil, plastics or cellophane, alone or in combination. Some drugs must be packaged in foil-to-foil wrappings to prevent the

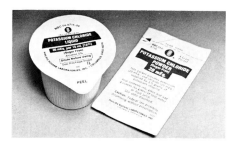
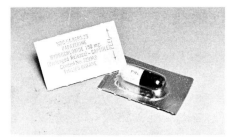
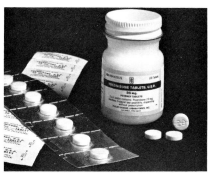

Fig. 2-10. *Examples of multiple-unit and single-unit packaging, including patient cup, unit dose of powder, blister packaging of single capsule, and strip packaging of tablets. (Courtesy of Philips Roxane Laboratories)*

deteriorating effects of light or the permeation of moisture. The packaging of solid dosage

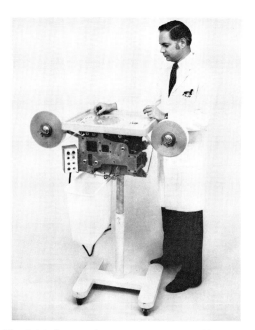

Fig. 2-11. *Strip packaging equipment capable of producing 50 packages per minute. Seals solid dosage units in a variety of wrapping materials and labels each package simultaneously. (Courtesy of Packaging Machinery Associates)*

forms in clear plastic blister wells is another popular method of single-unit packaging. Oral liquids are generally single-unit dispensed in paper, plastic, or foil cups, or pre-packaged and dispensed in glass containers having threaded caps or crimped aluminum caps (Fig. 2-12). A number of hospital pharmacies package oral liquids for pediatric use in disposable plastic syringes with rubber tips on the orifice for closure. In these instances the nursing staff must be fully aware of the novel packaging and special labeling used to indicate "not for injection." Medications which *are* used for injection may also be pre-packaged in syringes for direct administration to the patient. However, great care must be exercised in the preparation and packaging of parenteral products and appropriate laboratory tests performed to insure their sterility and stability. Other dosage forms, as suppositories, powders, ointments, creams, and ophthalmic solutions, are also commonly found in single-unit packages provided by large manufacturers. However, the relatively infrequent use of these dosage forms in a given hospital, extended care facility, or community pharmacy does not generally justify the expense of purchasing the specialized packaging machinery necessary for the small-scale packaging of these forms.

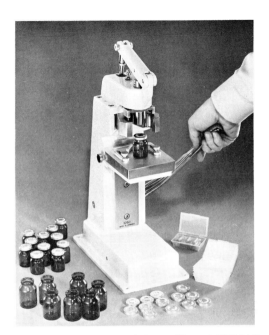

Fig. 2-12. *Components of Owens-Illinois' UNI-PAK System, including amber vials for oral liquids, aluminum closures, capper, and plastic hinged boxes for blister packaged solid dosage forms. Approximately 2,000 vials may be sealed per hour using the capper shown. (Courtesy of Owens-Illinois)*

Many pharmaceutical products require *light-resistant containers* to protect them from photochemical deterioration. In most instances a container made of a good quality of amber glass will reduce light transmission sufficiently to protect the light-sensitive pharmaceutical. The containers shown in Figure 2-13 are widely used for this purpose. In some instances opaque glass or glass rendered opaque by a special coating is employed. Opaque plastic containers are becoming increasingly popular in the packaging of pharmaceutical products. The use of outer wrappings or cartons can also be used to protect light-sensitive pharmaceuticals.

The official compendia provide tests and standards for glass and plastic containers with respect to their ability to prevent the transmission of light. Containers intended to provide protection from light or those offered as "light-resistant" containers must meet prescribed compendia standards which define the acceptable limits of light transmission at any wavelength of light between 290 and 450 nm.

The glass used in packaging pharmaceuticals is classified into four categories, depending upon the chemical constitution of the glass and its ability to resist deterioration. Table 2-3 presents the chemical make-up of the various glasses; types I, II, and III are intended for parenteral products and type NP is intended for nonparenteral products or those intended for oral or topical use.

Table 2-3. CONSTITUTION OF OFFICIAL GLASS TYPES

Type	General Description
I	Highly resistant, borosilicate glass
II	Treated soda-lime glass
III	Soda-lime glass
NP	General purpose soda-lime glass

Each type is tested according to its resistance to water attack. The degree of attack is determined by the amount of alkali released from the glass under the test conditions specified. Obviously the leaching of alkali from the glass into a pharmaceutical solution or preparation placed in the container could alter the pH and thus the stability of the product. Pharmaceutical manufacturers must select and utilize containers which do not adversely affect the composition or stability of their products. Type I is generally the most resistant glass of the four categories.

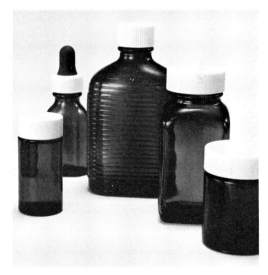

Fig. 2-13. *Examples of light-protective amber prescription containers for, from left to right: small numbers of solid dosage forms, as tablets and capsules; liquid preparations administered by drops; liquid preparations; powders, or large numbers of solid dosage forms; and semisolid preparations, such as ointments and pastes. (Courtesy of Armstrong Cork Company)*

Plastic containers are tested for suitability as containers of parenteral preparations. The object of the tests is to determine the reaction of living animal tissue and of normal animals to the presence of portions of the plastic and of injection extracts of it. On the basis of the biological test procedures, plastics intended for packaging parenteral products are also divided into classes of quality.

The interest and widespread use of plastic containers in the pharmaceutical industry has been generated by a number of factors including: (1) the advantage of plastic over glass containers in lightness of weight and resistance to impact and thus lower transporation costs and losses due to container damage; (2) the versatility in container design and in consumer acceptance afforded by plastics; (3) the interest and convenience in utilizing low and medium density polyethylene in the formation of squeeze bottles which serve a dual function of both package and applicator for preparations as ophthalmics, nasal solutions, and lotions; and (4) the advent of newer techniques in drug distribution, dispensing, and inventory control particularly in hospitals which required the development of packaging as the strip package, blister package, and plastic disposable syringe for unit-dose delivery.

Today a wide variety of dosage forms may be found packaged in plastic. The modern compact-type container used for oral contraceptives and which contain sufficient tablets for a monthly cycle of administration and permit the scheduled removal of one tablet at a time is a prime example of the imaginative packaging possible with plastics (Fig. 2-14). Plastic bags for intravenous fluids, plastic ointment tubes, plastic film protected suppositories and plastic tablet and capsule vials are other examples of the widespread use of plastics in pharmaceutical packaging.

The use of plastics in pharmaceutical packaging is a developing science and technology. Problems arise and indeed are resolved because of the nature and alterability of plastics. The term "plastic" does not apply to one type of material but rather to a vast number of existing and possible materials. Under specified experimental conditions monomers are added to each other forming long polymers. The desired properties of a plastic material may be produced by the right choice of the monomers, by the regulation of the synthesis, or by the addition of certain functional groups. For example, the addition of methyl groups to every other carbon atom in the polymer chains of polyethylene will give polypropylene a material which can be effectively autoclaved, whereas polyethylene cannot. If a chlorine atom is added to every other carbon in the polyethylene polymer, polyvinyl chloride is produced. This material is rigid and has good clarity making it a useful material in certain packaging situations. The placement of other functional groups on the main chain of polyethylene or added to other types of polymers

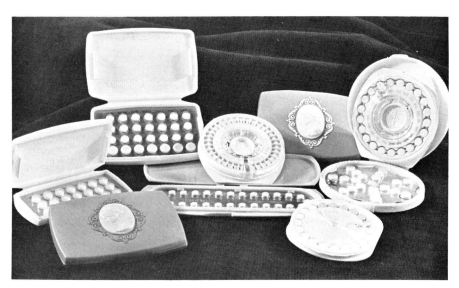

Fig. 2-14. *Examples of plastic packaging used for oral contraceptive products.*

can give a variety of alterations to the final plastic material. In addition, added agents may be employed to alter the properties of the plastic. These agents include plasticizers, stabilizers, anti-oxidants, fillers, anti-static agents, anti-mold agents, colorants, and others.

Among the problems associated with the use of plastics in packaging are (1) permeability of the containers to atmospheric gases and to moisture vapor; (2) leaching of the constituents of the container to the internal contents; (3) sorption of drugs from the contents to the container; (4) transmission of light through the container; and (5) alteration of the container upon storage.

True *permeability* is considered a process of solution and diffusion, with the penetrant initially dissolving in the plastic material on one side and diffusing through to the other side. Permeability should be contrasted with *porosity*, which is a condition in which minute holes or cracks are present in the plastic and through which gas or moisture vapor may move directly.

The permeability of a plastic is a function of several factors including the nature of the polymer itself, the amounts and types of plasticizers, fillers, lubricants, pigments and other additives used, the pressure conditions, and the temperature. Generally, increases in the temperature, pressure, and the use of additives to the polymer tend to increase the permeability of the plastic. In general, glass containers are less permeable than plastic containers. The closure plays as important a role in protecting pharmaceuticals as does the primary container. A tightly fitting closure can often be the difference between a protected or an unprotected drug product.

The movement of moisture vapor or gas, especially oxygen, through a pharmaceutical container can pose one of the greatest threats to the stability of a pharmaceutical product. For most pharmaceuticals which are dry powders or solid dosage forms, as tablets and capsules, moisture and gaseous penetration may be anticipated to occur predominantly from the environment toward the content. In the presence of moisture, these products may tend to cake or liquefy or in the case of solid dosage forms lose their color or physical integrity. A host of pharmaceutical adjuncts, especially those used in tablet formulations, as diluents, binders, and disintegrating agents, are affected by moisture. The majority of these adjuncts are carbohydrates, starches, and natural or synthetic gums, and because of their hygroscopicity they hold moisture and may even serve as nutrient media for the growth of microorganisms. Many of the tablet disintegrating agents fulfill their pharmaceutical function by swelling in an aqueous media, and, if exposed to high moisture vapor upon storage, the disintegrants may prematurely swell, and cause the tablets to become deformed. Further, many medicinal agents, as aspirin, some barbiturates, and vitamins, are quite prone to hydrolytic decomposition and dosage forms of these agents must be especially guarded against moisture penetration.

Drug substances which exhibit oxidation propensity may undergo a greater degree of degradation when packaged in plastic as compared to glass. In glass, the void space is filled with air which is in a confined space and presents only a limited amount of oxygen to the drug contents. On the other hand, a drug packaged in a gas-permeable plastic container may be constantly exposed to oxygen due to the replenished supply entering the container.

Liquid pharmaceutical products packaged in plastic which is permeable to the contents tend to lose molecules of solute (drug) or solvent (vehicle) outward toward the container. Such permeation can drastically alter the concentration of the drug in the pharmaceutical product thereby affecting its efficacy.

Leaching is a term used to describe the release or movement of components of a container into the contents. Compounds leached from plastic containers are generally the polymer additives as the plasticizers, stabilizers, or antioxidants. The leaching of these additives occurs predominantly when liquid or semi-solid dosage forms are packaged in plastic. Little leaching occurs when tablets or capsules are packaged in plastic.

Leaching may be influenced by temperature, excessive agitation of the filled container, and by the solubilizing effect of the contents on one or more of the polymer additives. The leaching of polymer additives from plastic containers of fluids intended for intravenous administration is an especially worrisome problem since the additive is injected along with the medication. The toxicologic effect of any leached additive is of prime concern and is presently an important area of investigation. Soft-walled plastic containers of polyvinyl chloride are frequently used to package various intravenous solutions as well as blood for transfusion. One of the plasticizers used in this plastic has been found to be leached from the plastic upon agitation and has been identified as the particulate matter found in these containers.[1] Leached material, whether dissolved in the contents or present as minute particles, poses a health hazard to the patient and sufficient studies should be performed on the leaching characteristics of each plastic material prior to its use in packaging a given pharmaceutical product.

Sorption is a term used to indicate the binding of molecules to polymer materials. Both *adsorption* and *absorption* may be considered within this term. Sorption occurs through chemical or physical means, or both, with the phenomena related to the chemical structure of the solute molecules and the physical and chemical properties of the polymer. Generally, the unionized species of a solute has a greater tendency to be bound than does the ionized species. Since the degree of ionization of a solute may be affected by the pH of the solution in which it is contained, the pH of a pharmaceutical solution may influence the sorption tendency of a particular solute. Further, the pH of a solution may affect the chemical nature of a plastic container in such a way to either increase or decrease the active bonding sites available to the solute molecules. Plastic materials with polar groups are particularly prone to the sorption process. Since the process of sorption is dependent upon the penetration or diffusion of a solute into the plastic, the pharmaceutical vehicle or solvent for the solute also plays a major role in the sorption process. Certain solvents may alter the plastic and increase its permeability to solute.

The process of sorption may be initiated by the adsorption of a solute to the inner surface of a plastic container. After the saturation of the surface, the solute may then diffuse into the plastic, perhaps with the assistance of the pharmaceutical solvent or vehicle, to be absorbed and bound to sites within the plastic. The sorption of a drug component from a pharmaceutical solution would naturally reduce the concentration of that agent in the solution and render the product unreliable as to potency and unacceptable for use. The sorption of antimicrobial preservatives or stabilizers from a pharmaceutical product would likewise render the product unsuitable for use. Even the sorption of

colorants and flavorants which would alter a preparation's color stability and taste would be unacceptable to a pharmaceutical manufacturer. Thus, each formulative ingredient must be examined in the proposed plastic packaging to ascertain its tendency for sorption and to insure the continued stability and potency of a product during its anticipated shelf life.

Insofar as the ability of plastic containers to protect pharmaceutical products from destructive light transmission, clear and uncolored plastic containers behave in much the same manner as clear and uncolored glass containers in allowing such transmissions. In fact, certain plastics allow permeability to short-waved rays that is even greater than for glass. Agents termed UV-absorbers may be added to the plastic to decrease the transmission of these short ultraviolet rays and thus may be used to protect drugs sensitive to these offending rays. As for glass, the official compendia set standards for the transmission of light through plastic containers intended to be "light resistant" for wavelengths of light between 290 and 450 nm. Many of the clear but colored plastic containers available to pharmacists meet these standards as do opaque containers.

Deformations, softening, hardening, and other physical changes in plastic containers have been observed. These changes may result from the permeation or sorption of the contents into the container changing its chemical or physical makeup. They may also result from the leaching of a component of the container into the contents, or from changes in temperature or physical stress placed upon the container in handling, shipping or storage.

In summary, each pharmaceutical preparation must be considered separately with respect to packaging and type of container selected. The container must be suited to the prolonged stability of the pharmaceutical preparation and must be conducive to the safe and effective utilization by the patient. A good guideline for the practicing pharmacist is to utilize the original or the same type of container in which the drug product was supplied originally by the manufacturer. For prescribed mixtures of drugs, especially liquid preparations and products containing volatile substances, a tightly closed, light-resistant glass container is usually the most protective container to use. Perhaps the best example which may be cited for the protective packaging of a volatile drug is that for

[1]Needham, T. E. Jr., and Luzzi, L. A.; "Particulate Matter in Polyvinyl Chloride Intravenous Bags," *New England Journal of Medicine*, 289, 1256, 1973.

nitroglycerin tablets, which must be dispensed in the original unopened (glass) container and must be maintained in this container by the patient to prevent the loss of potency due to the volatilization of nitroglycerin.

Safety Closures

In an effort to reduce the occurrence of accidental poisonings through the ingestion of drugs and other household chemicals, the Poison Prevention Packaging Act was passed into law in 1970. The responsibility for the administration and enforcement of the Act, originally with the Food and Drug Administration, was transferred to the Consumer Product Safety Commission in 1973 when this agency was created through the enactment of the Consumer Product Safety Act. The initial regulations called for the use of "child-proof" closures for aspirin products and certain household chemical products shown to have a significant potential for causing accidental poisoning in youngsters. As the technical capability in producing effective closures was developed, the regulations were extended to include the use of such safety closures in the packaging of both legend and over-the-counter medications. Presently, all legend drugs intended for oral use must be dispensed by the pharmacist to the patient in containers having safety closures unless the prescribing physician or the patient specifically requests otherwise. Examples of commonly used safety closures in dispensing medication are presented in Figures 2-15 and 2-16. Some manufacturers provide the safety closures with the smaller size packages of their prescription products which lend themselves directly to use as a dispensing quantity.

The Consumer Product Safety Commission may propose the exemption of certain drugs and drug products from the safety closure regulation based on toxicologic data or on practical considerations. For instance, certain cardiac drugs, as nitroglycerin, are exempt from the regulations because of the importance to the welfare of the patient for direct and immediate access to his medication. The few extra seconds required to open a safety container might be dangerously extended should the heart patient panic in his manipulative efforts with the closure. Exemptions are also permitted in the case of over-the-counter medications for one package size or

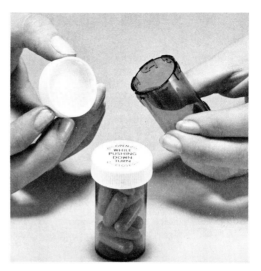

Fig. 2-15. *Example of child-resistant safety closure on a prescription container. (Courtesy of Owens-Illinois.)*

specially marked package to be available to consumers for whom safety closures might be unnecessary or too difficult to manipulate. These consumers would include childless persons, arthritic patients, and the debilitated.

Drugs which are utilized or dispensed in inpatient institutions, as hospitals, nursing homes, and extended care facilities, need not be dispensed with safety closures unless they are intended for patients who are leaving the confines of the institution (outpatients).

Labeling

The labeling of all drug products distributed in the United States must meet the specific labeling requirements as set forth in the federal regulations. These labeling requirements apply not only to proprietary products sold over-the-counter, but also to prescription drugs distributed to various health practitioners for ultimate dispensing to the patient. The labeling regulations are changed from time to time to meet the changing informational needs of the health professional and the patient. The federal labeling requirements for drug products may be further enhanced by state and local drug laws. The contents of the label that the pharmacist affixes to dispensed medication is another topic, but it too is subject to specific requirements of the federal, state, and local regulations.

According to federal regulations, drug labeling includes not only the labels placed on the

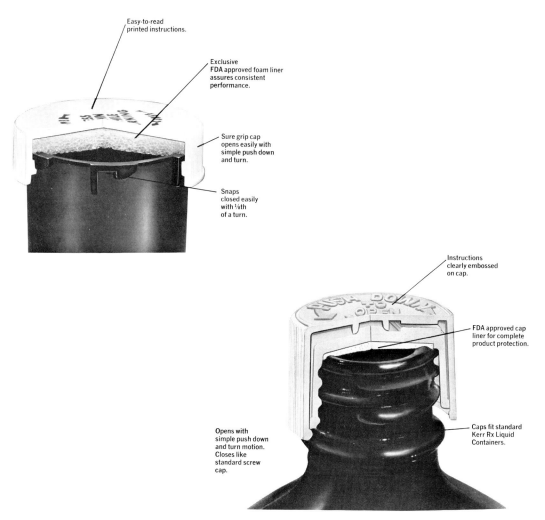

Easy-to-read
printed instructions.

Exclusive
FDA approved foam liner
assures consistent
performance.

Sure grip cap
opens easily with
simple push down
and turn.

Snaps
closed easily
with ⅛th
of a turn.

Instructions
clearly embossed
on cap.

FDA approved cap
liner for complete
product protection.

Opens with
simple push down
and turn motion.
Closes like
standard screw
cap.

Caps fit standard
Kerr Rx Liquid
Containers.

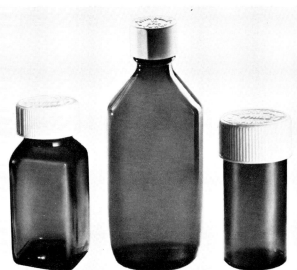

Fig. 2-16. *Gross and cut-away views of child-resistant prescription containers. (Courtesy of Kerr Glass Manufacturing Corporation.)*

immediate container and packaging, but also the package inserts accompanying the product as well as all company literature and advertising or promotional material pertaining to the drug product. This includes such things as brochures, booklets, mailing pieces, file cards, bulletins, price lists, catalogs, sound recordings, film strips, motion-picture films, lantern slides, exhibits, displays, literature reprints and any other material containing product information provided by the manufacturer or distributor.

The essential information on a prescription-only drug is generally provided to the health professional through the product's package insert. This insert must provide *full disclosure;* that is, it must contain a full and balanced presentation of the positive as well as the negative aspects of the drug product to enable the prescriber to utilize the drug most safely and effectively.

Included among the information usually appearing on the manufacturer's or distributor's label affixed to the container of Legend drugs are the following:

1. The nonproprietary name(s) of the drug(s) present and the trademark name of the product if one is used.
2. The name and address of the manufacturer or distributor of the product.
3. A quantitative statement of the amount of each drug present per unit of weight, volume, or dosage unit, whichever is most appropriate.
4. The pharmaceutical type of dosage form constituting the product.
5. The net amount of drug product contained in the package, in units of weight, volume or number of dosage units, as is appropriate.
6. The Federal Legend: "Caution—Federal law prohibits dispensing without prescription," or a similar statement.
7. The Usual Dose of the product including special dosage guidelines for children or for other patients under certain conditions, when appropriate.
8. A label reference to see the accompanying package insert or other product literature for additional information.
9. Special storage instructions, when applicable.
10. The National Drug Code identification number for the product.

11. The manufacturer's control number identifying the batch or lot of the drug.
12. An expiration date if required or applicable.
13. For controlled drug substances, the DEA symbol ("C") together with the schedule assigned (e.g. III). The statement: "Warning—May be habit forming" may appear also.

The label on the container of products sold over-the-counter without prescription usually contains much of the same type of product information as the prescription-only items with the exception of the Federal Legend and the DEA symbol. However, to insure the safe and proper use of over-the-counter medications, the pharmacologic category of the product follows any proprietary name and additional patient-oriented information is included in the labeling. Generally, this includes the following:

1. Statements of all conditions, purposes, or uses for which the drug is intended or commonly used.
2. Quantity of dose, including usual quantities for each of the uses for which it is intended and the usual quantities for persons of different ages and physical conditions, if pertinent.
3. Frequency of administration, if used internally, or application, if used externally.
4. Maximum duration of administration or application prior to consulting a physician.
5. Time of administration or application, with respect to meals, onset of symptoms, or other time factors.
6. Route of administration or application.
7. Preparation for use—shaking, dilution, adjustment of temperature, or other manipulations or processes.

In addition, over-the-counter package labeling must include appropriate warning statements whenever the medication is such that indiscriminate use may lead to serious medical complications or mask a condition more serious than that for which the medication was intended. For example, the use of laxatives is a dangerous practice when symptoms of appendicitis are present and can result in an intensification of the problem and even a rupturing of the appendix. For this reason the following statement is required by law to appear on laxative preparations:

"Warning: Do not use when abdominal pain, nausea, or vomiting are present. Frequent or prolonged use of this preparation may result in dependence on laxatives."

The seriousness of a cough may be underestimated by a patient if a proprietary cough syrup temporarily relieves the cough; however, coughing is a symptom of many serious conditions requiring specific treatment. Cough remedies sold over-the-counter must therefore bear the following warning statement:

"Warning: Persons with a high fever or persistent cough should not use this preparation unless directed by physician."

These are but two examples of the statements required on various types of proprietary products. The statements themselves and the types of preparations requiring them are written into the law and are available through the government literature. The labels of drugs sold directly to the layman should recommend their use against only those conditions that have been shown scientifically to be treated effectively by the drug. Serious conditions that cannot be diagnosed or successfully treated by the layman should not be mentioned in the labeling. In addition, the label must be perfectly clear in meaning and must not contain any false or misleading statement.

These labeling requirements apply to all drugs of commerce, not only to official drugs. A drug not recognized in the official compendia is considered adulterated and misbranded if its strength differs from, or its purity falls below, that which it purports to have or is represented to possess through advertising or labeling.

When a drug or pharmaceutical preparation is especially liable to deterioration, an expiration date may also be required in the package labeling. This date usually represents a specific time following the manufacture and packaging or distribution of the drug after which period the product is likely to have reduced potency. Biological and antibiotic products generally bear an expiration date. In the case of Insulin injection, the USP states that the expiration date on the package must be "not later than 24 months after the immediate container was filled." The expiration dates vary with the stability of the drug and the dosage form in which it is prepared. Penicillin G potassium crystalline drug powder has an official expiration date of 5 years, whereas a sterile aqueous solution of the same chemical intended for parenteral use is stable under refrigeration for only 3 days after preparation without significant loss of potency.

Storage

To insure the stability of a pharmaceutical preparation for the period of its intended shelf life, the product must be stored under proper conditions. The labeling of each product generally includes the desired conditions of storage for that particular product. The terms generally employed in such labeling have definite meaning, as defined by the official compendia:

Cold—Any temperature not exceeding 8°C (46°F). A *refrigerator* is a cold place in which the temperature is maintained thermostatically between 2° and 8°C (36° and 46°F). A *freezer* is a cold place in which the temperature is maintained thermostatically between −10° and −20°C (14° and −4°F).

Cool—Any temperature between 8° and 15°C (46° and 59°F). An article for which storage in a cool place is directed may, alternatively, be stored in a refrigerator unless otherwise specified in the individual monograph.

Room Temperature—The temperature prevailing in a working area. *Controlled room temperature* is a temperature maintained thermostatically between 15° and 30°C (59° and 86°F).

Warm—Any temperature between 30° and 40°C (86° and 104°F).

Excessive Heat—Any temperature above 40°C (104°F).

Protection from Freezing—Where in addition to the risk of breakage of the container, freezing subjects a product to loss of strength or potency, or to destructive alteration of the dosage form, the container label bears an appropriate instruction to protect the product from freezing.

When no specific storage or limitations are provided, it is understood that the storage conditions include protection from moisture, freezing, and excessive heat.

Standards for Good Manufacturing Practice

To insure high standards for drug product quality, the Food and Drug Administration enforces compliance with the requirements of its Current Good Manufacturing Practice (GMP) regulations. The first GMP regulations were promulgated in 1963 under one of the provisions of the Kefauver-Harris Drug Amendments of 1962. Since that time they have been revised periodically. An adaptation of the GMP regulations which became effective in 1971 is presented in Table 2-4.[1] As may be seen from this table, the GMP regulations establish standards for the manufacturing facilities, equipment, personnel, components or raw materials, production and control records and procedures, product containers, packaging and labeling, laboratory controls, distribution records, product stability, expiration dating, and complaint files for all pharmaceutical products manufactured in this country. Compliance with these standards is our best assurance that the products dispensed by the pharmacist to the patient is of appropriate high quality.

[1] These regulations were being revised as this text went to press. Revised regulations are expected to become effective during 1977 or 1978.

Some Definitions

Raw material or *component*—any material used in the manufacture of drugs in dosage forms, including those which may not be present in the finished product.

Batch—a specific quality of a drug of uniform specified quality produced according to a single manufacturing order during the same cycle of manufacture.

Lot—a batch or any portion of a batch having uniform specified quality and a distinctive identifying "lot number."

Lot number or *control number*—any distinctive combination of letters and/or numbers from which the complete history of the manufacture, control, packaging, and distribution of a batch or lot of a drug may be determined.

Active ingredient—any component which is intended to furnish pharmacological activity or other direct effect in the diagnosis, cure, mitigation, treatment or prevention of disease or to affect the structure or function of the body.

Inactive ingredient—substance(s) other than the active ingredients in a drug product.

Table 2-4. ADAPTION OF CURRENT GOOD MANUFACTURING PRACTICE REGULATIONS[*]

1. Finished pharmaceuticals; manufacturing practice.

(a) The criteria herein presented shall apply in determining whether the methods used in, or the facilities or controls used for, the manufacture, processing, packing, or holding of a drug conform to or are operated or administered in conformity with current good manufacturing practice to assure that a drug meets the requirements of the act as to safety and has the identity and strength and meets the quality and purity characteristics which it purports or is represented to possess.

(b) The regulations in this part permit the use of precision automatic, mechanical, or electronic equipment in the production and control of drugs when adequate inspection and checking procedures are used to assure proper performance.

2. Buildings.

Buildings shall be maintained in a clean and orderly manner and shall be of suitable size, construction, and location to facilitate adequate cleaning, maintenance, and proper operations in the manufacturing, processing, packing, labeling, or holding of a drug. The buildings shall:

(a) Provide adequate space for:

(1) Orderly placement of equipment and materials to minimize any risk of mixups between different drugs, drug components, in-process materials, packaging materials, or labeling, and to minimize the possibility of contamination.

(2) The receipt, storage, and withholding from use of components pending sampling, identification, and testing prior to release by the materials approval unit for manufacturing or packaging.

(3) The holding of rejected components prior to disposition to preclude the possibility of their use in manufacturing or packaging procedures for which they are unsuitable.

(4) The storage of components, containers, packaging materials, and labeling.

(5) Any manufacturing and processing operations performed.

(6) Any packaging or labeling operations.

(7) Storage of finished products.

(8) Control and production-laboratory operations.

(b) Provide adequate lighting, ventilation, and screening and, when necessary for the intended production or control purposes, provide facilities for adequate air-pressure, microbiological, dust, humidity, and temperature controls to:

[*] Adapted from Title 21 of the Code of Federal Regulations Part 133. U.S. Government Printing Office, Washington, D.C., 1973.

Table 2-4. ADAPTION OF CURRENT GOOD MANUFACTURING PRACTICE REGULATIONS* (*Cont.*)

(1) Minimize contamination of products by extraneous adulterants, including cross-contamination of one product by dust or particles of ingredients arising from the manufacture, storage, or handling of another product.

(2) Minimize dissemination of microorganisms from one area to another.

(3) Provide suitable storage conditions for drug components, in-process materials, and finished drugs in conformance with stability information.

(c) Provide adequate locker facilities and hot and cold water washing facilities, including soap or detergent, air drier or single service towels, and clean toilet facilities near working areas.

(d) Provide an adequate supply of potable water under continuous positive pressure in a plumbing system free of defects that could cause or contribute to contamination of any drug. Drains shall be of adequate size and, where connected directly to a sewer, shall be equipped with traps to prevent back-siphonage.

(e) Provide suitable housing and space for the care of all laboratory animals.

(f) Provide for safe and sanitary disposal of sewage, trash, and other refuse within and from the buildings and immediate premises.

3. Equipment.

Equipment used for the manufacture, processing, packing, labeling, holding, testing, or control of drugs shall be maintained in a clean and orderly manner and shall be of suitable design, size, construction, and location to facilitate cleaning, maintenance, and operation for its intended purpose. The equipment shall:

(a) Be so constructed that all surfaces that come into contact with a drug product shall not be reactive, additive, or absorptive so as to alter the safety, identity, strength, quality, or purity of the drug or its components beyond the official or other established requirements.

(b) Be so constructed that any substances required for operation of the equipment, such as lubricants or coolants, do not contact drug products so as to alter the safety, identity, strength, quality, or purity of the drug or its components beyond the official or other established requirements.

(c) Be constructed and installed to facilitate adjustment, disassembly cleaning and maintenance to assure the reliability of control procedures uniformity of production and exclusion from the drugs of contaminants from previous and current operations that might affect the safety, identity, strength, quality, or purity of the drug or its components beyond the official or other established requirements.

(d) Be of suitable type, size, and accuracy for any testing, measuring, mixing, weighing, or other processing or storage operations.

4. Personnel.

(a) The personnel responsible for directing the manufacture and control of the drug shall be adequate in number and background of education, training, and experience, or combination thereof, to assure that the drug has the safety, identity, strength, quality, and purity that it purports to possess. All personnel shall have capabilities commensurate with their assigned functions, a thorough understanding of the manufacturing or control operations they perform, the necessary training or experience, and adequate information concerning the reason for application of pertinent provisions of this part to their respective functions.

(b) Any person shown at any time (either by medical examination or supervisory observation) to have an apparent illness or open lesions that may adversely affect the safety or quality of drugs shall be excluded from direct contact with drug products until the condition is corrected. All employees shall be instructed to report to supervisory personnel any conditions that may have such an adverse effect on drug products.

5. Components.

All components and other materials used in the manufacture, processing, and packaging of drug products, and materials necessary for building and equipment maintenance, upon receipt shall be stored and handled in a safe, sanitary, and orderly manner. Adequate measures shall be taken to prevent mixups and cross-contamination affecting drugs and drug products. Components shall be withheld from use until they have been identified, sampled, and tested for conformance with established specifications and are released by a materials approval unit. Control of components shall include the following:

(a) Each container of component shall be examined visually for damage or contamination prior to use, including examination for breakage of seals when indicated.

(b) An adequate number of samples shall be taken from a representative number of component containers from each lot and shall be subjected to one or more tests to establish the specific identity.

(c) Representative samples of components liable to contamination with filth, insect infestation, or other extraneous contaminants shall be appropriately examined.

(d) Representative samples of all components intended for use as active ingredients shall be tested to determine their strength in order to assure conformance with appropriate specifications.

(e) Representative samples of components liable to microbiological contamination shall be subjected to microbiological tests prior to use. Such components shall not contain microorganisms that are objectionable in view of their intended use.

Table 2-4. ADAPTION OF CURRENT GOOD MANUFACTURING PRACTICE REGULATIONS* (*Cont.*)

(f) Approved components shall be appropriately identified and retested as necessary to assure that they conform to appropriate specifications of identity, strength, quality, and purity at time of use. This requires the following:

(1) Approved components shall be handled and stored to guard against contaminating or being contaminated by other drugs or components.

(2) Approved components shall be rotated in such a manner that the oldest stock is used first.

(3) Rejected components shall be identified and held to preclude their use in manufacturing or processing procedures for which they are unsuitable.

(g) Appropriate records shall be maintained, including the following:

(1) The identity and quantity of the component, the name of the supplier, the supplier's lot number, and the date of receipt.

(2) Examinations and tests performed and rejected components and their disposition.

(3) An individual inventory and record for each component used in each batch of drug manufactured or processed.

(h) An appropriately identified reserve sample of all active ingredients consisting of at least twice the quantity necessary for all required tests, except those for sterility and determination of the presence of pyrogens, shall be retained for at least 2 years after distribution of the last drug lot incorporating the component has been completed or 1 year after the expiration date of this last drug lot, whichever is longer.

6. Master production and control records; batch production and control records.

(a) To assure uniformity from batch to batch, a master production and control record for each drug product and each batch size of drug product shall be prepared, dated, and signed or initialed by a competent and responsible individual and shall be independently checked, reconciled, dated, and signed or initialed by a second competent and responsible individual. The master production and control record shall include:

(1) The name of the product, description of the dosage form, and a specimen or copy of each label and all other labeling associated with the retail or bulk unit, including copies of such labeling signed or initialed and dated by the person or persons responsible for approval of such labeling.

(2) The name and weight or measure of each active ingredient per dosage unit or per unit of weight or measure of the finished drug, and a statement of the total weight or measure of any dosage unit.

(3) A complete list of ingredients designated by names or codes sufficiently specific to indicate any special quality characteristic; an accurate statement of the weight or measure of each ingredient regardless of

whether it appears in the finished product, except that reasonable variations may be permitted in the amount of components necessary in the preparation in dosage form provided that provisions for such variations are included in the master production and control record; an appropriate statement concerning any calculated excess of an ingredient; an appropriate statement of theoretical weight or measure at various stages of processing; and a statement of the theoretical yield.

(4) A description of the containers, closures, and packaging and finishing materials.

(5) Manufacturing and control instructions, procedures, specifications, special notations, and precautions to be followed.

(b) The batch production and control record shall be prepared for each batch of drug produced and shall include complete information relating to the production and control of each batch. These records shall be retained for at least 2 years after the batch distribution is complete or at least 1 year after the batch expiration date, whichever is longer. These records shall identify the specific labeling and lot or control numbers used on the batch and shall be readily available during such retention period. The batch record shall include:

(1) An accurate reproduction of the appropriate master formula record checked, dated, and signed or initialed by a competent and responsible individual.

(2) A record of each significant step in the manufacturing, processing, packaging, labeling, testing, and controlling of the batch, including: Dates; individual major equipment and lines employed; specific identification of each batch of components used; weights and measures of components and products used in the course of processing; in-process and laboratory control results; and identifications of the individual(s) actively performing and the individual(s) directly supervising or checking each significant step in the operation.

(3) A batch number that identifies all the production and control documents relating to the history of the batch and all lot or control numbers associated with the batch.

(4) A record of any investigation made.

7. Production and control procedures.

Production and control procedures shall include all reasonable precautions, including the following, to assure that the drugs produced have the safety, identity, strength, quality, and purity they purport to possess:

(a) Each significant step in the process, such as the selection, weighing, and measuring of components, the addition of ingredients during the process, weighing and measuring during various stages of the processing, and the determination of the finished yield, shall be performed by a competent and responsible individual and checked by a second competent and responsible

Table 2-4. ADAPTION OF CURRENT GOOD MANUFACTURING PRACTICE REGULATIONS* (*Cont.*)

individual; or if such steps in the processing are controlled by precision automatic, mechanical, or electronic equipment, their proper performance is adequately checked by one or more competent and responsible individuals. The written record of the significant steps in the process shall be identified by the individual performing these tests and by the individual charged with checking these steps. Such identifications shall be recorded immediately following the completion of such steps.

(b) All containers, lines, and equipment used during the production of a batch of a drug shall be properly identified at all times to accurately and completely indicate their contents and, when necessary, the stage of processing of the batch.

(c) To minimize contamination and prevent mixups, equipment, utensils, and containers shall be thoroughly and appropriately cleaned and properly stored and have previous batch identification removed or obliterated between batches or at suitable intervals in continuous production operations.

(d) Appropriate precautions shall be taken to minimize microbiological and other contamination in the production of drugs purporting to be sterile or which by virtue of their intended use should be free from objectionable microorganisms.

(e) Appropriate procedures shall be established to minimize the hazard of cross-examination of any drugs while being manufactured or stored.

(f) To assure the uniformity and integrity of products, there shall be adequate in-process controls, such as checking the weights and disintegration times of tablets, the adequacy of mixing, the homogeneity of suspensions, and the clarity of solutions. In-process sampling shall be done at appropriate intervals using suitable equipment.

(g) Representative samples of all dosage form drugs shall be tested to determine their conformance with the specifications for the product before distribution.

(h) Procedures shall be instituted whereby review and approval of all production and control records, including packaging and labeling, shall be made prior to the release or distribution of a batch. A thorough investigation of any unexplained discrepancy or the failure of a batch to meet any of its specifications shall be undertaken whether or not the batch has already been distributed. This investigation shall be undertaken by a competent and responsible individual and shall extend to other batches of the same drug and other drugs that may have been associated with the specific failure. A written record of the investigation shall be made and shall include the conclusions and follow-up.

(i) Returned goods shall be identified as such and held. If the conditions under which returned goods have been held, stored, or shipped prior to or during their return, or the condition of the product, its container, carton, or labeling as a result of storage or shipping, cast doubt on the safety, identity, strength, quality, or purity of the drug, the returned goods shall be destroyed or subjected to adequate examination or testing to assure that the material meets all appropriate standards or specifications before being returned to stock for warehouse distribution or repacking. If the product is neither destroyed nor returned to stock, it may be reprocessed provided the final product meets all its standards and specifications. Records of returned goods shall be maintained and shall indicate the quantity returned, date, and actual disposition of the product. If the reason for returned goods implicates associated batches, an appropriate investigation shall be made in accordance with the requirements of paragraph (h) of this section.

8. Product containers and their components.

Suitable specifications, test methods, cleaning procedures, and, when indicated, sterilization procedures shall be used to assure that containers, closures, and other component parts of drug packages are suitable for their intended use. Product containers and their components shall not be reactive, additive, or absorptive so as to alter the safety, identity, strength, quality, or purity of the drug or its components beyond the official or established requirements and shall provide adequate protection against external factors that can cause deterioration or contamination of the drug.

9. Packaging and labeling.

Packaging and labeling operations shall be adequately controlled: To assure that only those drug products that have met the standards and specifications established in their master production and control records shall be distributed; to prevent mixups between drugs during filling, packaging, and labeling operations; to assure that correct labels and labeling are employed for the drug; and to identify the finished product with a lot or control number that permits determination of the history of the manufacture and control of the batch. An hour, day, or shift code is appropriate as a lot or control number for drug products manufactured or processed in continuous production equipment. Packaging and labeling operations shall:

(a) Be separated (physically or spatially) from operations on other drugs in a manner adequate to avoid mixups and minimize cross-contamination. Two or more packaging or labeling operations having drugs, containers, or labeling similar in appearance shall not be in process simultaneously on adjacent or nearby lines unless these operations are separated either physically or spatially.

(b) Provide for an inspection of the facilities prior

Table 2-4. ADAPTION OF CURRENT GOOD MANUFACTURING PRACTICE REGULATIONS* (*Cont.*)

to use to assure that all drugs and previously used packaging and labeling materials have been removed.

(c) Include the following labeling controls:

(1) The holding of labels and package labeling upon receipt pending review and proofing against an approved final copy by a competent and responsible individual to assure that they are accurate regarding identity, content, and conformity with the approved copy before release to inventory.

(2) The maintenance and storage of each type of label and package labeling representing different products, strength, dosage forms, or quantity of contents in such a manner as to prevent mixups and provide proper identification.

(3) A suitable system for assuring that only current labels and package labeling are retained and that stocks of obsolete labels and package labeling are destroyed.

(4) Restriction of access to labels and package labeling to authorized personnel.

(5) Avoidance of gang printing of cut labels, cartons, or inserts when the labels, cartons, or inserts are for different products or different strengths of the same products or are of the same size and have identical or similar format and/or color schemes. If gang printing is employed, packaging and labeling operations shall provide for added control procedures. These added controls should consider sheet layout, stacking, cutting, and handling during and after printing.

(d) Provide strict control of the package labeling issued for use with the drug. Such issue shall be carefully checked by a competent and responsible person for identity and conformity to the labeling specified in the batch production record. Said record shall identify the labeling and the quantities issued and used and shall reasonably reconcile any discrepancy between the quantity of drug finished and the quantities of labeling issued. All excess package labeling bearing lot or control numbers shall be destroyed. In event of any significant unexplained discrepancy, an investigation should be carried out according to established procedure.

(e) Provide for adequate examination or laboratory testing of representative samples of finished products after packaging and labeling to safeguard against any errors in the finishing operations and to prevent distribution of any batch until all specified tests have been met.

10. Laboratory controls.

Laboratory controls shall include the establishment of scientifically sound and appropriate specifications, standards, and test procedures to assure that components, in-processed drugs, and finished products conform to appropriate standards of identity, strength, quality, and purity. Laboratory controls shall include:

(a) The establishment of master records containing appropriate specifications for the acceptance of each lot of drug components, product containers, and their components used in drug production and packaging and a description of the sampling and testing procedures used for them. Said samples shall be representative and adequately identified. Such records shall also provide for appropriate retesting of drug components, product containers, and their components subject to deterioration.

(b) A reserve sample of all active ingredients.

(c) The establishment of master records, when needed, containing specifications and a description of sampling and testing procedures for in-process drug preparations. Such samples shall be adequately representative and properly identified.

(d) The establishment of master records containing a description of sampling procedures and appropriate specifications for finished drug products. Such samples shall be adequately representative and properly identified.

(e) Adequate provisions for checking the identity and strength of drug products for all active ingredients and for assuring:

(1) Sterility of drugs purported to be sterile and freedom from objectionable micro-organisms for those drugs which should be so by virtue of their intended use.

(2) The absence of pyrogens for those drugs purporting to be pyrogen-free.

(3) Minimal contamination of ophthalmic ointments by foreign particles and harsh or abrasive substances.

(4) That the drug release pattern of sustained release products is tested by laboratory methods to assure conformance to the release specifications.

(f) Adequate provision for auditing the reliability, accuracy, precision, and performance of laboratory test procedures and laboratory instruments used.

(g) A properly identified reserve sample of the finished product (stored in the same immediate container-closure system in which the drug is marketed) consisting of at least twice the quantity necessary to perform all the required tests, except those for sterility and determination of the absence of pyrogens, and stored under conditions consistent with product labeling shall be retained for at least 2 years after the drug distribution has been completed or at least 1 year after the drug's expiration date, whichever is longer.

(h) Provision for retaining complete records of all laboratory data relating to each batch or lot of drug to which they apply. Such records shall be retained for at least 2 years after distribution has been completed or 1 year after the drug's expiration date, whichever is longer.

(i) Provision that animals shall be maintained and controlled in a manner that assures suitability for their

Table 2-4. ADAPTION OF CURRENT GOOD MANUFACTURING PRACTICE REGULATIONS* (*Cont.*)

intended use. They shall be identified and appropriate records maintained to determine the history of use.

(j) Provision that firms which manufacture non-penicillin products (including certifiable antibiotic products) on the same premises or use the same equipment as that used for manufacturing penicillin products, or that operate under any circumstances that may reasonably be regarded as conducive to contamination of other drugs by penicillin, shall test such nonpenicillin products to determine whether any have become cross-contaminated by penicillin. Such products shall not be marketed if intended for use in man and the product is contaminated with an amount of penicillin equivalent to 0.05 unit or more of penicillin G per maximum single dose recommended in the labeling of a drug intended for parenteral administration, or an amount of penicillin equivalent to 0.5 unit or more of penicillin G per maximum single dose recommended in the labeling of a drug intended for oral use.

11. Distribution records.

(a) Finished goods warehouse control and distribution procedures shall include a system by which the distribution of each lot of drug can be readily determined to facilitate its recall if necessary. Records within the system shall contain the name and address of the consignee, date and quantity shipped, and lot or control number of the drug. Records shall be retained for at least 2 years after the distribution of the drug has been completed or 1 year after the expiration date of the drug, whichever is longer.

(b) To assure the quality of the product, finished goods warehouse control shall also include a system whereby the oldest approved stock is distributed first whenever possible.

12. Stability.

There shall be assurance of the stability of finished drug products. This stability shall be:

(a) Determined by reliable, meaningful, and specific test methods.

(b) Determined on products in the same container-closure systems in which they are marketed.

(c) Determined on any dry drug product that is to be reconstituted at the time of dispensing (as directed in its labeling), as well as on the reconstituted product.

(d) Recorded and maintained in such manner that the stability data may be utilized in establishing product expiration dates.

13. Expiration dating.

To assure that drug products liable to deterioration meet appropriate standards of identity, strength, quality, and purity at the time of use, the label of all such drugs shall have suitable expiration dates which relate to stability tests performed on the product.

(a) Expiration dates appearing on the drug labeling shall be justified by readily available data from stability studies.

(b) Expiration dates shall be related to appropriate storage conditions stated on the labeling wherever the expiration date appears.

(c) When the drug is marketed in the dry state for use in preparing a liquid product, the labeling shall bear expiration information for the reconstituted product as well as an expiration date for the dry product.

14. Complaint files.

Records shall be maintained of all written and oral complaints regarding each product. An investigation of each complaint shall be made in accordance with established procedures. The record of each investigation shall be maintained for at least 2 years after distribution of the drug has been completed or 1 year after the expiration date of the drug, whichever is longer.

Selected Reading

Preface, *United States Adopted Names,* USAN Division USP Convention, Inc., Rockville, Md., 1972.

Varsano, J. and Gilbert, S.: Pharmaceuticals in Plastic Packaging. *Drug and Cosmetic Industry, 104,* No. 1, 88; No. 2, 72; No. 3, 98, 1969.

United States Pharmacopeia, 19th Revision, The United States Pharmacopeial Convention, Inc., New York, 1975.

National Formulary, 14th Edition, American Pharmaceutical Association, Washington, D.C., 1975.

Chapter 3

General Considerations in Dosage Form Design

$\mathbf{D}$RUG SUBSTANCES are seldom administered in their natural or pure state, but rather as part of a formulation in combination with one or more nonmedicinal agents that serve varied and specialized pharmaceutical functions. Through selective use of these nonmedicinal agents, referred to as pharmaceutical aids, adjuncts, or necessities, pharmaceutical preparations of various types result. It is the pharmaceutical adjunct that serves to solubilize, suspend, thicken, dilute, emulsify, stabilize, preserve, color, flavor, and fashion the many and varied medicinal agents into efficacious and appealing pharmaceutical preparations. Each different type of preparation is unique in its physical and pharmaceutical characteristics and in the final form in which the drug is presented to the patient. These varied preparations, which provide the manufacturing pharmacist with the challenges of formulation and the physician with the choice of pharmaceutical types, are termed "dosage forms." The general area of study which concerns itself with the physical, chemical, and biological factors which influence the formulation, manufacture, stability, and effectiveness of pharmaceutical dosage forms is termed *pharmaceutics.*

The Need for Dosage Forms

The potent nature and low dosage of most of the drugs in use today precludes any expectation that the general public could safely obtain the appropriate dose of a drug from the bulk material. The vast majority of drug substances are administered in milligram amounts, much too small to be weighed on anything but a sensitive laboratory balance. For instance, how could the layman accurately obtain the 325 mg of aspirin found in the common aspirin tablet from a bulk supply of aspirin? He couldn't. Yet, compared with many other drugs, the dose of aspirin is formidable (Table 3-1). For example, the dose of ethinyl estradiol, 0.05 mg, is 1/6500 the amount of aspirin in an aspirin tablet. To put it another way, 6500 ethinyl estradiol tablets, each containing 0.05 mg of drug, could be made from an amount of ethinyl estradiol equal to the amount of aspirin in just one aspirin tablet. When the dose of the drug is minute, as that for ethinyl estradiol, solid dosage forms such as tablets and capsules must be prepared with fillers or diluents so that the size of the resultant dosage unit is large enough to pick up with the fingertips.

In addition to providing the mechanism for the safe and convenient delivery of accurate dosage, dosage forms are needed for the following and other reasons:

1. For the protection of a drug substance from the destructive influences of atmospheric oxygen or moisture (e.g. coated tablets, sealed ampules).
2. For the protection of a drug substance from the destructive influence of gastric acid after oral administration (e.g. enteric coated tablets).
3. To conceal the bitter, salty, or obnoxious taste or odor of a drug substance (e.g. capsules, coated tablets, flavored syrups)
4. To provide liquid preparations of substances that are either insoluble or unstable in the desired vehicle (e.g. suspensions).
5. To provide liquid dosage forms of substances soluble in the desired vehicle (e.g. solutions).
6. To provide extended drug action through controlled release mechanisms (e.g. various controlled release tablets, capsules and suspensions)
7. To provide optimal drug action from topical administration sites (e.g. ointments,

Table 3-1. EXAMPLES OF SOME DRUGS
WITH RELATIVELY LOW USUAL DOSES

Drug	Usual Dose mg	Category
Lithium Carbonate	300	Antidepressant
Ferrous Sulfate	300	Hematinic
Erythromycin	250	Antibacterial
Ampicillin	250	Antibacterial
Tetracycline HCl	250	Antibacterial
Nitrofurantoin	100	Antibacterial (urinary)
Digitalis	100	Cardiotonic
Pentobarbital Sodium	100	Hypnotic
Propoxyphene HCl	65	Analgesic
Hydrochlorothiazide	50	Diuretic
Codeine Phosphate	30	Analgesic
Phenobarbital	30	Sedative
Chlorpromazine HCl	25	Tranquilizer
Diphenhydramine HCl	25	Antihistaminic
Morphine Sulfate	10	Narcotic analgesic
Prednisolone	5	Adrenocortical steroid
Chlorpheniramine maleate	4	Antihistaminic
Colchicine	0.5	Gout Supressant
Diethylstilbestrol	0.5	Estrogen
Atropine Sulfate	0.4	Anticholinergic
Nitroglycerin	0.4	Antianginal
Ergonovine Maleate	0.2	Oxytocic
Digitoxin	0.1	Cardiotonic (maintenance)
Ethinyl Estradiol	0.05	Estrogen

creams, ophthalmic, ear, and nasal preparations).

8. To provide for the insertion of a drug into one of the body's orifices (e.g. rectal or vaginal suppositories).
9. To provide for the placement of drugs within body tissues (e.g. injections).
10. To provide for optimal drug action through inhalation therapy (e.g. inhalants and inhalation aerosols).

In addition to the above, many dosage forms permit ease of drug identification through distinctiveness of color, shape, or identifying markings.

The Variety of Dosage Forms

There are many different forms into which a medicinal agent may be placed for the conven-ient and efficacious treatment of disease. Drugs can be prepared for administration by every conceivable route, and the appropriate pharmaceutical preparation can be formulated to insure maximum therapeutic response. Drugs may be taken orally and swallowed or allowed to dissolve in the buccal cavity or under the tongue. They may be injected into the vein or muscle or under the skin. They may be inserted rectally or vaginally, instilled in the eye, placed in the ear or nose, applied to the skin, or taken by inhalation. For each of these routes of administration, drugs can be prepared in a variety of physical forms to achieve the proper effect. Drugs can be dissolved in a suitable solvent and employed as a solution. Drug substances can also be suspended in a suitable vehicle as solid particles or as tiny droplets or immiscible liquids. Most commonly, drugs are prepared in solid dosage forms as either tablets or capsules with or without various coatings. Drugs intended for topical application to the skin may be prepared as greasy or nongreasy ointments, creams, lotions, pastes, dusting powders, or aerosols. Drugs may also be prepared as suppositories for insertion into one of the body's orifices, or as sprays, drops, plasters, and other types, depending on the treatment required.

Each drug and each disease must be considered as one applies to the other before the proper combination of drug and dosage form can be prepared, for every body tissue is subject to disease, with each disease requiring a different type of drug therapy. Drugs may be administered for systemic action throughout the body or for limited or local effects on a selected body tissue.

Some individual medicinal agents are effective therapeutic agents for maladies of various parts of the body and are formulated into a half dozen or more dosage forms of varying strengths, each having the particular pharmaceutical characteristics which lend themselves best to a specific application. One such versatile drug is prednisolone, a synthetic adrenocortical steroid, used primarily for its anti-inflammatory activity on various parts of the body. In the USP XIX, prednisolone and its various chemical forms are officially recognized as:

(a) Prednisolone, the chemical powder used in pharmaceutical compounding, particularly in the preparation of (b) and (c).
(b) Prednisolone Tablets, used orally for the

systemic action of prednisolone. Tablets generally contain 1, 2.5, and 5 mg of prednisolone.

(c) Prednisolone Tebutate, a very slightly soluble in water compound, used in the form of a sterile suspension as an intra-articular, intrabursal, and soft-tissue injection.

(d) Prednisolone Acetate, the acetate ester form of prednisolone, used primarily in the preparation of (e).

(e) Sterile Prednisolone Acetate Suspension, employed as an intra-articular and intramuscular injection.

(f) Prednisolone Sodium Phosphate, a water soluble salt form of prednisolone, used primarily in the preparation of (g) and (h).

(g) Prednisolone Sodium Phosphate Injection, an aqueous solution used for intravenous or intramuscular injection.

(h) Prednisolone Sodium Phosphate Ophthalmic Solution, an aqueous solution for topical application to the eye.

(i) Prednisolone Succinate, a very slightly soluble in water compound, used in the preparation of (j).

(j) Prednisolone Sodium Succinate for Injection, a sterile powder, prepared from sodium succinate with the aid of sodium carbonate. At the time of use it is prepared into a solution and used by intramuscular or intravenous injection.

By creating special chemical forms of the basic chemical prednisolone, research pharmacists have facilitated the preparation of effective anti-inflammatory pharmaceuticals of prednisolone for use orally, by injection as a suspension or solution, and for topical application to the eye. The extreme insolubility in water of prednisolone acetate makes this chemical form useful in the preparation of a pharmaceutical suspension. Generally, an injection of a suspension is slowly absorbed from the site of injection, thereby decreasing its onset and increasing the duration of action within the body. On the other hand, prednisolone sodium phosphate is quite water soluble, and an injection of its solution results in a rapid onset of action, particularly if injected intravenously. However, a solution generally has a shorter duration of action than the corresponding suspension. From the various pharmaceutical forms of this one chemical the physician can select the proper preparation for an individual patient. When

further variation is desired, as with the strength of a preparation, the community pharmacist can skillfully employ his training to meet the particular needs of the physician and patient.

In addition to prednisolone, many other such versatile drugs are prepared in numerous dosage forms and strengths for the efficacious and convenient treatment of disease. Figure 3-1 depicts the various dosage forms of the antibiotic drug erythromycin manufactured by one pharmaceutical firm. Before a medicinal agent is formulated into one or more dosage forms by either the community or industrial pharmacist, many factors must be considered. These factors can be broadly grouped into three categories for consideration: (1) therapeutic considerations, including the nature of the illness, the manner in which it is generally treated, locally or through systemic action, and the age and anticipated condition of the patient; (2) drug considerations, including the chemical and physical properties of the drug substance; and (3) biopharmaceutic considerations, including the drug's inherent ability to be absorbed from various body sites, the nature of its subsequent distribution throughout the body, the manner of its detoxification and excretion from the body, and how factors of pharmaceutical formulation and manufacture may alter these processes. When these factors are considered together, as one relates to the other, the result is dosage forms that are appropriate and efficacious in terms of therapeutics, elegant and chemically and physically stable in terms of pharmaceutics, and acceptable and well tolerated by the patient. This is the goal in the creation of dosage forms.

Therapeutic Considerations in Dosage Form Design

The nature of the disease or illness against which the drug is intended is an essential consideration in deciding which dosage forms of a drug to prepare and market. Such basic questions as whether the disease is best treated systemically or locally must be answered, and the most appropriate dosage forms must be evaluated in clinical trials. Assessments must be made as to whether the illness is best treated with prompt-, slow-, short-, or long-acting pharmaceuticals. If there is the remotest chance that a given drug may have application to an

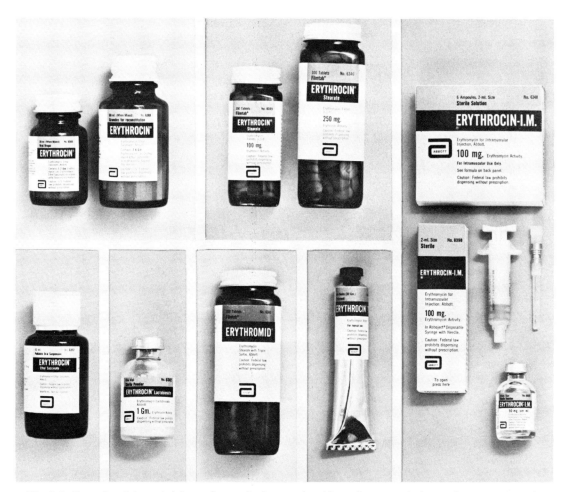

Fig. 3-1. *Examples of the varied dosage forms of a drug marketed by a pharmaceutical manufacturer to meet the special requirements of the patient. Clockwise, from upper left: oral drops (suspension prepared by pharmacist on reconstitution of granules) for pediatric patient; granules for reconstitution to prepare oral suspension administered by spoon; film-coated tablets of two strengths; solutions for intramuscular injection; ointment for topical use; combination tablet with another medicinal agent; sterile lyophilized powder for the preparation of an intravenous solution; and a prepared pediatric oral suspension. (Courtesy of Abbott Laboratories)*

emergency situation or one in which the patient is comatose, frantic, or simply uncooperative, a form suitable for parenteral administration may be developed. If the illness is one that can generally be treated safely through the self-administration of the drug, manufacturer's oblige by placing the drug in compact dosage units such as tablets or capsules or in easily administered liquid forms. In the vast majority of instances, drug manufacturers prepare a single medicinal agent into many dosage forms, partly to satisfy the personal preference of the physician or patient and partly to meet the peculiar needs or requirements of a certain situation. For instance, drugs used to combat nausea and vomit-

ing may be taken prophylactically in tablet form, as before boarding an airplane or for the morning sickness of pregnancy, but this form may be of little value if given during the course of the illness because it may be spewed with the vomitus. For this particular type of drug it is therefore not unusual to find suppositories marketed, to obviate the occasional ineffectiveness of orally administered medication. Many asthmatic patients are treated by inhalation therapy using finely powdered medication or aerosol mists from which the drug is absorbed into the systemic circulation after deep inhalation into the lungs. Patients suffering from angina pectoris, a painful condition resulting from an inadequacy of coronary circulation, are most rapidly treated by allowing a nitroglycerin tablet to dissolve under the tongue from which site it is rapidly absorbed. Thus although systemic effects are generally obtained through the oral and parenteral administration of drugs, other routes may be employed as the situation requires and the drug permits. Each drug has its own individual characteristics relating to drug absorption. Some may be well absorbed from a given route of administration, whereas others may be poorly absorbed. Each drug must be individually evaluated and the most efficacious routes determined.

Drugs intended to provide localized effects are applied directly to the site of their intended action. This would include most of the products utilized in the eye, ear, nose, throat, as well as those applied to the skin or placed in the vagina or rectum. Drugs intended for localized effects within the gastrointestinal tract generally are composed of insoluble materials which when swallowed result in little if any systemic absorption. Products of this type are commonly employed in treating gastric hyperacidity, diarrhea, and constipation.

The Age of the Patient

The age of the intended patient has a pronounced influence on the types of dosage forms prepared for a given drug. For infants, pharmaceutical liquids rather than solid dosage forms are preferred for oral administration. These liquids, which are generally aqueous solutions or suspensions, are usually administered by drops directly into the infant's mouth or incorporated with his food. Needless to say, the amount of drug in a pediatric preparation is less than would be present in an adult preparation of the same drug. However, by having drugs dissolved or suspended in liquid vehicles, the amount of drug administered may be adjusted by merely increasing or decreasing the volume given. A single pediatric preparation may be used for infants and children of all ages, with the dose of the drug and the volume administered being dependent upon the age, weight, and condition of the youngster. When an infant is in the throes of a vomiting crisis, is gagging, has a productive cough, or is simply rebellious, there may be some question as how much of the medicine administered is actually swallowed and how much is expectorated. In such in-

stances, injections and infant size suppositories play an important role in providing the means whereby drugs may be administered and retained in known amounts.

In early childhood a youngster may still have difficulty in swallowing an intact solid dosage form. For this reason most oral preparations intended for children are prepared either as pleasant tasting syrups or other liquids or as chewable tablets. Chewable tablets may be compared in texture with an after dinner mint: they readily dissolve in the mouth to a pleasant tasting creamy substance or may be chewed and easily swallowed.

Solid dosage forms for adults must be of a size and shape easily swallowed. Drugs effective only in extra large doses are generally prepared as chewable tablets or in liquid form. Adults are generally interested in convenience, and when drugs are to be carried about and taken away from home, solid dosage forms are preferred. With solid dosage forms there is no inconvenience of measuring spoons, sticky bottles, or large containers as there is with liquid pharmaceuticals. One tablet may be easily carried, but one teaspoon of medication may not. Unquestionably, solid dosage forms, and tablets in particular, are the most convenient and popular forms of pharmaceuticals. From a cost standpoint, tablets are probably the least expensive dosage form dispensed.

Drug Considerations
in Dosage Form Design

In dealing with the problem of formulating a new drug into a proper dosage form, research pharmacists employ knowledge that has been gained through experience with other similar drugs and through the proper utilization of the disciplines of the physical, chemical, and biological sciences. The early stages of any new formulation involve the collection of basic information of the physical and chemical characteristics of the drug substance to be incorporated into a pharmaceutical preparation.

The majority of drug substances in use today occur as solid materials. Most of them are pure chemical compounds of either crystalline or amorphous constitution. Some are powdered animal or vegetable drugs; others are powdered extractives from these same naturally occurring substances. Liquid drugs are used to a much lesser extent; gases, even less frequently. Of the official medicinal gases, nitrous oxide, cyclopropane, and ethylene are used as general anesthetics by inhalation and oxygen and carbon dioxide are respiratory aids. Several other gases used for pharmaceutical purposes are also official, as nitrogen, used as a replacement for air in hermetically sealed containers, helium, used as a diluent for medicinal gases, and trichloromonogluoromethane, one of the propellant gases used in aerosol packaging.

Liquid Medicinal Agents

Among the few official liquid medicinal agents are the following:

Alcohol, local anti-infective at 70% concentration

Amyl nitrite, vasodilator by inhalation

Castor oil, cathartic

Clofibrate, antihyperlipidemic

Dimercaprol, antidote for arsenic, gold, and mercury poisoning

Ether, general anesthetic by inhalation

Ethchlorvynol, hypnotic

Glycerin, cathartic in suppository form

Mineral oil, cathartic

Nikethamide, central and respiratory stimulant

Nitroglycerin (as tablets), anti-anginal

Paraldehyde, sedative-hypnotic

Paramethadione, anticonvulsant

Prochlorperazine, tranquilizer and antiemetic

Propylhexedrine, vasoconstrictor by nasal inhalation

Tetrachloroethylene, anthelmintic

Undecylenic acid, fungistatic agent

Liquid drugs pose an interesting problem in dosage form design. Many of them are volatile substances and as such must be physically sealed from the atmosphere to insure their continued presence. Amyl nitrite, for example, is a clear yellowish liquid that is volatile even at low temperatures and is also highly flammable. It is maintained for medicinal purposes in small sealed glass cylinders wrapped with gauze or another suitable material. When amyl nitrite is administered, the glass is broken between the fingertips and the liquid wets the gauze covering, producing vapors that are inhaled by the patient requiring vasodilation. Propylhexedrine provides another example of a volatile liquid drug that must be contained in a closed system to maintain its presence. This drug is used as a

nasal inhalant for its vasoconstrictor action. A cylindrical roll of fibrous material is impregnated with propylhexedrine, and the saturated cylinder is placed in a suitable, generally plastic, sealed nasal inhaler. The inhaler's cap must be securely tightened each time it is used. Even then, the inhaler maintains its effectiveness for only a limited period of time due to the volatilization of the drug.

Another problem associated with liquid drugs is that those intended for oral administration cannot generally be formulated into tablet form, the most popular form of oral medication, without undertaking major chemical modification of the drug. An exception to this is the liquid drug nitroglycerin which is formulated into tablet triturates which disintegrate within seconds after placement under the tongue. However, because the drug is volatile, it has a tendency to escape from the tablets during storage and it is critical that the tablets be stored in tightly sealed glass containers. For the most part, when a liquid drug is to be administered orally and a solid dosage form is desired, two approaches are used. First, the liquid substance may be sealed in a soft gelatin capsule. Paramethadione, ethchlorvynol, and clofibrate are examples of liquid drugs commercially available in capsule form.[1] Secondly, the liquid drug may be developed into a salt form that will be suitable for tableting or drug encapsulating. Arecoline, an anthelmintic used in veterinary medicine, and scopolamine, a central depressant, are liquid chemicals, the hydrobromide salt forms of which are solids used to prepare the respective tablet and injectable dosage forms.

For certain liquid drugs, especially those employed orally in large doses or applied topically, their liquid nature may be of some advantage in therapy. For example 15 ml doses of mineral oil may be administered conveniently as such, or as an emulsified product which serves to mask the unpleasant greasy nature of the oil. Also, the liquid nature of undecylenic acid certainly does not hinder but rather enhances its use topically in the treatment of fungus infections of the skin. However, for the most part, solid materials are preferred by pharmacists in formulation work because of their superior stability characteristics over liq-

---

[1] Paramethadione as Paradione (Abbott); ethchlorvynol as Placidyl (Abbott) and clofibrate as Atromid S (Ayerst)

uids, their ease of handling, and their amenability to the preparation of tablets and capsules. For these reasons, whenever possible, the medicinal chemist searches for and creates solid forms, which will be biologically active and will lend themselves well to the development and production of solid dosage forms.

Solid Medicinal Agents

Formulation and stability difficulties arise less frequently with solid dosage forms than with liquid pharmaceutical preparations, and for this reason many new drugs first reach the market as tablets or dry filled capsules. Later, when the pharmaceutical problems are resolved, a liquid form of the same drug may be marketed. This procedure, when practiced, is doubly advantageous, since for the most part physicians and patients alike prefer small, generally tasteless, accurately dosed tablets or capsules to the analogous liquid forms that may have an unpleasant taste and are likely to be measured by the patient with highly variable household spoons. Therefore, marketing a drug in solid form first is more practical for the manufacturer and also suits the majority of patients. It is estimated that tablets and capsules comprise the dosage form dispensed 70% of the time by community pharmacists, with tablets dispensed twice as frequently as capsules.

Some important relationships between the physical characteristics of certain solid medicinal agents (as particle size and crystalline or amorphous form and the resultant biologic availability of the drug from the prepared dosage form are presented later in this Chapter.

Drug Stability

The chemical problems of formulation generally are centered around the chemical stability of the medicinal agent and its compatibility with the other formulative ingredients.

Chemical instability of medicinal agents may take many forms, since the drugs in use today are of such diverse chemical constitution. Chemically, drug substances are alcohols, phenols, aldehydes, ketones, esters, ethers, acids, salts, alkaloids, glycosides, and others, each with reactive chemical groups having different susceptibilities toward chemical instability. Drugs of synthetic origin may contain chemical residues or by-products of the synthesis which might influence the chemical stability of the drug itself. Drugs of natural origin may be complex mixtures of chemicals of undefined chemical composition or may contain other substances extracted along with the drug during the process of separating the drug from its natural source. Drug purification and specific chemical characterization of all components used in a drug formulation are essential first steps if drug product stability is to be achieved and reasons for any chemical or physical instability identified and corrected.

In the usual processes of formulation and manufacture, medicinal agents are exposed to and come into contact with many other chemical agents, some of which remain in the completed dosage form and others which do not remain with the finished product. In each case, the formulative materials must be selected so as to not interfere with the chemical or physical stability of the therapeutic ingredient. If the medicinal agent is relatively unstable, it is the responsibility of the research pharmacist to find a way to increase its stability. This may entail the use of a new salt or ester form of the medicinal agent, the addition, deletion, or substitution of a formulative material, or an alteration in the usual method of manufacture whereby the drug is given special and lasting protection against decomposition.

Changes in a pharmaceutical preparation's stability may be noticed as precipitation from solution of a chemical agent, an evolution of a gas with resultant odor release or container explosion, an alteration in the color of a solid or liquid dosage form, a change in the fluid characteristics of a liquid preparation, a rancid smell of an ointment, and others. Chemically, the most frequently encountered destructive processes in drug formulation work are those of hydrolysis and oxidation.

Hydrolysis may be defined as that process in which (drug) molecules interact with water molecules to yield breakdown products of different chemical constitution. For example, aspirin or acetylsalicylic acid combines with a water molecule and hydrolyzes into one molecule of salicylic acid and one molecule of acetic acid:

Aspirin   Salicylic Acid   Acetic Acid

Among the other chemicals of pharmaceutical interest that may be decomposed by the hydrolytic process are atropine, barbituric acid derivatives, chloramphenicol, penicillin, procaine, the sulfonamide drugs, and the pharmaceutical adjuncts sucrose and chlorobutanol, the former employed in the preparation of pharmaceutical syrups and the latter used in preserving certain preparations from microbial contamination and growth.

The process of hydrolysis is probably the most important single cause of drug decomposition mainly because a great number of medicinal agents are esters or contain such other groupings as substituted amides, lactones, and lactams, which are susceptible to the hydrolytic process.

There are several approaches to the stabilization of pharmaceutical preparations containing drugs subject to deterioration by hydrolysis. Perhaps the most obvious is the reduction, or better yet, the elimination of water from the pharmaceutical system. Even solid dosage forms containing water-labile drugs must be protected from the humidity of the atmosphere. This may be accomplished by applying a waterproof protective coating over tablets or by enclosing and maintaining the drug in tightly closed containers. It is not unusual to detect hydrolyzed aspirin by noticing an odor of acetic acid upon opening a bottle of aspirin tablets. In liquid preparations, water can frequently be replaced or reduced in the formulation through the use of substitute liquids such as glycerin, propylene glycol, and alcohol. In certain instances, anhydrous vegetable oils may be used as the drug's solvent and thereby reduce the chance of hydrolytic decomposition. To cite an example, Isoflurophate Ophthalmic Solution, USP, is a solution of the drug, isoflurophate, used primarily in the treatment of glaucoma, in a suitable vegetable oil. The commercial preparation, Floropryl Solution (Merck Sharp & Dohme), is made with anhydrous peanut oil. The use of the anhydrous oil and the absence therefore of moisture inhibits the decomposition of isoflurophate and the release of hydrofluoric acid, a compound so corrosive it is employed in the etching of glass. Obviously the release of this agent would be quite damaging to the eye, and this occurrence must be avoided.

Decomposition by hydrolysis may be prevented for other drugs to be administered in liquid form by suspending them in an appropriate vehicle rather than by dissolving them in an

$$(CH_3)_2CHO—\overset{\overset{\displaystyle F}{|}}{\underset{\underset{\displaystyle O}{\|}}{P}}—OCH(CH_3)_2 \xrightarrow{\text{H}_2\text{O}}$$

Isoflurophate

$$(CH_3)_2CHO—\overset{\overset{\displaystyle OH}{|}}{\underset{\underset{\displaystyle O}{\|}}{P}}—OCH(CH_3)_2 + \qquad HF$$

Hydrofluoric Acid

aqueous solvent. In still other instances, particularly for certain unstable antibiotic drugs, when an aqueous preparation is desired, the drug may be supplied to the pharmacist in a dry form for reconstitution by adding a specified volume of purified water just before dispensing. The dry powder supplied commercially is actually a mixture of the antibiotic, suspending or solubilizing agents, flavorants, and colorants, which, when reconstituted by the pharmacist, remains a stable suspension or solution of the drug for the time period in which the preparation is normally consumed. Storage under refrigeration is advisable for most preparations considered unstable due to hydrolytic causes. In the instance of Penicillin G Potassium the USP is explicit in describing its instability:

"Its solutions retain substantially full potency for several days at temperatures below 15°, but are rapidly inactivated by acids, alkali hydroxides, glycerin, and oxidizing agents."

The monograph also states that Penicillin G Potassium must comply with the Food and Drug Administration requirements for its pH, moisture content, heat stability, potency, and other measures. Together with temperature, pH is a major determinant in the stability of a drug prone to hydrolytic decomposition. The hydrolysis of most drugs is dependent upon the relative concentrations of the hydroxyl and hydronium ions, and a pH at which each drug is optimally stable can be easily determined. For most hydrolyzable drugs the pH of optimum stability is on the acid side, somewhere between pH 5 and 6. Therefore, through judicious use of buffering agents, the stability of otherwise unstable compounds can be increased. In the USP, Sterile Penicillin G Potassium, if maintained in the dry state is considered stable for 5 years, whereas its solutions are stable under refrigeration for only 3 days. On the other hand, Penicillin G Potassium for Injection, USP, which is Penicillin G Potassium with a citrate buffer, is considered stable in solution under refrigeration for a period of 7 days. In the case of Penicillin G Potassium, acid or enzymatic hydrolysis may occur after oral administration due to the acidity of the gastric juice and to the activity of penicillinase, an enzyme produced by certain microorganisms in the intestinal tract. The result of each type of hydrolysis is the transformation of penicillin into penicilloic acid, an inactive compound. The destruction of penicillin G by enzymatic hydrolysis is so effective that pharmaceutical preparations of the enzyme are employed therapeutically to treat cases involving allergic reactions to penicillin therapy. Many of the newer synthetic penicillins have been developed to be resistant to both the acidity of the stomach and the activity of penicillinase, and these compounds generally produce clinical effects that are usually of greater magnitude and reliability than the older penicillin G. Other hydrolytic enzymes, in addition to penicillinase, exist in body fluids and are responsible for the hydrolytic conversion of many drugs into breakdown products.

In addition to water present, temperature, pH, and hydrolytic enzymes, the research pharmacist must carefully consider the possibility of other formulative agents acting as catalysts to a hydrolytic reaction. Whenever a hydrolyzable drug is formulated into a pharmaceutical preparation, it must be the aim to maintain that drug, in whatever form is required, at its optimum potency for the longest possible shelf life period and for efficient effective therapy upon its administration.

The official compendia permit the addition of "suitable substances" to pharmaceutical preparations to enhance their permanency and usefulness. One destructive process against which certain pharmaceuticals may be protected by the use of specific pharmaceutical stabilizers is oxidation. The oxidative process is destructive to many drug types, including aldehydes, alcohols, phenols, sugars, alkaloids, and unsaturated fats and oils. The formulation pharmacist is keenly aware of this process when he develops products containing such popular and oxidizable drugs as ascorbic acid, vitamin A, streptomycin, epinephrine, ferrous sulfate, resorcinol, and many others. Pharmaceutical additives employed to deter or inhibit the oxidative process are termed "antioxidants."

Pharmaceutically, the oxidation of a susceptible drug substance is most likely to occur when it is maintained in other than the dry state in the presence of oxygen, exposed to light, or carelessly combined in formulation with other chemical agents without proper regard to their influence on the oxidation process. The oxidation of a chemical in a pharmaceutical preparation is usually attendant with an alteration in the color of that preparation. It may also be made manifest by precipitation or a change in the usual odor of a preparation.

Chemically, oxidation involves the loss of electrons from an atom or a molecule. Each electron lost is accepted by some other atom or molecule, thereby accomplishing the reduction of the recipient. In inorganic chemistry, oxidation is accompanied by an increase in the positive valence of an element—for example, ferrous ($+2$) oxidizing to ferric ($+3$). In organic chemistry, oxidation is frequently considered synonymous with the loss of hydrogen (dehydrogenation) from a molecule. The oxidative process frequently involves free chemical radicals, which are molecules or atoms containing one or more unpaired electrons, as molecular (atmospheric) oxygen ($\cdot O{-}O \cdot$) and free hydroxyl ($\cdot OH$). These radicals tend to take electrons from other chemicals, thereby oxidizing the donor. Many of the oxidative changes in pharmaceutical preparations have the character of autoxidations. Autoxidations occur spontaneously under the initial influence of atmospheric oxygen and proceed slowly at first and then more rapidly as the process continues. The process has been described as a type of chain reaction commencing by the union of oxygen with the drug molecule and continuing with a free radical of this oxidized molecule participating in the destruction of other drug molecules and so forth.

The oxidative process is diverted, and the stability of the drug is preserved by antioxidants, which react with one or more compounds in the drug to prevent progress of the chain reaction. In general, antioxidants act by providing electrons and easily available hydrogen atoms that are accepted more readily by the free radicals than are those of the drug being protected. Various antioxidants are employed in pharmacy. Among those most frequently used in aqueous preparations are sodium sulfite (Na_2SO_3), sodium bisulfite ($NaHSO_3$), hypophosphorous acid (H_3PO_2), and ascorbic acid. In oleaginous (oily or unctuous) preparations, alphatocopherol, butylhydroxyanisole, and ascorbyl palmitate find application.

The proper use of antioxidants involves their specific application only after appropriate pharmaceutical studies. In certain instances other pharmaceutical additives have been found to inactivate a given antioxidant when used in the same formulation. In other cases certain antioxidants have been found to react chemically with the drugs they were intended to stabilize, without a noticeable change in the appearance of the preparation. The reaction of bisulfite with epinephrine to form colorless, pharmacologically inactive epinephrine sulfonate is an example of this type of easily unnoticed interference.[1]

Since the stability of oxidizable drugs may be adversely affected by oxygen, certain pharmaceuticals may require an oxygen-free atmosphere during their preparation and storage. Oxygen may be present in pharmaceutical liquids in the airspace within the container or may be dissolved in the liquid vehicle. To avoid these exposures, oxygen sensitive drugs may be prepared in the dry state and they, as well as liquid preparations, may be packaged in sealed containers with the air replaced by an inert gas such as nitrogen. This is common practice in the commercial production of vials and ampules of easily oxidizable preparations intended for parenteral use.

Trace metals originating in the drug, solvent, container, or stopper are a constant source of difficulty in preparing stable solutions of oxidizable drugs. The rate of formation of color in epinephrine solutions, for instance, is greatly increased by the presence of ferric, ferrous, cupric, and chromic ions. Great care must be taken to eliminate these trace metals from labile preparations by thorough purification of the source of the contaminant or by chemically complexing or binding the metal through the use of specialized agents that make it chemically unavailable for participation in the oxidative process. These agents are referred to as chelating agents and are exemplified by calcium disodium edetate and ethylenediaminetetraacetic acid (EDTA).

[1]Higuchi, T., and Schroeter, L. C.: Reactivity of Bisulfite with a Number of Pharmaceuticals. J. Amer. Pharm. Ass., Scientific Edition, 48:535–540, 1959.

Proposed calcium complex of EDTA

Light can also act as a catalyst to oxidation reactions. As a photocatalyst, light waves transfer their energy (photon) to drug molecules, making the latter more reactive through increased energy capability. As a precaution against the acceleration of the oxidative process, sensitive preparations are packaged in light-resistant colored glass or opaque containers.

Since most drug degradations proceed more rapidly with an advanced temperature, it is also advisable to maintain oxidizable drugs in a cool place. Another factor that could affect the stability of an oxidizable drug in solution is the pH of the preparation. Each drug must be maintained in solution at the pH most favorable to its stability. This, in fact, varies from preparation to preparation and must be determined on an individual basis for the drug in question.

Monographic statements, such as some presented in Table 3-2, warn of the oxidative decomposition of drugs and preparations. In some instances the specific agent to employ as a stabilizer is mentioned in the monograph, and in others the term "suitable stabilizer" is used. One instance in which a particular agent is designated is in the monograph for Potassium Iodide Solution, USP. Potassium iodide in solution is prone to photocatalyzed oxidation and the release of free iodine with a resultant brown discoloration of the solution. The use of light-resistant containers is essential to its stability. As a further precaution against decomposition if the solution is not to be used within a short time, the USP recommends the addition of 0.05% of sodium thiosulfate to the preparation. In the event free iodine is released during storage, the sodium thiosulfate converts it to colorless and soluble sodium iodide:

Table 3-2. Examples of Some Official Drugs
and Preparations Especially Subject to Chemical
or Physical Deterioration

Preparation	Category	Monograph Warning
Epinephrine Inhalation, USP Epinephrine Injection, USP Epinephrine Nasal Solution USP	Adrenergic	Do not use the inhalation, injection, or nasal solution if it is brown or contains a precipitate.
Ferrous Sulfate, USP	Hematinic	Do not use ferrous sulfate that is coated with brownish yellow basic ferric sulfate.
Isoproterenol Hydrochloride Inhalation, USP Isoproterenol Hydrochloride Injection, USP	Adrenergic (bronchodilator)	Do not use the inhalation or injection if it is brown in color or contains a precipitate.
Nitroglycerin Tablets, USP	Antianginal	To prevent loss of potency, keep these tablets in the original container. Close tightly immediately after each use.
Orange Oil, USP	Pharmaceutic aid (flavor)	Do not use orange oil that has a terebinthine odor.
Paraldehyde, USP	Hypnotic	Paraldehyde is subject to oxidation to form acetic acid.
Vinyl Ether, NF	General anesthetic	Do not use vinyl ether for anesthesia if the original container has been opened longer than 48 hours.

$$I_2 + 2Na_2S_2O_3 \longrightarrow 2\,NaI + Na_2S_4O_6$$

In summary, for easily oxidizable drugs, the formulation pharmacist may stabilize the respective preparations by the selective exclusion from the system of oxygen, oxidizing agents, trace metals, light, heat, and other chemical catalysts to the oxidation process. He may add antioxidants, chelating agents, and buffering agents to create and maintain a favorable pH.

In addition to oxidation and hydrolysis, other destructive processes such as polymerization, chemical decarboxylation, and deamination may occur in pharmaceutical preparations. However, these processes occur less frequently and are peculiar to only small groups of chemical substances. Drug polymerization involves a reaction between two or more identical molecules with resultant formation of a new and generally larger molecule. Formaldehyde is an example of a drug capable of polymerization. In solution it may polymerize to paraformaldehyde $(CH_2O)_n$, a slowly soluble white crystalline substance that may cause the solution to become cloudy. The formation of paraformaldehyde is enhanced by cool storage temperatures, especially in solutions with high concentrations of formaldehyde. The official formaldehyde solution contains approximately 37% formaldehyde and according to the USP should be stored at temperatures greater than 15°C (59°F). If the solution becomes cloudy upon standing in a cool place, it generally may be cleared by gentle warming. Formaldehyde is prepared by the limited oxidation of methanol (methyl alcohol), and the USP permits a residual amount of this material to remain in the final product, since it has the ability to retard the formation of paraformaldehyde. Formaldehyde solution must be maintained in tight containers because oxidation of the formaldehyde yields formic acid.

$$CH_3OH \xrightarrow{(O)} HCHO \xrightarrow{(O)} HCOOH$$
methanol   formaldehyde   formic acid

Other organic drug molecules may be degraded through processes in which one or more of their active chemical groups are removed. These processes may involve various catalysts, including light and enzymes. Decarboxylation and deamination are examples of such processes, with the former involving the decomposition of an organic acid $(R \cdot COOH)$ and the consequent release of carbon dioxide gas and the latter involving the removal of the nitrogen-containing group from an organic amine. Organic amines are organic compounds formed by replacing one or more of the hydrogen atoms of ammonia (NH_3) with carbon-containing radicals. The resulting compounds are classified as primary amines $(R-NH_2)$, secondary amines (R_2NH), and tertiary amines (R_3N).

Determining Drug Formulation Stability

Drug instability in pharmaceutical formulations may be detected in some instances by a change in the physical appearance, color, odor, taste or texture of the formulation whereas in other instances chemical changes may occur which are not self-evident and may only be ascertained through chemical analysis. Scientific data pertaining to the stability of a formulation leads to the prediction of the expected shelf-life of the proposed product and, when necessary, to the redesign of the drug (e.g. into a more stable salt or ester form) and to the reformulation of the dosage form. Obviously the *rate* or speed at which drug degradation occurs in a formulation is of prime importance. The study of the rate of chemical change and the way in which it is influenced by such factors as the concentration of the drug or reactant, the solvent employed, the conditions of temperature and pressure, and the presence of other chemical agents in the formulation is termed *reaction kinetics*.

In general a kinetic study begins by measuring the concentration of the drug being examined at given time intervals under a specific set of conditions including temperature, pH, ionic strength, light intensity, and drug concentration. The measurement of the drug's concentration at the various time intervals reveals the stability or instability of the drug under the specified conditions with the passage of time. From this starting point, each of the original conditions may be varied on an individual basis to determine the influence that such changes make on the drug's stability. For example, the pH of the solution may be changed, whereas the temperature, light intensity, and original drug concentration remain as they were in the original or baseline experiment.

The data collected may be presented graphically, by plotting the drug concentration as a function of time. From the experimental data, the reaction rate may be determined and a rate constant calculated.[1] The rate constant describes the rate at which a drug is degrading under the conditions of the experiment and may be expressed as for example "2.6 mg/day," "0.1%/hour," or "0.155 g/liter/day."

The data also may be utilized in determining the experimental half-life of the drug. The *half-life* of a drug is defined as the time required for the drug to degrade to one-half of its original concentration. The half-life of a drug is expressed as its $t_{1/2}$ or t_{50}. Other expressions of drug remaining with reference to the original concentration may be used, as t_{90} and t_{95} indicating the drug remaining is 90 and 95% respectively of the original concentration.

The use of *exaggerated* conditions of temperature, humidity, light, and others, to test the stability of drug formulations is termed *accelerated stability testing*. Accelerated temperature-stability studies, for example, are generally conducted at 37°, 50°, and 60°C (140°F), as well as at "room," refrigerator, and freezing temperatures. The use of short-term accelerated studies is for the purpose of determining the most stable of the proposed formulations for a drug product. Once the most stable formulation is ascertained, its long-term stability is predicted from the data generated from continuing stability studies. Depending upon the types and severity of conditions employed, it is not unusual to maintain samples under exaggerated conditions for periods of 1 month to 1 year. Such studies lead to the prediction of shelf-life for a drug product and may be utilized in the deter-

[1] For the mathematical treatment of this type of data, the student is referred to "Reaction Kinetics," by H. B. Kostenbauder in *Remington's Pharmaceutical Sciences*, 15th Ed., Easton, Pa., Mack Publishing Co., 1975, pp. 275–284.

mination of the product's labeled expiration date.

In addition to the accelerated stability studies, drug products are also stored under the usual conditions of transport and storage expected during product distribution. Samples maintained under these conditions may be retained for periods of 5 years or longer during which time they are observed for physical signs of deterioration and chemically assayed. These studies considered with the accelerated stability studies previously performed then lead to a more precise determination of drug product stability, actual shelf-life, and expiration dating.

Under usual circumstances, most manufactured products require a shelf-life of 2 or more years to insure their stability at the time of patient consumption. Commercial products corresponding to officially recognized monographs for dosage forms must bear an appropriate expiration date for the particular formulation. This date then identifies the time during which the product may be expected to meet the compendial requirements when maintained under the prescribed storage conditions. The expiration date officially limits the time during which the product may be dispensed by the pharmacist or used by the patient.

Prescriptions requiring extemporaneous compounding by the pharmacist generally do not require the extended shelf-life that commercially manufactured and distributed products do since they are intended to be utilized immediately upon their receipt by the patient and used only during the immediate course of the prescribed treatment. However, these compounded prescriptions must remain stable and efficacious during the course of their use and the compounding pharmacist must employ formulative components and techniques which will result in a stable product. He must also dispense the medication in a container conducive to stability and use and must advise the patient of the proper method of use and conditions of storage of the medication.

Preservation Against Microbial Contamination

In addition to the stabilization of pharmaceutical preparations against chemical and physical degradation due to changed environmental conditions within a formulation, certain liquid and semisolid preparations also must be preserved against microbial contamination. Although some types of pharmaceutical products like ophthalmic and injectable preparations are sterilized by physical methods (autoclaving for 20 minutes at 15 pounds pressure and 120°C, dry heat at 170°C for 1 hour, or by bacterial filtration) during their manufacture, many of them additionally require the presence of an antimicrobial preservative to maintain their aseptic condition throughout the period of their storage and use. Other types of preparations that are not sterilized during their preparation but are particularly susceptible to microbial growth because of the nature of their ingredients are protected by the addition of an antimicrobial preservative. Preparations that provide excellent growth media for microbes are most aqueous preparations, especially syrups, emulsions, suspensions, and some semisolid preparations, particularly creams. Certain hydroalcoholic and most alcoholic preparations may not require the addition of a chemical preservative when the alcoholic content is sufficient to prevent microbial growth. Generally, 15% alcohol will prevent microbial growth in acid media and 18% in alkaline media. Most alcohol-containing pharmaceuticals such as elixirs, spirits, and tinctures are self-sterilizing and do not require additional preservation. The same would apply to other pharmaceuticals on an individual basis, which by virtue of their vehicles or other formulative agents, including the main therapeutic agent, may not permit the growth of microorganisms.

Selection of Preservatives

When experience or shelf-storage experiments indicate that a preservative is required in a pharmaceutical preparation, its selection is based on many cross considerations including some of the following.

(1) The preservative is effective in preventing the growth of the type of microorganisms considered the most likely contaminants of the preparation being formulated.
(2) The preservative is soluble enough in water to achieve adequate concentrations in the aqueous phase of a two or more phase system.
(3) The proportion of preservative remaining undissociated at the pH of the preparation

makes it capable of penetrating the microorganism and destroying its integrity.

(4) The required concentration of the preservative does not affect the safety or comfort of the patient when the pharmaceutical preparation is administered by the usual or intended route.

(5) The preservative has adequate stability and will not be reduced in concentration due to chemical decomposition or volatilization during the desired shelf-life of the preparation.

(6) The preservative is completely compatible with all other formulative ingredients and does not interfere with them, nor do they interfere with the effectiveness of the preservative agent.

(7) The preservative does not adversely affect the preparation's container or the closure.

General Considerations

Pharmaceutical preparations may be contaminated by molds, yeasts, or bacteria, with the latter generally favoring a slightly alkaline medium and the others an acid medium. Although few microorganisms can grow below a pH of 3 or above pH 9, most aqueous pharmaceutical preparations are within the favorable pH range and therefore must be protected against microbial growth. To be effective, a preservative agent must be dissolved in sufficient concentration in the aqueous phase of a preparation. Further, only the undissociated fraction or molecular form of a preservative possesses preservative capability, since the ionized portion is incapable of penetrating the microorganism. Thus the preservative selected must be largely undissociated at the pH of the formulation being prepared. Acidic preservatives like benzoic, boric, and sorbic acids are more undissociated and thus more effective as the medium is made more acid. Conversely, alkaline preservatives are less effective in acid or neutral media and more effective in alkaline media. Thus, it is meaningless to suggest preservative effectiveness at specific concentrations unless the pH of the system is mentioned and the undissociated concentration of the agent is calculated or otherwise determined. Also, if formulative materials interfere with the solubility or availability of the preservative agent, its chemical concentration may be misleading, since it may not be a true measure of the effective concentration. Many incompatible combinations of preservative agents and other pharmaceutical adjuncts have been discovered in recent years, and undoubtedly many more will be uncovered in the future as new preservatives, pharmaceutical adjuncts, and therapeutic agents are combined for the first time. Many of the recognized incompatible combinations that result in preservative inactivation involve macromolecules such as various cellulose derivatives, polyethylene glycols, and natural gums such as tragacanth, which have been shown to attract and hold preservative agents, such as the parabens and phenolic compounds, rendering them unavailable for their preservative function. It is essential for the research pharmacist to examine all formulative ingredients as one affects the other to assure himself that each agent is free to do the job for which it was included in the formulation. In addition, the preservative must not interact with a container such as a metal ointment tube or a plastic medication bottle or with an enclosure such as a rubber or plastic cap or liner. Such an interaction could result in the decomposition of the preservative or the container closure, or both, with resultant product decomposition and contamination. Appropriate tests should be devised and conducted to insure against this type of preservative interaction.

Mode of Action for Preservatives

Preservatives are thought to interfere with microbial growth, multiplication, and metabolism by one or more of the following mechanisms:

(1) Modification of membrane permeability.
(2) Denaturation of enzymes or other cellular proteins.
(3) Oxidation of cellular constituents.
(4) Hydrolysis.

A few of the commonly used pharmaceutical preservatives and their possible mode of action are presented in Table 3-3.

Preservations for Official Preparations

The official compendia state that suitable substances may be added to an official preparation to enhance its permanency or usefulness.

Table 3-3. PROBABLE MODE OF ACTION OF SOME PRESERVATIVES

Preservative	Probable Mode of Action
Benzoic acid, boric acid, and p-hydroxybenzoates	Denaturation of proteins
Phenols, and chlorinated phenolic compounds	Lytic and denaturation action on membranes and for chlorinated preservatives, also by oxidation of enzymes
Alcohols	Lytic and denaturation action on membranes
Quaternary compounds	Lytic action on membranes
Mercurials	Denaturation of enzymes

Such additives are suitable only if they are nontoxic and harmless in the amounts administered and do not interfere with the therapeutic efficacy or tests or assays of the preparation. For the preservation of preparations intended for parenteral administration or topical application, suitable preservatives may be added unless interdicted in the monograph. Certain intravenous preparations given in large volumes as blood replenishers or as nutrients are not permitted to contain bacteriostatic additives, for the amounts required to preserve such large volumes would constitute a health hazard when administered to the patient. Thus preparations like Dextrose Injection, USP, and others commonly given as fluid and nutrient replenishers by intravenous injections in amounts of 500 to 1000 ml may not contain antibacterial preservatives. On the other hand, injectable preparations given in small volumes—for example, Morphine Sulfate Injection, USP, which provides a therapeutic amount of morphine sulfate in approximately a 1-ml volume—can be preserved with a suitable preservative without the danger of coadministering an excessive amount of the preservative to the patient. Certain monographs indicate the specific preservatives that must be used and the amounts to be employed. For instance, the monograph for Insulin Injection, USP, specifies that "0.1 to 0.25% (w/v) of either phenol or cresol" must be contained in the injection. Other preparations have similar preservative requirements. Examples of the preservatives and their concentrations commonly employed in pharmaceutical preparations are: benzoic acid (0.1 to 0.2%), sodium benzoate (0.1 to 0.2%), alcohol (15 to 20%), phenylmercuric nitrate and acetate (0.002 to 0.01%), phenol (0.1 to 0.5%), cresol (0.1 to 0.5%), chlorobutanol (0.5%), benzalkonium chloride (0.002 to 0.01%), and combinations of methylparaben and propylparaben (0.1 to 0.2%), the latter being especially good against fungus. The required proportion would vary with the factors of pH, dissociation, and others already indicated as well with the presence of other formulative ingredients with inherent preservative capabilities that contribute to the preservation of the preparation and require less additional preservation assistance.

For each type of preparation to be preserved, the research pharmacist must consider the influence of the preservative on the comfort of the patient. For instance, it is apparent that a preservative in an ophthalmic preparation would have to have an extremely low degree of irritant qualities, which is characteristic of chlorobutanol, benzalkonium chloride, and phenylmercuric nitrate, frequently used preservatives in ophthalmic preparations. In all instances, the preserved preparation must be biologically tested to determine its safety and efficacy and shelf-tested to determine its stability for the intended shelf life of the product.

Appearance and Palatability

Although most drug substances in use today are unpalatable and unattractive in their natural state, modern pharmaceutical preparations present them to the patient as colorful, flavorful formulations attractive to the sight, smell, and taste. These qualities, which today are the rule rather than the exception, have virtually eliminated the natural reluctance of many patients to take medications because of their disagreeable odor or taste. In fact, the inherent attractiveness of today's pharmaceuticals has caused them to acquire the dubious distinction of being a major source of accidental poisonings in the home, particularly among children who are lured by their organoleptic appeal.

There is a great psychologic basis to drug therapy, and the odor, taste, and color of a pharmaceutical preparation can play their own peculiar part. Although most patients prefer a palatable medication, there are some who equate the value of the drug with its disagreeable taste; the more disgusting the taste, the more potent the drug. Certain individuals consider a colorless or water-like preparation as being impotent, even though a pharmacist may advise to the contrary. To some, a black or purplish preparation may allude to the toxic or poisonous character of the medicine. Whatever the basis of belief, an appropriate drug will have its most beneficial effect when it is accepted, trusted, and believed in by the patient.

To the formulation pharmacist, the proper combination of color, fragrance, and taste of a pharmaceutical preparation is a challenging task requiring a specialized skill that must be applied with great care, since the success or commercial failure of the product depends upon physician and patient acceptance of the sensuous features of the preparation. This acceptance is also important to the community pharmacist, for he issues the medication to the patient and serves him best with pharmaceuticals that are not only efficacious but attractive and palatable as well. In addition, the colorful array of pharmaceutical products on the pharmacist's shelves, each with its characteristic features, permits their rapid recognition and identification. This ready recognition enables the patient to self-administer the proper drug when on multiple drug therapy and permits the pharmacist and physician to recognize a drug rapidly in instances of poisoning or whenever a question arises as to the drug being taken by an individual.

The flavoring of pharmaceuticals applies primarily to liquid dosage forms intended for oral administration. The 9000 taste buds of the mouth are located principally on the tongue and respond quickly and favorably or unfavorably to contact with medication. Medication in liquid form obviously comes into immediate and direct contact with these taste buds. By the addition of flavoring agents to liquid medication, the disagreeable taste of drugs may be successfully masked. Drugs placed in capsules or prepared as coated tablets may be easily swallowed with total avoidance of contact between the drug and the taste buds. Tablets containing drugs that are not especially distasteful may remain uncoated

and unflavored. Rapidly swallowing them with water usually is sufficient to avoid undesirable drug taste sensations. However, tablets of the chewable type as certain antacid, vitamin, and antibiotic products, which are intended for mastication in the mouth usually *are* sweetened and flavored to receive better patient acceptance.

The flavor sensation of a food or pharmaceutical is actually a complex blend of taste and smell with lesser influences of texture, temperature, and even sight. In flavor formulating a pharmaceutical product, the pharmacist must give consideration to the color, odor, texture, and taste of the preparation. It would be incongruous, for example, to color a liquid pharmaceutical red, give it a banana taste, and a mint odor. The color of a pharmaceutical must have a psychogenic balance with the taste, and the odor must also enhance that taste. Odor greatly affects the flavor of a preparation or foodstuff. If one's sense of smell is impaired, as during a head cold, the usual flavor sensation of food is similarly diminished.

Today, the tastes of foods and drugs are generally classified into four main groups—sweet, salty, bitter, and sour, with such additional tastes as metallic and alkaline sometimes given reference. Sweet and salty sensations are perceived by the taste buds located near the tip of the tongue; sour, at the sides of the tongue; and bitter, at the back.

Flavoring Agents

The medicinal chemist and the formulation pharmacist are well acquainted with the taste characteristics of certain chemical types of drugs and strive to mask effectively the unwanted taste through the appropriate use of flavoring agents. Although there are no dependable rules for unerringly predicting the taste sensation of a drug based upon its chemical constitution, experience permits the presentation of several observations. For instance, although we recognize and assume the salty taste of sodium chloride, the formulation pharmacist knows that all salts are not salty, but that their taste is a function of both the cation and anion. Whereas salty tastes are evoked by sodium, potassium, and ammonium chlorides and by sodium bromide, potassium and ammonium bromides elicit simultaneous bitter and salty sensations, and potassium iodide and magnesium sulfate (epsom salt) are predominantly bitter. In general, low molecular weight salts are salty, and higher molecular weight salts are bitter although certain lead salts are actually sweet. With organic compounds, an increase in the number of hydroxyl groups (-OH) seems to increase the sweetness of the compound. Sucrose, which has eight hydroxyl groups, is sweeter than glycerin, another pharmaceutical sweetener, which has but three hydroxyl groups. In general, the organic esters, alcohols, and aldehydes are pleasant to the taste, and since many of them are volatile, they also contribute to the odor and thus the flavor of preparations in which they are used. Many nitrogen-containing compounds are extremely bitter, especially the plant alkaloids (as quinine), but certain other nitrogen-containing compounds are extremely sweet (as saccharin). The medicinal chemist recognizes that even the most simple structural change in an organic compound can alter its taste. D-glucose is sweet, but L-glucose has a slightly salty taste; saccharin is very sweet, but N-methylsaccharin is tasteless:[1]

| Saccharin | N-Methylsaccharin |
| (Very sweet) | (Tasteless) |

Thus, the predicability of the taste characteristics of a new drug is only speculative. However, it is soon learned, and the formulation pharmacist is then put to the task of increasing the drug's palatability in the environment of other formulative agents. The proper selection of the appropriate flavoring agent depends upon several factors, but primarily upon the taste of the drug substance itself. Certain flavoring materials have been found through experience to be more effective than others in masking or disguising the particular bitter, salty, sour, or otherwise undesirable taste of medicinal agents. Although individuals' tastes and flavor preferences differ, cocoa-flavored vehicles are considered effective for masking the taste of bitter drugs. Fruit or citrus flavors are frequently used to combat sour or acid tasting drugs, and cin-

namon, orange, raspberry, and other flavors have been successfully employed to make preparations of salty drugs more palatable. A list of some official flavoring and sweetening agents is presented in Table 3-4. The solubility of the flavoring or sweetening agent in the vehicle selected for the preparation is a most important consideration as is the chemical stability of the flavorant in the presence of the other formulative ingredients. The age of the intended patient should also be considered in the selection of the flavoring agent, for certain age groups seem to prefer certain flavors. Children prefer sweet, candy-like preparations with fruity flavors, but adults seem to prefer less sweet preparations with a tart rather than a fruit flavor, and geriatric patients may favor the refreshing taste of mint or of a tasty wine. Many nonofficial flavors are employed commercially to achieve the particular distinctive quality desired for a preparation by its manufacturer. Regardless of the flavor employed, the goals are the same, that is, to make the preparation more palatable for the patient.

Most large pharmaceutical manufacturers have special laboratories for the taste-testing of proposed formulations of their products. Panels of employees or interested community participants become involved in evaluating the various formulations and their assessments become the basis for the firm's flavoring decisions.

In flavoring liquid pharmaceutical products, the flavoring agent is added to the solvent or vehicle-component of the formulation in which it is most soluble or miscible. That is, water-soluble flavorants are added to the aqueous component of a formulation and poorly water-soluble flavorants are added to the alcoholic or other non-aqueous solvent component of the formulation. In a hydroalcoholic or other multi-solvent system, care must be exercised to maintain the flavorant in solution. This is accomplished through experience in the order of mixing of the formulative components by constantly maintaining a sufficient level of solvent in which the flavorant is soluble.

Coloring Agents

The use of coloring principles in pharmaceutical preparations for purposes of esthetics, as sensory adjuncts to the flavors employed, and for purposes of product distinctiveness have already been pointed out. However, a distinc-

---

[1] Hornstein, I., and Teranishi, R.: The Chemistry of Flavor. Chem. Engin. News, 45:92–108, 1967.

Table 3-4. SOME OFFICIAL SWEETENING, FLAVORING, PERFUMING, AND COLORING AGENTS AND PREPARATIONS

Sweetening Agents and Preparations:

Saccharin	Compressible Sucrose (for tableting)
Sorbitol Solution	Confectioner's Sucrose
Sucrose	Syrup

Flavoring and Perfuming Agents and Preparations:

Acacia Syrup	Glycyrrhiza Fluidextract
Almond Oil	Iso-Alcoholic Elixir
Anethole	Lavender Oil
Anise Oil	Lemon Oil
Aromatic Elixir	Methyl Salicylate
Benzaldehyde	Nutmeg Oil
Compound Benzaldehyde Elixir	Orange Flower Oil
Cocoa	Orange Flower Water
Cocoa Syrup	Orange Oil
Caraway Oil	Sweet Orange Peel Tincture
Cardamom Oil	Compound Orange Spirit
Compound Cardamom Tincture	Orange Syrup
Cherry Juice	Peppermint
Cherry Syrup	Peppermint Oil
Cinnamon Oil	Peppermint Spirit
Clove Oil	Peppermint Water
Coriander Oil	Pine Needle Oil
Eriodictyon Fluidextract	Rose Oil
Aromatic Eriodictyon Syrup	Stronger Rose Water
Ethyl Acetate	Spearmint
Ethyl Vanillin	Spearmint Oil
Fennel Oil	Tolu Balsam Syrup
Glycyrrhiza	Tolu Balsam Tincture
Glycyrrhiza Elixir	Vanilla
Pure Glycyrrhiza Extract	Vanilla Tincture
	Vanillin

Coloring Agents and Preparations:

Amaranth*	Compound Amaranth Solution*
Amaranth Solution*	Caramel

* In January, 1976, the FDA issued a ban on the further use of FD&C Red No. 2 (amaranth) from foods, drugs, and ingested cosmetics as lipsticks, mouthwashes, and dentifrices. The basis for the action was a study that showed a statistically significant increase in a variety of malignant neoplasms among aged Osborne-Mendel rats to whom high dosages of Red No. 2 had been fed.

tion should be made between those materials that have inherent color but are used medicinally and those agents that by virtue of possessing color are employed as colorants. Certain medicinal agents—sulfur (yellow), cupric sulfate (blue), ferrous sulfate (bluish green), and red mercuric iodide (vivid red)—are used medicinally and are not thought of as pharmaceutical colorants in the usual sense of the term. The coloring principles employed in pharmacy are generally limited to agents having this sole function.

Although most pharmaceutical colorants in use today are of synthetic origin, a few are naturally occurring principles obtained from mineral, plant, and animal sources. For example, red ferric oxide is mixed in small proportions with zinc oxide powder to prepare calamine, giving the latter its characteristic pink color intended to match the skin tone upon application. Chlorophyll, present in green parts of plants, imparts its color to many pharmaceuticals prepared by extracting the soluble principles (active and inactive) from the dried leaves of such medicinal plants as digitalis and belladonna. Other plant colorants are separated and intentionally added to medicinal agents to impart color; red saunders, the dried heartwood of *Pterocarpus santalinus* is employed as a red coloring agent. Animals have been used as a source of coloring principles throughout the history of mankind. Insects, in particular, have served as a rich source of coloring principles. One such agent is cochineal, defined as consisting of the dried female insects, *Coccus cacti*, enclosing the young larvae. Cochineal is bright red, owing its color to a glucosidal anthraquinone, carminic acid.

The synthetic coloring agents used in pharmaceutical products were first prepared in the middle of the 19th century from principles of coal tar. Coal tar (*pix carbonis*), a thick, black, viscid liquid, is a by-product in the destructive distillation of coal. Its composition is extremely complex, and many of its constituents are separated from it by fractional distillation. Among the many products obtained from coal tar are anthracene, benzene, naphtha, creosote, phenol, and pitch. From the basic oil of coal tar are manufactured the aniline or so-called "coal-tar dyes." However, the miracle of synthetic chemistry has permitted the creation of a vast number of synthetic dyes from starting materials other than aniline or coal-tar precursors. These same dyes, which are so extensively used in the pharmaceutical industry, are also used in many other industries that require dyes and artistic materials.

Many coal-tar dyes were originally used indiscriminately in foods and beverages to enhance their appeal without regard to their toxic potential. It was only after careful scrutiny that some dyes were found to be hazardous to health due to either their own chemical nature or the impurities they carried. As more dyestuffs became available, it became apparent that some expert guidance and regulation was needed to insure the safety of the public. After passage of the Food and Drug Act in 1906, the United States Department of Agriculture established regulations by which a few colorants were *permitted* or *certified* for use in certain products. Today, the use of color additives in foods, drugs, and cosmetics is regulated by the Food and Drug Administration through the provisions of the Federal Food, Drug, and Cosmetic Act of 1938, as amended in 1960 with the Color Additive Amendments. A list of certified colors to be used as additives is maintained and made available by the Food and Drug Administration. These approved color additives are classified into three groups: (1) FD&C dyes, which may be legally used in foods, drugs, and cosmetics; (2) D&C dyes, which may be legally used only in drugs and cosmetics; and (3) External D&C dyes, which may be legally used only to color externally applied drugs and cosmetics. The selection of a synthetic color additive for use in a pharmaceutical preparation to be used internally would have to be from among the certified colors of the first two categories. The individual certified dyes are designated with a title such as FD&C Red No. 2, which indicates the color's certification status, its basic color, and the specific member of that color group. In this example, the dye is also known as amaranth, a powdered colorant which is official in the USP. For each certification category there is a variety of basic colors with various choices within each color group. One may select from a variety of FD&C, D&C, and External D&C reds, yellows, oranges, greens, blues, and even violets and blacks. By selective combinations of the colorants one can create unique colors for special effects such as mint green, lemon or lime, chocolate, raspberry, wine, and others.

The certification status of the colorants is continuously reviewed, and changes are made in the list of certified colors in accordance with toxicologic findings. These changes may involve (1) the withdrawal of certification, (2) the transfer of a colorant from one certification category to another, or (3) the addition of new colors to the list. Before gaining certification, a color additive must be demonstrated to be safe. In the case of pharmaceutical preparations, color additives, like all additives, must not interfere with the therapeutic efficacy of the product in which they are used nor may they interfere with the prescribed assay procedure for that preparation.

A colorant becomes an integral part of a pharmaceutical formulation, and its exact quantitative amount must be reproducible each time the formulation is prepared, or else the preparation would have a different appearance from batch to batch. This requires a high degree of pharmaceutical skill, for the amount of colorant generally added to liquid preparations ranges between 0.0005 and 0.001% depending upon the colorant and the depth of color desired. Because of their color potency, whenever possible dyes are added to pharmaceutical preparations in the form of diluted solutions rather than as concentrated dry powders. This permits greater accuracy in measurement and more consistent color production. Dry preparations such as tablets, capsules, and powders may also be colored, and special coloring techniques may be involved. In the case of tablets, the color may be sprayed on the formed tablet during the coating process, or the colorant may be admixed as part of the dry powder mixture for uncoated tablets. In the preparation of capsules, various colored empty gelatin capsule shells may be used to hold the powdered drug mixture. Many commercial capsules are prepared with capsule bodies of one color and a different colored capsule cap, resulting in a two-colored capsule. This makes certain commercial products even more readily identifiable than solid colored capsules. For powdered drugs dispensed as such or compressed into tablets, a generally larger proportion of dye is required (about 0.1%) to achieve the desired hue than with liquid preparations. For the most part, ointments, suppositories, and ophthalmic and parenteral products assume the color of their ingredients and do not contain color additives. Should a dye lose the certification status it held when a product was first formulated, manufactured, and marketed, the manufacturer must, within a reasonable length of time, reformulate, using only color additives certified at the new date of manufacture.

In addition to esthetics and the certification status of a dye, a formulation pharmacist must select the dyes to be used in a particular formula on the basis of the physical and chemical properties of the dyes available. Of prime importance is the solubility of a prospective dye in the vehicle to be used for a liquid formulation or in a solvent to be employed in conjunction with it during a pharmaceutical process, as when the dye is sprayed on a batch of tablets. In general, most dyes may be broadly grouped into those that are water-soluble and those that are oil-soluble; few, if any, dyes are both. Usually, a water-soluble dye is also adequately soluble in commonly used pharmaceutical liquids like glycerin, alcohol, and glycol ethers. Oil-soluble dyes may overlap somewhat and also be soluble to some extent in these three liquids, as well as in liquid petrolatum (mineral oil), fatty acids, fixed oils, and waxes. It should be remembered that generally a great deal of solubility is not required, for the concentration of dye in a given preparation is rather minimal. Even in the preparation of concentrated dye solutions to be used as stock solution and added in small proportions to color a final preparation, a high degree of solubility is not usually required.

Another important consideration when selecting a dye for use in a liquid pharmaceutical is the pH and pH stability of the preparation to be colored. Dyes can change color with a change in pH, and a dye must be selected for a product so that any anticipated pH change will not alter the color during the usual shelf life. Needless to say, the dye must be chemically stable in the environment of the other formulative ingredients and must not interfere with the stability of the other agents. Dyes must also be reasonably photostable; that is, they must not change color when exposed to light of reasonable intensities and wavelengths for a reasonable length of time. Here again, the product must be color stable under the usual conditions of shelf storage. Certain medicinal agents, particularly those prepared in liquid form, must be protected from light to maintain their chemical stability and their therapeutic effectiveness. These preparations are generally maintained and dispensed in dark amber or opaque containers, and the esthetic value of added coloring agents appears tenuous. However, it should be remembered that the patient will see the liquid medication upon its administration, and the value of the color in terms of balance with the flavor and product identification remains, even though the preparation does not reveal the color through its container. For solid dosage forms of photolabile drugs, a colored capsule shell (which may be prepared clear or opaque) may actually enhance the drug's stability by shielding out light rays.

Although the official compendia permit the use of color additives, few are official. The standards and regulations are already provided by law and their enforcement is a matter of record. There is no real need for the official compendia to duplicate the standards set for these materials.

Biopharmaceutic Considerations in Dosage Form Design

The biologic response to a drug is the result of an interaction between the drug substance and the living system. The response is made manifest by an alteration in the biologic processes (whether normal or abnormal) that were present prior to the drug's administration. Unlike living matter, which is in a high state of physical and chemical organization and difficult to rearrange, the physical properties of drugs can be rather easily changed through chemical and physical modification to suit the requirements of the biologic system. It is the responsibility and the challenge of the research pharmacist to determine the drug and dosage form modifications that will best serve the therapeutic requirement. The area of study embracing this relationship between the physical, chemical, and biological sciences as they apply to drugs, dosage forms, and to drug action has been given the descriptive term *biopharmaceutics.*

In general, in order for a drug to exert its biologic effect, it must be soluble in and transported by the body fluids, traverse the required biologic membrane barriers, escape widespread distribution to unwanted areas, endure metabolic attack, penetrate in adequate concentration to the sites of action, and interact in a specific fashion, causing an alteration of function which is termed the "action of the drug." A simplified diagram of this complex series of events between a drug's administration and its elimination is presented in Figure 3-2.

The absorption, distribution, biotransformation (metabolism), and elimination of a drug from the body are dynamic processes that continue from the time a drug is taken until all of the drug has been removed from the body. The rates at which these processes occur affect the onset, intensity, and the duration of the drug's action within the body. The area of study which elucidates these processes is termed *pharmacokinetics.*

Once a drug is administered and drug ab-

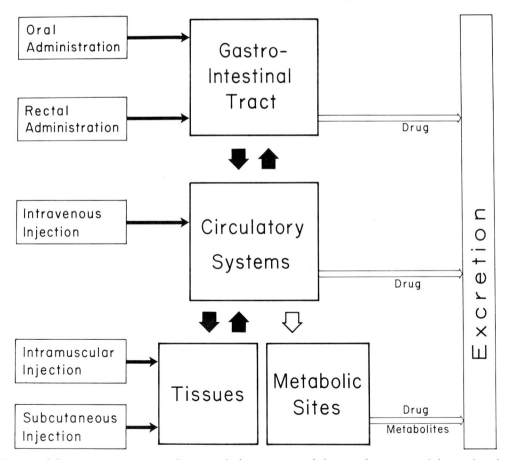

Fig. 3-2. *Schematic representation of events of absorption, metabolism, and excretion of drugs after their administration by various routes.*

sorption begins, the drug does not remain in a single body location, but rather is translocated throughout the body until its ultimate elimination. For instance, following the oral administration of a drug and its entry into the gastrointestinal tract, a portion of the drug is absorbed into the circulatory system from which it is distributed to the various other body fluids, tissues, and organs. From these sites the drug may return to the circulatory system and be eliminated through the kidney as such or the drug may be metabolized by the liver or other cellular sites and be eliminated as metabolites. As shown in Figure 3-2, drugs administered by intravenous injection are placed directly into the circulatory system, thereby avoiding the absorption process which is required from all other routes of administration.

The various body locations to which a drug travels may be viewed as separate compartments, each containing some fraction of the administered dose of drug. The transfer of drug from the blood to other body locations is referred to as drug *distribution*. The process is generally a rapid one and is reversible; that is, the drug may diffuse back into the circulation. The drug in the blood therefore exists in equilibrium with the drug in the other compartments. However, in this equilibrium state, the concentration of the drug in the blood may be quite different (greater or lesser) than the concentration of drug in the other compartments. This is due largely to the physicochemical properties of the drug and its resultant ability to leave the blood and traverse the biological membranes. Certain drugs may leave the circulatory system rapidly and completely, whereas other drugs may do so slowly and with difficulty. A number of drugs become bound to blood proteins, particularly the albumins, and only a small fraction of the drug administered may actually be found at locations outside of the circulatory system at a given time. The transfer of drug from one compartment to another is mathematically associated with a specific rate constant (k) describing that particular transfer. Generally, the rate of transfer of a drug from one compartment to another is proportional to the concentration of the drug in the compartment from which it exits; the greater the concentration, the greater is the amount of drug transfer. The mathematical relationship for a two-compartment system in which the drug transfer is assumed to be taking place in only one direction is:

$$\frac{dc}{dt} = -KC$$

in which dc/dt (change in drug concentration/ change in time) is the transfer rate, C is the drug concentration in the compartment from which the drug is leaving, and K is the rate constant associated with the process. Processes such as this in which the rate is dependent upon the drug concentration are termed *first order rate processes*.

The transfer of drug from the blood to the urine or other excretory compartments, as well as the *biotransformation* of the drug in the plasma or tissues to inactive metabolic products, is usually an irreversible process which culminates in the elimination or excretion of the drug from the body, usually via the urine. The pharmacokineticist may calculate an elimination rate constant (termed K_E) for a drug to describe its rate of elimination from the body. For drugs which are administered intravenously, and therefore involve no absorption process, the task is much less complex than for drugs administered by the other routes since the amount of drug in the blood at a given moment in the latter instances is a function of drug absorption and drug elimination, both of which are occurring simultaneously but at different rates.

The difference in the degree of a drug's absorption from the various routes of administration depends on the biological barriers (both biophysical and biochemical) encountered as well as on the nature of the drug substance and its dosage form. Indeed, the same chemical substance combined with different formulative materials in the preparation of various dosage forms may result in different therapeutic response due to differences in the degree of drug release from each dosage form and its subsequent availability for absorption. For example, a drug intended for oral administration may be administered in the form of a liquid, a suspension, a powder, a capsule, or a tablet. In each instance formulative materials may enhance or retard drug release. Also, tablets may be uncoated or coated with various materials of varying thickness and dissolution characteristics that may further impede drug release. In addition, tablets may be compressed during manufacture to various degrees of hardness, resulting in different dissolution rates for the drug substance. In general, the major types of orally administered dosage forms release their medicaments according to the following schedule.

Aqueous Solution—Suspension—Powder—
Capsule—Compressed Tablet—Sugar Coated
Tablet—Enteric Coated Tablet
(decreasing rate of drug release) $\longrightarrow$

Other preparations intended for the various routes of administration may be similarly characterized according to usual rate of drug release.

Often it is not the therapeutic desire to achieve drug absorption to any great extent, but rather to effect a local drug action at or proximate to the site of a drug's administration. In these instances the drug's incongruity with the biologic factors of drug absorption enables the desired local drug action with little, if any, systemic effects. Such local drug action is frequently desired at such body sites as the skin, eye, nose, ear, vagina, rectum, and even within the gastrointestinal tract through the use of drugs that are poorly absorbed or not absorbed at all.

General Principles
of Drug Absorption

Although it is not within the scope of this text to present an in-depth study of the theory of drug absorption and distribution, it is desirable for the beginning student in pharmacy to be introduced to this area of study which today is the object of a great deal of pharmaceutical research.

Before an administered drug can arrive at its site of action in effective concentrations, it must surmount a number of barriers. These barriers are chiefly a succession of biologic membranes such as those of the skin, gastrointestinal epithelium, lungs, and blood. Body membranes are generally classified as three main types: (a) those composed of several layers of cells, as the skin; (b) those composed of a single layer of cells, as the intestinal epithelium; and (c) those of less than one cell in thickness, as the membrane of a single cell. In most instances a drug substance must pass more than one of these membrane types before it reaches its site of action. For instance, a drug taken orally must first traverse the gastrointes-

tinal membranes (stomach, small and large intestine), gain entrance into the general circulation, pass to the organ or tissue with which it has affinity, gain entrance into that tissue, and then enter into its individual cells.

Although the chemistry of body membranes differs one from another, the membranes may be viewed in general as a bimolecular lipoid (fat-containing) layer attached on both sides to a protein layer. Substances such as drugs are thought to penetrate these biologic membranes in two general ways: (1) by passive diffusion and (2) through specialized transport mechanisms. Within each of these main categories, more clearly defined processes have been ascribed to drug transfer.

Passive Diffusion

The term *passive diffusion* is used to describe the passage of (drug) molecules through a membrane which behaves inertly in that it does not actively participate in the process. Drugs absorbed according to this method are said to be *passively absorbed*. The absorption process is driven by the concentration gradient (i.e., the differences in concentration) existing across the membrane, with the passage of drug molecules occurring primarily from the side of high drug concentration to the side of lower drug concentration.

Passive diffusion is described by *Fick's first law*, which states that the rate of diffusion or transport across a membrane (dc/dt) is proportional to the difference in drug concentration on both sides of the membrane:

$$-\frac{dc}{dt} = k_a(C_1 - C_2)$$

in which C_1 and C_2 refer to the drug concentrations on each side of the membrane and k_a is a proportionality constant. The term C_1 is customarily used to represent the compartment with the greater concentration of drug and thus the transport of drug proceeds from compartment one (e.g., absorption site) to compartment two (e.g., blood).

Since the concentration of drug at the site of absorption (C_1) is usually much greater than on the other side of the membrane, due to the rapid dilution of the drug in the blood and its subsequent distribution to the tissues, for practical purposes the value of $C_1 - C_2$ may be taken simply as that of C_1 and the equation written in the standard form for a first order rate equation:

$$-\frac{dc}{dt} = k_a C_1$$

The gastrointestinal absorption of most drugs from solution occurs in this manner in accordance with first order kinetics in which the rate is dependent upon drug concentration. The magnitude of the proportionality constant, k_a, depends on the diffusion coefficient of the drug, the thickness and area of the absorbing membrane, and the permeability of the membrane to the particular drug.

Because of the lipoid nature of the cell membrane, it is highly permeable to lipid soluble substances. The rate of diffusion of a drug across the membrane depends not only upon its concentration but also upon the relative extent of its affinity for lipid and rejection of water (a high lipid partition coefficient[1]). The greater its affinity for lipid and the more hydrophobic it is, the faster will be its rate of penetration into the lipid-rich membrane. Since biologic cells are also permeated by water and lipid-insoluble substances, it is thought that the membrane also contains water-filled pores or channels that permit the passage of these types of substances. As water passes in bulk across a porous membrane, any dissolved solute molecularly small enough to traverse the pores passes in by *filtration*. Aqueous pores vary in size from membrane to membrane and thus in their individual permeability characteristics for certain drugs and other substances.

The majority of drugs today are weak organic acids or bases. Knowledge of their individual ionization or dissociation characteristics is important, since their absorption is governed to a large extent by their degrees of ionization as they are presented to the membrane barriers. Cell membranes are more permeable to the unionized forms of drugs than to their ionized forms, mainly because of the greater lipid solubility of the unionized forms and to the highly charged nature of the cell membrane which results in the binding or repelling of the ionized drug and thereby decreases cell penetration. Also, ions become hydrated through

[1] Partition coefficients are determined by dissolving drugs in aqueous solution, shaking the solution with an organic solvent, and assaying each of the two phases for drug content. The partition coefficient is the organic solvent:water-drug concentration ratio.

association with water molecules, resulting in larger particles than the undissociated molecule and again decreased penetrating capability.

The degree of a drug's ionization depends both on the pH of the solution in which it is presented to the biologic membrane and on the pK_a, or dissociation constant, of the drug (whether an acid or a base). The concept of pK_a is derived from the Henderson-Hasselbalch equation and is:

For an acid:

$$pH = pK_a + \log \frac{\text{salt concentration (ionized)}}{\text{acid concentration (unionized)}}$$

For a base:

$$pH = pK_a + \log \frac{\text{base concentration (unionized)}}{\text{salt concentration (ionized)}}$$

Since the pH of body fluids varies (stomach, $\simeq$ pH 1; lumen of the intestine, $\simeq$ pH 6.6; blood plasma, $\simeq$ pH 7.4), the absorption of a drug from various body fluids will differ and may dictate to some extent the type of dosage form and the route of administration preferred for a given drug.

By rearranging the equation for an acid:

$$pK_a - pH = \log \frac{\text{acid concentration}}{\text{salt concentration}}$$

one can theoretically determine the relative extent to which a drug remains unionized under various conditions of pH. This is particularly useful when applied to conditions of body fluids. For instance, if a weak acid having a pK_a of 4 is assumed to be in an environment of gastric juice with a pH of 1, the left side of the equation would yield the number 3, which would mean that the ratio of unionized to ionized drug particles would be about 1000 to 1, and gastric absorption would be excellent. At the pH of plasma the reverse would be true, and in the blood the drug would be largely in the ionized form. Table 3-5 presents the effect of pH on the ionization of weak electrolytes, and Table 3-6 offers some representative pK_a values of common drug substances.

From the equation and from Table 3-5, it may be seen that a drug substance is half ionized at a pH value which is equal to its pK_a. For example, phenobarbital has a pK_a value of about 7.4, and in plasma (pH 7.4) it is present as ionized and unionized forms in equal amounts. However, a drug substance cannot reach the blood plasma for distribution throughout the body unless it is placed there directly

Table 3-5. THE EFFECT OF pH ON THE IONIZATION OF WEAK ELECTROLYTES*

| | %Unionized | |
pK_a-pH	If weak acid	If weak base
−3.0	0.100	99.9
−2.0	0.990	99.0
−1.0	9.09	90.9
−0.7	16.6	83.4
−0.5	24.0	76.0
−0.2	38.7	61.3
0	50.0	50.0
+0.2	61.3	38.7
+0.5	76.0	24.0
+0.7	83.4	16.6
+1.0	90.9	9.09
+2.0	99.0	0.99
+3.0	99.9	0.100

*From Doluisio, J. T., and Swintosky, J. V.; Amer. J. Pharm., *137*:149, 1965.

through intravenous injection or is favorably absorbed from a site along its route of entry, as the gastrointestinal tract, and allowed to pass into the general circulation. Utilizing Table 3-5 it may be easily seen that phenobarbital, a weak acid, with a pK_a of 7.4 would be largely undissociated in the gastric environment of pH 1, and would likely be well absorbed. A drug may enter the circulation rapidly and at high concentrations if membrane penetration is easily accom-

Table 3-6. pK_a VALUES FOR SOME ACIDIC AND BASIC DRUGS AT 25°C.*

Weak Acids	pK_a
Acetylsalicylic Acid	3.49
Barbital	7.91
Benzylpenicillin	2.76
Boric Acid	9.24
Phenobarbital	7.41
Phenol	10.0
Salicylic Acid	2.97
Sulfadiazine	6.48
Weak Bases	
Apomorphine	7.00
Atropine	9.65
Cocaine	8.41
Codeine	7.90
Ephedrine	9.36
Morphine	7.87
Procaine	8.8
Reserpine	6.6

*Adapted from Martin, A. N.: *Physical Pharmacy.* Philadelphia, Lea & Febiger, 1960, p. 218.

plished or at a low rate and low level if the drug is not readily absorbed from its route of entry. The pH of the drug's current environment influences the rate and the degree of its further distribution, since it becomes more or less unionized and therefore more or less lipid-penetrating under some condition of pH than under another. If an unionized molecule is able to diffuse through the lipid barrier and remain unionized in the new environment, it may return to its former location or go on to a new one. However, if in the new environment it is greatly ionized due to the influence of the pH of the second fluid, it likely will be unable to cross the membrane with its former ability. Thus a concentration gradient of a drug usually is reached at equilibrium on each side of a membrane due to different degrees of ionization occurring on each side.

Absorption from the various sites can be facilitated in certain instances by an adjustment of the pH at the absorbing surface. This may be accomplished by building into the pharmaceutical formulation buffering agents that have the capacity to maintain a certain pH. Buffering agents are frequently added to ophthalmic preparations and on occasion to orally administered drugs. Under proper guidance, a patient may be instructed to take an antacid along with certain medication in order to increase drug absorption (particularly for weak bases).

It is often possible for pharmaceutical scientists to make minor structural modifications in organic drugs and thereby favorably alter their lipid solubility, partition coefficients, and dissociation constants while maintaining the same basic pharmacologic activity. These efforts frequently result in increased absorption, better therapeutic response, and lower dosage.

Specialized Transport Mechanisms

In contrast to the passive transfer of drugs and other substances across a biologic membrane, certain substances, including some drugs and biologic metabolites, are conducted across a membrane through one of several postulated *specialized transport* mechanisms. This type of transfer seems to account for those substances, many naturally occurring as amino acids and glucose, that are too lipid-insoluble to dissolve in the boundary and too large to flow or filter through the pores. This type of transport is thought to involve membrane components that

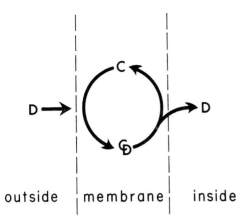

Fig. 3-3. *Active transport mechanism. D represents a drug molecule; C represents the carrier in the membrane. (After O'Reilly, W. J.: Aust. J. Pharm., 47:568, 1966.)*

may be enzymes or some other type of agent capable of forming a complex with the drug (or other agent) at the surface membrane, after which the complex moves across the membrane where the drug is released, with the carrier returning to the original surface. Figure 3-3 presents the simplified scheme of this process, which is still poorly understood. Specialized transport may be differentiated from passive transfer in that the former process may become "saturated" as the amount of carrier present for a given substance becomes completely bound with that substance resulting in a delay in the "ferrying" or transport process. Other features of specialized transport include the specificity by a carrier for a particular type of chemical structure so that if two substances are transported by the same mechanism one will competitively inhibit the transport of the other. Further, the transport mechanism is inhibited in general by substances that interfere with cell metabolism. The term *active transport*, as a subclassification of specialized transport, denotes a process with the additional feature of the solute or drug being moved across the membrane against a concentration gradient, that is, from a solution of lower concentration to one of a higher concentration or, if the solute is an ion, against an electrochemical potential gradient. In contrast to active transport, *facilitated diffusion* is a specialized transport mechanism having all of the above characteristics except that the solute is not transferred against a concentration gradient and may attain the same concentration inside the cell as that on the outside.

Dissolution and Drug Absorption

In order for a drug to be absorbed, it must first be dissolved in the fluid at the absorption site. For instance, a drug administered orally in tablet or capsule form cannot be absorbed until the drug particles are solubilized by the fluids at some point within the gastrointestinal tract. In instances in which the solubility of a drug is dependent upon either an acidic or basic medium, the drug would be solubilized in the stomach or intestines respectively (Fig. 3-4). The process by which a drug particle dissolves is termed *dissolution*.

As a drug particle undergoes dissolution, the drug molecules on the surface are the first to enter into solution creating a saturated layer of drug-solution which envelops the surface of the solid drug particle. This layer of solution is referred to as the *diffusion layer*. From this diffusion layer, the drug molecules pass throughout the dissolving fluid and make contact with the biologic membranes and absorption ensues. As the molecules of drug continue to leave the diffusion layer, it is replenished with dissolved drug from the surface of the drug particle and the process of absorption continues.

If the process of dissolution for a given drug particle is rapid, or if the drug is administered as a solution and remains present in the body as such, the rate at which the drug becomes absorbed would be primarily dependent upon its

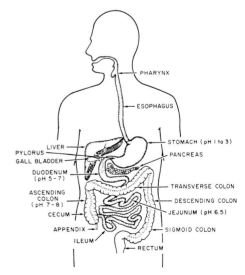

Fig. 3-4. *Anatomical diagram showing the digestive system including the locations involved in drug absorption and their respective pHs.*

ability to traverse the membrane barrier. However, if the rate of dissolution for a drug particle is slow, as may be due to the physicochemical characteristics of the drug substance or the dosage form, the dissolution process itself would be a rate-limiting step in the absorption process. Slowly soluble drugs may not only be absorbed at a slow rate, they may be incompletely absorbed, or, in some cases largely unabsorbed following oral administration, due to the natural limitation of time that they may remain within the stomach or the intestinal tract. Thus, poorly soluble drugs or poorly formulated drug products may result in a drug's incomplete absorption and its passage, unchanged, out of the system via the feces.

The dissolution of a substance may be described by the Noyes-Whitney equation[1]:

$$\frac{dC}{dt} = KS\,(C_s - C)$$

in which dC/dt is the rate of dissolution, K is the dissolution rate constant, S is the surface area of the dissolving solid, C_s is the concentration of drug in the diffusion layer (which may be approximated by the solubility of the drug in the solvent since the diffusion layer is considered saturated), and C is the concentration of the drug in the dissolution medium at time t. The rate of dissolution is governed by the rate of diffusion of solute molecules through the diffusion layer into the body of the solution. The equation reveals that the dissolution rate of a drug may be increased by increasing the surface area (reducing the particle size) of the drug, by increasing the solubility of the drug in the diffusion layer, and by factors embodied in the dissolution rate constant, K, including the intensity of agitation of the solvent and the diffusion coefficient of the dissolving drug. For a given drug, the diffusion coefficient and usually the concentration of the drug in the diffusion layer will increase with increasing temperature. Also, increasing the rate of agitation of the dissolving medium will increase the rate of dissolution. A reduction in the viscosity of the solvent employed is another means which may be used to enhance the dissolution rate of a drug. Changes in the pH or the nature of the solvent which influence the solubility of the drug may be used to advantage in increasing dissolution rate. Many manufacturers will utilize a particular amorphous, crystalline, salt or ester form of a drug that will exhibit the solubility characteristics needed to achieve the desired dissolution characteristics when administered. Some of these factors which affect drug dissolution will be briefly discussed in the following paragraphs, whereas others will be brought into the discussions of succeeding chapters in which they are relevant.

Surface Area

When a drug particle is reduced to a larger number of smaller particles, the total surface area created is increased. For drug substances that are poorly or slowly soluble, this generally results in an increase in the *rate* of dissolution. The actual solubility of a pure drug remains the same.

Increased therapeutic response to drugs due to smaller particle size has been reported for a number of drugs, among them tolbutamide, an oral hypoglycemic agent useful in the treatment of diabetes mellitus; griseofulvin, an antifungal antibiotic taken orally; the anti-infective sulfa drugs, sulfadiazine and sulfisoxazole; chloramphenicol, an antibiotic substance effective against a wide variety of pathogenic microorganisms; and phenothiazine, a tranquilizer.[1] To achieve increased surface area, pharmaceutical manufacturers frequently use *micronized* powders in their solid dosage form products. Micronized powders consist of drug particles reduced in size to about 5 microns and smaller.

Due to the different rates and degrees of absorption obtainable from drugs of various particle size, it is conceivable that products of the same drug substance prepared by two or more reliable pharmaceutical manufacturers may result in different degrees of therapeutic response in the same individual. It is generally advisable for a person to continue taking the same brand of medication, provided it produces satisfactory effects, rather than alternating companies' products. The pharmacist should see that this procedure is followed for his clientele.

Occasionally, a rapid rate of drug absorption is not desired in a pharmaceutical preparation. Research pharmacists, in providing sustained rather than rapid action in certain preparations, may employ agents of sufficiently large particle

[1] Noyes, A. A. and Whitney, W. R., *J. Am. Chem. Soc.*, 19:930, 1897.

[1] Lamy, P. P.: Importance of Particle Size in Pharmaceutical Practice, *Hospital Pharmacy*, 1:29–32, 1966.

size so that rapid dissolution is avoided in favor of a slow dissolution process.

Crystal or Amorphous Drug Form

Solid drug materials may occur as pure crystalline substances of definite identifiable shape or as amorphous particles without definite structure. The amorphous or crystalline character of a drug substance may be of considerable importance to its ease of formulation and handling, its chemical stability, and, as has been recently shown, even its biological activity. Certain medicinal agents may be produced to exist in either a crystalline or an amorphous state. Since the amorphous form of a chemical is usually more soluble than the crystalline form, different extents of drug absorption may result with consequent differences in the degree of pharmacologic activity obtained from each. Experiences with two antibiotic substances, novobiocin and chloramphenicol palmitate, have revealed that these materials are essentially inactive when administered in crystalline form, but when they are administered in the amorphous form, absorption from the gastrointestinal tract proceeds rapidly with good therapeutic response. In other instances, crystalline forms of drugs may be used because of greater stability than the corresponding amorphous forms. For example, the crystalline forms of Penicillin G as either the potassium or sodium salt are considerably more stable than the analogous amorphous forms. Thus, in formulation work involving Penicillin G, the crystalline forms are preferred and result in excellent therapeutic response.

The hormonal substance insulin presents another striking example of the different degree of activity that may result from the use of different physical forms of the same medicinal agent. Insulin is the active principle of the pancreas gland and is vital to the body's metabolism of glucose. The hormone, which is obtained from the pancreas glands of hogs, sheep, and cattle, is used by man as replacement therapy, by injection, when his body's production of the hormone is insufficient. Insulin is a protein, which, when combined with zinc in the presence of acetate buffer, forms an extremely insoluble zinc-insulin complex. Depending upon the pH of the acetate buffer solution, the complex may be an amorphous precipitate or a crystalline material. Each type is produced commercially to take advantage of their unique absorption characteristics. The amorphous form, referred to as *semilente insulin* or Prompt Insulin Zinc Suspension, USP, is rapidly absorbed upon intramuscular or subcutaneous (under the skin) injection. The larger crystalline material, called *ultralente insulin* or Extended Insulin Zinc Suspension, USP, is more slowly absorbed with a resultant longer duration of action. By combining the two types in various proportions, a physician is able to provide his patients with intermediate acting insulin of varying degrees of onset and duration of action. A physical mixture of 70% of the crystalline form and 30% of the amorphous form, called *lente insulin* or Insulin Zinc Suspension, USP, is commercially available and provides an intermediate acting insulin preparation that meets the requirements of many diabetics.

Some medicinal chemicals that exist in crystalline form are capable of forming different types of crystals, depending upon the conditions (temperature, solvent, time) under which crystallization is induced. This property, whereby a single chemical substance may exist in more than one crystalline form, is known as "polymorphism." It is known that only one form of a pure drug substance is stable at a given temperature and pressure with the other forms, called metastable forms, converting in time to the stable crystalline form. It is therefore not unusual for a metastable form of a medicinal agent to change form even when present in a completed pharmaceutical preparation, although the time required for a complete change may exceed the normal shelf-life of the product itself. However, from a pharmaceutical point of view, any change in the crystal structure of a medicinal agent may critically affect the stability and even the therapeutic efficacy of the product in which the conversion takes place.

The various polymorphic forms of the same chemical generally differ in many physical properties, including their solubility and dissolution characteristics, which are of prime importance to the rate and extent of drug absorption into the body's system. These differences are manifest so long as the drug is in the solid state. Once solution is effected, the different forms are indistinguishable one from another. Therefore, differences in drug action, pharmaceutically and therapeutically, can be expected from polymorphs contained in solid dosage forms as well as in liquid suspension. The use of metastable forms generally results in higher solubility and dissolution rates than the respective stable crystal forms of the same drug. If all other factors remain constant, more rapid and complete drug absorption will likely result from the metastable forms than from the stable form of the same drug. On the other hand, the stable polymorph is generally more resistant to chemical degradation and because of its lower solubility is frequently preferred in pharmaceutical suspensions of insoluble drugs. If metastable forms are employed in the preparation of suspensions, their gradual conversion to the stable form may be accompanied by an alteration in the consistency of the suspension itself, thereby affecting its permanency. In all instances, the advantages of the metastable crystalline forms in terms of increased physiologic availability of the drug must be balanced against the increased product stability when stable polymorphs are employed. Sulfur and cortisone acetate are two examples of drugs that exist in more than one crystalline form and are frequently prepared in pharmaceutical suspensions. In fact, cortisone acetate is reported to exist in at least five different crystalline forms. It is possible for the commercial products of two manufacturers to differ in stability and in the therapeutic effect, depending upon the crystalline form of the drug used in the formulation.

Salt Forms

The dissolution rate of a salt form of a drug is generally quite different from that of the parent compound. Sodium and potassium salts of weak organic acids and hydrochloride salts of weak organic bases dissolve much more readily than do the respective free acids or bases. The result is a more rapid saturation of the diffusion layer surrounding the dissolving particle and the consequent more rapid diffusion of the drug to the absorption sites.

There are numerous examples which could be cited to demonstrate the increased rate of drug dissolution due to the use of the salt form of the drug rather than the free acid or base, but the following will suffice: The sodium salt of phenobarbital has a dissolution rate which is about 800 times greater than that of phenobarbital in 0.1 N HCl and the sodium salt of tolbutamide has a dissolution rate of almost 10,000 times greater than that of the free acid, tolbutamide, also in 0.1 N HCl.[1,2]

Other Factors

The *state of hydration* of a drug molecule can affect its solubility and pattern of absorption. Usually the anhydrous form of an organic molecule is more readily soluble than the hydrated form. This characteristic was demonstrated recently with the drug ampicillin, when the anhydrous form was shown to have a greater rate of solubility than the trihydrate form.[3] It was also shown in the same study that the rate of absorption for the anhydrous form was greater than that for the trihydrate form of the drug.

Once swallowed, a drug is placed in the gastrointestinal tract where its solubility can be affected not only by the pH of the environment, but by the normal components of the tract and the foodstuffs which may be present. A drug may interact with one of the other agents present to form a chemical complex which may result in reduced drug solubility and decreased drug absorption. Also, if the drug becomes *ad*sorbed onto insoluble material in the tract, its availability for absorption may be correspondingly reduced.

Concept of Bioavailability

The availability to the biologic system of a drug substance formulated into a pharmaceutical product is integral to the goals of dosage form design and paramount to the effectiveness of the medication. The study of bioavailability depends upon the absorption of a drug into the general circulation and the subsequent measurement of the absorbed drug or its degraded metabolite. The term *bioavailability* is used to describe the *extent* and the *rate* of drug absorption from a dosage form as reflected by a concentration-time curve of the administered drug in biologic tissues or fluids, as blood or urine (Fig. 3-5). Bioavailability data are used to determine: (1) the amount or proportion of drug absorbed from a formulation or dosage form; (2)

[1] Nelson, E., *J. Am. Pharm. Assoc., (Sci. Ed.),* 47:297, 1958.
[2] Nelson, E., Wagner, J. G., *J. Pharm. Sci.,* 50:375, 1960.
[3] J. Poole, *Current Therapeutic Research, 10,* 292–303, 1968.

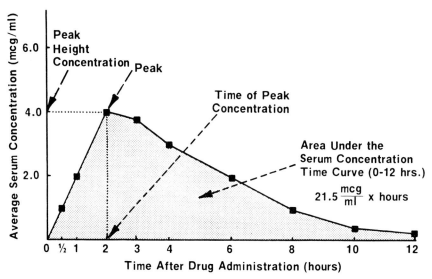

Fig. 3-5. *Serum concentration-time curve showing peak height concentration, time of peak concentration, and area under the curve. (Courtesy of D. J. Chodos and A. R. DiSanto, The Upjohn Company.)*

the rate or speed at which the drug was absorbed; (3) the duration of the drug's presence in the biologic fluid or tissue; and, when correlated with patient response, (4) the relationship between drug blood levels and therapeutic effectiveness or toxic effects.

During the product-development stages of a proposed drug product, pharmaceutical manufacturers may employ bioavailability studies in comparing different formulations of the drug substance to ascertain the one allowing the most desirable absorption pattern. Later, bioavailability studies may be used to compare the availability of the drug substance from different production batches of the product. They may also be used to compare the availability of the drug substance from different dosage forms (as tablets, capsules, elixir, etc.), or from the same dosage form produced by different (competing) manufacturers.

Until the present time, most of the bioavailability studies have been applied to drugs contained in solid dosage forms intended to be administered orally for systemic effects. The emphasis in this direction has been primarily due to the proliferation of competing products on the market in recent years, particularly the nonproprietary capsules and tablets, and the scientific revelation that certain drug entities when formulated and manufactured differently into solid dosage forms are particularly prone to variations in biologic availability. Thus, the present discussions will be centered around the

solid dosage form product. However, this is not to imply that systemic drug absorption is not intended from other routes of administration or other dosage forms, or that bioavailability problems do not exist from these products as well. Indeed, drug absorption from the parenteral, rectal, inhalation, and other routes is affected by the physicochemical properties of the drug and the formulative and manufacturing aspects of the dosage form design. General considerations of these routes of administration and applicable dosage forms will be discussed later in this section as well as in the subsequent chapters covering the specific dosage forms.

The Blood (or Serum or Plasma) Concentration-Time Curve

Following the administration of a medication, if blood samples are drawn from the patient at specific time intervals and analyzed for drug content, the resulting data may be plotted on ordinary graph paper to yield the type of drug blood level curve presented in Figure 3-5. The vertical axis of this type of plot characteristically presents the concentration of drug present in the blood (or serum or plasma) and the horizontal axis presents the time the samples were obtained following the administration of the drug. When the drug is first administered (time zero), the blood concentration of the drug should also be zero. As the drug passes into the stomach and/or intestine, it is released from the dosage form, eventually dissolves, and is absorbed. As the sampling and analysis continue, the blood samples reveal increasing concentrations of drug until the maximum (peak) concentration is reached. Then, the blood level of the drug progressively decreases and, if no additional dose is given, eventually falls to zero. The diminished blood level of drug after the peak height is reached indicates that the rate of drug elimination from the blood stream is greater than the rate of drug absorption into the circulatory system. It should be understood that drug absorption does not terminate after the peak blood level is reached, but may continue for some time. Similarly the process of drug elimination is a continuous one. It begins as soon as the drug first appears in the blood stream and continues until all of the drug has been eliminated. As will be discussed later, when the drug leaves the blood it may be found in various body tissues and cells for which it has an affinity until ultimately it is excreted as such or as drug metabolites in the urine or via some other route. The urinalysis for the drug or its metabolites may be used to indicate the extent of drug absorption and/or the rate of drug elimination from the body.

Parameters for Assessment and Comparison of Bioavailability

In discussing the important parameters to be considered in the comparative evaluation of the blood level curves following the oral administration of single doses of two formulations of the same drug entity, Chodos and DiSanto[1] list the following:

1. The Peak Height Concentration.
2. The Time of the Peak Concentration.
3. The Area Under the Blood (or serum or plasma) Concentration-Time Curve.

Using Figure 3-5 as an example, the height of the peak concentration is equivalent to 4.0 mcg/ml of drug in the serum; the time of the peak concentration is 2 hours following administration; and the area under the curve from 0 to 12 hours is calculated as 21.5 mcg/ml × hours. The meaning and use of these parameters are further explained as follows.

PEAK HEIGHT. The height of the peak of the blood level curve represents the highest concentration of drug reached in the blood following its administration. The amount of drug is usually expressed in terms of its concentration in relation to a specific volume of blood, serum, or plasma. For example, the concentration may be expressed as g/100 ml, mcg/ml or mg% (mg/100 ml). Figure 3-6 depicts concentration-time curves for two different formulations of an orally administered drug. The horizontal line drawn across the figure indicates that the minimum effective concentration (MEC) for the drug substance is 4.0 mcg/ml. This means that

[1] From "Basics of Bioavailability," by D. J. Chodos and A. R. DiSanto, The Upjohn Company, 1973.

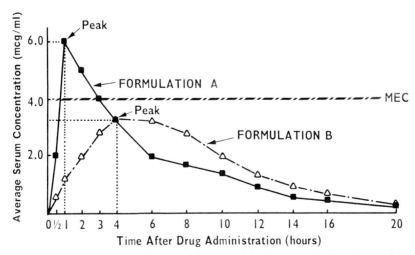

Fig. 3-6. *Serum concentration-time curve showing different peak height concentrations for equal amounts of drug from two different formulations following oral administration. (Courtesy of D. J. Chodos and A. R. DiSanto, The Upjohn Company.)*

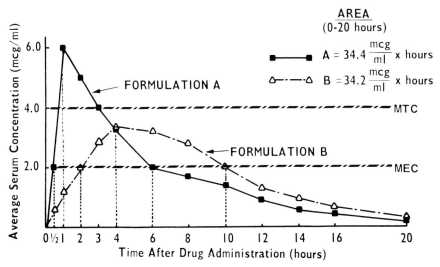

Fig. 3-7. *Serum concentration-time curve showing peak height concentrations, peak height times, times to reach minimum effective concentration (MEC) and areas under the curves for equal amounts of drug from two different formulations following oral administration. (Courtesy of D. I. Chodos and A. R. DiSanto, The Upjohn Company.)*

in order for the patient to elicit an adequate response to the drug, this concentration in the blood must be achieved. Comparing the blood levels of drug achieved after the oral administration of equal doses of formulations "A" and "B" in Figure 3-6, it is apparent that formulation "A" will achieve the required blood levels of drug to produce the desired pharmacologic effect whereas the administration of formulation "B" will not. On the other hand, if the minimum effective concentration for the drug was 2.0 mcg/ml and the minimum toxic concentration (MTC) was 4.0 mcg/ml as depicted in Figure 3-7, equal doses of the two formulations would result in toxic effects produced by formulation "A" but only desired effects by formulation "B". It should be understood that this example is hypothetical and used for explanatory purposes. Actual values for minimum effective and minimum toxic concentrations *have not* been determined for most drugs and would vary considerably from patient to patient. When these types of data do become available they will, in all likelihood, be expressed as *ranges* of concentrations rather than as single values. In the meantime, it is still worth recognizing that for the individual drug, in the individual patient and in a given circumstance, there is a blood level of drug, however unspecified and variable, which must be reached before the desired pharmacologic effects may be achieved, and a second level, if reached, which will elicit undesired toxic effects. The objective

in the individual dosing of a patient is to achieve the MEC but not the MTC.

TIME OF PEAK. The second parameter of importance in assessing the comparative bioavailability of two formulations is the time required to achieve the maximum level of drug in the blood. In Figure 3-6, the time required to achieve the peak serum concentration of drug is 1 hour for formulation "A" and 4 hours for formulation "B". This parameter is considered to be closely related to the *rate* of drug absorption from a formulation. It is primarily the rate or speed of drug absorption that determines the time needed for the minimum effective concentration to be reached and thus for the initiation of the desired pharmacologic effect. The rate of drug absorption also influences the period of time over which the drug enters the blood stream and therefore affects the duration of time that the drug is maintained in the blood. Looking at Figure 3-7, formulation "A" allows the drug to reach the MEC within 30 minutes following administration and a peak concentration in 1 hour. Formulation "B" has a slower rate of drug release. Drug from this formulation reached the MEC 2 hours after administration and its peak concentration 4 hours after administration. Thus formulation "A" permits the greater rate of drug absorption; it allows drug to reach both the MEC and its peak height sooner than drug from formulation "B". On the other hand, formulation "B" provides the greater duration of time for drug concentrations maintained above the MEC, 8 hours (from 2 to 10 hours following administration) to $5\frac{1}{2}$ hours (from 30 minutes to 6 hours following administration) for formulation "A". Thus, if a rapid onset of action is desired, a formulation similar to "A" would be preferred, but, if a longer duration of action is desired rather than a rapid onset of action, a formulation similar to "B" would be preferred.

AREA UNDER THE SERUM CONCENTRATION-TIME CURVE. The area under the curve (AUC) of a concentration-time plot (Fig. 3-5) is considered representative of the total amount of drug absorbed into the circulation following the administration of a single dose of that drug. The area under the curve may be measured mathematically, using a technique known as the trapezoidal rule, and is reported in $\frac{\text{amount of drug}}{\text{volume of fluid}}$ $\times$ time $\left(e.g., \frac{mcg}{ml} \times \text{hours}; \frac{g}{100} \times \text{hours; etc.} \right)$. Thus, two curves very much unlike in terms of peak height and time of peak, as those of Figure 3-7, may be very much alike in terms of area under the curve, and thus in the amount of drug absorbed from a formulation. As indicated in Figure 3-7, the area under the curve for formulation "A" is 34.4 $\frac{mcg}{ml} \times$ hours and for formulation "B" is 34.2 $\frac{mcg}{ml} \times$ hours, essentially the same. On the other hand, Figure 3-8

depicts concentration-time curves for three different formulations of the same drug with greatly different areas under the curve. In this example, formulation "A" delivers a much greater amount of drug to the circulatory system than do the other two formulations.

Bioequivalence of Drug Products

A great deal of discussion and scientific investigation has been devoted recently to the problem of determining the biological equivalence between proposed formulations for a drug product or between two or more existing drug products of competing manufacturers. Differences in the bioavailability of chemically equivalent drug products have been demonstrated for a number of products involving the following and other drugs: tetracycline, chloramphenicol, digoxin, phenylbutazone, and oxytetracycline. Not only has bio*in*equivalence been shown to exist in products of different manufacturers but there have also been substantial variations in the bioavailability of different batches of drug products from the same manufacturer. The extent to which the problem exists is still uncertain since only a small portion of the more than 20,000 prescription drug products have been subjected to the appropriate comparative studies; however, it is known that the variations in the bioavailability of certain drug products have resulted in some therapeutic failures in patients who have taken two inequivalent drug products in the course of their therapy.

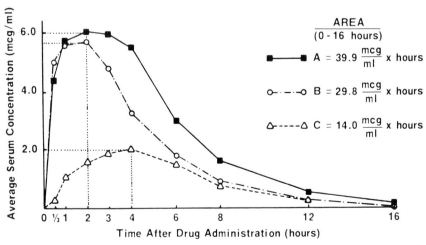

Fig. 3-8. *Serum concentration-time curve showing peak height concentrations, peak height times, and areas under the curves for equal amounts of drugs from three different formulations following oral administration. (Courtesy of D. J. Chodos and A. R. DiSanto, The Upjohn Company.)*

According to the Drug Bioequivalence Study Panel of the Office of Technical Assessment,[1] *bioequivalents* are *chemical equivalents which when administered to the same individuals in the same dosage regimen will result in comparable bioavailability.* It should be recalled from Chapter 1, that *chemical equivalents* are drug products that contain the same amounts of the same therapeutically active ingredients in the same dosage forms and that meet present (physicochemical) compendial standards.

The most common experimental plan for comparing the bioavailability of two drug products is the simple *crossover study.* By this method, each individual in a group of carefully selected subjects receives both drug products (in different sequence and at different times) so that there is a direct comparison of the absorption of each product in the same individual. Special care is exercised to allow sufficient time to elapse between the administration of the first and second drug products so that there are no carryover effects.

It should be recognized that there are inherent differences in individuals which result in different patterns of drug absorption, metabolism and excretion. These differences must be statistically analyzed to separate them from the factors of bioavailability related to the products themselves.

Absolute bioequivalency between drug products rarely, if ever, occurs. Such absolute equivalency would yield serum concentration-time curves for the products involved that would be exactly superimposable. This simply is not expected of products which are made at different times, in different batches, or indeed by different manufacturers. However, some expectations of bioequivalency are expected of products which are considered to be of equivalent merit for therapy.

In most studies of bioavailability, the originally marketed product is recognized as the established product of the drug and is utilized as the standard for the bioavailability comparative studies. A suggested rule for judging the bioequivalence between drug products considers the products bioequivalent if their differences are similar to that which one finds in the batch-to-batch variation of the original product.

[1]"Drug Bioequivalence," A Report of the Office of Technology Assessment, Drug Bioequivalence Study Panel, Congress of the United States, Washington D.C., 1974.

In comparing the concentration-time curves for two products the entire curves need not be equivalent, but rather only the portions of the curves that are considered of prime importance with regard to the type of drug being studied. Thus in comparing two products, the speed of absorption (peak time), maximum concentration (peak height), total amount absorbed (area under the curve), and the rate of drug absorption may not all be of equal importance. For instance, in comparing products containing a drug intended to induce sleep, the peak time and the peak height may be considered to be the prime parameters of evaluation, whereas for products intended to provide daytime sedation, the area under the curve may be considered the prime factor.

The differences in bioavailability between drug products manufactured from chemical equivalents may be due to differences in the formulative ingredients employed, the methods of product manufacture utilized, the rigor of in-process quality control procedures, and even the methods of handling, packaging, and storage. The variables which can contribute to the differences between products are many. For instance in the manufacture of a tablet, different materials or amounts of such formulative components as fillers, disintegrating agents, binders, lubricants, colorants, flavorants and coatings may be used. The particle size or crystalline form of a therapeutic or pharmaceutic component may vary between formulations. The tablet may vary in shape, size, and hardness depending upon the punches and dies selected for use by the manufacturer and the compression forces utilized in the process. During packaging, shipping and storage the integrity of the tablets may be altered by physical impact, or changes in conditions of humidity, temperature, or through interactions with the components of the container. Each of the factors noted may have an effect on the rate of tablet disintegration, drug dissolution, and consequently on the rate and extent of drug absorption. Although the bioequivalency problems are perhaps greater among tablets than for other dosage forms because of the multiplicity of variables, the same types of problems exist for the other dosage forms and must be considered in bioequivalency evaluations.

Since it is unlikely that all products will be subjected to bioequivalence studies, it remains important to identify those drug entities and products for which therapeutic failures have resulted and to be prudent in initial product selection and wary of product interchange.

Routes of Drug Administration

It should be apparent from the preceding discussion that drug substances are not just swallowed and automatically absorbed and transferred to their sites of action. Indeed, with the great diversity of chemical types constituting the modern stockpile of drugs, their absorption characteristics vary greatly one from another as well as from each potential route of administration. It is the combined responsibility of all involved in pharmaceutical research to determine the most effective and appropriate routes of administration for a drug substance. It is the particular responsibility of the research pharmacist to provide the drug in a suitable dosage form for proper absorption from each of the selected routes of administration. Commercially, most prescription drug substances are marketed in forms for more than a single route of administration, and frequently several appropriate dosage forms and drug strengths are offered for each route.

The following discussion will briefly treat the usual routes of drug administration and point out certain important characteristics of each and the most commonly used dosage forms prepared for each route. Although dosage forms are included, this is intended to serve merely as their introduction, since they will be discussed in greater detail in the individual chapters devoted to them.

Oral Route

Today, as throughout history, drugs are most frequently taken by oral administration. Although a few drugs taken orally are intended to be dissolved within the mouth and absorbed from the surface of the cavity, the vast majority of drugs taken orally are swallowed. Of these, the majority are taken for the systemic drug effects that result after absorption from the various surfaces along the gastrointestinal tract. A few drugs are swallowed for their local action within the confines of the gastrointestinal tract, made possible by their insolubility and/or poor absorbability from this route.

Most drugs may be effectively administered by the oral route for systemic effects and are preferred to be taken in this manner by most persons. Compared with alternate routes, the oral route is considered the most natural, uncomplicated, convenient, and safe means of administering drugs. Disadvantages of the oral route include slow drug response (when compared with parenterally administered drugs); irregular absorption of drugs, depending upon such factors as constitutional make-up, the amount or type of food present within the gastrointestinal tract; and the destruction of certain drugs by the acid reaction of the stomach or by gastrointestinal enzymes. Perhaps the most notable examples of the latter are the various preparations of insulin, all of which must be administered parenterally due to the destruction of this hormonal protein substance by the proteolytic enzymes of the gastrointestinal tract. The uncertainty of maintenance of the prescribed dosage regimen when the medication is in the hands of the patient is a distinct possibility, and undoubtedly many instances of overdosage or underdosage with self-administered drugs result. Although error in dosage is a disadvantage inherent in all types of self-administered drugs, not only the more common oral types, there is no realistic alternative. Faith must be placed in the individual's sincere desire to regain health, and adequate guidance in the proper use of drugs must be provided him by the physician and the pharmacist.

DOSAGE FORMS APPLICABLE. Drugs are administered by the oral route in a variety of pharmaceutical forms, each with inherent therapeutic advantages that result in their selective use by physicians. The most popular forms are tablets, capsules, suspensions, and various pharmaceutical solutions. Briefly, tablets are solid dosage forms prepared by compression or molding and contain medicinal substances with or without suitable diluents, disintegrants, coatings, colorants, and other pharmaceutical adjuncts. Diluents are necessary in preparing tablets of the proper size and consistency. Disintegrants are used when rapid separation of the tablet's compressed ingredients is desired. This insures prompt exposure of drug particles to the dissolution process thereby enhancing drug absorption. Tablet coatings are of several types and for several different purposes. Some called *enteric coatings* are employed to permit safe passage of a tablet through the acid environment of the stomach where certain drugs may be destroyed to the more suitable juices of the intestines where tablet dissolution safely takes place. Other coatings are employed to protect the drug substance from the destructive influences of moisture, light, and air throughout their period of storage or to conceal a bad or bitter taste from the taste buds of a patient. Commercial tablets, because of their distinctive shapes, colors, and frequently employed monographs of company symbols and drug strengths, facilitate identification by persons trained in their use and serve as an added protection to public health.

Capsules are solid dosage forms in which the drug substance and such appropriate pharmaceutical adjuncts as fillers are enclosed in either a hard or a soft "shell," which is generally composed of a form of gelatin. Capsules vary in size, depending upon the amount of drug to be administered, and are of distinctive shapes and colors when produced commercially. Generally speaking, drug materials are released from capsules faster than from tablets. Capsules of gelatin, a protein, are rapidly disfigured within the gastrointestinal tract, permitting the gastric juices to permeate and reach the contents.

Suspensions are preparations of finely divided drugs held in suspension throughout a suitable vehicle. Suspensions taken orally generally employ an aqueous vehicle, whereas those employed for other purposes may utilize a different vehicle. Suspensions of certain drugs to be used for intramuscular injection, for instance, may be maintained as a suspension in a suitable oil. To be suspended, the drug particles must be insoluble in the vehicle in which they are placed. Nearly all suspensions must be shaken before using because they tend to settle. This insures not only uniformity of the preparation but more importantly the administration of the proper dosage. Suspensions are a useful means of administering large amounts of solid drugs that would be inconveniently taken in tablet or capsule form. Also, a liquid preparation is more convenient to administer to those who are unable to swallow tablets or capsules or have difficulty swallowing them. In addition, suspensions have the advantage over solid dosage forms in that they do not have the delay characteristics of solid dosage forms but are presented to the body in fine particle size, ready for the dissolution process immediately upon administration. However, not all oral suspensions are intended to be dissolved and absorbed by the body. For instance, Kaolin Mixture with Pectin contains suspended kaolin, a

naturally occurring adsorbent material, which is useful in the treatment of diarrhea by virtue of its ability to resist dissolution and absorption and remain in the intestinal tract long enough to adsorb excessive intestinal fluid on the large surface area of its particles.

Drugs administered in solution are generally absorbed much more rapidly than those administered in solid form, since the process of dissolution is not required. Even if a drug administered in solution is precipitated from solution by the acidity of the stomach, the resultant particles, which likely would be redissolved upon entrance into the intestines, are available more rapidly to the body fluids than tablets requiring disintegration and capsules requiring the softening of the shell and permeation. For the most part, the pharmaceutical solutions differ in the type of solvent or vehicle employed and therefore in their fluidity characteristics. Several of the solutions frequently administered orally are elixirs, which are solutions in a sweetened hydroalcoholic vehicle and are generally more mobile than water; syrups, which generally utilize sucrose solutions as the sweet vehicle resulting in a viscous preparation; and solutions themselves, which officially are preparations in which the drug substance is dissolved predominantly in an aqueous vehicle and do not for reasons of their method of preparation (e.g., injections, which must be sterilized) fall into another category of pharmaceutical preparations.

ABSORPTION RATE. Absorption of drugs after oral administration may occur at the various body sites between the mouth and rectum. In general, the higher up a drug is absorbed along the length of the alimentary tract, the more rapid will be its action, a desirable feature in most instances. However, because of the differences in the chemical and physical nature among drug substances and in the forms in which they are presented to the body, a given drug may be better absorbed from the environment of one position than from another, irrespective of its relative location within the alimentary tract.

The oral cavity is used on certain occasions as the absorption site for certain drugs. The mucosal lining of the mouth behaves as a lipoid barrier to the passage of drugs and involves the same principles of drug absorption as described earlier, with the lipid/water distribution coefficient being a prime factor in the absorption capability of a drug substance. Physically, the oral absorption of drugs is managed by allowing the drug substance to be dissolved (if not presented as a solution) and withheld in the oral cavity with infrequent or no swallowing until the taste of the drug has dissipated. This process is accommodated pharmaceutically by providing the drug in a dissolved state (impregnated on a cotton swab, for instance) or as extremely soluble and rapidly dissolving uncoated tablets. Drugs capable of being absorbed in the mouth may present themselves to the absorbing surface in a much more concentrated form than when swallowed, since drugs become progressively more diluted with gastrointestinal secretions and contents as they pass along the alimentary tract. When these secretions adversely affect the stability of a drug substance, its absorption as an active molecule is further decreased, and oral absorption or parenteral administration may be required. Similar alternatives may be required for drugs that are especially susceptible to metabolic degradation by the liver, since on gastrointestinal absorption, drug substances enter the portal circulation and are exposed to the detoxification processes of the liver.

Currently the oral or sublingual (beneath the tongue) administration of drugs is regularly employed for only a few drugs, with nitroglycerin and certain steroid sex hormones being the best examples. Nitroglycerin, a coronary vasodilator used in the prophylaxis and treatment of angina pectoris, is administered in the form of tiny tablets which are allowed to dissolve under the tongue, producing therapeutic effects in 1 to 2 minutes after administration. The dose of nitroglycerin is so small (usually 400 mcg) that if it were swallowed the resulting dilute gastrointestinal concentration may not result in reliable and sufficient drug absorption. Even more important, however, is that nitroglycerin is rapidly destroyed by the liver, thereby further reducing its chances of reaching its site of action. Many sex hormones have been shown to be absorbed materially better from sublingual administration than when swallowed. Although the sublingual route is probably an effective absorption route for many other drugs, it has not been extensively studied primarily because other routes have proven satisfactory and more convenient for the patient. Retaining drug substances in the mouth presents a psychological barrier to some, is unattractive to others because of the bitter taste of most drugs, and would be difficult to manage with certain patients, as infants. However, with each passing year a greater number of so-called "chewable" tablets of vitamins, antibiotics, and other drugs are made commercially available to facilitate ease of administration to pediatric patients, and although they are intended to be swallowed, they do dissolve in the mouth and may result in oral absorption. It may be that these tablets, which when chewed become creamy and pleasant tasting and dissolve readily, may provide the incentive for further studies of oral absorption, which in turn may result in increased drug administration by this little used route.

Absorption from the gastrointestinal tract follows the general principles of drug absorption already outlined; indeed, many of these principles are based on findings of studies of the alimentary tract. Several specific features of gastrointestinal absorption should be mentioned, since this route is most frequently employed in the administration of drugs.

In general, it may be stated that the oral administration of drugs by swallowing is the route of first choice except when the drug is ineffective by this route or when an extremely rapid onset of action is desired, in which case administration by intravenous injection is usually preferred. Lack of effectiveness after oral administration may be due to the destruction of the drug substance by the enzymes or environmental conditions of the gastrointestinal tract, or it may be due to poor or little absorption through the membrane barriers.

Drugs may be altered within the gastrointestinal tract into forms that render them less or more slowly available for absorption. This alteration may be the result of the drug's association with or binding to some other agent, which may be a normal constituent of the gastrointestinal tract or a foodstuff or even another drug. For instance, the absorption of the tetracycline group of antibiotics is greatly interfered with by the simultaneous presence of calcium. Because of this, tetracycline drugs must not be taken with milk or other calcium-containing foods, and for further assurance they are generally taken an hour or two before or after meals. In the case of the tetracyclines, and for other drugs as well, it is of vital concern that the pharmaceutical adjuncts, such as the fillers and diluents employed in the preparation of capsules and tablets, be inert with respect to their effects, not only on the chemical stability of the medicinal agents but also on their physiologic availability once administered. It is the responsibility of the research pharmacist to assess carefully the total compatibility of all formulative materials prior to production and distribution, and to reevaluate a formulation periodically for reassurance of its pharmaceutical correctness. In some instances it is the intent of the pharmacist to prepare a formulation that releases the drug slowly over an extended period of time. There are many commercial and patented methods by which slow release is accomplished, including the complexation or combination of the medicinal agent with another material, the combination of which is only slowly released from the dosage form, or only slowly soluble or absorbable once released. Although current medical practice has embraced the extended-type medication as a useful method of achieving prolonged blood levels of drugs with less frequent dosage, it is not within the realm of the official compendia to endorse one method over another for achieving this type of effect. Thus, many official medicinal agents are commercially available in forms unique with their manufacturer, with many of these providing drug absorption at various rates and with various durations of drug action.

Whether or not a drug truly interacts with food present in stomach, the intermingling of food and drug generally results in delayed absorption for the latter. The stomach contents tend to dilute the drug concentration, with a greater dilution and decreased absorption resulting from an increased proportion of food present. Since most drugs are absorbed more effectively from the intestines than from the stomach, when rapid absorption is intended, it is generally desirable to have the drug pass from the stomach into the intestines as rapidly as possible. Therefore, gastric emptying time is an important factor in effecting drug action dependent upon intestinal absorption. Also, slow gastric emptying time is especially detrimental to drugs that may be destroyed by the gastric environment if permitted lengthy exposure. Gastric emptying time may be increased by a number of factors, including the presence of fatty foods (more effect than proteins, which in turn have more effect than carbohydrates), lying on the back when bedridden (lying on the right side facilitates passage in many instances), and the presence of drugs (for example, morphine) that have a quieting effect on the movements of the gastrointestinal tract. If a drug is administered in the form of a solution, it may be expected to pass into the intestines more rapidly than drugs administered in solid form. However, it should be borne in mind that drugs administered in solution may precipitate rapidly and entirely from solution upon entrance into the stomach, in which event drug absorption may not be as rapid as for a drug administered in solid form which disintegrates and dissolves rapidly and completely in the stomach. As a rule, large volumes of water taken with medication facilitate gastric emptying and passage into the intestines.

The pH of the gastrointestinal tract increases progressively along its length from a pH of about 1 in the stomach to approximately pH 8 at the far end of the intestines. As pointed out earlier, pH has a definite bearing on the degree of ionization of most drugs, and this in turn effects lipid solubility and membrane permeability. Since most drugs are absorbed by passive diffusion through the lipoid barrier, the lipid/water partition coefficient and the pK_a of the drugs are of prime importance to both their degree and site of absorption within the gastrointestinal tract. As a general rule, weak acids are largely unionized in the stomach and are absorbed fairly well from this site, whereas weak bases are highly ionized in the stomach and are not significantly absorbed from the gastric surface. Alkalinization of the gastric environment by artificial means (simultaneous administration of alkaline or antacid drugs) would be expected to decrease the gastric absorption of weak acids and to increase that of weak bases. Strong acids and bases are generally poorly absorbed due to their high degrees of ionization.

The small intestine serves as the major absorption pathway for drugs because of its suitable pH and the great surface area available for drug absorption within its approximate 20-foot length extending from the pylorus at the base of the stomach to the junction with the large intestine at the cecum. The pH of the lumen of the intestine is about 6.5, and both weakly acidic and weakly basic drugs are well absorbed from the intestinal surface, which behaves in the ionization and distribution of drugs between it and the plasma on the other side of the membrane as though its pH were about 5.3.

The degree to which a drug is absorbed from a particular route of administration has a great deal to do with the dose that must be given to achieve the proper drug concentration at the sites of action. For this reason, doses of the same drug may differ, depending upon the intended route of administration. It should also be remembered that even by the same route the effective dose of a drug may vary, depending upon its physical characteristics, such as particle size and crystal form. The rate of drug absorption also differs between the routes of administration and must be considered in selecting the proper route as well as in determining the frequency of dose administration. Drugs that are absorbed readily may also be eliminated from the body more readily than drugs that are more slowly absorbed (although this is not necessarily true) and therefore would require more frequent dose administration to maintain the desired blood level of the drug. For this reason some drugs are taken once daily; others, four or more times a day. Although most drugs are absorbed faster and to a greater extent if taken on an empty stomach, certain drugs that are irritating to the gastrointestinal tract are frequently administered with meals to reduce their concentration and irritant action.

Rectal Route

Drugs are frequently administered rectally for their local effects and less frequently for their systemic effects. Drugs given rectally are generally administered as solutions, suppositories, or ointments. Briefly, suppositories may be defined as solid bodies of various weights and shapes intended for introduction into a body orifice (usually rectal, vaginal, or urethral) where they soften or melt, release their medication, and exert their drug effects. These effects simply may be the promotion of laxation (as with glycerin suppositories), the soothing of inflamed tissues (as with various commercial suppositories used to relieve the discomfort of hemorrhoids), or the promotion of systemic effects (as the analgesic effects of aspirin suppositories commonly employed in infants). The composition of the suppository base, or carrier of the medication, can greatly influence the degree and rate of drug release and should be selected on an individual basis for each drug to be prepared into a suppository. The use of rectal ointments is generally limited to the treatment of local conditions.

The rectum and the colon are capable of absorbing many soluble drugs, and administration rectally for drugs intended for systemic

action may be preferred for those destroyed or inactivated by the environments of the stomach and intestines. The administration of drugs by the rectal route may also be indicated when the oral route is precluded by vomiting or when the patient is unconscious or incapable of swallowing drugs safely without choking. Also, drugs absorbed rectally do not pass through the liver before entry into the systemic circulation, an important factor when considering drugs that are rapidly destroyed in the liver. On the negative side, compared with oral administration, rectal administration of drugs is inconvenient, and the absorption of drugs from the rectum is frequently irregular and difficult to predict.

Parenteral Route

The term *parenteral* is derived from the Greek words *para*, meaning beside, and *enteron*, meaning intestine, which together indicate something done outside of the intestine and not by way of the alimentary tract. A drug administered parenterally is one injected through the hollow of a fine needle into the body at various sites and to various depths. The three primary routes of parenteral administration are subcutaneous, intramuscular (I.M.), and intravenous (I.V.) although there are others such as intracardiac and intraspinal.

Drugs destroyed or inactivated in the gastrointestinal tract or too poorly absorbed to provide satisfactory response may be administered parenterally. The parenteral route is also preferred when rapid absorption is essential, as in emergency situations. Absorption by the parenteral route is not only faster than after oral administration, but the blood levels of drug that result are far more predictable, since little is lost after subcutaneous or intramuscular injection, and virtually none by intravenous injection; this also generally permits the administration of smaller doses. The parenteral route of administration is especially useful in treating patients who are uncooperative, unconscious, or otherwise unable to accept medication orally.

One disadvantage of parenteral administration is that once the drug is injected, there is no retreat. That is, once the substance is within the tissues or is placed directly into the blood stream, removal of the drug warranted by an untoward or toxic effect or an inadvertent overdose is virtually impossible. By other means of administration, there is more of an element of time between drug administration and drug absorption, which in essence becomes a safety factor in allowing time for the extraction of unabsorbed drug, as by the induction of vomiting after an orally administered drug. Also, because of the strict sterility requirements for all injections, they are generally more expensive than other dosage forms and require competent trained personnel for their proper administration.

DOSAGE FORMS APPLICABLE. Pharmaceutically, injectable preparations are usually either sterile suspensions or solutions of a drug substance in water or in a suitable vegetable oil. In general, drugs in solution act faster than drugs in suspension, with an aqueous vehicle providing faster action in each instance than an oleaginous vehicle. As in other instances of drug absorption, a drug must be in solution to be absorbed, and a suspended drug must first submit to the dissolution process. Also, since body fluids are aqueous, they are more receptive to drugs in an aqueous vehicle than those in an oily one. For these reasons, the rate of drug absorption can be varied in parenteral products by selective combinations of drug state and supporting vehicle. For instance, a suspension of a drug in a vegetable oil likely would be much more slowly absorbed than an aqueous solution of the same drug. Slow absorption generally means prolonged drug action, and when this is achieved through pharmaceutical means, the resulting preparation is referred to as a *depot* or *repository* injection, since it represents a storage reservoir of the drug substance within the body from which it is slowly removed into the systemic circulation. In this regard, even more sustained drug action may be achieved through the use of subcutaneous implantation of compressed tablets, termed pellets in these instances, which are only slowly dissolved from their site of implantation, releasing their medication at a rather constant rate over a period of several weeks to many months. The repository type of injection is mainly limited to the intramuscular type. It is obvious that drugs injected intravenously do not encounter absorption barriers and thus produce only rapid drug effects. From a pharmaceutical standpoint, preparations for intravenous injection must not interfere in any way with the blood components or with circulation and therefore are limited in type to aqueous solutions of drugs.

SUBCUTANEOUS INJECTIONS. The subcutaneous (hypodermic) administration of drugs involves their injection through the layers of skin into the loose subcutaneous tissue. Generally, subcutaneous injections are prepared as aqueous solutions or as suspensions and are administered in a lesser dosage than the corresponding oral dose for the drug. Insulin, which cannot be given orally, is an example of a drug administered in its various forms by the subcutaneous route. Subcutaneous injections are generally given in the forearm, arm, thigh, or nates. After injection, the drug comes into the immediate vicinity of blood capillaries and permeates them by diffusion or filtration. The capillary wall is an example of a membrane that behaves as a lipid pore barrier, with lipid-soluble substances penetrating the membrane at rates varying with their oil/water partition coefficients. Lipid-insoluble (generally more water-soluble) drugs penetrate the capillary membrane at rates which appear to be inversely related to their molecular size, with smaller molecules penetrating much more rapidly than larger ones. All substances, whether lipid-soluble or not, cross the capillary membrane at rates that are much more rapid than the rates of their transfer across other body membranes. The blood supply to the site of injection is an important factor in considering the rate of drug absorption, since the more proximal capillaries are to the site of injection, the more prompt will be the drug's entrance into the circulation. Also, the more capillaries, the more surface area for absorption, and the faster the rate of absorption. Some substances have the capability of modifying the rate of drug absorption from a subcutaneous site of injection. The addition of a vasoconstrictor to the injection formulation (or its prior injection) will generally diminish the rate of drug absorption by causing constriction of the blood vessels in the area of injection and thereby reducing blood flow and the capacity for absorption. This principle is frequently utilized in the administration of local anesthetics by employing the vasoconstrictor epinephrine, which is additionally effective in delaying drug absorption because of its own resistance to destruction after injection. Conversely, vasodilators may be employed to enhance subcutaneous absorption by increasing blood flow to the area.

INTRAMUSCULAR INJECTIONS. Intramuscular injections are performed deep into the skeletal muscles, generally the gluteal or lumbar muscles. Aqueous or oleaginous solutions or suspensions may be used intramuscularly with rapid effects or depot activity selected to meet the requirements of the patient. Injections of the various types of penicillin are largely administered by the intramuscular route. Certain drugs, because of their inherent low solubilities, provide sustained drug action after an intramuscular injection of a suspension of the drug. For instance, one intramuscular injection of a suspension of benzathine penicillin G results in detectable blood levels of the drug for seven to ten days.

INTRAVENOUS INJECTIONS. In the intravenous administration of drugs, an aqueous solution is injected directly into the vein at a rate commensurate with efficiency, safety, comfort to the patient, and the desired duration of drug response. The latter point refers mainly to drugs administered as a slow drip during intravenous feeding of nutrients and drugs to a patient after surgery. Intravenous injections are usually made into the veins of the forearm and are especially useful in emergency situations where immediate drug response is desired. It is essential that the drug be maintained in solution after injection and not be precipitated within the circulatory system, an event that might result in circulatory blockage and failure. Injections prepared with an oleaginous base are not given intravenously, as they might result in pulmonary embolisms. After intravenous injection, the optimum blood level of the drug may be obtained with an accuracy and immediacy not possible by any other means. However, when an immediate drug effect is not required and when oral administration is ruled out, another route of parenteral administration is preferred for the protection of the patient against an unexpected reaction to the drug. It should be remembered that a dose of a drug that is satisfactorily tolerated by one or many individuals may prove excessive with others, and by using administration means other than intravenous there is a greater opportunity to select and administer a proper antidote or otherwise provide restorative action.

Topical Route

Drugs are administered topically, or applied to the skin, chiefly for their action at the site of application rather than for systemic drug effects. This is not to imply that drugs may not be absorbed into the general circulation following topical application; indeed they may. However, such percutaneous absorption is generally poor and uncertain; when it does occur, it is usually unintended, undesirable, and viewed with dismay. In general, drug absorption via the skin follows the same basic pattern and criteria previously discussed for drug passage through biologic membranes. In essence, percutaneous absorption is enhanced if the drug substance is in solution, if it has a favorable lipid/water partition coefficient, and if it is a nonelectrolyte. Drugs that are absorbed enter the skin by way of the sweat glands, hair follicles, sebaceous glands, and other anatomic structures of the skin's surface. Since blood capillaries are present just below the epidermal cells, a drug that penetrates the skin and is able to traverse the capillary wall finds ready access to the general circulation. Naturally, absorption is facilitated by drug application to abraded or broken skin.

For the most part, pharmaceutical preparations applied to the skin are intended to serve some local action and as such are formulated to provide prolonged local contact with minimal absorption. One means of insuring such limited action is through the use of drugs in powdered or solid form rather than in solution. When drugs are applied to the skin in solution, as are many skin antiseptics, they are either prepared in an alcoholic vehicle, which rapidly evaporates after application, leaving the drug distributed over the skin in fine residue of particles, or the drug itself is of such a nature to be poorly absorbed through the skin. Generally, drugs applied to the skin are employed for their local action as antiseptics, antifungal agents, antiinflammatory agents, local anesthetic agents, skin emollients, or for their protective action against environmental conditions, including the effects of the sun, wind, pests, and chemical irritants as found, for example, in dishwashing detergents. For these purposes drugs are most commonly administered in the form of ointments and related semisolid preparations such as creams and pastes, as solid dry powders, or as liquid preparations such as solutions and lotions. The administration of drugs for topical application through the use of aerosol spray remains popular, especially in the proprietary consumer product market. However, increasing concern of the effects of the aerosol propellants on the health of the individual and the environment has prompted some recent reevaluations of their utility.

Pharmaceutically, ointments, creams, and pastes are semisolid preparations in which the drug is contained in a suitable base (ointment base) which is itself semisolid and either hydrophilic or hydrophobic in character. These bases play an important role in the proper formulation of semisolid preparations, and there is no single base universally suitable as a carrier of all drug substances or for all therapeutic indications. The proper base for a drug must be determined individually to provide the desired drug release rate, staying qualities after application, and texture. Briefly, ointments are simple mixtures of drug substances in an ointment base, whereas creams are semisolid emulsions and are generally less viscid and lighter than ointments. Creams are considered to have greater esthetic appeal due to their nongreasy character and their ability to "vanish" into the skin upon rubbing. Pastes contain more solid materials than do ointments and are therefore stiffer and less penetrating. Pastes are usually employed for their protective action and for their ability to absorb serous discharges from skin lesions. Thus when protective rather than therapeutic action is desired, the formulation pharmacist will favor a paste, but when therapeutic action is required, he will prefer ointments and creams. Commercially, many therapeutic agents are prepared in both ointment and cream form and are dispensed and used according to the particular preference of the patient and the prescribing practitioner.

Medicinal powders are simply intimate mixtures of medicinal substances usually in an inert base like talcum powder. Depending upon the particle size of the resulting blend, the powder will have varying dusting and covering capabilities. In any case, the particle size should be small enough to insure against grittiness and consequent skin irritation. Powders are most frequently applied topically to relieve such conditions as diaper rash, chafing, and athlete's foot.

When topical application is desired in liquid form other than solution, lotions are most frequently employed. Lotions are generally suspensions of solid materials in an aqueous vehicle, although certain emulsions and even some true solutions have been designated as lotions because of either their appearance or application. Lotions may be preferred over semi-solid preparations because of their nongreasy character and their increased spreadability over large areas of skin.

In addition to skin, drugs are frequently applied topically to other surfaces such as those of the eye, ear, and the mucous membranes of the nose. In these instances, the same general types of pharmaceutical preparations are employed—ointments, suspensions, and solutions. Usually, ophthalmic solutions and suspensions are aqueous preparations with maintained sterility and other qualities that are essential to the safety and comfort of the patient as well as to the therapeutic effectiveness of the preparation. These qualities include pH and buffer capacity, viscosity and lasting characteristics, tonicity, and non-gritty character of any suspended particles, which will be mentioned later during the general discussion of ophthalmic solutions and suspensions. In a similar fashion, ophthalmic ointments must be sterile, free of grittiness, and have other qualities essential for their total effectiveness. Nasal preparations are usually solutions or suspensions administered by drops or as a fine mist from a nasal spray container. Otic, or ear preparations are usually viscid so that they have prolonged contact with the affected area. They may be employed simply to soften ear wax, to relieve an earache, or to combat an ear infection. Eye, ear, and nose preparations are not employed for systemic effects, and although ophthalmic and otic preparations are not usually absorbed to any great extent, nasal preparations may be absorbed and systemic effects after the intranasal application of solution are not unusual.

Other Routes

The lungs provide an excellent absorbing surface for the administration of gases and for aerosol mists of very minute particles of liquids or solids. The gases employed are mainly oxygen and the common general anesthetic drugs administered to patients entering surgery. The rich capillary area of the alveoli of the lungs, which in man covers nearly a thousand square feet, provides rapid absorption and drug effects comparable in speed to those following an intravenous injection. In the case of drug particles, their size largely determines the depth to which they penetrate the alveolar regions; their solubility, the extent to which they are absorbed. After contact with the inner surface of the lungs, an insoluble drug particle is caught in the mucus and is moved up the pulmonary tree by ciliary action. Soluble drug particles that are approximately 0.5 to 1.0 micron in size reach the minute alveolar sacs and are most prompt and efficient in providing systemic effects. Particles that are smaller than 0.5 micron are expired to some extent, and thus their absorption is not total but variable. Particles from 1 to 10 microns in size effectively reach the terminal bronchioles and to some extent the alveolar ducts and are favored for local therapy. Therefore, in the pharmaceutical manufacture of aerosol sprays for inhalation therapy, the manufacturers not only must attain the proper drug particle size but also must insure their uniformity for consistent penetration of the pulmonary tree and uniform effects.

In certain instances and generally for local effects, drugs are inserted into the vagina and the urethra. Drugs are generally presented to the vagina in tablet form, as suppositories, ointments, or solutions, and to the urethra as suppositories or solutions. Systemic drug effects, which may result after the vaginal or urethral application of drugs due to absorption of the drug from the mucous membranes of these sites, are an undesirable feature of this type of drug administration.

Fate of Drug after Absorption

After absorption into the general circulation from any route of administration, a drug may become bound to blood proteins and delayed in its passage into the surrounding tissues. The drug-protein complex is reversible and generally involves albumin, although globulins are also involved in the binding of drugs, particularly some of the hormones. The binding capacity of blood proteins is limited, and once they are saturated, additional drug absorbed into the blood stream remains unbound unless bound drug is released, creating a vacant site for another drug molecule to attach. However, once the binding proteins are saturated, there can be no additional net increase in bound drug, so the unbound portion of drug remains free to leave the blood and enter the surrounding tissues. Additional drug being absorbed into the blood stream must also remain free and may result in a sudden upsurge in the concentration of free or unbound drug in the blood. Bound drug is nei-

ther exposed to the body's detoxication processes nor is it filtered through the renal glomeruli. Bound drug is therefore referred to as the inactive portion in the blood, and unbound drug, with its ability to penetrate cells, is termed the active blood portion. The bound portion of drug serves as a drug reservoir or a depot, from which the drug is released as the free form when the level of free drug in the blood no longer is adequate to insure protein saturation. The free drug may be only slowly released, thereby increasing the duration of the drug's stay in the body. For this reason a drug that is highly protein bound may remain in the body for longer periods of time and require less frequent dosage administration than another drug that may be only slightly protein bound and may remain in the body for only a short period of time. In addition to the normal complexities, drug binding to proteins is further complicated by the fact that certain drugs are capable of influencing the binding capabilities of other drugs to protein. Their simultaneous presence may result in drug effects or durations of drug action quite dissimilar to that found when each is administered alone. Salicylates, for instance, have the effect of decreasing the binding capacity of thyroxin, the thyroid hormone, to proteins.

In the same manner as they are bound to blood proteins, drugs may become bound to specific components of certain cells. Thus drugs are not distributed uniformly among all cells of the body, but rather tend to pass from the blood into the fluid bathing the tissues and may accumulate in certain cells according to their permeability capabilities and chemical and physical affinities. This affinity for certain body sites influences their action, for they may be brought into contact with reactive tissues (their receptor sites) or deposited in places where they may be inactive. Many drugs, because of their affinity for and solubility in lipids, are found to be deposited in fatty body tissue, thereby creating a storage place or drug reservoir from which they are slowly released to other tissues.

Biologic Half-Life

The *biologic half-life* of a drug describes the time required for a drug's blood level of activity to be one-half of its original high or desired level. The term may also be used to describe the time required for the body to eliminate, by metabolism or excretion or both, one-half of the administered dose of a drug.

The biologic half-life of a drug in the blood may be determined by administering the drug intravenously, drawing blood samples from the patient at given time intervals, and assaying these samples for drug content. The amount of time required for the quantity of drug in the blood to decrease to one-half of its peak level is considered its biologic half-life. The same type of determination may be made following drug administration by routes other than intravenous.

The biologic half-life varies widely between drugs; for some drugs it may be 30 minutes or less, whereas for other drugs it may be 8 hours or more. Data on a drug's biologic half-life are useful in determining the most appropriate dosage regimen to achieve and maintain the desired blood level of drug. Such determinations usually result in such recommended dosage schedules for a drug, as the drug to be taken every 4 hours, 6 hours, 8 hours, etc. Although these types of recommendations generally suit the requirements of most patients, they do not suit all patients. The most exceptional patients are those with reduced or impaired ability to metabolize or excrete drugs. These patients, generally suffering from liver dysfunction or kidney disease, retain the administered drug in the blood or tissues for extended periods of time due to their decreased ability to eliminate the drug. The resulting extended biologic half-life of the drug generally necessitates an individualized dosage regimen calling for less frequent drug administration than that called for in patients with normal processes of drug elimination.

The biologic half-life of a drug in the blood stream may also be affected by a change in the extent to which it is bound to blood protein or cellular components. Such a change in a drug's binding pattern may be brought about by the administration of a second drug having a greater affinity than the first drug for the same binding sites. The result is the displacement of the first drug from these sites by the second drug and the sudden availability of free (unbound) drug which may pass from the blood stream to other body sites, including those concerned with its elimination. It should be noted that the displacement of one drug from its binding sites by another is generally viewed as an undesired event, since the amount of free drug resulting is greater than the level normally achieved during single drug therapy and may result in untoward drug effects.

Biotransformation

Although some drugs are excreted from the body in their original form, many drugs undergo biotransformation prior to excretion. Biotransformation is a term used to indicate the chemical changes that occur with drugs within the body as they are metabolized and altered by various biochemical mechanisms. Generally, the biotransformation of a drug results in its conversion to a compound that is more water soluble, more ionized, less capable of binding to proteins of the plasma and tissues, less capable of being stored in fat tissue, and less able to penetrate cell membranes, thereby resulting in a less active compound. Because of its new characteristics, a drug so transformed is rendered less toxic and is more readily excreted. It is for this reason that the process of biotransformation is also commonly referred to as the "detoxication" or "inactivation" process.

The exact metabolic processes (pathways) by which drugs are transformed represent an active area of biomedical research. Much work has been done with the processes of animal degradation of drugs and in many instances the biotransformation in the animal is thought to parallel that in man. There are four principal chemical reactions involved in the metabolism of drugs: oxidation, reduction, hydrolysis, and conjugation. The liver plays a dominant role in drug metabolism, and impaired liver function must be considered by the physician when prescribing drugs dependent upon proper hepatic function for detoxication. The prolongation of a drug within the body because of nonfunctioning detoxication processes may result in the accumulation of a drug to toxic levels. Many infant deaths in years past, after the administration of certain drugs in usual amounts and at regular intervals, have since been attributed to the rise of the drug concentration to accumulated toxic levels due to underdeveloped liver enzyme systems, now recognized as common during the neonatal period. Liver enzyme systems incapable of adequately detoxifying certain drugs would be presumed for infants born prematurely.

In recent years, much interest has been shown in the metabolites of drug biotransformation. It is known that certain metabolites may be as active or even more active pharmacologically than the original compound. Occasionally an active drug may be converted into an active metabolite, which must be excreted as such or undergo further biotransformation to an inactive metabolite. In other instances of drug therapy, an inactive parent compound may be converted to an active therapeutic agent by chemical transformation in the body. The possible use of these active metabolites as "original" drugs represents a new area of drug investigation and a vast reservoir of potential therapeutic agents.

Several examples of biotransformations occurring within the body are as follows:[1]

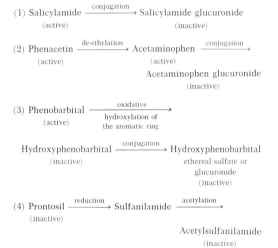

The active compound acetaminophen, in reaction 2, is commonly administered as an analgesic-antipyretic agent, thereby avoiding the biotransformation process required for its formation when phenacetin is administered. It should be pointed out that phenacetin is itself an active compound and is also administered for its capacity to act as an analgesic; however, it does have a higher incidence of severe toxic effects in patients than does acetaminophen, and its use in medical practice has diminished in recent years.

Excretion of Drugs

The excretion of drugs and their metabolites terminates their activity and presence in the

[1] Fingl, E. and Woodbury, D. M.: General Principles. In *The Pharmacological Basis of Therapeutics*, 5th ed. L. S. Goodman, and A. Gilman, eds. New York, The Macmillan Company, 1975, Chapter 1.

body. They may be eliminated by various routes, with the kidney playing the dominant role by eliminating drugs via the urine. Drug excretion with the feces is also important, especially for drugs that are poorly absorbed and remain in the gastrointestinal tract after oral administration. Exit through the bile is significant only when the drug's reabsorption from the gastrointestinal tract is minimal. The lungs provide the exit for many volatile drugs through the expired breath. The sweat glands, saliva, and milk play only minor roles in drug elimination. However, it should be recognized that if a drug gains access to the milk of a mother during lactation, it could easily exert its drug effects in the nursing infant. It is generally good practice for the mother to abstain from taking medication during the period of time she is nursing her infant. If she must take medication, she should abide by a dosage regimen and nursing schedule that permit her own therapy yet insure the safety of her child. Not all drugs gain entrance into the milk; nevertheless, caution is advisable.

The unnecessary use of medications during the early stages of pregnancy is likewise being more strictly prohibited by physicians, since certain drugs are known to have the ability to cross the placental barrier and gain entrance to the tissues and blood of the fetus. Among the many drugs known to do so after administration to an expectant mother are all of the anesthetic gases, many barbiturates, sulfonamides, salicylates, and a number of other potent agents like quinine, meperidine, and morphine, the latter two drugs being narcotic analgesics with great addiction liabilities. In fact, it is not unusual for a newborn infant to be born an addict due to the narcotic addiction of its mother and the passage of the narcotic drugs across the placental barrier.

The kidney, as the main organ for the elimination of drugs from the body, must be functioning adequately if drugs are to be efficiently eliminated. Drugs are concentrated at the site of their excretion, and thus many symptoms of poisoning are manifested in the organs of elimination. For example, in instances of mercury poisoning severe renal damage and colitis occur due to the excretion of this metal by the kidneys and colon. For this reason, many useful drugs intended for a variety of body maladies are contraindicated in the presence of impaired renal function.

Some drugs may be reabsorbed from the renal tubule even after having been sent there for excretion. Since the rate of reabsorption is proportional to the concentration of drug in unionized form, it is possible to modify this rate by adjusting the pH of the urine. By acidifying the urine, as with the oral administration of ammonium chloride, or by alkalinizing it, as with the administration of sodium bicarbonate, one can increase or decrease the ionization of the drug and thereby alter its prospect of being reabsorbed. Alkalinization of the urine has been shown to enhance the urinary excretion of weak acids such as salicylates, sulfonamides, and phenobarbital. The opposite effect can be achieved by acidifying the urine. Thus, the duration of a drug's stay within the body may be materially altered by changing the pH of the urine.

The urinary excretion of drugs may also be retarded by the concurrent administration of agents capable of inhibiting their tubular secretion. A well-known example is the use of probenecid to inhibit the tubular secretion of various types of penicillin, thereby reducing the frequency of dosage administrations usually necessary to maintain adequate therapeutic blood levels of the antibiotic drug. In this particular instance, the elevation of penicillin blood levels, by whatever route the antibiotic is administered, to twofold and even fourfold levels has been demonstrated by adjuvant therapy with probenecid. The effects are completely reversible upon withdrawal of the probenecid from concomitant therapy.

The fecal excretion of drugs appears to lag behind the rate of urinary excretion partly because a day or so elapses before the feces reach the rectum. It should be easily seen that drugs administered orally for local activity within the gastrointestinal tract and not absorbed will be eliminated completely via the feces. Unless the drug is particularly irritating to the gastrointestinal tract (in which case diarrhea or vomiting would likely occur), there is generally no urgency in removing unabsorbable drugs from the system by means other than the normal defecation process. Some drugs that are only partially absorbed after oral administration will naturally be partly eliminated by the rectum.

Selected Reading

Brest, A. N.: *The Scientific Evaluation of Drug Equivalency*, Princeton, *Exerpta Medica*, 1974.

Chodos, D. J. and DiSanto, A. R.: *Basics of Bioavailability*, Kalamazoo, The Upjohn Company, 1973.

Chun, A. H. C. and Seitz, J. A.: Drug Bioavailability Information and its Utility, *J. Am. Pharm. Assoc.*, NS14:407–414, 1974.

Dittert, L. W. and DiSanto, A. R.: The Bioavailability of Drug Products, *J. Am. Pharm. Assoc.*, NS13:421–432, 1973.

Gibaldi, M.: *Introduction to Biopharmaceutics.* Philadelphia, Lea & Febiger, 1971.

Lachman, L. and Roemer, W. C.: Pharmaceutical Properties of Drugs and Dosage Forms Affecting Physiological Availability, *J. Am. Pharm. Assoc.* NS12:215–224, 1972.

Lamy, P. P.: Importance of Particle Size in Pharmaceutical Practice, *Hosp. Pharm.* 1:29–32, 1966.

_____:*Drug Bioequivalence: A Report of the Office of Technology Assessment Drug Bioequivalence Study Panel*, Washington, D.C., U.S. Government Printing Office, 1974.

Chapter 4

Oral Solutions, Syrups, and Elixirs

IN PHYSICOCHEMICAL terms, solutions may be prepared from any combination of solid, liquid, and gas, the three states of matter. For example, a solid solute may be dissolved in either another solid, a liquid, or a gas, and with the same being true for a liquid solute and for a gas, nine types of homogeneous mixtures are possible. In pharmacy, however, interest in solutions is for the most part limited to preparations of a solid, a liquid, and less frequently a gas solute dissolved in a liquid solvent.

In pharmaceutical terms, solutions are defined as "liquid preparations that contain one or several soluble chemical substances usually dissolved in water and that do not, by reasons of their ingredients or method of preparation, fall into another group of products." Indeed, many pharmaceutical products, which from a physicochemical standpoint are solutions in that they are homogeneous mixtures of solute dissolved in solvent, are, from a pharmaceutical standpoint, classified as other product types. For example, aqueous pharmaceutical solutions containing a sugar are classified as *syrups;* sweetened hydroalcoholic (combinations of water and ethyl alcohol) solutions are termed *elixirs;* solutions of aromatic materials may be termed *spirits* if the solvent is alcoholic or *aromatic waters* if the solvent is aqueous. Solutions prepared by extracting active constituents from crude drugs

may be termed *tinctures* or *fluidextracts,* depending upon their method of preparation and their concentration. *Tinctures* may also be solutions of chemical substances dissolved in alcohol or in a hydroalcoholic solvent. Certain solutions prepared to be sterile and pyrogen-free and intended for parenteral administration are classified as *injections.* Although other examples could be cited, it is apparent that a solution, as a distinct type of pharmaceutical preparation, is much more limited in its meaning than is the physicochemical definition of the term *solution.*

This chapter will deal with the general area of solution preparation and concentrate on the oral solution and the two other dosage forms most frequently utilized in the administration of oral medication in solution, the syrup and elixir. Solutions employed topically, by injection, ophthalmically, and by other means will be covered in subsequent chapters.

Oral solutions, syrups, and elixirs are prepared and utilized for the specific effects of the medicinal agents present. In these preparations the medicinal agents are generally expected to provide systemic effects. The fact that they are administered in solution form usually means that their absorption from the gastrointestinal tract into the systemic circulation may be expected to occur more rapidly than from suspension or solid dosage forms of the same medicinal agent.

Solutes other than the medicinal agent are usually present in orally administered solutions. These additional agents usually are included to provide color, flavor, sweetness, or stability to the solution. In formulating or compounding a pharmaceutical solution, the pharmacist must utilize information on the solubility and stability of each of the solutes present with regard to the solvent or solvent system employed. He must guard against using combinations of medicinal or pharmaceutic agents which will result in chemical or physical interactions affecting the therapeutic quality or pharmaceutic stability of the product.

For single-solute solutions and especially for multiple-solute solutions, the pharmacist must be keenly aware of the solubility characteristics of the solutes and the solubulizing features of the common pharmaceutical solvents. Each chemical agent has its own individual extent of solubility in a given solvent. For many medicinal agents, their exact solubilities in the usual solvents are stated in the official monographs;

for others, their degree of solubility is expressed by such terms as "freely soluble" or "slightly soluble."

Solubility

The solubility of an agent in a particular solvent indicates the maximum concentration to which a solution may be prepared with that agent and that solvent. When a solvent, at a given temperature, has dissolved all of the solute it can, it is said to be *saturated*. In order to emphasize the possible variation in solubility between two chemical agents and therefore in the amounts of each required to prepare a saturated solution, two official aqueous saturated solutions are cited as examples, Calcium Hydroxide Solution, USP, and Potassium Iodide Solution, USP. The first solution, prepared by agitating an excess amount of calcium hydroxide with purified water, contains only about 140 mg of dissolved solute per 100 ml of solution at 25°, whereas the latter solution contains about 100 g of solute per 100 ml of solution, over 700 times as much solute as present in the Calcium Hydroxide Solution, USP. It is apparent from this comparison that the maximum possible concentration to which a pharmacist may prepare a solution varies greatly and is dependent, in part, on the chemical constitution of the solute. Through selection of a different solubilizing agent or a different chemical salt form of the medicinal agent, alteration in the pH of a solution, or substitution, in part or in whole, of the solvent, a pharmacist can in certain instances dissolve greater quantities of a solute than would otherwise be possible. For example, iodine granules are soluble in water only to the extent of 1 g in about 3000 ml of water. Using only these two agents, the maximum concentration possible would be approximately 0.03% of iodine in aqueous solution. However, through the use of an aqueous solution of potassium or sodium iodide as the solvent, much larger amounts of iodine may be dissolved as the result of the formation of a water-soluble complex with the iodide salt. This reaction is taken advantage of, for example, in the preparation of the two official aqueous iodine solutions, Iodine Solution USP, and Strong Iodine Solution, USP, with the first solution prepared to contain about 2% of iodine and the second solution about 5% of iodine.

Temperature is an important factor in determining the solubility of a drug and in preparing its solution. Most chemicals absorb heat when they are dissolved and are said to have a *negative heat of solution*, resulting in increased solubility with a rise in temperature. A few chemicals have a *positive heat of solution* and exhibit a decrease in solubility with a rise in temperature. Other factors, in addition to temperature, affect solubility. These include the various chemical and other physical properties of both the solute and the solvent, factors of pressure, the acidity or basicity of the solution, the state of subdivision of the solute, and the physical agitation applied to the solution during the dissolving process. The solubility of a pure chemical substance at a given temperature and pressure is constant; however, its *rate of solution*, that is, the speed at which it dissolves, depends upon the particle size of the substance and the extent of agitation. The finer the powder, the greater the surface area that comes in contact with the solvent, and the more rapid the dissolving process. Also, the greater the agitation, the more unsaturated solvent passes over the drug, and the faster the formation of the solution.

The solubility of a substance in a given solvent may be determined by preparing a saturated solution of it at a specific temperature and determining by chemical analysis the amount of chemical dissolved in a given weight of solution. By simple calculation, the amount of solvent required to dissolve the amount of solute can be determined. The solubility may then be expressed as grams of solute dissolving in milliliters of solvent—for example, "1 g of sodium chloride dissolves in 2.8 ml of water." When the exact solubility has not been determined, general expressions of relative solubility may be used. These terms are defined in the USP and NF as follows:

Descriptive Term	Parts of Solvent Required for 1 Part of Solute
Very soluble	Less than 1
Freely soluble	From 1 to 10
Soluble	From 10 to 30
Sparingly soluble	From 30 to 100
Slightly soluble	From 100 to 1000
Very slightly soluble	From 1000 to 10,000
Practically insoluble, or Insoluble	More than 10,000

A great many of the important organic medicinal agents are either weak acids or weak bases, and their solubility is dependent to a large measure upon the pH of the solvent. These drugs react either with strong acids or strong bases to form water-soluble salts. For instance, the weak bases, including many of the alkaloids (atropine, codeine, and morphine), antihistamines (diphenhydramine and tripelennamine), local anesthetics (cocaine, procaine, and tetracaine), and other important drugs are not very water-soluble,[1] but they are soluble in dilute solutions of acids. Pharmaceutical manufacturers have prepared many acid salts of these organic bases to enable the pharmacist to prepare aqueous solutions of them. It must be recognized, however, that if the pH of the aqueous solutions of these salts is changed by the addition of alkali, the free base may separate from solution unless it has adequate solubility in water. Organic medicinals that are weak acids include the barbiturate drugs (as phenobarbital and pentobarbital) and the sulfonamides (as sulfadiazine and sulfacetamide). These and other weak acids form water-soluble salts in basic solution and may separate from solution by a lowering of the pH. Table 4-1 presents the comparative solubilities of some typical examples of weak acids and weak bases and their salts.

Although there are no exact rules for predicting unerringly the solubility of a chemical agent in a particular liquid, experienced pharmaceutical chemists utilize the type of information presented in Table 4-1 in estimating the solubility features of a similar chemical compound. The information gathered on a great number of individual chemical compounds has led to the characterization of the solubilities of groups of compounds, and though there may be an occasional inaccuracy with respect to an individual member of a group of compounds, the generalizations nonetheless serve a useful function. As demonstrated by the data in Table 4-1 and other similar data, salts of organic compounds are generally more soluble in water than are the corresponding organic bases. Conversely, the organic bases are generally more soluble in organic solvents, including alcohol, than are the corresponding salt forms. Perhaps

Table 4-1. WATER AND ALCOHOL SOLUBILITIES OF SOME SELECTED WEAK ACIDS, WEAK BASES, AND THEIR SALTS

| Drug | *Number of ml of Solvent Required to Dissolve 1 g of Drug* | |
	Water	*Alcohol*
Atropine	455	2
Atropine sulfate	0.5	5
Codeine	120	2
Codeine sulfate	30	1280
Codeine phosphate	2.5	325
Morphine	5000	210
Morphine sulfate	16	565
Phenobarbital	1000	8
Phenobarbital sodium	1	10
Procaine	200	soluble
Procaine hydro-chloride	1	15
Sulfadiazine	13,000	sparingly soluble
Sodium sulfa-diazine	2	slightly soluble

the most written guideline for the prediction of solubility is that "like dissolves like," meaning that a solvent having a chemical structure most similar to that of the intended solute will be most likely to dissolve it. Thus, organic compounds are more soluble in organic solvents than in water. Organic compounds may, however, be somewhat water-soluble if they contain polar groups capable of forming hydrogen bonds with water.[1] In fact, the greater the number of polar groups present, the greater will likely be the organic compound's solubility in water. Further, the introduction of halogen atoms into a molecule tends to decrease water-solubility because of an increase in the molecular weight of the compound without a proportionate increase in polarity. An increase in the molecular weight of an organic compound without a change in polarity generally results in decreased solubility in water. Table 4-2 demonstrates some of these generalities through the use of specific chemical examples.

As with organic compounds, the pharmacist

---

[1] However, they are usually more soluble in the less polar solvents as alcohol and the various organic solvents.

[1] Polar groups include OH, CHO, COH, CHOH, CH_2OH, COOH, NO_2, CO, NH_2 and SO_3H.

Table 4-2. SOLUBILITIES OF SELECTED ORGANIC COMPOUNDS IN WATER AS A DEMONSTRATION OF CHEMICAL STRUCTURE-SOLUBILITY RELATIONSHIP*

Compound	Formula	Number of ml of Water Required to Dissolve 1 g of Compound
Benzene	C_6H_6	1430
Benzoic acid	C_6H_5COOH	275
Benzyl alcohol	$C_6H_5CH_2OH$	25
Phenol	C_6H_5OH	15
Pyrocatechol	$C_6H_4(OH)_2$	2.3
Pyrogallol	$C_6H_3(OH)_3$	1.7
Carbon Tetra-chloride	CCl_4	2000
Chloroform	$CHCl_3$	200
Methylene Chloride	CH_2Cl_2	50

*Adapted from *Remington's Pharmaceutical Sciences*, 13th ed. E. W. Martin, ed. Easton, Pa., Mack Publishing Company, 1965, p. 210.

is aware of some general patterns of solubility that apply to inorganic compounds. For instance, most salts of monovalent cations such as sodium, potassium, and ammonium are water soluble, whereas the divalent cations like calcium, magnesium, and barium usually form water soluble compounds with nitrate, acetate, and chloride anions but not with carbonate, phosphate, or hydroxide anions.[1] To be sure, there are certain combinations of anion and cation which would seem to be quite similar in make-up but which do not have similar solubility characteristics. For instance, magnesium sulfate (Epsom salt) is soluble, but calcium sulfate is only slightly soluble; barium sulfate is very insoluble (1 g dissolves in about 400,000 ml of water) and is used as an opaque media for x-ray observation of the intestinal tract, but barium sulfide and barium sulfite are not as insoluble, and their use results in poisoning; mercurous chloride (HgCl) is insoluble and is used effectively as a cathartic, but mercuric chloride ($HgCl_2$) is soluble in water and is a deadly poison if taken internally. There are many instances in which the solubilities of certain drugs and their differentiation from other drugs are critical to the pharmacist in order that he might avoid compounding failures or therapeutic disasters.

For organic as well as for inorganic solutes, the ability of a solvent to dissolve them depends upon its effectiveness in overcoming the electronic forces that hold the atoms of the solute together and the corresponding lack of resolute on the part of the atoms themselves to resist the solvent action. During the dissolution process, the molecules of the solvent and the solute become uniformly mixed and cohesive forces of the atoms are replaced by new forces due to the attraction of the solute and solvent molecules for one another.

The student may find the following general rules of solubility useful.

A. For Inorganic Molecules

1. If *both* the cation and anion of an ionic compound are *monovalent*, the solute-solute attractive forces are usually easily overcome, and therefore, these compounds are generally water soluble. (Examples: NaCl, LiBr, KI, NH_4NO_3, $NaNO_2$)
2. If only *one* of the two ions in an ionic compound is *monovalent*, the solute-solute interactions are also usually easily overcome and the compounds are generally water soluble. (Examples: $BaCl_2$, MgI_2, Na_2SO_4, Na_3PO_4)
3. If *both* the cation and anion are *multivalent* the solute-solute interaction may be too great to be overcome by the solute-solvent interaction and the compound may have poor water solubility. (Examples: $CaSO_4$, $BaSO_4$, $BiPO_4$; Exceptions: $ZnSO_4$, $FeSO_4$)
4. Common salts of alkali metals (Na, K, Li, Cs, Rb) are usually water soluble (Exception: Li_2CO_3)
5. Ammonium and quaternary ammonium salts are water soluble.
6. Nitrates, nitrites, acetates, chlorates, and lactates are generally water soluble. (Exceptions: silver and mercurous acetate)
7. Sulfates, sulfites, and thiosulfates are generally water soluble. (Exceptions: calcium and barium salts)
8. Chlorides, bromides, and iodides are generally water soluble. (Exceptions: salts of silver and mercurous ions)
9. Acid salts corresponding to an insoluble salt

[1] An excellent chart depicting the solubility characteristics of inorganic salts may be found in *Husa's Pharmaceutical Dispensing*, 6th ed. E. W. Martin, ed. Easton, Pa., Mack Publishing Company, 1966. p. 549.

will be more water soluble than the original salt.

10. Hydroxides and oxides of compounds other than alkali metal cations and the ammonium ion are generally water insoluble.

11. Sulfides are water insoluble except for their alkali metal salts.

12. Phosphates, carbonates, silicates, borates, and hypochlorites are water insoluble except for their alkali metal salts and ammonium salts.

B. For Organic Molecules

1. Molecules having one polar functional group are usually soluble to total chain lengths of five carbons.

2. Molecules having branched chains are more soluble than the corresponding straight-chain compound.

3. Water solubility decreases with an increase in molecular weight.

4. Increased structural similarity between solute and solvent is accompanied by increased solubility.

It is the pharmacist's knowledge of the chemical characteristics of drugs that permits him to select the proper solvent for a particular solute. However, in addition to the factors of solubility, the selection is based on such additional solvent characteristics as clarity, low toxicity, viscosity, compatibility with other formulative ingredients, chemical inertness, palatability, odor, color, and economy. In most instances, and especially for solutions to be taken orally, used ophthalmically, or injected, water is the preferred solvent, since it comes the closest in meeting the majority of the above criteria than the other available solvents. In many instances, when water is used as the primary solvent, an auxiliary solvent is also employed to augment the solvent action of water or to counter any of its deficiencies. Alcohol, glycerin, and propylene glycol, perhaps the most used auxiliary solvents, have been quite effective in contributing to the desired characteristics of pharmaceutical solutions and in maintaining their stability and permanency.

Other solvents, as acetone, ethyl oxide, and isopropyl alcohol, are too toxic to be permitted in pharmaceutical preparations to be taken internally, but they are useful as reagent solvents in organic chemistry and in the preparatory stages of drug development, as in the extraction or removal of active constituents from medicinal plants. For purposes such as this, certain solvents are officially recognized in the compendia. A number of fixed oils, as corn oil, cottonseed oil, peanut oil, and sesame oil, serve useful solvent functions particularly in the preparation of oleaginous injections and are recognized in the official compendia for this purpose.

Some Official Solvents

The following official agents find use as solvents in the preparation of oral solutions, syrups, and elixirs.

Alcohol, USP (Ethyl Alcohol, Ethanol, Spiritus Vini Rectificatus, S.V.R.)

Next to water, alcohol is the most useful solvent in pharmacy. It is used as a primary solvent for many organic compounds. Together with water it forms a hydroalcoholic mixture that dissolves both alcohol-soluble and water-soluble substances, a feature especially useful in the extraction of active constituents from crude drugs. By varying the proportion of the two agents, the active constituents may be selectively dissolved and extracted or allowed to remain behind according to their particular solubility characteristics in the menstruum. Alcohol, USP, is 94.9 to 96.0% C_2H_5OH by volume (i.e., v/v) when determined at $15.56°$, the U.S. Government's standard temperature for alcohol determinations. Diluted Alcohol, USP, is prepared by mixing equal portions of Alcohol, USP, and purified water. The final volume of such mixtures is not the sum of the individual volumes of the two components, but due to contraction of the liquids upon mixing, the final volume is generally about 3% less than what would normally be expected. Thus when 50 ml of each component is combined, the resulting product measures approximately 97 ml. It is for this reason that the strength of Diluted Alcohol, USP, is not exactly half that of the more concentrated alcohol, but slightly greater, approximately 49%. Diluted alcohol is a useful hydroalcoholic solvent in various pharmaceutical processes and preparations. Dehydrated alcohol (absolute alcohol) is practically free of water and is employed mainly in analytical work and in organic synthesis.

Glycerin, USP (Glycerol)

Glycerin is a clear syrupy liquid with a sweet taste. It is miscible both with water and alcohol. As a solvent, it is comparable with alcohol, but because of its viscosity, solutes are slowly soluble in it unless it is rendered less viscous by heating. Glycerin has preservative qualities and is often used as a stabilizer and as an auxiliary solvent in conjunction with water or alcohol. It is used in many internal preparations.

Propylene Glycol, USP

Propylene glycol, a viscous liquid, is miscible with water and alcohol. It is a useful solvent with a wide range of application and is frequently substituted for glycerin in modern pharmaceutical formulations.

Purified Water, USP

Naturally occurring water exerts its solvent effect on most substances it contacts and thus is impure and contains varying amounts of dissolved inorganic salts, usually sodium, potassium, calcium, magnesium, and iron, chlorides, sulfates, and bicarbonates, as well as dissolved and undissolved organic matter and microorganisms. Water found in most cities and towns where water is purified for drinking purposes usually contains less than 0.1% of total solids, determined by evaporating a 100-ml sample of water to dryness and weighing the residue (which would weigh less than 100 mg). Drinking water must meet the United States Public Health Service regulations with respect to bacteriological purity. Acceptable drinking water should be clear, colorless, odorless, and neutral or only slightly acid or alkaline, the deviation from neutral being due to the nature of the dissolved solids and gases (carbon dioxide contributing to the acidity and ammonia to the alkalinity of water).

Ordinary drinking water obtained from the tap is not generally acceptable for the manufacture of most aqueous pharmaceutical preparations or for the extemporaneous compounding of prescriptions because of the chemical incompatibilities that may result from the combination of dissolved solids present and the medicinal agents being added. Signs of such incompatibilities are precipitation, discoloration, and occasionally effervescence. Its use is permitted in the washing and in the extraction of crude vegetable drugs, in the preparation of certain products for external use, and in other instances in which the difference between the use of water and purified water is of no consequence. Naturally, when large volumes of water are required to clean pharmaceutical machinery and equipment, tap water may be economically employed so long as a residue of solids is prevented by using purified water as the final rinse or by wiping the water dry with a meticulously clean cloth.

Purified Water, USP is obtained by distillation, ion exchange treatment, reverse osmosis, or other suitable process. It is prepared from water complying with the United States Public Health Service with respect to drinking water. Compared to ordinary drinking water, Purified Water, USP is more free of solid impurities. When evaporated to dryness, it must not yield greater than 0.001% of residue (1 mg of total solids per 100 ml of sample evaporated). Thus purified water is 100 times more free of dissolved solids than is water. Purified water is employed in the preparation of all aqueous pharmaceuticals intended for oral administration as well as in other preparations that require purity. When sterility is additionally required, purified water is further treated to satisfy that requirement. Sterile waters are used principally for parenteral and ophthalmic preparations and are discussed in Chapter 8.

The main methods used in the preparation of purified water are distillation and ion-exchange; these methods are described briefly as follows.

DISTILLATION METHOD. The USP does not describe a method for preparing purified water by any of the recognized processes. However, there are many commercially available stills in various sizes and styles with various capacities of from about one-half to 100 gallons of distillate per hour. Generally the first portion of aqueous distillate (about the first 10 to 20%) must be discarded, since it contains many foreign volatile substances usually found in urban drinking water, the usual starting material in the preparation of purified water. Also, the last portion of water (about 10% of the original volume of water) remaining in the distillation apparatus must be discarded and not subjected to further distillation because distillation to dryness would undoubtedly result in the decomposition of the remaining solid impurities to volatile substances that would distill and contaminate the previously collected portion of distillate.

ION-EXCHANGE METHOD. On a large or small scale, the ion-exchange method for the preparation of purified water offers a number of advantages over the distillation method. For one thing, the requirement of heat is eliminated and with it costly and troublesome maintenance frequently encountered in the operation of the more complex distillation apparatus. Because of the simpler equipment and the nature of the method, the ion-exchange process permits ease of operation, minimal maintenance, and a more mobile facility. Many pharmacies and small laboratories which purchase large volumes of distilled water from commercial suppliers for use in their work would no doubt benefit financially and in convenience through the installation of an ion-exchange demineralizer in their work area.

The ion-exchange equipment in use today generally involves the passage of water through a column of cation and anion exchangers, consisting of water-insoluble, synthetic, polymerized phenolic, carboxylic, amino, or sulfonated resins of high molecular weight. These resins are mainly of two types: (a) the cation, or acid exchangers, which permit the exchange of the cations in solution (in the tap water) with hydrogen ion from the resin; (b) the anion, or base exchange resins, which permit the removal of anions. These two processes are successively or simultaneously employed to remove both cations and anions from water. The processes are indicated as follows, with M^+ indicating the metal or cation (as Na^+) and the X^- indicating the anion (as Cl^-).

(a) *Cation Exchange:*
$$H\text{-Resin} + M^+ + X^- + H_2O \rightarrow$$
$$M\text{-Resin} + H^+ + X^- + H_2O$$

(b) *Anion Exchange:*
$$Resin\text{-}NH_2 + H^+ + X^- + H_2O \rightarrow$$
$$Resin\text{-}NH_2 \cdot HX + H_2O \text{ (pure)}$$

Water purified in this manner is referred to as *demineralized* or *de-ionized water*, and may be used in any pharmaceutical preparation or prescription calling for distilled water (aqua destillata).

Preparation of Solutions

Most of the official solutions and, indeed, most liquid pharmaceutical preparations of all classifications are unsaturated with solute. Thus the amounts of solute to be dissolved are usually well below the capacity of the volume of solvent employed. The strengths of pharmaceutical preparations are usually expressed in terms of *% strength*, although for very dilute preparations, expressions of *ratio strength* or *mg%* may be used. These expressions and examples are shown in Table 4-3.

The term %, when used without qualification (as with w/v, v/v, or w/w) means %weight-in-volume for solutions or suspensions of solids in liquids; % weight-in-volume for solutions of gases in liquids; % volume-in-volume for solutions of liquids in liquids; and, weight-in-weight for mixtures of solids and semisolids.

Some chemical agents that may be soluble in a given solvent are only slowly soluble and require an extended time for dissolving. To hasten the dissolution process, a pharmacist may employ one or several techniques. He may apply heat, reduce the particle size of the solute, utilize a solubilizing agent, or subject the ingredients to rigorous agitation during the preparation of the solution. Normally, most chemical agents are more soluble in solvents at elevated temperatures than at room temperature or below because an endothermic reaction between the solute and solvent utilizes the energy of the heat to enhance the dissolution process. However, elevated temperatures cannot be maintained for pharmaceuticals, and the net effect of heat is simply an increase in the *rate* of solution rather than an increase in solubility. An increased rate is satisfactory to the pharmacist, since most of his solutions are unsaturated anyhow and do not require the presence of solute above the normal capacity of the solvent at room temperature. Pharmacists are generally reluctant to employ heat to facilitate solution, and when they do, they are very careful not to exceed the minimally required temperature, for many medicinal agents are destroyed at elevated temperatures, and the advantage of rapid solution may be completely offset by drug deterioration. If volatile solutes are to be dissolved or if the solvent is volatile (as alcohol), the heat would encourage the loss of these agents to the atmosphere and must therefore be avoided. Pharmacists are aware that certain chemical agents, particularly calcium salts, undergo exothermic reactions as they dissolve and give off heat. For such materials the use of heat would actually discourage the formation of a solution. The best pharmaceutical example of this type of chemical is calcium hydroxide, which is used in the preparation of Calcium Hydroxide Solution,

Table 4-3. COMMON METHODS OF EXPRESSING THE STRENGTHS
OF PHARMACEUTICAL PREPARATIONS

Expression	Abbreviated Expression	Meaning and Example
Percent weight in volume	% w/v	number of grams of a constituent in 100 ml of preparation (e.g., 1% w/v = 1 g of constituent in 100 ml of preparation).
Percent volume in volume	% v/v	number of ml of a constituent in 100 ml of preparation (e.g., 1% v/v = 1 ml of constituent in 100 ml of preparation).
Percent weight in weight	% w/w	number of grams of a constituent in 100 g of preparation (e.g., 1% w/w = 1 g of constituent in 100 g of preparation).
Ratio strength, weight in volume	__:_____ w/v	number of grams of constituent in stated number of ml of preparation (e.g., 1:1000 w/v = 1 g of constituent in 1000 ml of preparation).
Ratio strength, volume in volume	__:_____ v/v	number of ml of constituent in stated number of ml of preparation (e.g., 1:1000 v/v = 1 ml of constituent in 1000 ml of preparation).
Ratio strength, weight in weight	__:_____ w/w	number of grams of constituent in stated number of grams of preparation (e.g., 1:1000 w/w = 1 g of constituent in 1000 g of preparation).
Milligram percent	mg %	number of mg of constituent in 100 ml of preparation (e.g. 5 mg% = 5 mg of constituent in 100 ml of preparation).

USP. This solute is soluble in water to the extent of 140 mg per 100 ml of solution at 25° (about 77°F) and 170 mg per 100 ml of solution at 15° (about 50°F). Obviously the temperature at which the solution is prepared or stored can affect the concentration of the resultant solution. This preparation will be discussed at greater length later in this chapter.

In addition to, or instead of, raising the temperature of the solvent to increase the rate of solution, a pharmacist may choose to decrease the particle size of the solute. This may be accomplished by the *comminution* (grinding a solid to a fine state of subdivision) of the solute with a mortar and pestle. The reduced particle size causes an increase in the surface area of the substance exposed to the solvent. If the powder is placed in a suitable vessel (as a beaker, graduate cylinder, or bottle) with a portion of the solvent and is stirred or shaken, as suited to the container, the rate of solution may be increased due to the continued circulation of fresh solvent to the drug's surface and the con-

stant removal of newly formed solution from the drug's surface.

Most solutions prepared for oral administration are prepared by simple solution of the solutes in the solvent or solvent mixture. A few, as Magnesium Citrate Solution, NF, are prepared by chemical reaction of the formulative components. As will be discussed in succeeding chapters, some solutions (as tinctures) may be prepared by extraction and others (as injectable solutions) require sterilization prior to use.

Oral Solutions
and Preparations
for Oral Solution

Solutions intended for oral administration usually contain flavorants and colorants to make the medication more attractive and palatable for the patient. When needed, they may also contain stabilizers to maintain the chemical and physical stability of the medicinal agents and preservatives to prevent the growth of microorganisms in the solution. The formulation pharmacist must be wary of chemical interactions which may occur between the various components of a solution which may result in an alteration in the preparation's stability and/or potency. For instance, it has recently been demonstrated that esters of p-hydroxybenzoic acid (methyl-, ethyl-, propyl-, and butylparabens), the most frequently used preservatives in oral preparations, have a tendency to partition into certain flavoring oils.[1] This partitioning effect could reduce the effective concentration of the preservatives in the aqueous medium of a pharmaceutical product below the level needed for preservative action.

Liquid pharmaceuticals for oral administration are usually formulated such that the patient receives the usual dose of the medication in a conveniently administered volume, as 5 ml (one teaspoonful), 10 ml, or 15 ml (one tablespoonful). A few solutions have unusually large doses, as Magnesium Citrate Solution, NF, with a usual adult dose of 200 ml. On the other hand many solutions used in pediatric patients are given by drop, utilizing a calibrated dropper usually furnished by the manufacturer in the product package.

A number of medicinal agents, particularly certain antibiotics, have insufficient stability in aqueous solution to meet extended shelf-life periods. Thus, commercial manufacturers of these products provide them to the pharmacist in dry powder or granule form for reconstitution with a prescribed amount of purified water immediately before dispensing to the patient. The dry powder mixture contains all of the formulative components including drug, flavorant, colorant, buffers, and others, except for the solvent. Once reconstituted by the pharmacist the resultant solutions remain stable when stored in the refrigerator for periods of from 7 to 14 days depending upon the preparation. This is generally a sufficient period of time for the patient to complete the volume of medication usually prescribed. However, if medication remains after the patient completes his course of therapy, he should be instructed to discard the remaining portion which would be unfit for use at a later date.

Among the official dry powder mixtures intended for reconstitution to oral solutions are the following:

Cloxacillin Sodium for Oral Solution, USP [Corresponding Commercial Product: Tegopen (Bristol)]

Nafcillin Sodium for Oral Solution, USP [Unipen (Wyeth)]

Oxacillin Sodium for Oral Solution, USP [Prostaphlin (Bristol)]

Penicillin V Potassium for Oral Solution, USP [Pen-Vee K (Wyeth); V-Cillin K (Lilly); various others]

Clindamycin Palmitate HCl for Oral Solution, NF [Cleocin Pediatric (Upjohn)]

Vancomycin HCl for Oral Solution, NF [Vancocin HCl (Lilly)]

Each of the above is an antibacterial agent used for the systemic treatment of infection and is formulated to contain the usual dose of the medication in each 5 ml of reconstituted solution. For optimal absorption, most antibiotic preparations are taken 1 hour before or 2 hours after meals. All but clindamycin palmitate and vancomycin HCl are derivatives of penicillin and should be avoided in patients having a known allergy to penicillin. The prescribing physician should be notified of patients who develop a skin rash during the use of these or any other medications. Such a reaction usually indicates an allergic or sensitivity response to the drug and a change of medication is usually warranted. As a matter of professional practice, all important untoward drug effects should be promptly reported to the prescribing physician. In the case of clindamycin, the occurrence of diarrhea is an important warning of adverse drug effects. Severe and persistent diarrhea has been associated with the use of clindamycin preparations and may be accompanied by blood and mucus. It is interesting to note that diarrhea may actually occur several weeks following normal cessation of therapy with clindamycin. The diarrhea may be associated with changes in the large bowel mucosa diagnosed as "pseudomembranous colitis." Mild cases may respond to the discontinuance of the drug. More severe cases require treatment for the mucosal impairment.

[1]Chemburkar, P. B. and Joslin, R. S.: "Effect of Flavoring Oils on Preservative Concentrations in Oral Liquid Dosage Forms," *J. Pharm. Sci.*, 64:414–41, 1975.

Official Oral Solutions

Most of the official oral solutions are prepared commercially by pharmaceutical manufacturers and made available to pharmacists for dispensing to their patients. Thus the concern of the pharmacist with these products is generally not in the area of their specific manufacture, but rather in their therapeutic and pharmaceutic characteristics so that he can advise the patient of the proper use, dosage, method of administration, and storage of the product. Knowledge of the solubility and stability characteristics of the medicinal agents and the solvents employed in the commercial products are useful to the pharmacist in informing the patient of the advisability of mixing the solution with juice, milk, or other beverages upon administration. Information regarding the solvents used in each commercial product appears on the product label and in the accompanying package insert. Table 4-4 presents these official solutions and some pertinent information regarding their composition and use.

There are several official oral solutions which are commonly prepared by the community pharmacist and others which by virtue of their characteristics or method of manufacture are of especial interest to the pharmacy student. A few of these solutions are described below.

Potassium Iodide Solution, USP

This is a saturated solution of potassium iodide in purified water. It is commonly prescribed as "SSKI." A liter of the solution is prepared by dissolving 1000 g of KI in 680 ml of hot purified water, cooling to about 25°, and adding sufficient purified water to make the product measure 1000 ml. The solution is filtered, if necessary. The fact that the solution is saturated can be easily shown: since potassium iodide is soluble in water to the extent of 1 g of KI in 0.7 ml of water, the amount of water required to dissolve 1000 g of KI is obviously 700 ml. The specific gravity of the resultant solution is 1.700, and therefore a liter of solution weighs 1700 g. Since 1000 g of KI were used, the remainder of the weight, or 700 g must be the weight of water present. It follows that 700 ml of water are present, the precise volume required to dissolve 1000 g of KI.

If the solution is not to be used within a short period of time, the USP recommends the addition of 500 mg of sodium thiosulfate to each liter of solution. Potassium iodide is prone to oxidation with the liberation of free iodine, which colors the solution yellow. As free iodine is formed, the sodium thiosulfate converts it to colorless, soluble sodium iodine. To reduce the occurrence of this oxidative decomposition, the solution is best stored in tight, light-resistant containers.

The solution is categorized as an expectorant and source of iodine (antigoitrogenic) with a usual dose of 0.3 ml. The pharmacist should issue the medication with a calibrated dropper service and recommend that the dose be diluted with a glassful of water prior to its oral administration.

Strong Iodine Solution, USP

This solution, commonly known as Lugol's solution, contains about 5% of iodine and about 10% of potassium iodide, the latter used to solubilize the iodine. The solution is prepared by dissolving the solutes in a portion of the purified water, and when the solution is effected, the product is diluted to the proper volume with additional purified water. Strong Iodine Solution, USP, is usually administered internally for the systemic effect of iodine, as in the treatment of thyrotoxicosis. For this purpose, the usual dose of the solution is 0.3 ml, diluted well with water or milk, 3 times a day. Since the dose is so small, the pharmacist generally dispenses the solution in a dropper bottle precalculated to deliver the dose in a specified number of drops.[1] Because of the high concen-

---

[1] The USP medicine dropper is 3 mm in external diameter at its delivery end and when held vertically delivers water in drops each of which weighs between 45 mg and 55 mg. However, in using a medicine dropper, one should keep in mind that few liquids have the same surface and flow characteristics as water, and therefore the size of the drops varies materially from one preparation to another. Further, the dimensions of the medicine dropper employed may not be the same dimensions as the USP dropper described above. Thus, for the determination of the number of drops equivalent to a specified volume, most droppers must be calibrated with the liquid involved. This is easily done by the pharmacist. He generally uses a small 10-ml graduate cylinder to collect the liquid as he drops the liquid from the dropper, counting each drop. When a sufficient volume is collected, to ensure accuracy, he compares the volume collected and the number of drops issued. For instance, if in collecting 5 ml of liquid, he issued 120 drops, that particular dropper will deliver 24 drops of that liquid per ml. Therefore, if the liquid were Strong Iodine Solution and the dose 0.3 ml, then about 7 drops from that dropper would supply the dose of that liquid.

Table 4-4. Official Oral Solutions by Category

Official Oral Solution	Some Representative Commercial Products	Concentration of Official or Commercial Product	Comments
Antibacterial			
Neomycin Sulfate Oral Solution, USP	Mycifradin Sulfate Oral Solution (Upjohn)	125 mg neomycin sulfate/5 ml	Used in treating hepatic coma, infectious diarrhea, and for preoperative prophylaxis in abdominal surgery.
Anticonvulsants			
Paramethadione Oral Solution, USP	Paradione Solution (Abbott)	300 mg paramethadione/ml in diluted alcohol.	The solution is administered with a calibrated dropper, usually in amounts of 0.5 to 1 ml in the treatment of petit mal epilepsy.
Trimethadione Oral Solution, USP	Tridione Solution (Abbott)	40 mg trimethadione/ml	This is an aqueous solution used for the same purpose as paramethadione solution. One teaspoonful of the commercial preparation provides 200 mg of drug, an amount frequently given to young children.
Antidepressant			
Nortriptyline HCl Solution, NF	Aventyl HCl Liquid (Lilly)	10 mg nortriptyline HCl/5 ml in aqueous solution with 4% alcohol.	Indicated for relief of symptoms of depression. The usual adult dose is 25 mg with smaller dosages usually given to the elderly and adolescent patients.
Anticholinergic			
Mepenzolate Bromide Solution, NF	Cantil Liquid (Lakeside)	25 mg mepenzolate bromide/5 ml	Indicated for use as adjunctive therapy in treatment of peptic ulcer.
Antiperistaltic			
Diphenoxylate HCl and Atropine Sulfate Solution, USP	Lomotil Liquid (Searle)	2.5 mg of diphenoxylate HCl and 0.025 mg of atropine sulfate/5 ml	This preparation is indicated in the management of diarrhea. Diphenoxylate is related structurally and pharmacologically to the narcotic meperidine. Atropine sulfate is added to the solution in subtherapeutic amounts to discourage (by virtue of side effects) deliberate overdosage. A calibrated dropper is used to measure dosage for children.
Antipsychotics			
Prochlorperazine Edisylate Solution, USP	Compazine Concentrate (Smith Kline & French)	10 mg prochlorperazine edisylate/ml.	This concentrated solution is used primarily in severe neuropsychiatric conditions when oral medication is preferred and other oral dosage

Table 4-4. OFFICIAL ORAL SOLUTIONS BY CATEGORY (*Cont.*)

Official Oral Solution	Some Representative Commercial Products	Concentration of Official or Commercial Product	Comments
Antipsychotics (cont.)			
			forms (as tablets and capsules) are considered impractical. The concentrated solution is not intended for use in children. In addition to its use in psychotic disorders, the drug is also used to control severe nausea and vomiting. The concentrated solution is employed by adding the desired amount of the concentrate by calibrated dropper to 60 ml of soup or a beverage as tomato or fruit juices, milk, coffee, tea, or carbonated beverages. Since the concentrate is light sensitive, it must be protected from light and dispensed in amber bottles.
Carphenazine Maleate Solution, NF	Proketazine Maleate Concentrate (Wyeth)	50 mg carphenazine maleate/ml	
Haloperidol Solution, USP	Haldol Concentrate (McNeil)	2 mg haloperidol/ml	
Perphenazine Solution NF	Trilafon Concentrate (Schering)	16 mg perphenazine/ 5 ml	Use and administration similar to those of *Prochlorperazine Edisylate Solution.*
Promazine HCl Solution, NF	Sparine Concentrate (Wyeth)	30 mg and 100 mg promazine HCl/ml	
Thioridazine HCl Solution, USP	Mellaril HCl Solution (Sandoz)	30 and 100 mg thioridazine HCl/ml	
Thiothixene Solution, NF	Navane Concentrate (Roerig)	equivalent of 5 mg thiothixene/ml	
Cathartics			
Magnesium Citrate Solution, NF	—	amount of magnesium citrate equivalent to between 1.55 g and 1.9 g of magnesium oxide	Discussed in text.
Sodium Phosphate and Biphosphate Oral Solution, USP	Phospho-Soda (Fleet)	18 g sodium phosphate and 48 g sodium biphosphate/100 ml	Works as laxative within 1 hour when taken before meals or overnight when taken at bedtime. Usual dose is 10 to 20 ml of solution, best taken diluted with one-half glass of water and followed with a full glass of water.
Sodium Phosphate Solution, NF	—	7.5 g sodium phosphate/10 ml	Citric acid is present in the official solution to prevent the crystallization of sodium

Table 4-4. OFFICIAL ORAL SOLUTIONS BY CATEGORY (*Cont.*)

Official Oral Solution	Some Representative Commercial Products	Concentration of Official or Commercial Product	Comments
Cathartics (cont.)			
			phosphate, probably through the formation of sodium acid citrate and sodium acid phosphate. The citric acid also adds a pleasant tart taste to the solution. Glycerin is present in the preparation as an antimicrobial preservative and to add sweetness and viscosity to the solution. The solution is used as a pleasant tasting mild saline cathartic with a dose of 10 ml.
Diagnostic Aid			
Diatrizoate Sodium Oral Solution, USP	Hypaque Sodium Oral Liquid (Winthrop)	41.7% diatrizoate sodium.	The solution which contains organically bound iodine is employed in the radiographic examination of the gastrointestinal tract following oral or rectal administration.
Electrolyte Replenisher			
Potassium Chloride Oral Solution, USP	Kaochlor Liquid (Warren-Teed); Potassium Chloride Liquid (Philips Roxane)	5% KCl (20 mEq of K/30 ml); 10% KCl (40 mEq of K/30 ml); 20% KCl (80 mEq of K/30 ml)	Used in conditions of hypopotassemia (low level of potassium in the blood). Condition may be prompted by severe or chronic diarrhea, a low level of potassium intake in the diet, increased renal excretion of potassium, and other causes. The solution is diluted with water or fruit juice before taking.
Expectorant			
Potassium Iodide Solution, USP	SSKI (Upsher-Smith)	300 mg KI/0.3 ml	Discussed in text.
Fecal Softener			
Dioctyl Sodium Sulfosuccinate Solution, NF	Doxinate Solution (Hoechst-Roussel); Colace Liquid (Mead Johnson)	50 mg dioctyl sodium sulfosuccinate/ml (Doxinate) and 10 mg/ml (Colace)	Usually 50 to 200 mg of the drug is measured by calibrated dropper and mixed with milk, fruit juice, or other liquid (to mask the taste) before administration. The drug softens the fecal mass by lowering the surface tension, thus permitting normal bowel habits, particularly in geriatric, pediatric,

Table 4-4. OFFICIAL ORAL SOLUTIONS BY CATEGORY (*Cont.*)

Official Oral Solution	Some Representative Commercial Products	Concentration of Official or Commercial Product	Comments
Fecal Softener (*cont.*)			cardiac, obstetric, and surgical patients. Dosage is taken for several days or until bowel movements are normal.
Hematinic Ferrous Sulfate Solution, USP	Fer-In-Sol Drops (Mead Johnson); Mol-Iron Drops (Schering)	75 mg ferrous sulfate/ 0.6 ml	Used for prevention and treatment of iron deficiency anemias. Usual prophylactic dose of 0.3 or 0.6 ml measured by calibrated dropper and mixed with water, fruit juice, or vegetable juice before administration. Dosage form intended primarily for infants and children.
Iodine Source Strong Iodine Solution, USP	—	5% iodine and 10% potassium iodide	Discussed in text.
Vitamin D Source Ergocalciferol Solution, USP	Viosterol in Oil (Parke Davis); Drisdol (Winthrop)	250 µg (10,000 units) ergocalciferol/g	A solution of water-insoluble ergocalciferol (vitamin D_2) in vegetable oil or propylene glycol. The usual prophylactic dose of ergocalciferol is about 10 µg (400 units) and the therapeutic dose may be 5 mg (200,000 units) or as high as 25 mg (1,000,000 units) daily in treating rickets.

tration of free iodine present in this solution, it is also of great value externally as a germicide and fungicide.

Magnesium Citrate Solution, NF

Magnesium citrate solution is a colorless to slightly yellow, clear, effervescent liquid having a sweet, acidulous taste and a lemon flavor. It is commonly referred to as "Citrate" or as "Citrate of Magnesia." It is required to contain an amount of magnesium citrate equivalent to between 1.55 and 1.9 g of magnesium oxide in each 100 ml.

The solution is prepared by reacting official magnesium carbonate with an excess of citric acid (equation 1), flavoring and sweetening the solution with lemon oil and syrup, filtering with talc, and then carbonating it by the addition of either potassium or sodium bicarbonate (equation 2). The solution may be further carbonated by the use of carbon dioxide under pressure.

$$(1)\ (MgCO_3)_4 \cdot Mg(OH)_2 + 5H_3C_6H_5O_7 \rightarrow$$
$$5MgHC_6H_5O_7 + 4CO_2 + 6H_2O$$

$$(2)\ 3KHCO_3 + H_3C_6H_5O_7 \rightarrow$$
$$K_3C_6H_5O_7 + 3CO_2 + 3H_2O$$

The solution provides an excellent media for the growth of molds, and any mold spores present during the manufacture of the solution must be killed if the preparation is to remain stable. For this reason, during the preparation of the solution the liquid is heated to boiling (prior to carbonation), boiled water is employed to bring the solution to its proper volume, and boiling water is used to rinse the final container. The NF permits the sterilization of the final solution.

Magnesium citrate solution has always been troublesome, since it has a tendency to deposit a crystalline solid upon standing. Apparently this is due to the formation of some almost insoluble, normal magnesium citrate (rather than the exclusively dibasic form as in equation 1). The cause of the problem has largely been attributed to the indefinite composition of the official magnesium carbonate, which by definition is "a basic hydrated magnesium carbonate or a normal hydrated magnesium carbonate" (see equation 1). It contains the equivalent of 40 to 43.5% of magnesium oxide. Apparently solutions prepared from magnesium carbonates with differing equivalents of magnesium oxide vary in stability, with the most stable ones being prepared from samples of magnesium carbonate having the lower equivalent of magnesium oxide. The official formula for the preparation of 350 ml of magnesium citrate solution calls for the use of 15 g of official magnesium carbonate, which corresponds to from 6.0 to 6.47 g of magnesium oxide. To increase the stability of the solution, the NF permits the use of a quantity of magnesium carbonate (not necessarily 15 g) which is equivalent to 6.0 g of magnesium oxide per 350 ml of product. An accompanying excess of citric acid is also advised. Sterilization also seems to reduce the likelihood of precipitation.

In the carbonation step in the preparation of the solution, the bicarbonate is generally added in tablet form rather than as a powder in order to delay the effervescence resulting from its contact with the citric acid. If the powder were used, the reaction would be immediate and violent, and it would be virtually impossible to close the bottle in time to prevent the loss of carbon dioxide or solution. Most of the magnesium citrate solutions prepared commercially today are packaged in the same type of bottles as "soft drink" carbonated beverages. They have replaced the special "citrate bottles" having a glass plunger-cap (rather than a metal cap), which clamps into place. The solution is generally packaged in bottles of two capacities, 350 ml, that of the official formula, and 200 ml, the volume of the official dose. Since the solution is carbonated, it loses some of its character if allowed to stand for a period of time after the container has been opened. For this reason, the single-dose packages are probably the more appealing and less wasteful. Magnesium citrate solution is generally stored in a cold place, preferably in a refrigerator, keeping the bottle on its side so the cork or rubber liners of the caps are kept moist and swollen, thereby maintaining the airtight seal between the cap and the bottle.

The solution is employed as a saline cathartic, with the citric acid, lemon oil, syrup, carbonation, and the low temperature of the refrigerated solution all contributing to the patient's acceptance of the large volume of medication. For many patients it represents a pleasant way of taking an otherwise bitter saline cathartic.

Sodium Citrate and Citric Acid Solution, USP

This solution is generally prepared extemporaneously by the pharmacist upon receipt of a prescription. The official solution contains 100 mg of sodium citrate and 60 mg of citric acid in each ml of aqueous solution. The solution is administered orally in doses of 10 to 30 ml as frequently as four times daily as a systemic alkalinizer. Systemic alkalinization is useful in patients having conditions in which long term maintenance of an alkaline urine is desirable, such as patients with uric acid and cystine calculi of the urinary tract. The solution is also a useful adjuvant when administered with uricosuric agents in gout therapy since urates tend to crystallize out of an acid urine.

Syrups

Syrups are concentrated, aqueous preparations of a sugar with or without added flavoring agents and medicinal substances. Syrups containing flavoring agents but not medicinal substances are called *nonmedicated* or *flavored vehicles* (syrups). Official nonmedicated syrups are presented in Table 4-5. These syrups are intended to serve as pleasant tasting vehicles for medicinal substances to be added later, either in the extemporaneous compounding of prescriptions or in the preparation of a standard formula for a *medicated syrup*, which is a syrup

Table 4-5. OFFICIAL NONMEDICATED SYRUPS

Nonmedicated Syrup	Comments
Acacia Syrup, NF	A sucrose-based syrup flavored with vanilla tincture. The syrup is especially viscous due to the thickening effect of acacia. It is useful in administering unpleasant tasting drugs since its viscous nature reduces the proportion of dissolved drug making contact with the taste buds.
Cherry Syrup, NF	A sucrose-based syrup containing about 47% by volume of cherry juice. The syrup's tart and fruit flavor is attractive to most patients and the acidic pH of the syrup makes it useful as a vehicle for drugs requiring an acid medium.
Cocoa Syrup, USP	This syrup is a suspension of cocoa powder in an aqueous vehicle sweetened and thickened with sucrose, liquid glucose, and glycerin, and flavored with vanillin and sodium chloride. The syrup is particularly effective in administering bitter tasting drugs to children.
Aromatic Eriodictyon Syrup, NF	This syrup, prepared from eriodictyon fluidextract, is sucrose-based and contains lemon oil, clove oil, and compound cardamom tincture as adjunct flavors. The syrup has an alkaline pH and must be used as a vehicle only for those drugs stable in this medium. The syrup is recommended as a mask for bitter drugs.
Orange Syrup, NF	This sucrose-based syrup utilizes sweet orange peel tincture, and citric acid as the source of flavor and tartness. The syrup resembles orange juice in taste and is a good vehicle for drugs stable in an acidic medium.
Syrup, USP	This is an 85% solution of sucrose in purified water. This "simple syrup" may be used as the basis for the preparation of flavored or medicated syrups.
Tolu Balsam Syrup, NF	This sucrose-based syrup is prepared from tolu balsam tincture and possesses the flavor and expectorant qualities of the tolu balsam.

containing a therapeutic or medicinal agent. Medicated syrups may also be prepared from the starting materials; that is, by combining each of the individual components of the syrup, as sucrose, purified water, flavoring agents, coloring agents, the therapeutic agent, and other necessary and desirable ingredients. Naturally, medicated syrups are employed in therapeutics for the value of the medicinal agent present in the syrup.

Syrups provide a pleasant means of administering a liquid form of a disagreeable tasting drug. They are particularly effective in the administration of drugs to youngsters, since their pleasant taste usually dissipates any reluctance on the part of the child to take the medicine. The fact that syrups contain little or no alcohol adds to their favor among parents.

Any water-soluble drug that is stable in aqueous solution may be added to a flavored syrup. However care must be exercised to insure the compatibility between the medicinal drug substance and the other formulative components of the syrup. Also, certain flavored syrups have an acidic medium, whereas others may be neutral or slightly basic and the proper selection must be made to insure the stability of any added medicinal agent. Perhaps the most frequently found types of medications administered as medicated syrups are antitussive agents and antihistamines. This is not to imply that other types of drugs are not formulated into syrups; indeed, a wide variety of medicinal substances can be found in syrup form in the official compendia and among the many commercial products. The official medicated Syrups are presented in Table 4-6.

Components of Syrups

Generally speaking most syrups contain the following components in addition to the purified water and any medicinal agents present: (1) the sugar, usually sucrose, or sugar-substitutes used to provide sweetness and viscosity, (2) antimicrobial preservatives, (3) flavorants, and (4) colorants. Also, certain syrups, especially those prepared commercially, may contain special solvents, solubilizing agents, thickeners, or stabilizers.

Table 4-6. OFFICIAL MEDICATED SYRUPS BY CATEGORY

Official Syrup	Some Representative Commercial Products	Concentration of Official Commercial Product*	Comments
Adrenergic			
Pseudoephedrine HCl Syrup, NF	Sudafed Syrup (Burroughs Wellcome)	30 mg pseudoephedrine HCl/5 ml	Orally effective nasal decongestant
Analgesic			
Meperidine HCl Syrup, NF	Demerol Elixir (Winthrop)	50 mg meperidine HCl/5 ml	Narcotic analgesic indicated for relief of moderate to severe pain and as an adjunct to general anesthesia.
Anthelmintic			
Piperazine Citrate Syrup, USP	Antepar Syrup (Burroughs Wellcome)	Equivalent of 500 mg piperazine hexahydrate/5 ml	Treatment of roundworm and pinworm infections. Dosage range from 250 mg to 3.5 g in a single daily dose depending on age and weight of the patient.
Antiamebic			
Paromycin Sulfate Syrup, NF	Humatin Syrup Pediatric (Parke Davis)	125 mg paromycin sulfate/5 ml	Poorly absorbed drug used for acute and chronic amebiasis. Usual adult dose is 500 mg of paromycin every 6 hours.
Antibacterials			
Isoniazid Syrup, USP	Nydrazid Syrup (Squibb)	50 mg isoniazid/5 ml	Used in treatment of tuberculosis. Usual dose is 5 mg/kg of body weight once a day, up to 300 mg
Lincomycin HCl Syrup, NF	Lincocin Syrup (Upjohn)	Equivalent of 125 mg and 250 mg lincomycin/5 ml	Antibiotic effective against most common gram-positive pathogens. Usual adult dose is 500 mg three to four times a day.
Minocycline HCl Syrup, NF	Minocin Syrup (Lederle)	Equivalent of 50 mg minocycline/5 ml	A derivative of the antibiotic tetracycline with activity against a broad range of gram-negative and gram-positive pathogens. Usual adult dose is 200 mg initially and 100 mg every 12 hours.
Anticholinergic			
Dicyclomine HCl Syrup, USP	Bentyl Syrup (Merrell National)	10 mg dicyclomine HCl/5 ml	Used as adjunctive therapy in treatment of peptic ulcer.
Antiemetics			
Chlorpromazine HCl Syrup, USP	Thorazine Syrup (Smith Kline and French)	10 mg chlorpromazine HCl/5 ml	Used to control nausea and vomiting.
Dimenhydrinate Syrup, USP	Dramamine Liquid (Searle)	15 mg dimenhydrinate/5 ml	Used to control nausea, vomiting, and motion sickness.
Prochlorperazine Edisylate Syrup, USP	Compazine Syrup (Smith Kline and French)	5 mg prochlorperazine edisylate/5 ml	Used to control nausea and vomiting.

*The amount per stated volume of syrup constitutes a usual single dose of the medication unless otherwise stated.

Table 4-6. OFFICIAL MEDICATED SYRUPS BY CATEGORY (*Cont.*)

Official Syrup	Some Representative Commercial Products	Concentration of Official Commercial Product*	Comments
Antiemetics (cont.)			
Promethazine HCl Syrup, USP	Phenergan Syrup (Wyeth)	6.25 mg, 12.5 mg, and 25 mg promethazine HCl/ 5 ml	Used to control nausea, vomiting, motion sickness, and allergic reactions.
Antihistamines			
Chlorpheniramine Maleate Syrup, USP	Chlor-Trimeton Syrup (Schering)	2 mg chlorpheniramine maleate/ 5 ml	
Cyproheptadine HCl Syrup, NF	Periactin Syrup (Merck Sharp & Dohme)	2 mg cyproheptadine HCl/5 ml	
Dexchlorpheniramine Maleate Syrup, NF	Polaramine Syrup (Schering)	2 mg dexchlorpheniramine maleate/ 5 ml	
Dimethindene Maleate Syrup, NF	Forhistal Syrup (Ciba)	1 mg dimethindene maleate/5 ml	All of the antihistamines listed are used for prevention and treatment of allergic reactions.
Doxylamine Succinate Syrup, NF	Decapryn Syrup (Merrell-National)	6.25 mg doxylamine succinate/ 5 ml	
Methapyrilene Fumarate Syrup, NF	Histadyl Syrup (Lilly)	30 mg methapyrilene fumarate/5 ml	
Triprolidine HCl Syrup, NF	Actidil Syrup (Burroughs Wellcome)	1.25 mg triprolidine HCl/5 ml	
Hydroxyzine HCl Syrup, NF	Atarax Syrup (Roerig)	10 mg hydroxyzine HCl/5 ml	
Antipruritics			
Methdilazine HCl Syrup, NF	Tacaryl Syrup (Westwood)	4 mg methdilazine HCl/5 ml	These antipruritics are used for relief of itching in urticaria.
Trimeprazine Tartrate Syrup, USP	Temaril Syrup (Smith Kline and French)	2.5 mg trimeprazine tartrate/5 ml	
Antipsychotics			
Trifluoperazine HCl Syrup, NF	Stelazine Syrup (Smith Kline and French)	2 mg trifluoperazine HCl/0.2 ml	These agents are used in the management of psychotic disorders.
Promazine HCl Syrup NF	Sparine Syrup (Wyeth)	10 mg promazine HCl/5 ml	
Antitussive			
Dextromethorphan HBr Syrup, NF	Romilar Syrup (Block)	15 mg dextromethorphan HBr/5 ml	For relief of cough.
Antiviral			
Amantadine HCl Syrup, NF	Symmetrel Syrup (Endo)	50 mg amantadine HCl/5 ml	Prevention of respiratory infections caused by A_2 (Asian) viral strains.
Cathartic			
Senna Syrup, NF	—	25% senna fluidextract	Dose is 2 ml as a laxative.

Table 4-6. OFFICIAL MEDICATED SYRUPS BY CATEGORY (*Cont.*)

Official Syrup	Some Representative Commercial Products	Concentration of Official Commercial Product*	Comments
Cholinergic			
Pyridostigmine Bromide Syrup, USP	Mestinon Syrup (Roche)	60 mg pyridostigmine bromide/5 ml	Used in treatment of myasthenia gravis.
Emetic			
Ipecac Syrup, USP	—	21 mg ether-soluble alkaloids of ipecac/15 ml	Used to induce vomiting in poisoning. The dose of 15 ml may be repeated in 20 minutes if vomiting does not occur. If after the second dose, vomiting does not occur, the stomach should be emptied by gastric lavage.
Expectorant			
Glyceryl Guaiacolate Syrup, NF	Robitussin Syrup (Robins); 2/G (Dow)	100 mg glyceryl guaiacolate/5 ml	For symptomatic relief of respiratory conditions associated with cough and bronchial congestion.
Fecal Softener			
Dioctyl Sodium Sulfosuccinate Syrup, NF	Colace Syrup (Mead Johnson)	20 mg dioctyl sodium sulfosuccinate/5 ml	Stool softener by surface-action.
Glucocorticoids			
Betamethasone Syrup, NF	Celestone Syrup (Schering)	600 μg betamethasone/5 ml	These are adrenocortical steroids useful in treating inflammatory conditions and those resulting from adrenocortical insufficiency.
Triamcinolone Diacetate Syrup	Aristocort Syrup (Lederle)	2 and 5 mg triamcinolone diacetate/5 ml	
Hemostatic			
Aminocaproic Acid Syrup, NF	Amicar Syrup (Lederle)	1.25 g aminocaproic acid/5 ml	Used in treatment of excessive bleeding resulting from systemic hyperfibrinolysis and urinary fibrinolysis.
Hypnotic/Sedative			
Chloral Hydrate Syrup, USP	Kessodrate Syrup (McKesson); Noctec	250 mg and 500 mg chloral hydrate/5 ml	Sedative in doses of 250 mg and hypnotic to induce sleep at doses of 500 mg. Alcoholic beverages should be avoided when taking this syrup. The syrup is usually diluted with water or other beverage before taking.
Iron Supplement			
Ferrous Sulfate Syrup, NF	—	400 mg ferrous sulfate/10 ml	Used to treat iron deficiency anemia.

The Sugar or Sugar Substitutes

Sucrose is the sugar most frequently employed in syrups although in certain instances it may be replaced in part or totally by some other agent. For instance, dextrose is employed in "hydriodic acid syrup" since the acid character of the syrup tends to caramelize sucrose, resulting in the syrup's discoloration. By using dextrose, the discoloration is avoided. For reasons of enhancing the solubility of other formulative ingredients or for overall stability purposes, a pharmaceutical manufacturer occasionally may employ an auxiliary solvent or sweetener possessing the desired qualities. Such materials include glycerin, sorbitol, and propylene glycol. In still other instances, all glycogenetic substances (materials converted to glucose in the body), including those agents mentioned above, are replaced by nonglycogenetic substances such as methylcellulose or hydroxyethylcellulose. These two materials are not hydrolyzed and absorbed into the blood stream, and their use results in an excellent syrup-like vehicle for medications intended for use by diabetic patients and others whose diets must be controlled and restricted to nonglycogenetic substances. The viscosity generally resulting from the use of these cellulose derivatives is very much like that of a sucrose syrup. The addition of one or more artificial sweeteners usually produces an excellent facsimile of a true syrup.

The characteristic "body" that the sucrose and the substitutive agents seek to impart to the syrup is essentially the result of attaining the proper viscosity. This quality, together with the sweetness and the flavorants generally added, results in a type of pharmaceutical preparation that is quite effective in masking the taste of added medicinal agents. When the syrup is swallowed, only a portion of dissolved drug actually makes contact with the taste buds, the remainder of the drug being carried past them and down the throat in the containment of the viscous syrup. This type of physical concealment of the taste is not possible for a solution of a drug in an unthickened, mobile, aqueous preparation. In the case of antitussive syrups, the thick sweet syrup has a soothing effect on the irritated tissues of the throat as it passes over them.

Most syrups contain a high proportion of sucrose, usually 60 to 80%, not only because of the desirable sweetness and viscosity of such solutions but also because of their inherent stability in contrast to the unstable character of dilute sucrose solutions. The aqueous sugar medium of dilute sucrose solutions is an efficient nutrient medium for the growth of microorganisms, particularly yeasts and molds. On the other hand, concentrated sugar solutions are quite resistant to microbial growth, due to the unavailability of the water required for the growth of microorganisms. This aspect of syrups is best demonstrated by the simplest of all syrups, Syrup, USP, which has the synonym of "simple syrup" and is prepared by dissolving 85 g of sucrose in enough purified water to make 100 ml of syrup. The resulting preparation requires no additional preservation; in fact, preservatives may not be added to this official syrup. When properly prepared and maintained, the syrup is inherently stable and resistant to the growth of microorganisms. An examination of this syrup reveals its concentrated nature and the relative absence of available water for microbial growth. Syrup, USP, has a specific gravity of about 1.313, which means that each 100 ml of syrup weighs 131.3 g. Since 85 g of sucrose are present, the difference between 85 g and 131.3 g or 46.3 g, represents the weight of the purified water present. Thus, 46.3 g, or ml, of purified water are used to dissolve the 85 g of sucrose. The solubility of sucrose in water is 1 g in 0.5 ml of water; therefore, to dissolve 85 g of sucrose, about 42.5 ml of water would be required. Thus, only a very slight excess of water (about 3.8 ml per 100 ml of syrup) is employed in the preparation of Syrup, USP. Although not enough to be particularly amenable to the growth of microorganisms, the slight excess of water permits the syrup to remain physically stable under conditions of varying temperatures. If the syrup were completely saturated with sucrose, under cool storage conditions some sucrose might crystallize from solution and, by acting as nuclei, initiate a type of chain reaction that would result in the separation of an amount of sucrose disproportionate to its solubility at the storage temperature. The syrup would then be very much unsaturated and probably suitable for microbial growth. As formulated, the official syrup is both stable and resistant to crystallization as well as to microbial growth. However, many of the other official syrups and a host of commercial syrups are not intended to be as nearly saturated as Syrup, USP, and therefore must employ added preservative agents to prevent microbial growth and to ensure their stability during their period of use and storage.

Antimicrobial Preservative

The amount of a preservative required to protect a syrup against microbial growth would vary with the proportion of water available for growth, the nature and inherent preservative activity of some formulative materials (as many flavoring oils that are inherently sterile and possess antimicrobial activity), and the capability of the preservative itself. Among the preservatives commonly used in the preservation of syrups with the usually effective concentrations are benzoic acid (0.1 to 0.2%), sodium benzoate (0.1 to 0.2%), and various combinations of methyl-, propyl-, and butylparabens (totaling about 0.1%). Frequently alcohol is used in the preparation of syrups to assist in the dissolving of alcohol-soluble ingredients, but normally it is not present in the final product in amounts that would be considered to be adequate for preservation (15 to 20%). However, there is some feeling among pharmacists that even a small amount of alcohol contributes to the preservation of syrups by means of its vapor filling the airspace of the container and preventing the surface growth of microorganisms.

Flavorants

Most syrups are flavored with synthetic flavorants or with naturally occurring materials as volatile oils (e.g. orange oil), vanillin, cocoa, cherry juice, and others, to render the syrup pleasant tasting. Since syrups are aqueous preparations, these flavorants must possess sufficient water-solubility. However, sometimes a small amount of alcohol is added to a syrup to ensure the continued solution of a poorly water-soluble flavorant.

Colorant

To enhance the appeal of the syrup, a coloring agent is generally used which correlates with the flavorant employed (i.e. green with mint, brown with chocolate, etc.). The colorant used is generally water soluble, nonreactive with the other syrup components, and color-stable at the pH range and under the intensity of light that the syrup is likely to encounter during its shelf-life.

Preparation of Syrups

Syrups are most frequently prepared by one of four general methods, depending upon the physical and chemical characteristics of the ingredients. Broadly stated, these methods are (1) solution of the ingredients with the aid of heat, (2) solution of the ingredients by agitation without the use of heat, or the simple admixture of liquid components, (3) addition of sucrose to a prepared medicated liquid or to a flavored liquid, and (4) by percolation of either the source of the medicating substance or of the sucrose. In certain instances a syrup may be successfully prepared by more than one of the above methods, and the selection may simply be a matter of preference on the part of the pharmacist. It should be pointed out that the methods, as stated, are general methods; and it is not intended to convey that they are the only methods or that variations within them are not permitted or undertaken.

Solution with the Aid of Heat

Syrups are prepared by this method when it is desired to prepare the syrup as quickly as possible and when the syrup's components are not damaged or volatilized by heat. In this method the sugar is generally added to the purified water, and heat is applied until solution is effected. Then, other required heat-stable components are added to the hot syrup, the mixture is allowed to cool, and its volume is adjusted to the proper level by the addition of purified water. In instances in which heat-labile agents or volatile substances, as volatile flavoring oils and alcohol, are to be added, they are generally added to the syrup after the solution of the sugar is effected by heat, and the solution is rapidly cooled to room temperature.

The use of heat facilitates the rapid solution of the sugar as well as certain other components of syrups; however, caution must be exercised against becoming impatient and using excessive heat. Sucrose, a disaccharide, may be hydrolyzed into monosaccharides, dextrose (glucose), and fructose (levulose). This hydrolytic reaction is referred to as *inversion,* and the combination of the two monosaccharide products is *invert sugar.* When heat is applied in the preparation of a sucrose syrup, some inversion of the sucrose is almost certain. The speed of inversion is greatly increased by the presence of acids, the hydrogen ion acting as a catalyst to the reaction. Should inversion occur, the sweetness of the syrup is altered, since invert sugar is sweeter than sucrose; and the normally colorless syrup darkens due to the effect of heat on the levulose portion of the invert sugar. When the syrup is greatly overheated, it becomes amber colored due to the caramelization of the sucrose. Syrups so decomposed are more susceptible to fermentation and to microbial growth than the stable, nondecomposed syrups. Because of the prospect of decomposition by heat, syrups cannot be sterilized by autoclaving. The use of boiled purified water in the preparation of a syrup can enhance its permanency, and the addition of preservative agents, when permitted, can protect it during its shelf life. Storage in tight containers is a requirement for all syrups.

Among the official syrups prepared by solution with the aid of heat are the following:

Acacia Syrup, NF

Acacia Syrup, NF, contains 10% of powdered or granular acacia, 80% of sucrose, 0.1% of benzoic acid, 0.5% of vanilla tincture, and purified water. It is prepared by mixing the acacia, sucrose, and benzoic acid together and then adding purified water and heating the mixture over a steam bath until solution is effected. When the preparation is cool, the scum is removed from the top, and the vanilla tincture is added. Enough purified water is then added to make the proper volume, and the syrup is strained if necessary.

The mixing of the sucrose and the acacia before adding water helps to distribute the acacia and prevents its lumping when the water is added. The heating coagulates the albuminous material from the acacia, which is a dried gummy exudate from the stems and branches of *Acacia senegal* and other related species. Aqueous preparations of acacia and other plant materials are susceptible to mold growth, and the sodium benzoate is added as a preservative to prevent this occurrence. The vanilla tincture is added after the mixture is cool in order to prevent the loss of the volatile components of the tincture.

The syrup represents a colloidal type of product that is rather viscous because of the high proportion of sucrose present and the thickening effect of the acacia. The syrup is categorized as a flavored vehicle. It is particularly useful in administering unpleasant tasting drugs, since its viscous nature reduces the proportion of dissolved drug that makes contact with the taste buds.

Cocoa Syrup, USP

Cocoa Syrup, USP, is a suspension of cocoa powder in an aqueous vehicle sweetened with sucrose, liquid glucose, and glycerin and flavored with vanillin and sodium chloride. The syrup is preserved with 0.1% of sodium benzoate. It is prepared by agitating a mixture of the sucrose and the cocoa in an already prepared solution of the other ingredients in hot purified water. The entire mixture is boiled for 3 minutes, allowed to cool, and made to volume with additional purified water.

Official cocoa powder contains between 10 and 22% of nonvolatile, ether-soluble extractive ("fat"). However, the USP states that cocoa containing not more than 12% of this material yields a syrup having a minimum tendency to separate. So-called "breakfast cocoa" contains over 22% of "fat". Thus, since the cocoa contains water-insoluble components, the resulting syrup is not a clear solution, but rather a suspension. The viscosity created by the sucrose, glycerin, and liquid glucose prevents the rapid settling of the suspended particles.

The syrup is used as a sweetened, flavored vehicle and is particularly effective in administering bitter tasting drugs to children. The syrup is also called "Chocolate Syrup."

Syrup, USP

As noted earlier, Syrup, USP, is an 85% w/v solution of sucrose in purified water. It may be prepared by simple solution with agitation, usually with the aid of heat, or by percolation. These two processes, with respect to the preparation of this syrup, were formerly referred to as the "hot process" and the "cold process," respectively. As already pointed out, this syrup is nearly saturated, and so long as its concentration is maintained, it is relatively stable against microbial growth. A syrup prepared by percolation is colorless, but one prepared with heat generally has a yellowish tint due to the caramelization of a portion of the sucrose.

This syrup is employed as a pharmaceutic aid in the preparation of medicated syrups. Being sweet, but unflavored and uncolored, it is generally combined with flavorants and colorants, as well as other pharmaceutical adjuncts when used as a vehicle.

Solution by Agitation without the Aid of Heat

To avoid heat-induced inversion of sucrose, a syrup may be prepared without heat by agitation. On a small scale, sucrose and other formulative agents may be dissolved in purified water by placing the ingredients in a bottle of greater capacity than the volume of syrup to be prepared, thus permitting the thorough agitation of the mixture. This process is more time-consuming than that utilizing heat to facilitate the solution of sucrose, but the product has maximum stability. Huge glass-lined or stainless steel tanks affixed with mechanical stirrers or agitators are employed in the large-scale preparation of syrups.

Sometimes simple syrup or some other nonmedicated syrup, rather than sucrose, is employed as the sweetening agent and vehicle. In instances such as this, other liquids that are soluble in the syrup or miscible with it may be added and thoroughly mixed to form a uniform product. When solid agents are to be added to a syrup, it is best to dissolve them in a minimal amount of purified water and then incorporate the resulting solution into the syrup. When solid substances are added directly to a syrup, they generally dissolve slowly because the viscous nature of the syrup does not permit the solid substance to distribute readily throughout the syrup to the available solvent and also because a limited amount of available water is present in concentrated syrups.

An example of an official syrup prepared by agitation without the aid of heat is Ferrous Sulfate Syrup, NF:

Ferrous Sulfate Syrup, NF

Ferrous Sulfate Syrup, NF, contains about 4 g of ferrous sulfate per 100 ml of syrup. It is prepared by dissolving ferrous sulfate, citric acid, peppermint spirit, and about one-fourth the required sucrose in purified water and filtering until clear. A portion of the sucrose is added to provide a reducing environment, thereby inhibiting the oxidation of ferrous ion to ferric ion which would likely precipitate from solution as a basic ferric salt. The entire amount of sucrose is not used initially in order that the

solution may be readily filtered. The remainder of the sucrose is added to the filtrate, and sufficient purified water is used to bring the syrup to the required volume. Citric acid is employed in the syrup to chelate the ferric ions normally present in the ferrous sulfate to prevent them from forming insoluble ferric hydroxide. In this manner citric acid prevents the discoloration of the syrup from its normal green to a reddish brown tint. The peppermint spirit disguises the ferruginous taste of the ferrous sulfate.

Ferrous sulfate syrup is used as a hematinic, particularly for children since the dose can easily be varied. The usual dose is 10 ml, which contains about 400 mg of ferrous sulfate.

Addition of Sucrose to a Medicated Liquid or to a Flavored Liquid

Occasionally a medicated liquid, as a tincture of fluidextract, is employed as the source of medication in the preparation of a syrup. Many such tinctures and fluidextracts contain alcohol-soluble constituents and are prepared with alcoholic or hydroalcoholic vehicles. If the alcohol-soluble components are desired medicinal agents to be present in the corresponding syrup, some means of rendering them water-soluble is generally employed. However, if the alcohol-soluble components are undesirable or unnecessary components of the corresponding syrup, they are generally removed by mixing the tincture or fluidextract with water, allowing the mixture to stand until separation of the water-insoluble agents is complete, and filtering them from the mixture. The filtrate then represents the medicated liquid to which the sucrose is added in the preparation of the syrup. In other instances when the tincture or fluidextract is miscible with aqueous preparations, it may be added directly to simple syrup or to a flavored syrup to medicate it.

An example of an official medicated syrup prepared by the addition of sucrose to a medicated liquid is Senna Syrup, NF:

Senna Syrup, NF

This syrup is prepared by adding purified water to a mixture of senna fluidextract and coriander oil, and allowing this mixture to stand for 24 hours in order that the water-insoluble resins and other inert and insoluble components of the fluidextract may precipitate. The mixture is then filtered, and the sucrose is dissolved in the filtrate. By encouraging the separation of the water-insoluble constituents in this manner, the prospect of the syrup remaining clear during a usual shelf life is excellent.

Senna is the dried leaflet of *Cassia acutifolia* (Alexandria Senna) or *Cassia angustifolia* (Tinnevelly Senna) and, due to the presence of aloe-emodin, rhein, their glycoside derivatives, and other components, it exerts a strong cathartic effect, which results in the thorough evacuation of the bowels within 6 hours after taking the medication. The fluidextract, which is a hydroalcoholic preparation, contains these active constituents of senna and passes them along to the syrup. The coriander oil is added to the syrup both for its flavoring effects and its ability to moderate the pain and griping effects of the senna cathartics on the intestines. The dose of senna syrup is 8 ml.

In a limited number of instances, sucrose is dissolved in a flavoring liquid to prepare a flavoring syrup. Perhaps the most representative of these syrups are Cherry Syrup, NF and Orange Syrup, NF:

Cherry Syrup, NF

Cherry syrup is prepared from Cherry Juice, NF, which is the liquid expressed from the fresh ripe fruit of *Prunus cerasus.*

The cherry juice is obtained by crushing washed, stemmed, unpitted, sour cherries in a grinder so as to break the pits but not mash the kernels. To prevent fermentation, 0.1% benzoic acid is added. The crushed cherries are allowed to stand at room temperature for several days to permit the naturally occurring pectin to hydrolyze to insoluble pectic acid. This reaction, which is catalyzed by the enzyme pectase, is desired, since a syrup prepared from a juice containing pectin is likely to gel on standing. The juice is declared void of pectin when a clear portion of the filtered juice remains clear for 30 minutes after mixing with one half of its volume of alcohol. The pectin-free juice is then separated from the crude mixture with a press and is filtered. Cherry juice is red to reddish orange in color, but the color tends to fade when the juice is exposed to sunlight. Therefore the juice and the corresponding syrup should be stored in light-resistant containers. Cherry juice is required to contain not less than 1.0% of the

naturally occurring malic acid. The juice has a pH of between 3 and 4.

Cherry syrup is prepared by dissolving sucrose in the cherry juice with the aid of heat from a steam bath. The product is permitted to cool, and the foam and solids that float to the top and are composed of coagulated organic matter are removed. Then, a small volume of alcohol is added mainly to maintain the clarity of the product by preventing the separation of any alcohol-soluble but water-insoluble components on standing. Finally, sufficient purified water is added to prepare the prescribed volume of syrup.

Since 47.5 ml of cherry juice and 80 g of sucrose are used in the preparation of each 100 ml of syrup, the product is rather sweet and assumes much of the pleasantly tart and fruity flavor of the juice. Cherry syrup is employed as a flavored vehicle and is especially useful as a vehicle for drugs requiring an acid media.

Cherry syrup has the advantage over wild cherry syrup in that it does not contain tannins, which are present in the latter syrup and cause troublesome incompatibilities with a number of drugs, particularly iron salts and alkaloidal salts, that are frequently precipitated from aqueous solution if tannins are present.

Orange Syrup, NF

Orange syrup is prepared by dissolving sucrose in a saturated aqueous solution of orange oil, the latter being prepared by using sweet orange peel tincture as the source of the oil and talc as the distributing agent to increase the surface area of the oil, thus facilitating its dissolution in the purified water. Sweet orange peel tincture is an alcoholic solution of the aromatic principles extracted from the outer rind of the non-artificially colored fresh, ripe fruit of *Citrus sinensis.* When the tincture-talc mixture is added to the purified water, some of the poorly and slowly soluble oil separates from solution. However, upon standing and with agitation the purified water soon becomes saturated, and the excess oil is filtered out along with the talc. The final product, which also contains added citric acid to impart a tart taste resembling orange juice, has between 2 to 5% of alcohol to stabilize it. Heat must be avoided in the preparation of this syrup, since the orange oil and the alcohol are volatile.

This syrup, which is employed as a flavored vehicle, must not be used if it is has a terebinthine odor or taste or shows other signs of deterioration.

Percolation

In the percolation method, either sucrose may be percolated to prepare the syrup, or the source of the medicinal component may be percolated to form an extractive to which sucrose or syrup may be added. This latter method really is two procedures: first the preparation of the fluidextract of the drug and then the preparation of the syrup. As such, it may be just as appropriately classified under the addition method discussed on page 129.

In the preparation of a syrup by the percolation of sucrose, purified water or an aqueous solution of a medicating or flavoring liquid is allowed to pass slowly through a column of crystalline sucrose to dissolve it. The percolate is collected and returned to the percolator as required until all of the sucrose has been dissolved.

For percolation either a cylindrical or a cone-shaped percolator may be employed. Generally a coarsely granulated sucrose rather than finely granulated or powdered sucrose is used in order to prevent the column of sugar from being packed too tightly, in which case the solvent would be unable to permeate the column and dissolve the sugar. A pledget of cotton is placed at the base of the column firmly enough to prevent the undissolved sugar from passing into the lower orifice yet loosely enough to permit the free passage of the dissolved sucrose. The flow of the percolate may be adjusted by regulating the stopcock at the orifice. When all of the sucrose has dissolved, additional purified water or the required aqueous liquid is passed over the cotton in the percolator to wash the remainder of the syrup from the impregnated cotton into the percolate and to bring the final product to the required volume. Syrup, USP, and Tolu Balsam Syrup, NF, may be prepared in this manner.

Tolu Balsam Syrup, NF

Tolu Balsam Syrup, NF, may be prepared by either of two methods: (1) by triturating tolu balsam tincture with magnesium carbonate and a portion of the required amount of sucrose, adding purified water with continued stirring, filtering the mixture until clear, dissolving the remainder of the sucrose in the filtrate with gentle heating, straining the syrup while warm, and adding sufficient purified water through the strainer to make the required volume of product; or (2) instead of using heat to dissolve the remaining portion of sucrose, the sucrose may be packed in a suitable percolator, and the filtrate (as prepared above) may be poured upon the sucrose and the percolate collected, returning it to the percolator as necessary until all of the sucrose has dissolved and sufficient purified water has passed through the percolator to wash the cotton of its sucrose and make the product the required volume.

Tolu balsam tincture is an alcoholic preparation containing the alcohol-soluble components of tolu balsam, a brown or yellow-brown plastic solid balsam obtained from *Myroxylon balsamum*. If this tincture were added directly to purified water, it would precipitate into a sticky mass that could not be induced to enter into aqueous solution. By distributing the tincture throughout the magnesium carbonate and sucrose, a maximum surface area is exposed for solution by the water. Further, the magnesium carbonate, because of its alkalinity, converts the benzoic and cinnamic acids present in the balsam to their more soluble salts and renders some of the resins soluble by saponifying them. The sucrose in the original mixture also assists in the solubility of the resins, thereby ensuring a more concentrated syrup. All of the sucrose is not added initially because of the high viscosity that would make the filtration and the removal of the magnesium carbonate extremely difficult. The use of heat in the first process may result in some loss of volatile constituents, particularly if heat over 50°C is used. To avoid the use of heat, the second process may be employed. It has the disadvantage of being the slower of the two methods.

Tolu balsam syrup is a flavored vehicle. It is also claimed to possess expectorant properties.

If a vegetable drug, rather than sucrose, is to be extracted by percolation, it is ground into uniform particles that are neither too fine to cause caking or plugging nor too coarse to permit the menstruum to flow too freely past them. The drug is premoistened with a portion of the menstruum and packed firmly and evenly in the percolator to permit uniform passage of the extracting menstruum.[1] To the percolate may be added the sucrose or simple syrup to prepare the

[1] The process of percolation of drugs will be discussed at greater length in Chapter 7.

final product. Ipecac Syrup, USP is prepared in this manner.

Ipecac Syrup, USP

Ipecac syrup is prepared from powdered ipecac, with glycerin being added as an auxiliary solvent and stabilizer and syrup being used as the vehicle. The drug ipecac consists of the dried rhizome and roots of *Cephaëlis ipecacuanha* and contains the medicinally active alkaloids, emetine, cephaeline, and psychotrine. These alkaloids are extracted from the powdered ipecac by percolation with a hydroalcoholic menstruum. Plant resins are also extracted in the percolate and are removed by exposing them to large volumes of water in which they are insoluble and precipitate. The alkaloids are converted to their water-soluble hydrochloride salts by the addition of hydrochloric acid. Glycerin is added to the liquid extract as an auxiliary solvent which has the ability to maintain the stability of the final product by preventing the separation of certain plant components after the percolate is added to the syrup and upon standing during the shelf life. The final syrup is assayed for its alkaloidal content and is required to contain between 123 and 157 mg of ether-soluble alkaloids of ipecac for each 100 ml of syrup. If the syrup were prepared from an already standardized ipecac fluidextract, no such assay for the syrup would be required. However, ipecac fluidextract is no longer an official product, and thus the syrup must bear the assay requirement.

The syrup is categorized as an emetic with a usual dose of 15 ml. This amount of syrup is commonly used in the management of poisoning in children when the evacuation of the stomach contents is desirable. About 80% of children given this dose will vomit within a half hour. For a household emetic in event of poisoning, 1-oz. bottles of the syrup may be sold without the requirement of a prescription. Ipecac syrup must not be confused with ipecac fluidextract which has a dose of about 0.5 to 1.0 ml. Ipecac syrup also has some application as a nauseant expectorant, in doses smaller than the emetic dose.

For many of the official syrups there is no officially designated method for their preparation. This is due to the fact that most of the official syrups are available on a commercial basis and are not prepared extemporaneously by the pharmacist.

Elixirs

Elixirs are clear, sweetened, hydroalcoholic solutions intended for oral use, and are usually flavored to enhance their palatability. *Nonmedicated* elixirs are employed as vehicles and *medicated* elixirs for the therapeutic effect of the medicinal substances they contain. Compared to syrups, elixirs are usually less sweet and less viscous since they contain a lower proportion of sugar and consequently less effective than syrups in masking the taste of medicinal substances. However, because of their hydroalcoholic character, elixirs are better able than the aqueous syrups to maintain both water-soluble and alcohol-soluble components in solution. Also because of their stability characteristics and the ease with which they are prepared (by simple solution), from a manufacturing standpoint, elixirs are preferred over syrups.

The proportion of alcohol present in elixirs varies widely since the individual components of the elixirs have different water and alcohol solubility characteristics. Each elixir requires a specific blend of alcohol and water to maintain all of the components in solution. Naturally, for those elixirs containing agents which have poor water-solubility the proportion of alcohol required is greater than for elixirs prepared from components having good water solubility. Among the medicated elixirs presently official, the alcoholic strengths vary from a low of 3% in Brompheniramine Maleate Elixir, NF to a high of 41% in Terpin Hydrate Elixir, NF. Most of the official medicated elixirs contain between 5 and 15% alcohol. One nonmedicated elixir, High Alcoholic Elixir, NF contains 75% alcohol; however, it is used after mixing with Low Alcoholic Elixir, NF, containing 9% alcohol, to prepare an Iso-Alcoholic Elixir, NF of intermediate alcoholic strength which is used as a vehicle or elixir diluent. This preparation will be discussed in greater detail later in this section. In addition to alcohol and water, other solvents, as glycerin and propylene glycol, are frequently employed in elixirs as adjunct solvents.

Although many elixirs are sweetened with sucrose or with a sucrose-syrup, some utilize sorbitol, glycerin and/or artificial sweeteners as saccharin for this purpose. Elixirs having a high alcoholic content usually utilize an artificial sweetener as saccharin, which because of its great sweetness is required only in small amounts, rather than sucrose which is only slightly soluble in alcohol and requires greater quantities for equivalent sweetness.

All of the official elixirs for which formulas are indicated in the compendia have one or more flavoring materials to increase the palatability of the preparation. In addition most elixirs have coloring agents in their formulas to enhance their appearance. Elixirs containing volatile oils and perhaps over 10 to 12% of alcohol are usually self-preserving and do not require the addition of an antimicrobial agent for their preservation. In each instance an appropriate shelf-life study will reveal the stability characteristics of an elixir formulation. Since elixirs contain alcohol and usually some volatile oils that deteriorate in the presence of air and light, they are best stored in tight, light-resistant containers protected against extremes of temperature.

Medicated elixirs are formulated such that a patient receives the usual adult dose of the drug in a convenient measure of elixir. For most elixirs, one or two teaspoonfuls (5 or 10 ml) provide the usual adult dose of the drug. Table 4-7 presents the official medicated elixirs and shows the amounts of the various elixirs required to provide the usual adult dose of the related drugs. One advantage of elixirs over their counterpart drugs in solid dosage forms is the flexibility and ease of dosage administration, particularly to children. A parent can administer a half-teaspoonful of medication, for instance, to a child with much greater ease than would be required by the breaking of a corresponding tablet or by separating and dividing a capsule of medication. In instances in which elixir medication is intended for children, commercial packages often contain a calibrated measuring device, as a dropper or spoon, to enable the parent to measure the medication accurately according to the amounts recommended for the child's age, weight, or condition.

Preparation of Elixirs

Elixirs are usually prepared by simple solution with agitation and/or by the admixture of two or more liquid ingredients. Alcohol-soluble and water-soluble components are generally dissolved separately in alcohol and in purified water, respectively. Then the aqueous solution is added to the alcoholic solution, rather than the reverse, in order to maintain the highest possible alcoholic strength at all times so that minimal separation of the alcohol-soluble com-

ponents occurs. When the two solutions are completely mixed the mixture is made to volume with the specified solvent or vehicle. Frequently the final mixture will not be clear, but cloudy, due principally to the separation of some of the flavoring oils by the reduced alcoholic concentration. If this occurs, the elixir is usually permitted to stand for a prescribed number of hours, to ensure the saturation of the hydroalcoholic solvent and to permit the oil globules to coalesce so that they may be more easily removed by filtration. Talc, a frequent filter aid in the preparation of elixirs, has the ability to absorb the excessive amounts of oils and therefore assist in their removal from the solution. Care must be exercised not to employ an excessive amount of a filter aid, as an excess might result in the excessive removal of oils and colorants from solution and also in the increased filtration time required to achieve clarity. Only one official elixir specifies the filter aid and the amount to be employed. Aromatic Elixir, USP, includes 3% of talc in its official formula as an aid to filtration. It should be remembered that the alcoholic content of each of the elixirs is of great importance to the continued solubility of its ingredients, and thus during the filtration process, the filter paper should be wetted with a hydroalcoholic solution having the same alcoholic strength as the elixir being filtered, and the filter and collection flask should either be rinsed with the same alcoholic solution or should be employed dry. The presence of glycerin, syrup, sorbitol, and propylene glycol in elixirs generally contributes to the solvent effect of the hydroalcoholic vehicle, assists in the dissolution of the solute, and enhances the stability of the preparation. However, the presence of these materials adds to the viscosity of the elixir and slows the rate of their filtration.

Nonmedicated Elixirs

The only presently official nonmedicated elixirs are Aromatic Elixir, USP, Compound Benzaldehyde Elixir, NF, and Iso-Alcoholic Elixir, NF. Nonmedicated elixirs are useful to the pharmacist in the extemporaneous filling of prescriptions involving: (1) the addition of a therapeutic agent to a pleasant tasting vehicle, and (2) the dilution of an existing medicated elixir. In selecting a liquid vehicle for a drug substance, the pharmacist concerns himself with the solubility and stability of the drug

Table 4-7. OFFICIAL MEDICATED ELIXIRS BY CATEGORY

Official Elixir	Some Representative Commercial Products	Usual Adult Dose of Drug/Volume of Official or Commercial Elixir	Comments
Adrenocortical Steroid			
Dexamethasone Elixir, USP	Decadron Elixir (Merck Sharpe & Dohme)	500 μg/5 ml	Dexamethasone is a synthetic analogue of hydrocortisone that is considered to be about 30 times more potent than the latter drug. The commercial dexamethasone elixir is packaged with a calibrated dropper for the accurate measurement of small doses and is intended primarily for children, but also has utility for adults who may have trouble swallowing tablets. The elixir is used for many indications, including the treatment of rheumatoid arthritis, skin diseases, allergies and inflammatory conditions.
Analgesic/Antipyretic			
Acetaminophen Elixir, USP	Tylenol Elixir (McNeil)	300 mg/10 ml	Use for reduction of pain and lowering of fever particularly in patients sensitive to or unable to take aspirin. Elixir especially useful for pediatric patients.
Antibacterial (Urinary)			
Methenamine Elixir, NF	Uritone Elixir (Parke Davis)	880 mg/10 ml	Urinary tract antiseptic which acts by liberating formaldehyde in an acid urine.
Anticholinergic			
Homatropine Methylbromide Elixir, NF	Mesopin Elixir (Endo)	5 mg/5 ml	Used as adjunctive therapy in peptic ulcer, spastic and irritable colon, mucous colitis and other gastrointestinal disorders requiring a reduction of spasms and hyperactivity.
Antihistamines			
Bromodiphenhydramine HCl Elixir, NF	Ambodryl HCl Elixir (Parke Davis)	25 mg/10 ml	These elixirs are employed for a variety of allergic reactions including: perennial and seasonal allergic rhinitis, vasomotor rhinitis, allergic skin manifestations of urticaria, reactions to insect bites, and others.
Brompheniramine Maleate Elixir, NF	Dimetane Elixir (Robins)	4 mg/10 ml	
Carbinoxamine Maleate Elixir, NF	Clistin Elixir (McNeil)	4 mg/5 ml	
Diphenhydramine HCl Elixir, USP	Benadryl Elixir (Parke Davis)	25 mg/10 ml	
Tripelennamine Citrate Elixir, USP	Pyribenzamine Elixir (Ciba)	25 mg/5 ml	

Table 4-7. OFFICIAL MEDICATED ELIXIRS BY CATEGORY (*Cont.*)

Official Elixir	Some Representative Commercial Products	Usual Adult Dose of Drug/Volume of Official or Commercial Elixir	Comments
Antiparkinsonian			
Trihexyphenidyl HCl Elixir, USP	Artane Elixir (Lederle)	2 mg/5 ml	Has a potent antispasmodic effect on smooth muscles with therapeutic effect similar to atropine. Used as an adjunct in management of parkinsonism.
Antipsychotic			
Fluphenazine HCl Elixir, USP	Prolixin Elixir (Squibb)	2.5 mg/5 ml	Used in the management of psychotic disorders.
Bronchodilator			
Oxtriphylline Elixir, NF	Choledyl Elixir (Warner-Chilcott)	200 mg/10 ml	Used in treatment of bronchial asthma and in other conditions requiring bronchodilation.
Cardiotonic			
Digoxin Elixir, USP	Lanoxin Pediatric Elixir (Burroughs Wellcome)	50 μg/ml	Among other effects, digoxin increases the force of myocardial contraction. Used in congestive heart failure, atrial fibrillation and other cardiac conditions. See text for additional discussion.
Central Stimulant			
Dextroamphetamine Sulfate Elixir, USP	Dexedrine Elixir (Smith Kline & French)	5 mg/5 ml	Used in instances of narcolepsy, hyperkinesia, and exogenous obesity.
Electrolyte Replenisher			
Potassium Gluconate Elixir, NF	Kaon Elixir (Warren-Teed)	20 mEq K (782 mg)/15 ml	Used for the prevention and treatment of hypokalemia which may occur secondary to diuretic or corticosteroid administration. Elixir is mixed with water prior to taking.
Expectorants			
Terpin Hydrate Elixir, NF	—	170 mg/10 ml	
Terpin Hydrate and Codeine Elixir, NF	—	170 mg terpin hydrate and 20 mg codeine/10 ml	Terpin hydrate has expectorant action. The addition of codeine and dextromethorphan provides antitussive action as well. See text for additional discussion.
Terpin Hydrate and Dextromethorphan HBr Elixir, NF	—	170 mg terpin hydrate and 20 mg dextromethorphan HBr/10 ml	

Table 4-7. OFFICIAL MEDICATED ELIXIRS BY CATEGORY (*Cont.*)

Official Elixir	Some Representative Commercial Products	Usual Adult Dose of Drug/Volume of Official or Commercial Elixir	Comments
Sedative/Hypnotics			
Amobarbital Elixir, NF	Amytal Elixir (Lilly)	22 mg/5 ml	
Butabarbital Sodium Elixir, NF	Butisol Sodium Elixir (McNeil)	30 mg/5 ml	
Pentobarbital Elixir, NF	Nembutal Elixir (Abbott)	18 mg/5 ml	The barbiturate elixirs are utilized in low dosage as sedatives and in higher dosage as hypnotics. See text for additional discussion.
Pentobarbital Sodium Elixir, USP	—	20 mg/5 ml	
Phenobarbital Elixir, USP	—	20 mg/5 ml	
Secobarbital Elixir, USP	Seconal Elixir (Lilly)	22 mg/5 ml	
Smooth Muscle Relaxant			
Theophylline Sodium Glycinate Elixir, NF	Synophylate Elixir (Central)	330 mg/15 ml	Used in bronchial asthma and other conditions requiring smooth muscle relaxation; said to be less irritating to gastric mucosa than other forms of theophylline.

substance in water and alcohol. If a hydroalcoholic vehicle is selected, the proportion of alcohol present should be only slightly above that amount which is needed to effect and maintain the drug's solution. When a pharmacist is called upon to dilute an existing medicated elixir, the nonmedicated elixir he selects as the diluent should have the approximate alcoholic concentration as the elixir being diluted. Also, the flavor and color characteristics of the diluent should not be in conflict with the medicated elixir and all components should be chemically and physically compatible.

Aromatic Elixir, USP

Aromatic Elixir, USP, is probably the most widely used of all of the nonmedicated elixirs. Because of its attractive taste, provided by compound orange spirit and syrup, it is employed as the main vehicle in other elixirs. One feature of aromatic elixir not true for many other elixirs is that it may be diluted with water or with an aqueous solution without becoming turbid due to the separation of solute. The elixir is therefore a versatile vehicle for the pharmacist in his extemporaneous compounding of prescriptions requiring a pleasant tasting hydroalcoholic ve-

hicle to be incorporated with an aqueous solution.

Aromatic elixir is prepared by mixing the compound orange spirit with the required alcohol, adding the syrup gradually with agitation, and then adding enough purified water to prepare the proper volume of product. Some of the oils from the compound orange spirit become separated from solution, and talc is added to the mixture in an effort to absorb the separated oils and to act as a filter aid. The time required to filter this elixir is quite lengthy when the product is prepared on a small scale, as it would be in a pharmacy, due to the viscosity of the elixir caused by the presence of the syrup. It is not considered unusual for a pharmacist to lose over 10% of his product during the process of filtration, as the filtrate must be returned to the filter several times in order to achieve clarity. The viscous elixir is lost because it adheres to the container in which it was prepared, on the filter paper, and on the filter itself. Since the product is made to volume with purified water prior to the filtration process, no additional water may be added to the filtrate to restore the volume, since more water would alter the required concentration of each of the ingredients. Before the elixir is filtered, all glassware should be dried, and the filter paper should be wetted with diluted alcohol. If water were used to wet the filter paper, further separation of oils from the elixir would probably occur as the first portion of elixir contacted the wet paper.

Pharmacists generally purchase aromatic elixir as they require it from large pharmaceutical manufacturers who employ more efficient filtration apparatus to achieve the desired clarity.

Compound Benzaldehyde Elixir, NF

Compound Benzaldehyde Elixir, NF, is a nonmedicated elixir, flavored with vanillin, orange flower water, and benzaldehyde, the latter agent imparting an almond-like odor and taste to the preparation. A small amount of alcohol is present to dissolve the vanillin and the benzaldehyde, and syrup is added for sweetness.

The elixir is used as a flavored vehicle.

Iso-Alcoholic Elixir, NF

Under the monograph for iso-alcoholic elixir, the NF contains two separate formulas: one for a "Low-Alcoholic Elixir" and the other for a "High-Alcoholic Elixir." Each is flavored with compound orange spirit and contains glycerin. The low-alcoholic elixir contains between 8 and 10% alcohol and is prepared by combining the alcohol glycerin, purified water, and compound orange spirit, allowing the mixture to stand for 24 hours to ensure the saturation of the mixture with the oils and the separation and coalescing of the excess oils, then filtering until clear, dissolving sucrose in the filtrate by agitation or percolation, and making the product to volume with additional purified water. The high-alcoholic elixir, which contains between 73 and 78% of alcohol, is prepared by dissolving the compound orange spirit and saccharin, the sweetening agent, in alcohol, adding the glycerin and sufficient additional alcohol to make the required volume, mixing thoroughly, and then filtering. Because of the high alcoholic content of the latter elixir, it is impossible to dissolve an appreciable amount of sucrose; thus, saccharin, which is sufficiently alcohol-soluble, is employed as the sweetening agent.

Iso-Alcohol Elixir, NF, is intended to serve as a general vehicle for medicinal substances which, because of their nature, require a solvent of a specific alcoholic strength. In such instances, the two elixirs are combined in a proportion that yields the required alcoholic strength. If iso-alcoholic elixir is used to dilute another liquid preparation, the strength of the iso-alcoholic elixir is adjusted to be the same as that of the liquid being diluted. For instance, if phenobarbital elixir is to be diluted with iso-alcoholic elixir, the alcoholic strength of the latter should be adjusted to about 12 to 15%, the alcoholic content of the phenobarbital elixir, by combining the high- and the low-alcoholic elixirs in the proper proportion (in this example, 1 ml of the high-alcoholic elixir added to each 10 ml of the low-alcoholic elixir would produce an iso-alcoholic elixir of about 15% alcoholic strength). Table 4-8 presents examples of the proportions of low-alcoholic and high-alcoholic elixirs which may be mixed in preparing iso-alcoholic elixirs of various alcoholic strengths. The method by which such calculations are made is termed "alligation alternate," and the student may wish to refer to a text on pharmaceutical calculations to familiarize himself with this type of calculation.

Medicated Elixirs

As noted previously, medicated elixirs are employed for the therapeutic benefit of the medicinal agent present. In most instances, the official and commercial elixirs contain a single therapeutic agent. However, there are exceptions, as Terpin Hydrate and Codeine Elixir, NF, which contains the two therapeutic agents mentioned in the title of the elixir. The main advantage of having only a single therapeutic agent present is that the dosage taken of that single drug may be increased or decreased by simply taking more or less of the elixir, whereas when two or more therapeutic agents are present in the same preparation, it is impossible to increase or decrease the amount taken of one without an automatic and corresponding adjustment in the dose taken of the other; a change which may not be desired. Thus, for patients required to take more than a single medication, many physicians prefer them to take separate preparations of each drug so that if an adjustment in the dosage of one is desired, it may be accomplished without the concomitant adjustment of the other.

Table 4-7 presents the official medicated elixirs. It is easily seen that although a variety

Table 4-8. Examples of the Mix Proportions of Low-Alcoholic
and High-Alcoholic Elixirs Utilized in the Preparation
of Iso-alcoholic Elixirs of Various Alcoholic Concentrations

Desired Alcoholic Strength of Iso-Alcoholic Elixir %	Approximate ml of Low-Alcoholic Elixir (9% Alcohol) Used to Prepare each 100 ml of Iso-Alcoholic Elixir	Approximate ml of High-Alcoholic Elixir (75% Alcohol) Used to Prepare Each 100 ml of Iso-Alcoholic Elixir
10	98*	2
20	83	17
30	68	32
40	53	47
50	38	62
60	23	77
70	7	93

* For practical purposes, unaltered Low-Alcoholic Elixir would suffice. The NF states that
Low-Alcoholic Elixir contains between 8.0 and 10.0% alcohol.

of therapeutic categories of drugs are official in elixir form, the antihistamine and the sedative/hypnotic elixirs predominate.

Antihistamine Elixirs

As indicated in Table 4-7, antihistamines are useful primarily in the symptomatic relief of certain allergic disorders. In their action, they suppress symptoms caused by histamine, one of the chemical agents released during the antigen-antibody reaction of the allergic response. Although only minor differences exist in the properties of most antihistamines, one or another may be preferred by a prescriber through his experience in managing a specific type of allergic reaction. A prescriber's preference may also be based on the incidence of adverse effects which may be expected to occur. The incidence and severity of these effects do vary somewhat with the drug and the dose of each drug. The most common untoward effect is sedation, and patients taking antihistamines should be warned against engaging in activities requiring mental alertness, as driving an automobile or tractor or operating machinery. Other common adverse effects include dryness of the nose, throat, and mouth, dizziness and disturbed concentration. Included among the most sedating antihistamines are diphenhydramine, doxylamine, and methapyrilene. The latter agent is commonly found in popular over-the-counter preparations promoted as agents to overcome insomnia.

Most antihistaminic agents are basic amines. By forming salts through interaction with acid, the compounds are rendered water soluble. These salt forms are generally used in elixirs and thus the elixirs of the antihistamines are not required to contain a large proportion of alcohol. Since the acid salts of the antihistamines are used, the pH of these elixirs is on the acid side and must remain so if the drugs are to remain freely soluble in water. A pharmacist should keep this in mind when utilizing one of these elixirs in the compounding of a prescription involving adding or mixing other components.

Barbiturate Sedative/Hypnotic Elixirs

The barbiturates are sedative/hypnotic agents which are used to produce various degrees of central nervous system depression. As the dose of these drugs is increased, the effects go from sedation to hypnosis to respiratory depression, the latter being the cause of death in fatal barbiturate overdosage.

Barbiturates are administered in small doses in the daytime hours as sedatives to reduce restlessness and emotional tension. The appropriate dose for this purpose is that amount which alleviates anxiety or tension but does not produce drowsiness or lethargy. Greater doses of the barbiturates may be given before bedtime as hypnotics to relieve insomnia.

Barbiturates have been classified according to the duration of their (hypnotic) effects; that is, *long-acting, intermediate-acting, short-acting,* or *ultrashort-acting* agents. The long-acting barbiturates including phenobarbital are considered most useful in maintaining daytime sedation and in treating some convulsive states and least useful in acting as hypnotics. The intermediate-acting barbiturates include amobarbital and are used primarily for short-term daytime sedation and are effective in treating insomnia. The barbiturates classified as short-acting include pentobarbital and secobarbital and are used similarly to the intermediate-acting barbiturates. The ultrashort-acting barbiturates, as thiopental, are given intravenously to induce anesthesia.

The most common untoward effect noticed in patients taking barbiturates is drowsiness and lethargy. Large doses may produce residual sedation resembling the hangover following alcohol intoxication. Prolonged use of barbiturates may lead to psychic or physical dependence. This dependence, in susceptible individuals, leads to compulsive abuse of the drug with severe withdrawal symptoms following abstinence. In heavy chronic users, abrupt withdrawal may lead to convulsions, delirium, and occasionally to coma and death.

Some pharmaceutic aspects of Phenobarbital Elixir, USP, Pentobarbital Sodium Elixir, USP, and Secobarbital Elixir, USP are presented below.

Phenobarbital Elixir, USP

Phenobarbital elixir is probably the most used of all of the medicated elixirs. It is required to contain about 0.4% of phenobarbital, which provides about 20 mg of drug per teaspoonful of elixir. The elixir is pleasantly flavored by orange oil, colored red with an FDA-approved colorant, and sweetened with syrup. The elixir contains about 14% of alcohol, which is used to dissolve the phenobarbital. However, this amount represents almost the very minimum required to keep the phenobarbital in solution. Although 45% of glycerin is added to enhance the solubility of phenobarbital in the alcohol, the addition of water or an aqueous solution or an alcoholic solution of lower strength to the elixir may result in the precipitation of some of the phenobarbital.

Phenobarbital is a long-acting barbiturate with a duration of action of about 4 to 6 hours and a usual adult dose as a sedative of about 30 mg and a hypnotic dose of about 100 mg. The strength of the elixir permits the convenient adjustment of dosage to achieve the proper degree of sedation in the treatment of infants, children, and certain adult patients.

The elixir is commercially available from a variety of manufacturers under its nonproprietary name.

Secobarbital Elixir, USP

The USP does not specify directions for the preparation of secobarbital elixir; however, both the official elixir and its commercial counterpart contain about 440 mg of secobarbital in each 100 ml of elixir.

Secobarbital is a short-acting barbiturate employed primarily as a hypnotic administered at bedtime. Its pharmacologic effects are induced within a short period after oral administration, usually between 15 and 30 minutes, and last for a rather short duration, between 2 and 4 hours. The short duration of action makes this barbiturate attractive to many and of an advantage over the longer acting barbiturates, which because of their duration of action produce barbiturate "hangover" or postsomnial lassitude the next morning. As a hypnotic, the usual adult dose of secobarbital is about 100 mg. About half the hypnotic dose may be employed as a sedative.

The commercial product [Seconal Elixir (Lilly)] employs 12% of alcohol along with purified water and glycerin as the vehicle.

Pentobarbital Sodium Elixir, USP

Pentobarbital Sodium Elixir, USP, contains about 400 mg of sodium pentobarbital in each 100 ml of product. Aqueous solutions of pentobarbital sodium, like aqueous solutions of other barbiturate salts, are not stable but decompose on standing. In the preparation of this elixir, the sodium salt of pentobarbital is employed for its ease of solution in purified water and not for its permanency, for after being dissolved and the required amounts of alcohol, glycerin, syrup, orange oil, and caramel added, the pentobarbital sodium is converted to the alcohol-soluble pentobarbital base by the addition to the mixture of a small amount of diluted hydrochloric acid. The elixir is more readily prepared by this method than by using pentobarbital base directly.

Pentobarbital is a short-acting barbiturate used primarily as a hypnotic with an oral dose of about 100 mg, taken at bedtime.

Terpin Hydrate Elixirs

As indicated in Table 4-7, there are three terpin hydrate elixirs, Terpin Hydrate Elixir, NF, Terpin Hydrate Elixir with Codeine, NF, and Terpin Hydrate Elixir with Dextromethorphan Hydrobromide, NF. The latter two are solutions of the antitussive agents codeine and dextromethorphan HBr respectively in Terpin Hydrate Elixir, NF. Codeine is a narcotic antitussive agent, whereas dextromethorphan hydrobromide is a nonnarcotic antitussive agent. Each is effective in blocking the coughing reflex. Elixir Terpin Hydrate with Codeine is commonly referred to as "ETH&C."

Terpin Hydrate Elixir, NF represents an elixir that contains as the therapeutic agent a material that has a low water solubility but a high alcohol solubility. Therefore, the elixir requires a rather high final alcoholic strength (39 to 44%) and is prepared with an "order of mixing" of the components that assures the highest possible alcoholic content throughout its preparation. This is accomplished by delaying to the end, the addition of components having substantial proportions of water. The formula for the elixir is as follows:

Terpin Hydrate . . . . 17 g
Sweet Orange Peel Tincture . . . . 20 ml
Benzaldehyde . . . . 50 μl
Glycerin . . . . 400 ml
Alcohol . . . . 430 ml
Syrup . . . . 100 ml

Purified Water, a sufficient
    quantity, to make . . . . 1000 ml

The terpin hydrate is first dissolved in the alcohol, and the sweet orange peel tincture, which contains 67% alcohol, is added next. Then comes the benzaldehyde, glycerin, and syrup in that order, and finally the purified water. Because the elixir is composed of 40% of glycerin and 10% of syrup, it is quite viscous. Terpin hydrate elixir and its companion elixirs are not miscible with water, as the alcohol-soluble components separate.

Terpin hydrate is categorized as an expectorant, with an effective dose considered to be about 125 to 300 mg.

Digoxin Elixir, USP

No official method of preparation is indicated for Digoxin Elixir, USP; however, it is required to contain about 5 mg of digoxin per 100 ml of elixir or about 0.25 mg per teaspoonful. The usual oral adult dose of digoxin as a cardiotonic agent is about 1.5 mg on initial therapy and about 0.5 mg for maintenance therapy.

Digoxin is a cardiotonic glycoside obtained from the leaves of *Digitalis lanata*. It is a white crystalline powder that is insoluble in water, but soluble in dilute alcohol solutions. The official elixir contains about 10% of alcohol. Digoxin is a poisonous drug, and its dose must be carefully determined and administered to each individual patient. Adults generally take digoxin tablets rather than the elixir, which must be measured by the highly variable household teaspoon. The elixir is generally employed in pediatric practice, and the commercial product available for this purpose is packaged with a calibrated dropper to facilitate accurate dosage measurements.

Digoxin is one of many drugs which is available to the prescriber in more than a single type of dosage form. The prescriber frequently has the choice of selecting a solid dosage form, as a tablet or capsule, or a liquid form of the medication for his patient. The advantages of each have been noted in the previous chapter, but it is important here to point out again that drugs administered in different dosage forms may exhibit different bioavailability characteristics with varying patterns of drug release and rates and extents of drug absorption. Such differences have been noted for digoxin, between tablets from different manufacturers, as well as between tablets and oral liquid dosage forms.[1-3] Figure 4-1 shows the differences noted in one study of the serum digoxin levels following administration of 0.5 mg of digoxin by oral tablet and oral solution having an elixir-like vehicle. It can be readily seen that the serum digoxin levels following administration of the oral solution were considerably greater than from the oral tablet.

[1] Huffman, D. H. and Azarnoff, D. L., "Absorption of Orally Given Digoxin Preparations," *J.A.M.A*, 222:957–960, 1972.
[2] Lindenbaum, J., *et al.*, "Variation in Biologic Availability of Digoxin from Four Preparations," *New Engl. J. Med.* 285:1344–1347, 1971.
[3] Wagner, J., *et al.*, "Equivalence Lack in Digoxin Plasma Levels," *J.A.M.A.*, 224:199–204, 1973.

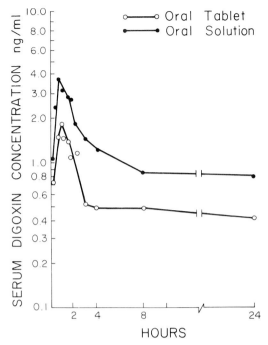

Fig. 4-1. *Serum digoxin concentrations following administration of 0.5 mg of digoxin by oral tablet and elixir-like oral solution. (Adapted from D. H. Huffman and D. L. Azarnoff: Absorption of Orally Given Digoxin Preparations, J.A.M.A., 222:957, 1972.)*

A patient taking a drug known to exhibit bioavailability problems, and whose therapeutic dosage regimen has been successfully established with a particular drug product, should not be changed to another product. It is the responsibility of health professionals to be familiar with drugs and drug products exhibiting bioavailability differences and to protect the patient from problems relating thereto. In most instances, problems with bioavailability exists among the solid dosage forms or suspension types of products rather than with the solution forms. Absorption from pharmaceutical solutions, including the elixirs, generally occurs satisfactorily. The bioavailability problems occurring with digoxin have been largely with the tablets and recent action by the Food and Drug Administration assuring that all currently marketed digoxin tablets meet the USP standards for tablet dissolution have been fruitful.[1] Among the other drugs and dosage forms identified by the FDA as exhibiting bioavailability problems are the following:[2] acetazolamide (tablets); acetylsalicylic acid (tablets and enteric coated tablets); ampicillin trihydrate (capsules); chloramphenicol (capsules); diphenylhydantoin (pediatric suspension); nitrofurantoin (tablets); oxytetracycline (capsules); phenylbutazone (tablets); riboflavin (sugar coated tablets); tetracycline HCl (capsules); trisulfapyrimidine (pediatric suspension).[2]

Selected Reading

"AMA Drug Evaluations," 2nd Ed., Chicago, The American Medical Association, 1973.

Daoust, R. G., and Lynch, M. J.: Sorbitol in Pharmaceutical Liquids, *Drug Cosmetic Ind.*, 90:689, 1962.

Huyck, C. L., and Maxwell, J. L.: Diabetic Syrups, *J. Amer. Pharm. Assoc., Pract. Ed.*, 19:142, 1958.

[1]*FDA Drug Bulletin*, January, 1974.
[2]Weekly Pharmacy Reports, "The Green Sheet," 23, No. 8, February 25, 1974.

Chapter 5

Oral Suspensions, Emulsions, Magmas, and Gels

Largely because of their greater size, dispersed particles in a coarse dispersion have a greater tendency to separate from the dispersion medium than do the particles of a fine dispersion. Most solids in dispersion tend to settle to the bottom of the container because of their greater density than the dispersing medium, whereas most emulsified liquids for oral use are oils and generally have a lesser density than the aqueous medium in which they are dispersed and tend to rise toward the top of the preparation. Complete and uniform redistribution of the disperse phase is essential to the accurate administration of uniform doses. For a properly prepared dispersion, this should be accomplished by the moderate agitation of the container.

While the focus of this chapter is on dispersions of drugs administered orally, the same basic pharmaceutical characteristics apply to those disperse systems administered by other routes and discussed later in this text. Included among these are lotions for topical application to the skin, ophthalmic suspensions, and sterile suspensions for injection.

THIS CHAPTER includes the main types of liquid preparations containing undissolved drug distributed throughout a vehicle and intended for oral administration. In these preparations, the substance distributed is referred to as the *disperse* or *dispersed phase* and the vehicle is termed the *dispersing phase* or *dispersion medium.* For most oral preparations of this type, the dispersion medium is aqueous.

The particles of the disperse phase are usually solid materials which are insoluble in the dispersion medium. In the case of emulsions, the disperse phase is a liquid substance which is neither soluble nor miscible with the liquid of the dispersing phase. The emulsification process results in the dispersion of liquid drug as fine droplets throughout the dispersing phase.

The particles of the disperse phase vary widely in size, from large particles visible to the naked eye down to particles of colloidal dimension, falling between 1 millimicron (mμ) and about 500 millimicrons or 0.5 micron (μ) in size. Dispersions containing coarse particles, usually 1 to 100 microns in size, are referred to as *coarse dispersions* and include the *suspensions* and *emulsions.* Dispersions containing particles of smaller size are termed *fine dispersions*, and, if the particles are in the colloidal range, *colloidal dispersions. Magmas* and *gels* represent such fine dispersions.

Oral Suspensions

Suspensions may be defined as preparations containing finely divided drug particles (referred to as the *suspensoid*) distributed somewhat uniformly throughout a vehicle in which the drug exhibits a minimum degree of solubility. Some suspensions are official and commercially available in ready-to-use form—that is, already distributed through a liquid vehicle with or without stabilizers and other pharmaceutical additives. Figure 5-1 presents examples of some commercial oral suspensions. Other preparations are available as dry powders intended for suspension in liquid vehicles. This type of product generally is a powder mixture containing the drug and suitable suspending and dispersing agents, which upon dilution and agitation with a specified quantity of vehicle (generally purified water) results in the formation of a suspension suitable for administration. Figure 5-2 demonstrates the preparation of this type of product. Drugs that are unstable if maintained for extended periods of time in the presence of an aqueous vehicle (for example, many antibiotic drugs) are most frequently supplied as dry powder mixtures for reconstitution at the time

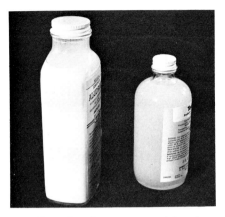

Fig. 5-1. *Examples of some commercial oral suspensions.*

of dispensing. This type of preparation is designated in the official compendia by a title of the form "... for Oral Suspension". Prepared suspensions not requiring reconstitution at the time of dispensing are simply designated as "... Oral Suspension."

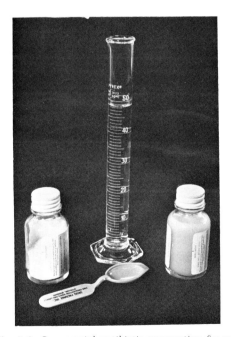

Fig. 5-2. *Commercial antibiotic preparation for oral suspension following reconstitution with purified water. On the left is the dry powder mixture, and on the right the suspension after reconstitution with the specified amount of purified water.*

Reasons for Oral Suspension

The reasons for having the oral suspension are several. For one thing, certain drugs are chemically unstable when in solution but stable when suspended. In instances such as this, the oral suspension insures chemical stability while permitting liquid therapy. For many patients, the liquid form is preferred over the solid form (tablets or capsules) of the same drug because of the ease of swallowing liquids, the flexibility in the administration of doses, the greater convenience in the administration of unusually large doses, and the safety and convenience of liquid doses for infants and children. The disadvantage of the disagreeable taste of certain drugs when given in solution form is negligible when the drug is administered as undissolved particles of a suspension. In fact, special chemical forms of certain poor tasting drugs have been specifically developed for their insolubility in a desired vehicle for the sole purpose of preparing a palatable liquid dosage form. For example, the water-insoluble ester form of chloramphenicol, chloramphenicol palmitate, was developed in order to prepare a palatable liquid dosage form of the chloramphenicol, the result being the development of Chloramphenicol Palmitate Oral Suspension, USP. By the creation of insoluble forms of drugs for use in suspensions, the difficult taste-masking problems of developmental pharmacists are greatly reduced, and the selection of the flavorants to be used in a given suspension may be based on taste preference rather than on a particular flavorant's ability to act as a masking agent for an unpleasant tasting drug. For the most part, oral suspensions are aqueous preparations with the vehicle flavored and sweetened to suit the anticipated taste preferences of the intended patient.

Features Desired in a Pharmaceutical Suspension

There are many considerations in the development and preparation of a pharmaceutically elegant suspension. In addition to therapeutic efficacy, chemical stability of the components of the formulation, permanency of the preparation, and esthetic appeal of the preparation—desirable qualities in all pharmaceutical preparations—a few other features apply more specifically in the pharmaceutical suspension:

1. A properly prepared pharmaceutical suspension should settle slowly and should be readily redispersed upon the gentle shaking of the container.
2. The characteristics of the suspension should be such that the particle size of the suspensoid remains fairly constant throughout long periods of undisturbed standing.
3. The suspension should pour readily and evenly from its container.

These main features of a suspension, which depend upon the nature of the dispersed phase, the dispersion medium, and pharmaceutical adjuncts, will be discussed briefly.

Sedimentation Rate of the Particles of a Suspension

The various factors involved in the rate of velocity of settling of the particles of a suspension are embodied in the equation of Stokes' law:

$$V = \frac{d^2(\rho_1 - \rho_2)g}{18\eta}$$

where V = the velocity of the fall of a spherical particle,

g = the gravitational constant,
d = the diameter of the sphere,
ρ_1 = the density of the sphere,
ρ_2 = the density of the liquid, and
η = the viscosity of the dispersion medium.

Stokes' equation was derived for an ideal situation in which uniform, perfectly spherical particles in a very dilute suspension settle without effecting turbulence in their downward course, without collision of the particles of the suspensoid, and without chemical or physical attraction or affinity for the dispersion medium. Obviously Stokes' equation does not apply precisely to the usual pharmaceutical suspension in which the suspensoid is irregularly shaped, of various particle diameters, and not spherical, in which the fall of the particles *does* result in both turbulence and collision, and also in which there may be a reasonable amount of affinity of the particles for the suspension medium. However, the basic concepts of the equation do give a valid indication of the factors that are important to the suspension of the particles and a clue to the possible adjustments that can be made to

a formulation to decrease the rate of particle sedimentation.

From the equation it is apparent that the velocity of fall of a suspended particle is greater for larger particles than it is for smaller particles, all other factors remaining constant. By reducing the particle size of the dispersed phase, one can expect a slower rate of descent of the particles. Also, the greater the density of the particles, the greater the rate of descent, provided the density of the vehicle is not altered. Since aqueous vehicles are generally used in pharmaceutical oral suspensions, the density of the particles is generally greater than that of the vehicle, a desirable feature, for if the particles were less dense than the vehicle, they would tend to float, and floating particles would be quite difficult to distribute uniformly in the vehicle. The rate of sedimentation may be appreciably reduced by increasing the viscosity of the dispersion medium, and within limits of practicality this may be done. However, a product having a high viscosity is not generally desirable, since it pours with difficulty and it is equally difficult to redisperse the suspensoid. Therefore, if the viscosity of a suspension is increased, it is done so only to a modest extent in order to avoid the aforementioned difficulties. For the most part, the physical stability of a pharmaceutical suspension appears to be most appropriately adjusted by an alteration in the dispersed phase rather than through great changes in the dispersion medium. In most instances, the dispersion medium is supportive to the adjusted dispersed phase. These adjustments mainly are concerned with particle size, uniformity of particle size, and separation of the particles so that they are not likely to become greatly larger or to form a solid cake on standing.

Physical Features of the Dispersed Phase of a Suspension

Probably the most important single consideration in a discussion of suspensions is the size of the drug particles.[1] In most good pharmaceutical suspensions, the particle diameter is between 1 and 50 microns.[2]

[1] The area of particle technology has come to be known as *micromeritics.*
[2] From a therapeutic standpoint, small particle size is perhaps of greater importance in the formulation of parenteral and ophthalmic suspensions than in the

Particle size reduction is generally accomplished by dry-milling prior to the incorporation of the dispersed phase into the dispersion medium. One of the most rapid, convenient, and inexpensive methods of producing fine drug powders of about 10 to 50 micron size is *micropulverization*. Micropulverizers are high-speed, attrition or impact mills which are efficient in reducing powders to the size acceptable for most oral and topical suspensions. For still finer particles, under 10 microns, the process of *fluid energy* grinding, sometimes referred to as *jet-milling* or *micronizing*, is quite effective. By this process, the shearing action of high velocity compressed air streams on the particles in a confined space produces the desired ultrafine or micronized particles. The particles to be micronized are swept into violent turbulence by the sonic and supersonic velocity of the air streams. The particles are accelerated into high velocities and collide with one another, resulting in fragmentation and a decrease in the size of the particles. This method may be employed in instances in which the particles are intended for parenteral or ophthalmic suspensions. Particles of extremely small dimensions may also be produced by *spray-drying* techniques. A spray dryer is a cone-shaped piece of apparatus into which a solution of a drug is sprayed and rapidly dried by a current of warmed, dry air circulating in the cone. The resulting dry powder is then collected. It is not possible for a community pharmacist to achieve the same degree of particle-size reduction with such simple comminuting equipment as the mortar and pestle. However, many micronized drugs are commercially available and when needed may be purchased by the pharmacist in bulk quantities.

As shown earlier, the reduction in the particle size of a suspensoid is beneficial to the stability of the suspension in that the rate of sedimentation of the solid particles is reduced as the particles are decreased in size. The reduction in particle size produces slow, more uniform rates of settling. However, one should avoid reducing the particle size to too great a degree of fineness, since fine particles have a tendency to form a compact cake upon settling to the bottom of the container. The result may be that the cake resists breakup upon shaking, and forms rigid aggregates of particles which are of larger dimension and less suspendable than the original suspensoid.

To avoid the formation of a cake, measures must be taken to prevent the agglomeration of the particles into larger crystals or into masses. One common method of preventing the rigid cohesion of small particles of a suspension is through the intentional formation of a less rigid or loose aggregation of the particles held together by comparatively weak particle-to-particle bonding forces. Such an aggregation of particles is termed a *floc* or a *floccule*, with flocculated particles forming a type of lattice structure that resists complete settling (although flocs settle more rapidly than fine, individual particles) and thus are less prone to compaction than unflocculated particles. The flocs settle to form a higher sediment volume than unflocculated particles, the loose structure of which permits the aggregates to break up easily and distribute readily with a small amount of agitation.

There are several methods of preparing flocculated suspensions, the choice depending on the type of drug involved and the type of product desired. For instance, in the preparation of an oral suspension of a drug, clays such as diluted bentonite magma are commonly employed as the flocculating agent. The structure of the bentonite magma and of other clays used for this purpose also assists the suspension by helping to support the floc once formed. When clays are unsuitable as agents, as in a parenteral suspension, frequently a floc of the dispersed phase can be produced by an alteration in the pH of the preparation (generally to the region of minimum drug solubility). Electrolytes can also act as flocculating agents, apparently by reducing the electrical barrier between the particles of the suspensoid and forming a bridge so as to link them together. The carefully determined concentration of nonionic and ionic surface-active agents (surfactants) can also induce the flocculation of particles in suspension and increase the sedimentation volume.

preparation of oral suspensions. In the injection of a suspension, drug particles below 10 microns in size are reported to produce considerably less pain and tissue irritation than drug particles of greater dimension. Also, a suspension intended for injection must have a reasonable "syringeability," that is, the ability to flow freely through the bore of the hypodermic needle. Ophthalmic suspensions are similarly less irritating to the tissues when the dispersed phase is finely divided. As mentioned in Chapter 3, drug particle size can have a bearing on the therapeutic efficacy or effectiveness of a drug preparation.

Dispersion Medium

Oftentimes, as with highly flocculated suspensions, the particles of a suspension settle too rapidly to be consistent with what might be termed a pharmaceutically elegant preparation. The rapid settling hinders the accurate measurement of dosage and from an esthetic point of view produces too unsightly a supernatant layer. In many of the commercial suspensions, suspending agents are added to the dispersion medium to lend it a structure to assist in the suspension of the dispersed phase. Carboxymethylcellulose, methylcellulose, and bentonite are a few of the agents employed to thicken the dispersion medium and help suspend the suspensoid. When polymeric substances and hydrophilic colloids are used as suspending agents, appropriate tests must be performed to show that the agent does not interfere with the availability for therapeutic effects of the suspension's medicinal substance. These materials have been found to bind certain medicinal agents, rendering them unavailable or more slowly available for their therapeutic function. Also, the amount of the suspending agent must not be such to render the suspension too viscous to agitate (to distribute the *suspensoid*) or to pour. The study of the flow characteristics is termed *rheology*.

Support of the suspensoid by the dispersion medium may depend upon several factors: the density of the suspensoid, whether it is flocculated, and the amount of material requiring support.

The solid content of a suspension intended for oral administration may vary considerably, depending on the dose of the drug to be administered, the volume of product desired to be administered, and also on the ability of the dispersion medium to support the concentration of drug while maintaining desirable features of viscosity and flow. The usual adult oral suspension is frequently designed to supply the dose of the particular drug in a convenient measure of 5 ml or one teaspoonful. Pediatric suspensions of many drugs intended for infant use are formulated to deliver the appropriate dose of drug by administering a relatively small number of drops, the amount usually determined by the body size and therapeutic requirements of the individual patient. Figure 5-3 shows commonly packaged oral suspensions administered as pediatric drops. Some are ac-

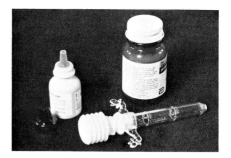

Fig. 5-3. *Examples of oral pediatric suspensions showing package designs of a built-in dropper device and a calibrated dropper accompanying the medication container.*

companied by a calibrated dropper, whereas other packages have the drop capability built into the container. On administration the drops may be placed directly into the infant's mouth or mixed with a small portion of food. Since many of the suspensions of antibiotic drugs intended for pediatric use are prepared in a highly flavored, sweetened, colored base, they are frequently referred to by their manufacturers and also popularly as "syrups," even though in fact they are suspensions.

In some instances it is not possible to prepare a suspension so that the usual dose is available in a teaspoonful measure, simply because of the large amount of drug usually taken. An example of this type of medication is Trisulfapyrimidines Oral Suspension, USP, a product containing about 10 g of total sulfapyrimidines in each 100 ml, which has an official usual dose of 40 ml initially (containing 4 g of drug) and 10 ml every 4 hours thereafter. The high volume of dosage is necessary, since it would be difficult to produce a more concentrated suspension and still meet desired qualities such as suspendability and pourability.

The Preparation of the Suspension

In the actual preparation of a suspension, the pharmacist must be acquainted with the characteristics of both the intended dispersed phase and the dispersion medium. In some instances the dispersed phase has an affinity for the vehicle to be employed and is readily "wetted" by it upon its addition. Other drugs are not penetrated easily by the vehicle and have a tendency to clump together or to float on top of the vehicle. In the latter case, the powder must first be wetted by a so-called "wetting agent" to make

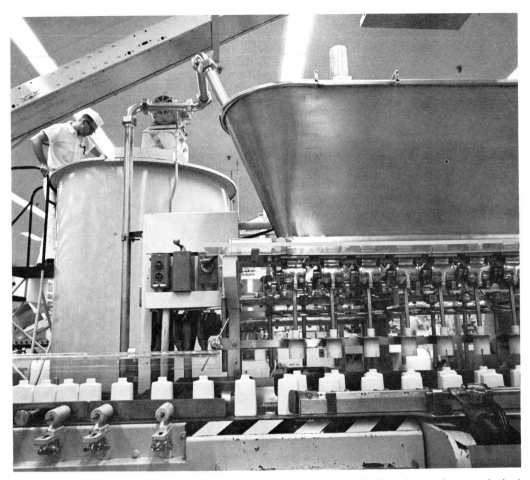

Fig. 5-4. *Liquid filling. The 1000-gallon portable storage tank holding the bulk product is shown in the background. The fluid preparation is pumped from the bottom of the tank through sanitary piping to the large stainless steel hopper located in the foreground. Immediately below the hopper are eight piston-type filling cylinders. Extending from the filling heads are eight filling tubes, each with a bottle-centering bell. On the left, bottles are shown being conveyed after cleaning. As they pass through an indexing worm, the bottles are then spaced accurately for transfer by a pusher bar to the filling position. After filling, incoming bottles push those filled onto the conveyor to the bottle-capping operation. (Courtesy of The Upjohn Company)*

the powder more penetrable by the dispersion medium. Alcohol, glycerin, and other hygroscopic liquids are employed as wetting agents when an aqueous vehicle is to be used as the dispersion phase. They function by displacing the air in the crevices of the particles, dispersing the particles, and subsequently allowing the penetration of dispersion medium into the powder. In the large-scale preparation of suspensions the wetting agents are mixed with the particles by an apparatus such as colloid mill; on a small scale in the pharmacy, they are mixed with a mortar and pestle. Once the powder is wetted, the dispersion medium (to which have been added all of the formulation's soluble components such as colorants, flavorants, and preservatives) is added in portions to the powder, and the mixture is thoroughly blended before subsequent additions of vehicle. A portion of the vehicle is used to wash the mixing equipment free of suspensoid, and this portion is used to make the suspension to final volume and insure that the suspension contains the desired concentration of solid matter. The final product is then passed through a colloid mill or other blender or mixing device to insure uniformity.

Preservation, Packaging, and Storage of Suspensions

Whenever appropriate, suitable preservatives should be included in the formulation of suspensions to preserve against bacterial and mold contamination.

All suspensions should be packaged in containers having adequate airspace above the liquid to permit adequate shaking, and oral suspensions should be provided in wide-mouthed containers to permit the prompt and unhindered removal of the suspension.

Most suspensions should be stored in tight containers protected from freezing, excessive heat, and light. It is important that suspensions be shaken before each use to ensure a uniform distribution of solid in the vehicle and thereby uniform and proper dosage.

Official Oral Suspensions

The official oral suspensions are presented in Table 5-1. Although a variety of therapeutic categories of drugs are represented, the antacid, anthelmintic, and antibacterial preparations are of especial therapeutic and pharmaceutic interest and will be discussed separately here.

Antacid Oral Suspensions

Antacids are intended to counteract the effects of gastric hyperacidity and as such are employed by persons, as peptic ulcer patients, who must reduce the level of acidity in the stomach. They are also widely employed and sold over-the-counter to patients suffering from conditions popularly referred to as "acid indigestion," "heartburn," and "sour stomach." Many patients belch or otherwise reflux acid from the stomach to the esophagus and take antacids to counter the acid brought to the esophagus and throat.

Most antacid preparations are composed of water-insoluble materials which act within the confines of the gastrointestinal tract to counteract the acid and/or soothe the irritated or inflamed linings of the gastrointestinal tract. There are a few water-soluble agents employed, as sodium bicarbonate, but for the most part, water-insoluble salts of aluminum, calcium, and magnesium are employed, as aluminum hydroxide, aluminum phosphate, dihydroxyaluminum aminoacetate, calcium carbonate, calcium phosphate, magaldrate, magnesium carbonate,

magnesium oxide, magnesium hydroxide and magnesium trisilicate. The ability of each of these to neutralize gastric acid varies with the chemical agent. For instance sodium bicarbonate, calcium carbonate, and magnesium hydroxide neutralize acid effectively, whereas magnesium trisilicate and aluminum hydroxide do so less effectively and much more slowly. In selecting an antacid, it is also important to consider the possible adverse effects of each agent in relation to the individual patient being treated. Each agent has its own peculiar potential for adverse effects. For instance, sodium bicarbonate possesses the capability for sodium overload and systemic alkalosis which is of potential hazard to patients on sodium-restricted diets. Magnesium preparations may lead to severe diarrhea and are dangerous to patients with renal failure due to the patients' inability to excrete all of the magnesium which may be absorbed (the gastric acid converts insoluble magnesium hydroxide to magnesium chloride which is water-soluble and is partially absorbed). Calcium carbonate carries the hazards of hypercalcemia, renal impairment, and stimulation of gastric secretion and acid production, the latter effect known as "acid rebound." Aluminum hydroxide may lead to phosphate depletion with consequent muscle weakness, bone resorption, and hypercalciuria.

The use to which an antacid is to be put is a major consideration in its selection. For instance, in the occasional treatment of heartburn, or other infrequent episodes of gastric distress, a single dose of sodium bicarbonate or a magnesium hydroxide preparation may be desired, but for the treatment of acute peptic ulcer or duodenal ulcer in which the therapeutic regimen usually includes the administration of hourly doses of antacids during the waking hours, sodium bicarbonate would provide too great an amount of sodium and the magnesium hydroxide would induce diarrhea. Thus, in the treatment of ulcerative conditions, a combination of magnesium hydroxide and aluminum hydroxide is frequently used since the latter agent possesses some constipating effects which counter the diarrhea effects of the magnesium hydroxide.

In instances in which frequent dosage administration is required, and in cases in which esophagitis is being treated, liquid antacids frequently are preferred over tablet forms. For one thing, the liquid suspensions assert more imme-

Table 5-1. OFFICIAL ORAL SUSPENSIONS BY CATEGORY

Official Oral Suspension	Some Representative Commercial Products	Concentration of Respective Drug in Official or Commercial Oral Suspension	Comments
Analgesic			
Propoxyphene Napsylate Oral Suspension, NF	Darvon N Suspension (Lilly)	50 mg/5 ml	Propoxyphene napsylate is a water-insoluble agent that differs from propoxyphene HCl (Darvon) in solubility (the HCl salt is water-soluble) and allows more stable liquid dosage forms and tablet formulations. The drug is employed as an analgesic in the relief of mild to moderate pain. It is related structurally to the narcotic methadone.
Antacids			
Alumina and Magnesia Oral Suspension, USP	Aludrox Oral Suspension (Wyeth)	Aluminum hydroxide, hydrated aluminum oxide, and magnesium hydroxide, equivalent to between 3.6 and 4.0% of aluminum oxide (Al_2O_3) and 1.7 to 2.2% of magnesium hydroxide ($Mg(OH)_2$); in total: between 5.3 and 6.2% combined Al_2O_3 and $Mg(OH)_2$	
Magaldrate Oral Suspension, USP	Riopan Oral Suspension (Ayerst)	Equivalent of between 2.5 and 3% magnesium oxide and 1.5 to 2.0% aluminum oxide (magaldrate is a chemical combination of aluminum hydroxide and magnesium hydroxide corresponding to the approximate formula: $Al_2H_{14}Mg_4O_{14} \cdot 2H_2O$).	These preparations are used to counteract gastric hyperacidity and to relieve distress in the upper gastrointestinal tract. See text for additional discussion.
Magnesia and Alumina Oral Suspension, USP	Maalox Suspension (Rorer)	Magnesium hydroxide, aluminum hydroxide, and hydrated aluminum oxide, equivalent to between 3.4 and 4.2% of magnesium hydroxide and 2.0 to 2.4% of aluminum oxide, with a total of between 5.4 and 6.6% combined $Mg(OH)_2$ and Al_2O_3	

Table 5-1. OFFICIAL ORAL SUSPENSIONS BY CATEGORY (*Cont.*)

Official Oral Suspension	Some Representative Commercial Products	Concentration of Respective Drug in Official or Commercial Oral Suspension	Comments
Anthelmintics			
Pyrantel Pamoate Oral Suspension, USP	Antiminth Oral Suspension (Roerig)	250 mg/5 ml	
Pyrvinium Pamoate Oral Suspension, USP	Povan Suspension (Parke Davis)	50 mg/5 ml	These anthelmintics are employed to rid the body of worm infections. See text for additional discussion.
Thiabenzadole Oral Suspension, USP	Mintezol Oral Suspension (Merck Sharp & Dohme)	500 mg/5 ml	
Antibacterials (*Antibiotics*)			
Chloramphenicol Pamitate Oral Suspension, USP	Chloromycetin Palmitate Oral Suspension (Parke Davis)	150 mg/5 ml	A broad-spectrum antibiotic reserved for serious infections by susceptible organisms when less potentially hazardous agents are ineffective or contraindicated. Serious and fatal blood dyscrasias (aplastic anemia, hypoplastic anemia, thrombocytopenia, and granulocytopenia) are known to occur following administration of chloramphenicol. The tasteless palmitate ester of chloramphenicol is hydrolyzed in the gut to chloramphenicol before absorption.
Demeclocycline Oral Suspension, NF	Declomycin Pediatric Drops (Lederle)	60 mg/ml	
Methacycline HCl Oral Suspension, NF	Rondomycin "Syrup" (Wallace)	75 mg/5 ml	Tetracycline derivatives effective against a wide range of gram-positive and gram-negative microorganisms.
Oxytetracycline Calcium Oral Suspension, NF	Terramycin Syrup and Terramycin Pediatric Drops (Pfizer)	125 mg/5 ml syrup; 100 mg/ml drops	
Penicillin V Hydrabamine Oral Suspension, NF	Compocillin V Oral Suspension (Ross)	180 mg/5 ml	This is an aqueous suspension of a water-insoluble salt of penicillin V (phenoxymethyl penicillin). It acts through the inhibition of biosynthesis of cell wall mucopeptide. It is effective against a wide variety of pathogenic organisms.

See text for additional discussion of antibacterial oral suspensions. |

Table 5-1. OFFICIAL ORAL SUSPENSIONS BY CATEGORY (*Cont.*)

Official Oral Suspension	*Some Representative Commercial Products*	*Concentration of Respective Drug in Official or Commercial Oral Suspension*	*Comments*
Antibacterials (Antibiotics) (cont.)			
Tetracycline Oral Suspension, USP	Achromycin Pediatric Drops and Achromycin Syrup (Lederle)	100 mg/ml (drops); 125 mg/ 5 ml (syrup)	Tetracycline antibiotics act by inhibiting microorganisms' protein synthesis. They are effective against a wide range of gram-positive and gram-negative microorganisms.
			See text for additional discussion of antibacterial oral suspensions.
Antibacterials (Non-antibiotic Anti-infectives)			
Methenamine Mandelate Oral Suspension, USP	Mandelamine Suspension and Mandelamine Suspension Forte (Warner/Chilcott)	250 and 500 mg (Forte)/5 ml	Methenamine mandelate oral suspension is prepared with an oleaginous vehicle because of the water solubility of methenamine mandelate. Methenamine mandelate is a chemical combination of approximately equal parts of methenamine and mandelic acid which is effective in destroying most of the pathogens commonly found to infect the urinary tract. It is an effective urinary antibacterial. An acid urine is essential for the activity of the drug, with maximum efficacy occurring at pH 5.5. The methenamine component of the drug in an acid urine is hydrolyzed to ammonia and the bactericidal agent, formaldehyde. The mandelic acid component meantime exerts its antibacterial action and contributes to the acidification of the urine. The usual dose of the drug is 1 g, up to four times a day.
			The suspension form of the drug is especially useful in treating pediatric patients as well as those adults who cannot or will not swallow a tablet (also official and commercially available).

Table 5-1. OFFICIAL ORAL SUSPENSIONS BY CATEGORY (*Cont.*)

Official Oral Suspension	Some Representative Commercial Products	Concentration of Respective Drug in Official or Commercial Oral Suspension	Comments
Antibacterials (Non-antibiotic Anti-infectives) (cont.)			
Nitrofurantoin Oral Suspension, USP	Furadantin Oral Suspension (Eaton)	25 mg/5 ml	The aqueous suspension of nitrofurantoin is a urinary tract antibacterial agent. Because nitrofurantoin is discolored by alkalies and by exposure to light and is decomposed upon contact with metals other than stainless steel and aluminum, the pharmacist should make certain that these offending environments are avoided in preparing and packaging of the drug. Amber glass containers are normally used in the packaging of the suspension.
			The usual adult dose of the drug is 100 mg (four times a day) corresponding to about 4 teaspoonfuls (20 ml) of the suspension. The nausea sometimes associated with nitrofurantoin therapy can usually be minimized by administering the drug during meals or before retiring with milk or other food snack.
			The suspension is particularly useful in treating children in which case the dose of nitrofurantoin is based on body weight, between 2.2 to 3.2 mg of drug being given per day (in divided doses) per pound of body weight. Infants less than 1 month of age should not be given the drug because of their inability, due to immature enzyme systems, to detoxify the drug.
Sulfamethoxazole Oral Suspension, NF	Gantanol Suspension (Roche)	500 mg/5 ml	These sulfa-drug suspensions are bacteriostatic agents particularly useful in the treatment of urinary tract infections. Sulfonamides competitively inhibit bacterial synthesis of folic acid and para-aminobenzoic acid.
Sulfisoxazole Acetyl Oral Suspension, USP	Gantrisin Syrup and Gantrisin Pediatric Suspension (Roche)	500 mg/5 ml	

Table 5-1. OFFICIAL ORAL SUSPENSIONS BY CATEGORY (*Cont.*)

Official Oral Suspension	Some Representative Commercial Products	Concentration of Respective Drug in Official or Commercial Oral Suspension	Comments
Antibacterials (Non-antibiotic Anti-infectives) (cont.)			
Trisulfapyrimidines Oral Suspension, USP	Neotrizine Suspension (Lilly); Sulfose suspension (Wyeth); Syrasulfas Syrup (Upjohn); Terfonyl Suspension (Squibb); Trisem Suspension (Massengill)	500 mg/5 ml (167 mg each of sulfadiazine, sulfamerazine, and sulfamethazine.	The advantage of taking the combination of three sulfa drugs rather than a greater amount of a single sulfa drug is to increase the amount of total drug solubilized by body fluids (each drug exerts its individual solubility) thereby enhancing therapy and reducing the chance of crystalluria (precipitation of sulfa-crystals in the urine with the potential to block the kidney tubules) during the drug's elimination process.
Anticonvulsants			
Phensuximide Oral Suspension, NF	Milontin Suspension (Parke Davis)	62.5 mg/ml	This anticonvulsant agent is used primarily in the treatment of patients with petit mal epilepsy.
Primidone Oral Suspension, USP	Mysoline Suspension (Ayerst)	250 mg/5 ml	This drug is useful in the management of grand mal epilepsy and psychomotor attacks.
Antiflatulent			
Simethicone Oral Suspension, NF	Mylicon Drops (Stuart)	40 mg/0.6 ml	Used for the symptomatic treatment of gastrointestinal distress due to entrapment of gas. The drug acts by reducing the surface tension of gas bubbles, enabling them to coalesce and to be released through belching or passing flatus.
Antifungal			
Nystatin Oral Suspension, USP	Mycostatin Oral Suspension (Squibb)	100,000 units/ml	Mycostatin is an antibiotic with antifungal activity. The suspension is held in the mouth as long as possible before swallowing in the treatment of infections of the oral cavity caused by *Candida* (Monilia) *albicans* and other Candida species.
Antipsychotics			
Chlorprothixene Oral Suspension, NF	Taractan Concentrate (Roche)	100 mg/5 ml	Used in the control of moderate to severe agitation, anxiety, and tension, when

Table 5-1. OFFICIAL ORAL SUSPENSIONS BY CATEGORY (*Cont.*)

Official Oral Suspension	Some Representative Commercial Products	Concentration of Respective Drug in Official or Commercial Oral Suspension	Comments
Antipsychotics (cont.)			
			such symptoms are manifestations of schizophrenia.
Triflupromazine Oral Suspension, NF	Vesprin Suspension (Squibb)	50 mg/5 ml	Useful in the treatment of psychotic disorders and for the control of nausea and vomiting.
Antitussive			
Levopropoxyphene Napsylate Oral Suspension, NF	Novrad Suspension (Lilly)	50 mg/5 ml	Used in the symptomatic relief of cough.
Diuretic			
Chlorothiazide Oral Suspension, USP	Diuril Oral Suspension (Merck Sharp & Dohme)	250 mg/5 ml	Acts as a diuretic by interfering with the renal tubular mechanism of electrolyte reabsorption (increases excretion of sodium and chloride).
Tranquilizers			
Hydroxyzine Pamoate Oral Suspension, NF	Vistaril Oral Suspension (Pfizer)	25 mg/5 ml	Used in the management of anxiety, tension, and psychomotor agitation.
Meprobamate Oral Suspension, NF	Equanil Suspension (Wyeth)	200 mg/5 ml	Skeletal muscle relaxant used in the management of anxiety and tension.

diate action—they do not require the time needed for tablets to disintegrate. It is important that an antacid preparation have a reasonably fast onset of action since its presence in the stomach may not last long due to gastric emptying into the intestines. It has been shown by endoscopic studies that on a fasting stomach very little antacid remains in the stomach 1 hour following administration. It is for this reason that the FDA has set the requirement that antacid tablets that are not intended to be chewed upon administration must disintegrate within 10 minutes in simulated gastric conditions. Frequent food snacks generally prolong the time an antacid remains in the stomach and can prolong its action.

Since many antacid materials, especially aluminum and calcium-containing products, interfere with the absorption of other drugs, especially the tetracycline group of antibiotics,

pharmacists must caution their patients against taking such drugs concomitantly.

In addition to the suspension forms of antacids, a number of liquid antacid preparations of the magma and gel type are official and commercially available and will be mentioned later in this chapter. All of these liquid forms are usually pleasantly flavored (generally with peppermint) to enhance their palatability and patient appeal. Since liquid antacid preparations characteristically contain a large amount of solid material, they must be shaken vigorously to redistribute the antacid material prior to administration. Since large doses of antacids are frequently required, many patients would prefer to swallow one or two tablespoonfuls of a liquid antacid preparation than to swallow whole or chew the corresponding number of tablets (commonly 3 to 6) for the equivalent dose of drug.

Anthelmintic Oral Suspensions

The anthelmintic oral suspensions presented in Table 5-1 exert their activity against worm infestations directly within the intestinal tract. Thiabenzadole is vermicidal against pinworm, roundworm, threadworm, and hookworm. Pyrantel pamoate, which is thought to exert its action through its neuromuscular blocking property, is employed chiefly for the treatment of roundworm and pinworm infections. Pyrvinium pamoate appears to act by preventing the parasite from using exogenous carbohydrate (from the host) and when the parasite's endogenous (its own) reserves are depleted, it perishes.

Pinworm infections can pass easily from person to person by the transfer of eggs through direct contact, handling contaminated objects, and even by breathing the airborne eggs in dust. Thus, if a pinworm infection is detected in one member of a family or institution group, it is generally advised that all members be simultaneously treated. Doses for patients vary, depending upon their body weight. For instance, for pyrvinium pamoate, the recommended dosage is 5 mg of the drug per kg of body weight, administered in a single dose. The commercial product is so formulated that a 5-ml teaspoonful will contain the dose per 10 kg (22 lb) of body weight. Since the gastrointestinal tract of adults does not appreciably increase in size with increased weight gain, the recommended maximum dosage is for patients weighing 154 lbs and above.

Pyrvinium pamoate is an interesting substance the features of which should be known by the pharmacist. It is a deep red powder that is practically insoluble in water. The drug will stain most materials including cloth that it may be spilled upon. It also stains the feces, and patients should be advised not to become concerned if the stool carries a bright red color during treatment with the drug. Also, since one of the most prominent of the adverse effects to anthelmintic therapy is nausea and vomiting, patients must be alerted to this possibility, and again advised not to become concerned should the vomitus be red.

Antibacterial Oral Suspensions

The antibacterial oral suspensions include preparations of antibiotic substances (e.g., chloramphenicol palmitate, penicillin V derivatives, and tetracycline and its derivatives), sulfonamides (e.g., sulfamethazole, sulfasoxazole acetyl and trisulfapyramidines), and other chemotherapeutic agents (e.g., methenamine mandelate and nitrofurantoin).

Most antibiotic materials are unstable when maintained in solution for an appreciable length of time and therefore, from a stability standpoint, insoluble forms of the drug substances in aqueous suspension or as dry powders for reconstitution (discussed next) are attractive to pharmaceutical manufacturers. The antibiotic oral suspensions also provide a convenient means of administering dosages to infants and children as well as to adult patients who may prefer liquid preparations to solid dosage forms. Many of the oral suspensions which are intended primarily for infants are packaged with a calibrated dropper to assist in the delivery of the prescribed dose. Examples of some commercial pediatric antibiotic oral suspensions are pictured in Figure 5-3, and examples of calibrated droppers in Figure 5-5.

The dispersing phase of antibiotic suspensions is aqueous, and usually colored, sweetened and flavored to render the liquid more appealing and palatable. As noted previously, the palmitate form of chloramphenicol was selected for the suspension dosage form not only because of its water-insolubility, but also because of its quality of being flavorless, thereby eliminating the formulating problem of trying to mask the otherwise bitter taste of the chloramphenicol base.

Comments on a number of non-antibiotic antibacterial oral suspensions are presented in Table 5-1.

Official Dry Powders for Oral Suspension

A number of official and commercial preparations consist of dry powder mixtures or granules, which are intended to be suspended in water or some other vehicle prior to oral administration. As indicated previously, these official preparations have "for Oral Suspension" in their official title to distinguish them from already prepared suspensions.

The majority of drugs prepared as a dry mix for oral suspension are the antibiotic drugs. The dry products are prepared commercially to contain the antibiotic drug, colorants, flavorants,

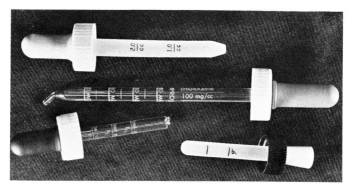

Fig. 5-5. *Examples of calibrated droppers utilized in the administration of pediatric medications.*

sweeteners and any stabilizing, suspending, or preserving agents that may be desired to enhance the stability of either the dry powder or granule mixture or the ultimate liquid suspension. When called upon to "reconstitute" and dispense one of these products, the pharmacist loosens the powder at the bottom of the container by lightly tapping it against a hard surface, and then adds the label-designated amount of purified water, usually in portions, and shakes until all of the dry powder has been suspended (Fig. 5-2). It is important for the pharmacist to add precisely the prescribed amount of purified water to the dry mixture if the proper drug concentration per dosage unit is to be achieved. Also, the use of purified water rather than tap water is needed to avoid the addition of possible offending impurities which could adversely affect the stability of the resulting preparation. Generally, manufacturers provide the dry powder or granule mixture in a slightly oversized container to permit the adequate shaking of the contents after the entire amount of purified water has been added. The pharmacist should advise the patient of this feature and instruct him to shake the contents thoroughly immediately prior to administration and to store the medication appropriately (usually under refrigeration). Among the official antibiotic drugs for oral suspension are the following:

Ampicillin for Oral Suspension, USP
   [Penbritin for Oral Suspension-Pediatric Drops (Ayerst)]
Cephalexin for Oral Suspension, NF
   [Keflex for Pediatric Drops (Lilly)]
Colistin Sulfate for Oral Suspension

   [Coly-Mycin S Oral Suspension (Warner/Chilcott)]
Doxycycline for Oral Suspension, USP
   [Vibramycin Monohydrate for Oral Suspension (Pfizer)]
Erythromycin Estolate for Oral Suspension, NF
   [Ilosone for Oral Suspension (Dista)]
Erythromycin Ethylsuccinate for Oral Suspension, USP
   [Erythrocin Ethylsuccinate for Oral Suspension (Abbott)]
Penicillin V for Oral Suspension, USP
   [V-Cillin Drops (Lilly)]
Tetracycline for Oral Suspension, USP
   [Achromycin for Oral Suspension (Lederle)]

Among the official drugs other than antibiotics prepared as dry powder mixtures for reconstitution to oral suspension are the following: Bephenium hydroxynaphthoate [Alcopara (Burroughs Wellcome)] an anthelmintic; ipodate calcium [Oragrafin Calcium (Squibb)], a diagnostic aid used in cholecystography; cholestyramine [Questran (Mead Johnson)], a drug used in the management of high cholesterol levels; and barium sulfate [Barosperse (Mallinckrodt)], used orally or rectally as a radiopaque contrast medium to visualize the gastrointestinal tract as an aid to diagnosis.

The most frequently used of these agents is barium sulfate. Barium sulfate was introduced into medicine about 1910 as a contrast medium in the roentgen-ray examination of the gastrointestinal tract. It is practically insoluble in water and thus its administration, even in the large doses required, is safe because it is not absorbed from the gastrointestinal tract. The pharmacist must be careful not to confuse "barium sulfate," with other forms of barium as the *sulfide* and *sulfite* which are soluble salts and *are* poisonous. Barium sulfate is a fine, non-gritty, white, odorless and tasteless powder. When prepared into a suspension and administered orally, it is used to diagnose conditions of the hypopharynx, esophagus, stomach, small intestine and colon. The barium sulfate renders the gastrointestinal tract opaque to the x ray so that it may be photographed, revealing any abnormality in the anatomic features of the tract. When administered rectally, the barium sulfate allows visualization of the features of the rectum and colon.

Commercially, barium sulfate for diagnostic use is available as a bulk powder containing the required suspending agents for effective reconstitution to an oral suspension or enema prior to administration. Enema units, which contain prepared suspension in a ready-to-use and disposable bag, are also available [Barosperse Disposable Barium Enema Unit (Mallinckrodt) and Fleet Barobag (Fleet)].

Emulsions

An emulsion is a dispersion in which the dispersed phase is composed of small globules of a liquid distributed throughout a vehicle in which it is immiscible. In emulsion terminology, the dispersed phase is referred to as the *internal phase*, and the dispersion medium as the *external* or *continuous phase*. Emulsions having an oleaginous internal phase and an aqueous external phase are referred to as *oil-in-water* emulsions and are commonly designated as "o/w" emulsions. Conversely, emulsions having an aqueous internal phase and an oleaginous external phase are termed *water-in-oil* emulsions and are referred to as "w/o" emulsions. Because the external phase of an emulsion is continuous, an oil-in-water emulsion may be diluted or extended with water or an aqueous preparation, and a water-in-oil emulsion with an oleaginous or oil-miscible liquid. Generally in order to prepare a stable emulsion, a third phase or part of the emulsion is necessary, that being an *emulsifying agent*. Depending upon their constituents, the viscosity of emulsions can vary greatly, and pharmaceutical emulsions may be prepared as liquids or semisolids. Based on the constituents and the intended application, liquid emulsions may be employed orally, topically, or parenterally;

semisolid emulsions, topically. Many pharmaceutical preparations that may actually be emulsions may not be classified as such because they seem to fit some other pharmaceutical category more appropriately. For instance, certain lotions, liniments, creams, ointments, and commercial vitamin drops may be emulsions but may be referred to in the terms indicated and will be discussed in this book under these various designations.

Purpose of Emulsions and of Emulsification

Pharmaceutically, the process of emulsification enables the pharmacist to prepare relatively stable and homogeneous mixtures of two immiscible liquids. It permits the administration of a liquid drug in the form of minute globules rather than in bulk. Therapeutically, this may be beneficial to the rate and degree of absorption of the drug after administration by any of the usual routes. It has recently been shown, that certain oil-in-water emulsions may also be useful as vehicles to potentiate the bioavailability of poorly absorbed drugs.[1] For orally administered emulsions, the oil-in-water type of emulsion permits the palatable administration of an otherwise distasteful oil by dispersing it in a sweetened, flavored aqueous vehicle in which it may be carried past the taste buds and into the stomach. The reduced particle size of the oil globules may render the oil more digestible and more readily absorbed, or if that is not the intent, more effective in its task, as for example the increased efficacy of mineral oil as a cathartic when in the emulsified form.

Emulsions to be applied externally to the skin may be prepared as o/w or w/o emulsions, depending upon such factors as the nature of the therapeutic agents to be incorporated into the emulsions, the desirability for an emollient or tissue softening effect of the preparation, and the condition of the skin surface. Medicinal agents that are irritating to the skin generally are less irritating if present in the internal phase of an emulsified topical preparation than in the external phase from which direct contact

[1] Bates, T. R. and Sequeira, J. A., "Bioavailability of Micronized Griseofulvin from Corn Oil-in-Water Emulsion, Aqueous Suspension, and Commercial Tablet Dosage Forms in Humans," *J. Pharm. Sci.*, 64:793–797, 1975.

with the skin is more prevalent. Naturally, the miscibility or the solubility in oil and in water of a medicinal agent to be used in an emulsified preparation would dictate to a great extent the solvent in which it must be present, and its nature would in turn suggest the phase of the emulsion that the resulting solution should become. On the unbroken skin, a water-in-oil emulsion can usually be applied more evenly since the skin is covered with a thin film of sebum, and this surface is more readily wetted by oil than by water. A water-in-oil emulsion is also more softening to the skin, since it resists drying out and is resistant to removal by contact with water. On the other hand, if it is desirable to have a preparation that is more easily removed from the skin with water, an oil-in-water emulsion would be preferred. As for absorption, absorption through the skin (percutaneous absorption) may be enhanced by the diminished particle size of the internal phase. Other aspects of topical preparations will be discussed in Chapter 10.

Theories of Emulsification

Many theories have been advanced in an attempt to explain how emulsifying agents act in promoting emulsification and in maintaining the stability of the resulting emusion. Although certain of these theories apply rather specifically to certain types of emulsifying agents and to certain conditions (as the pH of the phases of the system and the nature and relative proportions of the internal and external phases), they may be viewed in a general way to describe the possible manner in which emulsions may be produced and stabilized. Among the most prevalent theories are the *surface-tension theory*, the *oriented-wedge theory*, and the *plastic* or *interfacial film theory*.

All liquids have a tendency to assume a shape having the least amount of surface area exposed. For a drop of a liquid, that shape is spherical. In a spherical drop of liquid there are internal forces that tend to promote the association of the molecules of the substance to resist the distortion of the drop into a less spherical form. If two or more drops of the same liquid come into contact with one another, the tendency is for them to join or to *coalesce*, making one larger drop having a lesser surface area than the total surface area of the individual drops. This tendency of liquids may be measured quantitatively, and when the surrounding of the liquid is air, it is referred to as the liquid's *surface tension. When the liquid is in contact with a second liquid in which it is insoluble and immiscible, the force causing each liquid to resist breaking up into smaller particles is called interfacial tension.* Substances that can promote the lowering of this resistance to breakup can encourage a liquid to be reduced to smaller drops or particles. These tension-lowering substances are referred to as *surface-active* (surfactants) or *wetting agents.* According to the *surface-tension theory* of emulsification, the use of these substances as emulsifiers and stabilizers results in the lowering of the interfacial tension of the two immiscible liquids, reducing the repellent force between the liquids and diminishing each liquid's attraction for its own molecules. Thus the surface-active agents facilitate the breaking up of large globules into smaller ones, which then have a lesser than usual tendency to reunite or coalesce.

The *oriented-wedge* theory assumes monomolecular layers of emulsifying agent curved around a droplet of the internal phase of the emulsion. The theory is based on the presumption that certain emulsifying agents orient themselves about and within a liquid in a manner reflective of their solubility in that particular liquid. In a system containing two immiscible liquids, presumably the emulsifying agent would be preferentially soluble in one of the phases and would be imbedded more deeply and tenaciously into that phase than the other. Since many molecules of substances upon which this theory is based (for example, soaps) have a hydrophilic or water-loving portion and a hydrophobic or water-hating portion (but usually lipophilic or oil-loving), the molecules will position or orient themselves into each phase. Depending upon the shape and size of the molecules, their solubility characteristics, and thus their orientation, the wedge-shape arrangement envisioned for the molecules will cause the surrounding of either oil globules or water globules. Generally an emulsifying agent having a greater hydrophilic character than hydrophobic character will promote an oil-in-water emulsion, and a water-in-oil emulsion results through the use of an emulsifying agent that is more hydrophobic than hydrophilic. Putting it another way, the phase in which the emulsifying agent is more soluble will generally become the continuous or external phase of the emulsion. Although this theory may not represent a totally accurate depiction of the molecular arrangement of the emulsifier molecules, the concept that water-soluble emulsifiers generally do form oil-in-water emulsions is important and is generally found in practice.

The *plastic-* or *interfacial-film theory* places the emulsifying agent at the interface between the oil and water, surrounding the droplets of the internal phase as a thin layer of film adsorbed on the surface of the drops. The film prevents the contact and the coalescing of the dispersed phase; the tougher and more pliable the film, the greater the stability of the emulsion. Naturally, enough of the film-forming material must be available to coat the entire surface of each drop of internal phase. Here again, the formation of an oil-in-water or a water-in-oil emulsion is dependent upon the degree of solubility of the agent in the two phases, with water-soluble agents encouraging oil-in-water emulsions and oil-soluble emulsifiers the reverse.

In actuality, it is unlikely that a single theory of emulsification may be used to explain the means by which the many and varied emulsifiers promote emulsion formation and stability. It is more than likely that even within a given emulsion system, more than one of the aforementioned theories of emulsification is applicable and plays a part. For instance, lowering of interfacial tension is important in the initial formation of an emulsion, but the formation of a protective wedge of molecules or film of emulsifier is important for continued emulsion stability. No doubt certain emulsifiers are capable of both tasks.

Preparation of Emulsions

Emulsifying Agents

The initial step in preparation of an emulsion is the selection of the emulsifier. To be useful in a pharmaceutical preparation, the emulsifying agent must possess certain qualities. For one thing, it must be compatible with the other formulative ingredients and must not interfere with the stability or efficacy of the therapeutic agent. It should be stable and not deteriorate in the preparation. The emulsifier should be nontoxic with respect to its intended use and the amount to be consumed by the patient. Also, it should possess little odor, taste, or color. Perhaps of prime importance is the capability of the emulsifying agent to promote emulsification and to maintain the stability of the emulsion for the intended shelf life of the product.

Various types of materials have been used in pharmacy as emulsifying agents, with hundreds, if not thousands, of individual agents being tested for their emulsification capabilities. Although no attempt will be made here to try to discuss the merits of each of these agents in pharmaceutical emulsions, it would be well to point out the types of materials that are commonly used and their general application. Among the emulsifiers and stabilizers for pharmaceutical systems are the following:

1. Carbohydrate materials such as the naturally occurring agents acacia, tragacanth, agar, chondrus, and pectin. These materials form hydrophilic colloids when added to water and generally produce o/w emulsions. Acacia is perhaps the most frequently used emulsifier in the preparation of extemporaneous emulsions by the community pharmacist. Tragacanth and agar are commonly employed as thickening agents in acacia-emulsified products.

2. Protein substances such as gelatin, egg yolk, and casein. These substances produce o/w emulsions. The disadvantage of gelatin as an emulsifier is that the emulsions prepared from it frequently are too fluid and become more fluid upon standing.

3. High molecular weight alcohols such as stearyl alcohol, cetyl alcohol, and glyceryl monostearate. These are employed primarily as thickening agents and stabilizers for o/w emulsions of certain lotions and ointments used externally. Cholesterol and cholesterol derivatives may also be employed in externally used emulsions and promote w/o emulsions.

4. Wetting agents, which may be anionic, cationic, or nonionic. These agents contain both hydrophilic and lipophilic groups, with the lipophilic portion of the molecule generally accounting for the surface-activity of the molecule. In anionic agents, this lipophilic portion is negatively charged, but in the cationic agent it is positively charged. Owing to their opposing ionic charges, anionic and cationic agents tend to neutralize each other

if present in the same system and are thus considered incompatible with one another. Nonionic emulsifiers show no inclination to ionize. Depending upon their individual nature, certain of the members of these groups form o/w emulsions and others w/o emulsions. Anionic emulsifiers include various monovalent, polyvalent, and organic soaps such as triethanolamine oleate and sulfonates such as sodium lauryl sulfate. Benzalkonium chloride, known primarily for its bactericidal properties, may be employed as a cationic-type of emulsifier. Agents of the nonionic type include the sorbitan esters and the polyoxyethylene derivatives, some of which appear in Table 5-2.

5. Finely divided solids such as colloidal clays including bentonite, magnesium hydroxide, and aluminum hydroxide. These generally form o/w emulsions when the insoluble material is added to the aqueous phase if there is a greater volume of the aqueous phase than of the oleaginous phase. However, if the powdered solid is added to the oil and the oleaginous phase volume predominates, a substance like bentonite is capable of forming a w/o emulsion.

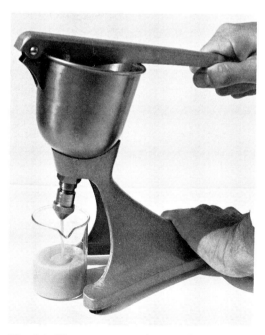

Fig. 5-6. *The preparation of an emulsion, using a hand homogenizer.*

The relative volume of internal and external phases of an emulsion is important, regardless of the type of emulsifier used. As the internal concentration of an emulsion is increased, there is an increase in the viscosity of the emulsion to a certain point, after which the viscosity decreases sharply. At this point the emulsion has undergone *inversion;* that is, it has changed from an o/w emulsion to a w/o, or vice versa. In practice, emulsions may be prepared without inversion with as much as about 75% of the volume of the product being internal phase.

The HLB System

Generally each emulsifying agent has a hydrophilic portion and a lipophilic portion with one or the other being more or less predominant and influencing in the manner already described the type of emulsion. A method has been devised[1] whereby emulsifying or surface-active agents may be categorized on the basis of their chemical make-up as to their hydrophile-lipophile balance or "HLB." By this method, each agent is assigned a HLB value or number which is indicative of the substance's polarity. Although the numbers have been assigned up to about 40, the usual range is between 1 and 20. Materials that are highly polar or hydrophilic have been assigned higher numbers than materials that are less polar and more lipophilic. Generally those surface-active agents having an assigned HLB value of from 3 to 6 are greatly lipophilic and produce water-in-oil emulsions, and those agents having HLB values of from about 8 to 18 produce oil-in-water emulsions. Examples of some assigned HLB values for some selected surfactants are shown in Table 5-2. The type of activity to be expected from surfactants of assigned HLB numbers is presented in Table 5-3.

In the HLB system, in addition to assigning values to the emulsifying agents, values are also assigned to oils and oil-like substances. In using the HLB concept in the preparation of an emulsion, one selects emulsifying agents having the same or nearly the same HLB value as the oleaginous phase of the intended emulsion. For example, mineral oil has an assigned HLB value of 4 if a w/o emulsion is desired and a value of 10.5 if a o/w emulsion is to be prepared. To

[1]Griffin, W. C.: *J. Soc. Cosmetics Chemists,* 1:311, 1949; *ibid,* 5:1, 1954.

Table 5-2. EXAMPLES OF ASSIGNED HLB VALUES FOR SOME SURFACTANTS*

Agent and Trademark Name	HLB
Sorbitan trioleate (Span 85†; Aracel 85†)	1.8
Sorbitan tristearate (Span 65†)	2.1
Propylene glycol monostearate	3.4
Sorbitan monooleate (Span 80†)	4.3
Acacia	8.0
Polyoxyethylene laurel ether (Brij 30†)	9.5
Gelatin	9.8
Methocel 15	10.5
Polyoxyethylene monostearate (Myrj 45†)	11.1
Triethanolamine oleate	12.0
Tragacanth	13.2
Polyoxyethylene sorbitan monostearate (Tween 60†)	14.9
Polyoxyethylene sorbitan mono-oleate (Tween 80†)	15.0
Polyoxyethylene sorbitan monolaurate (Tween 20†)	16.7
Sodium oleate	18.0
Sodium lauryl sulfate	40.0

* Adapted from Autian, J., in *Husa's Pharmaceutical Dispensing*, 5th ed. E. W. Martin, ed. Mack Publishing Co., Easton, Pa., 1966, p. 234. A more complete list is given in this reference.

† Atlas Powder Co., Wilmington, Del.

prepare a stable emulsion, the emulsifying agent selected should have an HLB value similar to the one for mineral oil, depending on the type of emulsion desired. When needed, two or more emulsifiers may be combined to achieve the proper HLB value.

Methods of Emulsion Preparation

Emulsions may be prepared by several methods, depending upon the nature of the emulsion components and the equipment available for use. On a small scale, emulsions may be prepared using a dry Wedgwood or porcelain mortar and pestle, a mechanical blender or mixer such as a Waring blender or a milk-shake mixer, a hand homogenizer, or in certain instances a simple prescription bottle. On a large scale, large volume mixing tanks may be used to form the coarse emulsion through the action of a high speed impeller, and the coarse product may be rendered fine by passage through a colloid mill, in which the particles are sheared between the small gap separating a high speed rotar and the stator, or by passage through a large homogenizer, in which the liquid is forced under great pressure through a small valve opening.

In the small-scale extemporaneous preparation of emulsions, three methods are generally used by the community pharmacist. They are the *continental* or *dry gum method*, the *English* or *wet gum method*, and the *bottle* or the *Forbes bottle method*. In the first method, the emulsifying agent (usually acacia) is mixed with the oil before the addition of water. In the second method, the emulsifying agent is added to the water (in which it is soluble) to form a mucilage, and then the oil is slowly incorporated to form the emulsion. The bottle method is reserved for volatile oils or less viscous oils and is a variation of the dry gum method.

CONTINENTAL OR DRY GUM METHOD. The method is also referred to as the "4:2:1" method because for every 4 parts (volumes) of oil, 2 parts of water and 1 part of gum are added in preparing the initial or *primary emulsion*. For instance, if 40 ml of oil are to be emulsified, 20 ml of water and 10 g of gum would be employed, with any additional water or other formulation ingredients being added afterward to the primary emulsion. In this method the acacia or other o/w emulsifier is triturated with the oil in a perfectly dry Wedgwood or porcelain mortar until thoroughly mixed. A mortar with a rough rather than smooth inner surface must be used to ensure proper grinding action and the reduction of the globule size during the preparation of the emulsion. A glass mortar has too smooth a surface to produce the proper size reduction of the internal phase. After the oil and gum have been mixed, the two parts of water are then added all at once, and the mixture is triturated immediately, rapidly, and continuously until the primary emulsion that forms is creamy white and produces a crackling sound to the movement of the pestle. Generally about 3 minutes of mixing are required to produce

Table 5-3. ACTIVITY AND HLB VALUE OF SURFACTANTS

Activity	Assigned HLB
Antifoaming	1 to 3
Emulsifiers (w/o)	3 to 6
Wetting Agents	7 to 9
Emulsifiers (o/w)	8 to 18
Solubilizers	15 to 20
Detergents	13 to 15

such a primary emulsion. Other liquid formulative ingredients that are soluble in or miscible with the external phase may then be added to the primary emulsion with mixing. Solid substances such as preservatives, stabilizers, colorants, and any flavoring material are usually dissolved in a suitable volume of water (assuming water is the external phase) and added as a solution to the primary emulsion. Any substances that might interfere with the stability of the emulsion or the emulsifying agent are added as near last as is practically possible. For instance, since alcohol has a precipitating action on gums such as acacia, alcohol or any solution containing alcohol should not be added directly to the primary emulsion, since the total alcoholic concentration of the mixture would be greater at that point than it would be after other diluents had been previously added. When all necessary agents have been added, the emulsion is transferred to a graduate and made to volume with water previously swirled about in the mortar to remove the last portion of emulsion.

ENGLISH OR WET GUM METHOD. By this method, the same proportions of oil, water, and gum are used as in the continental or dry gum method, but the order of mixing is different, and the proportion of ingredients may be varied during the preparation of the primary emulsion as is deemed necessary by the operator. Generally a mucilage of the gum is prepared by triturating granular acacia with twice its weight of water in a mortar. The oil is then added slowly in portions, and the mixture is triturated to emulsify the oil. Should the mixture become too thick during the process, additional water may be blended into the mixture before another successive portion of oil is added. After all of the oil has been added, the mixture is thoroughly mixed for several minutes to insure uniformity. Then, as with the continental or dry gum method, the other formulative materials are added, and the emulsion is transferred to a graduate and made to volume with water.

BOTTLE OR FORBES BOTTLE METHOD. For the extemporaneous preparation of emulsions from volatile oils or oleaginous substances of low viscosities, the bottle method is useful. In this method, powdered acacia is placed in a dry bottle, two parts of oil are then added, and the mixture is thoroughly shaken in the capped container. A volume of water approximately equal to the oil is then added in portions, the mixture being thoroughly shaken after each addition. When all of the water has been added, the primary emulsion thus formed may be diluted to the proper volume with water or an aqueous solution of other formulative agents.

This method is not suited for viscous oils, since they cannot be thoroughly agitated in the bottle when mixed with the emulsifying agent. In instances in which the intended dispersed phase is a mixture of part fixed oil and part volatile oil, the dry gum method is generally employed for emulsification.

AUXILIARY METHODS. Rather than use a mortar and pestle, the pharmacist can generally prepare an excellent emulsion using the dry gum method and an electric mixer or blender.

An emulsion prepared by either the wet gum or the dry gum methods can generally be increased in quality by passing it through a hand homogenizer. In this apparatus, the pumping action of the handle forces the emulsion through a very small orifice which reduces the globules of the internal phase to about 5 microns and sometimes less. The hand homogenizer is less efficient in reducing the particle size of very thick emulsions, and it should not be employed for emulsions containing a high proportion of solid matter because of possible damage to the valve.

Stability of Emulsions

Generally speaking, an emulsion is considered to be physically unstable if (a) the internal or dispersed phase upon standing tends to form aggregates of globules, (b) if large globules or aggregates of globules rise to the top or fall to the bottom of the emulsion to form a concentrated layer of the internal phase, and (c) if all or part of the liquid of the internal phase becomes "unemulsified" and forms a distinct layer on the top or bottom of the emulsion as a result of the coalescing of the globules of the internal phase. In addition, an emulsion may be adversely affected by microbial contamination and growth and by other chemical and physical alterations.

AGGREGATION AND COALESCENCE. Aggregates of globules of the internal phase have a greater tendency than do individual particles to rise to the top of the emulsion or fall to the bottom. Such a preparation of the globules is termed the "creaming" of the emulsion, and provided coalescence is absent, it is a reversible process. The term is taken from the dairy industry and is analogous to the creaming or the rising to the top of cream in milk that is allowed to stand. The creamed portion of an emulsion may be redistributed rather homogenously upon shaking, but if the aggregates are difficult to disassemble or if insufficient shaking is employed before each dose, improper dosage of the internal phase substance may result. Further, the creaming of a pharmaceutical emulsion is not esthetically acceptable to the pharmacist nor appealing to the consumer. More importantly, it increases the risk of the coalescing of the globules.

According to the Stokes' equation (page 144), the rate of separation of the dispersed phase of an emulsion may be related to such factors as the particle size of the dispersed phase, the difference in the density between the phases, and the viscosity of the external phase. It is important to recall that the rate of separation is increased by increased particle size of the internal phase, a larger density difference between the two phases, and a decreased viscosity of the external phase. Therefore, to increase the stability of an emulsion, the globule or particle size should be reduced as fine as is practically possible, the density difference between the internal and external phases should be minimal, and the viscosity of the external phase should be reasonably high. Thickeners like tragacanth and agar are frequently added to emulsions to increase the viscosity of the external phase. Upward creaming takes place in unstable emulsions of the o/w or w/o type in which the internal phase has a lesser density than the external phase. Downward creaming takes place in unstable emulsions in which the opposite is true.

Of greater destruction to an emulsion than creaming is the coalescence of the globules of the internal phase and the separation of that phase into a layer. The separation of the internal phase from the emulsion is called the "breaking" of the emulsion, and the emulsion is described as being "cracked" or "broken." This is irreversible, since the protective sheath about the globules of the internal phase no longer exists. Attempts to reestablish the emulsion by agitation of the two separate layers are generally unsuccessful. Additional emulsifying agent and reprocessing through appropriate machinery are usually necessary to reproduce an emulsion.

Generally, care must be taken to protect emulsions against the effects of cold and heat. Freezing and thawing result in the coarsening of an emulsion and sometimes in its breaking. Excessive heat has the same effect. Since emulsion products may be transported to and used in various geographic locations having varying climates and conditions of extremely high and low temperature, pharmaceutical manufacturers must have predetermined knowledge of their emulsion stability before they may be shipped. For most emulsions, the industry performs tests of evaluation under experimental conditions of 5°, 40°, and 50° to determine the product's stability. Stability at both 5° and 40° for 3 months is considered the minimal stability that an emulsion should possess. Shorter exposure periods at 50° may be used as an alternate test.

Since other environmental conditions such as the presence of light, air, and contaminating microorganisms can adversely affect the stability of an emulsion, appropriate formulative and packaging steps are usually taken to minimize such possible hazards to product stability. For light-sensitive emulsions, light-resistant containers are used. For emulsions susceptible to oxidative decomposition, antioxidants may be included in the formulation and adequate lable warning provided to ensure that the container is tightly closed to air after each use. Many molds, yeasts, and bacteria can bring about the decomposition of the emulsifying agent of an emulsion, thereby causing the disruption of the system. In cases in which the emulsifier is not affected by the microbes, the product can be rendered unsightly by their presence and growth and will of course not be efficacious from a pharmaceutical or therapeutic standpoint. Fungistatic preservatives are generally included in the aqueous phase of an o/w emulsion, since fungi (molds and yeasts) are more likely to contaminate emulsions than are bacteria. Combinations of methylparaben and propylparaben are frequently employed to serve this function. Alcohol in the amount of 12 to 15% based on the external phase volume is frequently added to orally used o/w emulsions for preservation.

Official Oral Emulsion

The only oral emulsion that is presently official is Mineral Oil Emulsion, NF. This emulsion, also referred to as liquid petrolatum emulsion, is an oil-in-water emulsion prepared from the following formula:

Mineral Oil.	500 ml
Acacia (finely powdered).	125 g
Syrup.	100 ml
Vanillin	40 mg
Alcohol	60 ml
Purified Water, a sufficient quantity, to make	1000 ml

The emulsion is prepared by the dry gum method (4:2:1), mixing the oil with the acacia and adding 250 ml of purified water all at once to effect the primary emulsion. To this is slowly added with trituration the remainder of the ingredients, with the vanillin dissolved in the alcohol. The NF permits the use of a substitute flavorant for the vanillin, a substitute preservative for the alcohol, and a substitute emulsifying agent for the acacia and an alternative method of emulsification.

The emulsion is employed as a lubricating cathartic with a usual dose of 30 ml. The usual dose of the plain (unemulsified) mineral oil for the same purpose is 15 ml. The emulsion is much more palatable than is the unemulsified oil. Both are best taken at bedtime. There are a number of commercial preparations of emulsified mineral oil, with many continuing additional cathartic agents as phenolphthalein, milk of magnesia, agar, and others.

Gels and Magmas

Gels are defined as semisolid systems consisting of dispersions made up of either small inorganic particles or large organic molecules enclosing and interpenetrated by a liquid. Gels in which the macromolecules are distributed throughout the liquid in such a manner that no apparent boundaries exist between them and the liquid are called *single-phase gels*. In instances in which the gel mass consists of floccules of small distinct particles, the gel is classified as a two-phase system and frequently called a *magma* or a *milk*. Gels and magmas are considered colloidal dispersions since they each contain particles of colloidal dimension.

Colloidal Dispersions

Many of the various types of colloidal dispersions have been given appropriate names. For instance, *sol* is a general term to designate a dispersion of a solid substance in either a liquid, a solid, or a gaseous dispersion medium. However, more often than not it is used to describe the solid-liquid dispersion system. To be more descriptive, a prefix such as *hydro-* for water (*hydrosol*) or *alco-* for alcohol (*alcosol*) may be employed to indicate the dispersion medium. The term *aerosol* has similarly been developed to indicate a dispersion of a solid or a liquid in a gaseous phase.

Although there is no precise point at which the size of a particle in a dispersion can be considered to be "colloidal," there is a generally accepted size range. A substance is said to be colloidal when its particles fall between 1 millimicron ($m\mu$) and about 500 millimicrons or 0.5 micron (μ).[1] Colloidal particles are usually larger than atoms, ions, or molecules and generally consist of aggregates of many molecules, although in certain proteins and organic polymers single, large molecules may be of colloidal dimension and form colloidal dispersions. One difference between colloidal dispersions and true solutions is the larger particle size of the disperse phase of the former type of preparation. Another difference is in the optical properties of the two systems. True solutions do not scatter light and therefore appear clear, but colloidal dispersions contain opaque particles that do scatter light and thus appear turbid. This turbidity is easily seen, even with dilute preparations, when the dispersion is observed at right angles to a beam of light passed through the dispersion (Tyndall effect). Although reference is made here to dilute colloidal dispersions, most pharmaceutical preparations contain high concentrations of particles within the colloidal size range, and in these instances there is no difficulty in observing turbidity. In fact, certain preparations may be quite opaque, depending upon the concentration of the disperse phase. Also, the particle size of the disperse phase in some pharmaceutical preparations may not be uniform, and a preparation may contain particles within and outside of the colloidal range, giving the preparation more of an opaque appearance than if all particles were uniformly colloidal.

Particle size is not the only important criterion for establishing the colloidal state. The nature of the dispersing phase with respect to the disperse phase is also of great importance.

[1] A micron, μ, is one-thousandth of a millimeter; a millimicron, $m\mu$, is one-thousandth of a micron or one-millionth of a millimeter.

The attraction or lack of attraction between the disperse phase and the dispersion medium affects the ease of preparation of a colloidal dispersion as well as the character of the dispersion. Certain terminology has been developed to characterize the various degrees of attraction between the phases of a colloidal dispersion. If the disperse phase interacts appreciably with the dispersion medium, it is referred to as being *lyophilic*, meaning "solvent-loving." If the degree of attraction is small, the colloidal is termed *lyophobic*, or "solvent-hating." These terms are more suitably used when reference is made to the specific dispersion medium, for a single substance may be lyophobic with respect to one dispersion medium and lyophilic with respect to another. For instance, starch is lyophilic in water but lyophobic in alcohol. Terms such as *hydrophilic* and *hydrophobic*, which are more descriptive of the nature of the colloidal property, have therefore been developed to refer to the attraction or lack of attraction of the substance to water. Generally speaking, because of the attraction to the solvent of lyophilic substances in contrast to the lack of attraction of lyophobic substances, lyophilic colloidal systems are usually easier to prepare and have the greater stability. A third type of colloidal sol, termed an *association* or *amphiphilic colloid*, is formed by the grouping or association of molecules that exhibit both lyophilic and lyophobic properties.

Lyophilic colloids are generally large organic molecules capable of being solvated or associated with the molecules of the dispersing phase. These substances disperse readily upon addition to the dispersion medium to form colloidal dispersions. As more molecules of the substance are added to the sol, the viscosity is characteristically increased and when the concentration of molecules is sufficiently high, the liquid sol may become a semisolid or solid dispersion, termed a *gel*. Gels owe their rigidity to an intertwining network of the disperse phase which entraps and holds the dispersion medium. A change in the temperature can cause certain gels to resume the sol or liquid state. Also, some gels may become fluid after agitation only to resume their solid or semisolid state after remaining undisturbed for a period of time, a phenomenon known as *thixotropy*.

Lyophobic colloids are generally composed of inorganic particles. When these are added to the dispersing phase, there is little if any interaction between the two phases. Unlike lyophilic colloids, lyophobic materials do not spontaneously disperse but must be encouraged to do so by special individualized procedures. Their addition to the dispersion medium does not greatly affect the viscosity of the vehicle. Amphiphilic colloids form dispersions in both aqueous and nonaqueous media. Depending upon their individual character and the nature of the dispersion medium, they may or may not become greatly solvated. However, they generally cause an increase in the viscosity of the dispersion medium with an increase in concentration.

For the most part, the colloidal sols and gels used in pharmacy are aqueous preparations. The various preparations composed of colloidal dispersions are prepared, not according to any general method but according to the means best suited to the individual preparation. Some substances such as acacia are termed *natural colloids* because they are self-dispersing upon addition to the dispersing medium. Other materials that require special means for prompt dispersion are termed *artificial colloids*. They may require fine pulverization of coarse particles to colloidal size by a colloid mill or a micropulverizer, or colloidal size particles may be formed by chemical reaction under highly controlled conditions.

Preparation of Magmas and Gels

Many magmas and gels are prepared by freshly precipitating the disperse phase in order to achieve a fine degree of subdivision of the particles and a gelatinous character to those particles. The desired gelatinous precipitate results when solutions of inorganic agents react to form an insoluble chemical having a high attraction for water. As the microcrystalline particles of the precipitate develop, they attract water strongly to yield gelatinous particles, which combine to form the desired gelatinous precipitate. Other magmas and gels may be prepared by the direct hydration in water of the inorganic chemical, the hydrated form constituting the disperse phase of the dispersion.

Because of the high degree of attraction between the disperse phase and the aqueous medium in both magmas and gels, these preparations remain fairly uniform on standing with little settling of the disperse phase. However, on long standing a supernatant layer of the dispersion medium develops, but the uniformity of the preparation is easily reestablished by moderate shaking. To ensure uniform dosage, magmas and gels should be shaken before use, and a statement to that effect must be included on the label of such preparations. The medicinal magmas and gels are used orally for the value of the disperse phase.

Official Magmas and Gels

One official magma, Bentonite Magma, USP, is used as a suspending agent and finds application in the extemporaneous compounding of prescriptions calling for the suspension of medicinal agents. Sodium Fluoride and Orthophosphoric Acid Gel, NF is applied topically to the teeth as a dental care prophylactic. The remainder of the official magmas and gels are employed as antacids, namely: Aluminum Phosphate Gel, NF; Aluminum Hydroxide Gel, USP; Dihydroxyaluminum Aminoacetate Magma, NF; Milk of Bismuth (Bismuth Magma), NF; and Milk of Magnesia (Magnesia Magma), USP. Some of these preparations are discussed briefly below.

Bentonite Magma, USP

Bentonite magma is a preparation of 5% bentonite, a native, colloidal hydrated aluminum silicate, in purified water. It may be prepared mechanically in a blender with the bentonite added directly to the purified water while the machine is running, or it may be prepared by sprinkling the bentonite, in portions, upon hot purified water, allowing each portion to become thoroughly wetted without stirring before another portion is added. By the latter method, the mixture must be allowed to stand for 24 hours before it may be stirred. The standing period ensures the complete hydration and swelling of the bentonite. Bentonite, which is insoluble in water, swells to approximately twelve times its volume upon addition to water. The USP monograph for bentonite contains a test for "swelling power," in which 2 g of a bentonite sample is added in portions to 100 ml of water contained in a 100-ml glass-stoppered cylinder. At the end of a 2-hour period, the mass at the bottom of the cylinder is required to occupy an apparent volume of not less than 24 ml. Other required tests are for gel formation, fineness of powder, and pH, the latter being between 9 and 10. After bentonite magma

has been allowed to stand undisturbed for some period of time, it sets to a gel. Upon agitation, the sol form returns. The process may be repeated indefinitely. As mentioned earlier, this phenomenon is termed *thixotropy*,[1] and bentonite magma is termed a *thixotropic gel*. The thixotropy occurs only when the bentonite concentration is somewhat above 4%.

Bentonite magma is employed as a suspending agent. Its alkaline pH must be considered, since this might be undesirable for certain drugs. Since the suspending capacity of the magma is drastically reduced if the pH is lowered to about pH 7, another suspending agent should be selected for drugs requiring a less alkaline medium rather than make bentonite magma more acidic.

Aluminum Hydroxide Gel, USP

Aluminum Hydroxide Gel, USP, is an aqueous suspension of a gelatinous precipitate composed of insoluble aluminum hydroxide and the hydrated aluminum oxide, equivalent to about 4% of aluminum oxide. The disperse phase of the gel is generally prepared by chemical reaction, using various reactants. Usually the aluminum source of the reaction is aluminum chloride or aluminum alum, which yields the insoluble aluminum oxide and aluminum hydroxide precipitate. To the gel, the USP permits the addition of peppermint oil, glycerin, sorbitol, sucrose, saccharin, or other flavorants and sweeteners as well as suitable preservatives.

This antacid preparation is a white, viscous suspension, each g of which is required to neutralize between 12.5 ml and 25.0 ml of 0.1 N hydrochloric acid by the test described in the USP. It is effective in neutralizing a portion of the gastric hydrochloric acid and by virtue of its gelatinous, viscous, and insoluble character, coats the inflamed and perhaps ulcerated gastric surface and is useful in the treatment of hyperacidity and peptic ulcers. The main disadvantage to its use is its constipating effects. The usual dose is 10 ml, four or more times a day. The preparation should be stored in tight containers, and freezing should be avoided. An analogous commercial product is Amphojel (Wyeth). Dried aluminum hydroxide gel is also official and is used in the form of tablets.

----

[1] From the Greek, meaning "to change by touching."

Aluminum Phosphate Gel, NF

Aluminum Phosphate Gel, NF, is an aqueous suspension of between 4 and 5% of aluminum phosphate. It may also contain flavorants, sweeteners, and preservatives as indicated for the aluminum hydroxide gel. Although the latter gel interferes with phosphate absorption from the intestines, aluminum phosphate gel does not and is preferred for use by patients with peptic ulcer who also suffer from chronic diarrhea and other conditions which may lead to potassium deficiency.

Each g of aluminum phosphate gel is required to neutralize between 6 and 11 ml of 0.1 N hydrochloric acid under the conditions of the test described in the NF. The usual dose of the preparation is 15 ml. The commercial counterpart is Phosphaljel (Wyeth).

Dihydroxyaluminum Aminoacetate Magma, NF

Dihydroxyaluminum Aminoacetate Magma, NF, is a suspension of the antacid, dihydroxyaluminum aminoacetate, in purified water. The commercial products contain flavoring agents, stabilizers, and preservatives as desired by the manufacturer. The preparation is not required by the NF to contain a specific amount of the antacid drug, but the commercially available products contain 10% of active constituent.

The usual dose of the preparation is 5 ml, or that amount containing about 500 mg of drug. It is generally employed in the treatment of hyperacidity and peptic ulcers. Commercial products include: Alzinox Magma (Smith, Miller & Patch) and Robalate Liquid (Robins)

Milk of Magnesia, USP

Milk of Magnesia, USP, is a preparation containing between 7 and 8.5% of magnesium hydroxide. Although there is no method of preparation indicated in the USP for this preparation, it may be prepared by a reaction between sodium hydroxide and magnesium sulfate (1), diluted solutions being used to ensure a fine, flocculent, gelatinous precipitate of magnesium hydroxide. The precipitate so produced is washed with purified water to remove the sodium sulfate prior to its incorporation with additional purified water to prepare the required volume of product. Commercially, the product is more economically produced by the direct hydration of magnesium oxide (2).

(1) $2NaOH + MgSO_4 \rightarrow Mg(OH)_2 + Na_2SO_4$
(2) $MgO + H_2O \rightarrow Mg(OH)_2$

Irrespective of its method of preparation, milk of magnesia is a white, opaque, viscous preparation from which varying proportions of water separate on standing. For this reason it should be shaken before use. The preparation has a pH of about 10, which may bring about a reaction between the magma and the glass container imparting a bitter taste to the preparation. To minimize such an occurrence, the USP permits the addition of 0.1% citric acid to the preparation. Also, flavoring oils at a concentration not exceeding 0.05% may be added to enhance the palatability of the preparation.

Milk of magnesia is a popular antacid, 5 ml being taken as a dose, four times a day if necessary. Larger doses, 30 to 60 ml, may be taken as a laxative.

The preparation is best stored in tight containers preferably at a temperature above freezing and below 35°. Freezing results in a coarsening of the disperse phase, and temperatures above 35° decrease the gel structure.

Milk of Bismuth, NF

Milk of Bismuth, NF (Bismuth Magma) is an aqueous preparation containing bismuth hydroxide and bismuth subcarbonate in the form of a gelatinous precipitate prepared by chemical reaction. The reactants are bismuth subnitrate, nitric acid, ammonium carbonate, and strong ammonia solution. The reactions occurring may be shown as follows:

(1) $Bi(OH)_2NO_3 + 2HNO_3 \rightleftharpoons Bi(NO_3)_3 2H_2O$
(2) $NH_4HCO_3 \cdot NH_4NH_2CO_2 + NH_4OH \rightleftharpoons$
$$2(NH_4)_2CO_3$$
(3) $Bi(NO_3)_3 + 3NH_4OH \rightarrow Bi(OH)_3 + 3NH_4NO_3$
(4) $4Bi(NO_3)_3 + 6(NH_4)_2CO_3 + H_2O \rightarrow$
$$[(BiO)_2CO_3]_2 \cdot H_2O + 12NH_4NO_3 + 4CO_2$$

Initially the insoluble bismuth subnitrate is converted to the soluble normal bismuth nitrate (1) by nitric acid, agitation, and gentle heat. Next, the official ammonium carbonate, which is a combination of the ammonium bicarbonate and ammonium carbamate, is converted to the normal ammonium carbonate by a strong ammonia solution diluted with water (2). The two solutions thus formed are mixed; the reaction takes place, yielding the gelatinous precipitate of bismuth hydroxide and bismuth subcarbonate (3, 4). After the precipitate settles, the supernatant liquid is siphoned off, the precipitate is washed first by decantation and then through a fine strainer with purified water. Finally it is made to volume with purified water and shaken to mix thoroughly.

The magma is a thick, white, opaque suspension from which water separates on standing. It may be prepared by a method other than indicated above as long as the monographic requirements are met, including a bismuth oxide equivalent of about 5.5%. It is employed as an antacid and astringent in a usual dose of about 5 ml. Because of its thickness, it is best dispensed in wide-mouthed containers to permit entrance of a spoon for convenient and rapid removal of the medication. To preserve the quality of the preparation, it should be stored in tight containers and protected from freezing. It should be shaken before use.

Selected Reading

Bates, T. R., and Sequeira, J. A.: Bioavailability of Micronized Griseofulvin from Corn Oil-in-Water Emulsion, Aqueous Suspension, and Commercial Tablet Dosage Forms in Humans, *J. Pharm. Sci.,* 64:793–797, 1975.

Cram, R. F.: General Considerations Concerning Drug Particle Size and Particle Size Determination, *Bull. Parenteral Drug,* Ass., 19:110–114, 1965.

duBan, G.: Apparatus for Small Scale Production of Emulsions, *Boll. Chim. Farm.,* 104:752–761, 1965.

Ecanow, B., Grundman, R., and Wilson, R.: Flocculation and Coagulation. *Amer. J. Hosp. Pharm.,* 23:404, 1966.

Frederick, K. J.: Performance and Problems of Pharmaceutical Suspensions, *J. Pharm. Sci.,* 50:531–535, 1961.

Garrett, E. R.: Stability of Oil-in-Water Emulsions, *J. Pharm. Sci.,* 54:1557–1570, 1965.

Griffin, W. C., Lynch, M. J., and Lathrop, L. B.: Emulsions, Part 1: Properties, Theory, and Emulsifier Selection, *Drug Cosmetic Ind.,* 101:No. 4, 41, 1967; Part II: Laboratory Preparation, Equipment and Potential, *ibid.:* No. 5, 52, 1967.

Haines, B. A., and Martin, A. N.: Interfacial Properties of Powdered Material. Caking in Liquid Dispersions I. Caking and Flocculation Studies. *J. Pharm. Sci.,* 50:228–232, 1961.

Hiestand, E. N.: Theory of Coarse Suspension Formulation. *J. Pharm. Sci.,* 53:1–18, 1964.

McCarthy, W. W.: Ultrasonic Emulsification. *Drug Cosmetic Ind.,* 94:821, 1964.

Marshall, K.: The Manufacture of Dispersions. *Soap, Perfumery, Cosmetic,* 38:759–768, 1965.

Martin, A. N.: Physical Chemical Approach to the Formulation of Pharmaceutical Suspensions. *J. Pharm. Sci.,* 50:513–517, 1961.

Nash, R. A.: The Pharmaceutical Suspension, Part I. *Drug Cosmetic Ind.,* 97:843, 1965; Part 2. *ibid.,* 98:39, 1966.

Oldshue, J. Y.: Mixing of Solid-Liquid Suspensions, *J. Pharm. Sci.,* 50:523–530, 1961.

Patel, B. N.: Hydrocolloids in Cosmetic and Pharmaceutical Dispersions. Part I: *Drug Cosmetic Ind.,* 95:337, 1964; Part II: *ibid.,* 95:509, 1964; Part III: *ibid.,* 95:898, 1964.

Peck, G. E., DeKay, G. and Banker, G. S.: A Comparative Study of Pharmaceutical Emulsification Equipment, *J. Amer. Pharm. Assoc., Sci. Ed.,* 49:75–79, 1960.

Rowe, E. L.: Effect of Emulsifier Concentration and Type on the Particle Size Distribution of Emulsions, *J. Pharm. Sci.,* 54:160–164, 1965.

Samyn, J. C.: An Industrial Approach to Suspension Formulation, *J. Pharm. Sci.,* 50:517–522, 1961.

Schlossman, M. L.: Clear Gel Systems, *Drug Cosmetic Ind.,* 98:32, 1966.

Sherman, P.: Flow Properties of Emulsions, *J. Pharm. Pharmacol.,* 16:1–25, 1964.

Soenen, F.: Stability of Oral Pharmaceutical Suspensions, *Sciences Et Techniques Pharmaceutiques,* 2:63–91, 1973.

Smith, E. A.: Some Practical Aspects of Colloids, *Mfg. Chem. Aerosol News,* 36:759–768, 1965.

Chapter 6

Powders, Granules, and Solid Dosage Forms for Oral Administration: Capsules and Tablets

Wwhen medications are to be administered orally in dry form, capsules and tablets are most frequently used. They are effective and provide the patient with convenience of handling, identification, and administration. From a pharmaceutic standpoint, solid dosage forms are generally more stable than are their liquid counterparts and thus are preferred for poorly stable drugs. Dry powders are taken orally (usually after mixing in water) to a much lesser extent than are capsules and tablets, but are preferred by some patients who are unable to swallow the solid dosage forms. However, most medicated powders are utilized as external applications to the skin. While the use of powders *per se* in therapeutics is limited, the use of powders in dosage form preparation is exten-

sive. Most of the medicinal substances in use today occur in crystalline or powdered form and are blended with other powdered materials, as inert fillers and disintegrants, prior to fabrication into solid dosage forms. Powdered drugs are also frequently added to ointments, pastes, suppositories, and other dosage forms during their preparation. Similarly, granules, which are agglomerates of powdered materials prepared into larger free flowing particles, are utilized chiefly in the preparation of tablets and in dry preparations intended to be reconstituted to liquid forms prior to use by the addition of the appropriate vehicle. The pharmacy student must be knowledgeable about the processes involved in the preparation of powders, powder mixtures, and granules, and in their utilization in the manufacture of other dosage forms.

Powders

As a pharmaceutical preparation, a *powder* (Latin, *pulvis*) is a mixture of finely divided drugs and/or chemicals in dry form. This then is in contrast to the general use of the term "powder" or "powdered" which frequently describes the physical state of a single chemical substance or a single drug.

A powder may be a finely subdivided preparation, a coarsely comminuted product, or a product of intermediate particle size. It may be prepared from a naturally occurring dried vegetable drug adjusted to the proper potency with a diluent or with a powdered drug of greater potency, or it may be a physical admixture of two or more powdered pure chemical agents present in definite proportions. Powders may contain small proportions of liquids dispersed thoroughly and uniformly over the solid components of the mixture, or the powder may be composed entirely of solid materials.

Some powders are intended to be used internally; others, externally. Certain powders are dispensed by the pharmacist to the patient in bulk quantities; others, in divided, individually packaged portions, depending primarily on the dose, or potency of the powder.

The disadvantages of powders as a dosage form include the undesirability of taking bitter or unpleasant tasting drugs in this manner, the difficulty of protecting from decomposition powders containing hydroscopic, deliquescent, or aromatic materials, and the time and expense required in the preparation of uniform powders.

To be of high efficacy, the powder must be a homogeneous blend of all of the components and must be of the most advantageous particle size. As noted earlier (Chapter 3), the particle size of a drug not only contributes to its rate of solubility in a glass of water or within the stomach or intestine, but also may influence its biological activity or therapeutic performance.

Preparation of Powders

Particle Size

Generally speaking, the particles of pharmaceutical powders may be very coarse, of the dimensions of about 10,000 microns or 10 mm, or they may be extremely fine, approaching colloidal dimensions of 1 micron or less. In order to standardize the particle size of a given powder, the USP and the NF employ descriptive terms such as "Very Coarse, Coarse, Moderately Coarse, Fine, and Very Fine," which for vegetable and animal drugs and for chemical substances are related to the proportion of powder that is capable of passing through the openings of standardized sieves of varying dimensions in a specified time period under shaking, generally in a *mechanical sieve shaker*. Table 6-1 presents the Standard Sieve Numbers and the sieve openings in each, expressed in millimeters and in micrometers. For the specified wire diameters for these sieves as well as the permissible variations in the maximum openings, the USP XIX or the NF XIV should be consulted. Sieves for such pharmaceutical testing and measurement are generally made of wire cloth woven from brass, bronze, or other suitable wire. They are not coated or plated.

Powders of vegetable and animal drugs are officially defined as follows:

Very Coarse (or a No. 8) powder—All particles pass through a No. 8 sieve and not more than 20% through a No. 20 sieve.
Coarse (or a No. 20) powder—All particles pass through a No. 20 sieve and not more than 40% through a No. 60 sieve.
Moderately Coarse (or a No. 40) powder—All particles pass through a No. 40 sieve and not more than 40% through a No. 80 sieve.
Fine (or a No. 60) powder—All particles pass through a No. 60 sieve and not more than 40% through a No. 100 sieve.

Table 6-1. OPENINGS OF STANDARD SIEVES[*]

	Sieve Opening	
Sieve Number	mm	µm
2	9.52	9520
4	4.76	4760
8	2.38	2380
10	2.00	2000
20	0.84	840
30	0.59	590
40	0.42	420
50	0.297	297
60	0.250	250
70	0.210	210
80	0.177	177
100	0.149	149
120	0.125	125
200	0.074	74

[*] Adapted from Table in USP XIX, p. 656 and NF XIV, p. 946.

Very Fine (or a No. 80) powder—All particles pass through a No. 80 sieve. There is no limit as to greater fineness.

The powder fineness for chemicals is defined as follows. It should be noted that there is no "Very Coarse" category.

Coarse (or a No. 20) powder—All particles pass through a No. 20 sieve and not more than 60% through a No. 40 sieve.
Moderately Coarse (or a No. 40) powder—All particles pass through a No. 40 sieve and not more than 60% through a No. 60 sieve.
Fine (or a No. 80) powder—All particles pass through a No. 80 sieve. There is no limit as to greater fineness.
Very Fine (or a No. 120) powder—All particles pass through a No. 120 sieve. There is no limit as to greater fineness.

Granules typically fall within the range of 4- to 12-sieve size, although granulations of powders prepared in the 12- to 20-sieve range are not uncommon when used in tablet making.

Particle size determination and distribution studies of powders may be performed by *sieving;* that is, by passing the powder by mechanical shaking through a series of sieves of known and successively smaller size, and determining the proportion of powder passing through or being withheld on each sieve. Other methods of particle size determinations include the measurement of the particles under the microscope through the use of a calibrated grid background or other measuring device, determination of sedimentation rates and the application of the Stokes' equation, electrical conductivity methods, and others.[1-3] The study of particle size is referred to as *micromeritics.*

Comminution of Drugs

On a small scale, as in the community pharmacy, the pharmacist usually reduces the size of chemical substances by exposing them to the rigor of the mortar and pestle. Generally a finer grinding action is accomplished in a mortar with a rough surface (as a porcelain mortar) than one with a smooth surface (as a glass mortar). The process of grinding a drug in a mortar to reduce its particle size is termed *trituration.*[4] On a large scale, various types of mills and pulverizers may be used to reduce powder fineness. Figure 6-1 shows one such piece of equipment. The type shown is the Stokes Tornado Mill. This machine is employed to pulverize, granulate, and disperse materials presented to it in the dry or wet state.

A process termed *levigation* is commonly employed in the reduction of particle size particularly in the small-scale preparation of ointments. This is done in order to prevent the feeling of grittiness in the preparation due to the solid drug present. In the process, a mortar and pestle is generally used, and a paste formed of the solid material and a small amount of liquid (the levigating agent) in which the solid material is insoluble. The paste is then triturated, effecting a reduction in particle size. The levigated paste may then be added to the oint-

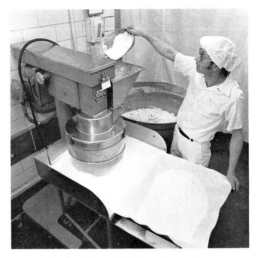

Fig. 6-1. *Stokes Tornado Mill used to pulverize, granulate, and disperse materials presented to it in the dry or wet state. (Courtesy of Eli Lilly and Company)*

ment and the mixture made uniform and smooth, usually by rubbing them together with a spatula on a porcelain or glass plate. The entire levigation procedure may be performed with the spatula, usually employing a "figure 8" track to incorporate and levigate the materials. Mineral oil is a commonly used levigating agent.

The Mixing of Powders

Generally speaking, when two or more substances are to be mixed together to form a uniform powder mixture, it is best to reduce the particle size of each individually before weighing and blending. Depending upon the nature of the ingredients, the amount of powder to prepare, and the equipment available, powders may be prepared by *spatulation, trituration, sifting, tumbling* or by *mechanical mixers.*

Spatulation is a method by which small amounts of powders may be blended by the movement of a pharmaceutical spatula through the powders on a sheet of paper or a pill tile. The method is not generally suitable for large quantities of powders or for powders containing one or more potent substances, since homogeneous blending is not as certain as with other methods. Very little compression or compacting of the powder results from this method, which is especially suited to the mixing of those solid substances that liquify or form *eutectic* mixtures when in close and prolonged contact with one another. These substances include phenol,

[1] Orr, C., and Dallavalle, J. M.: *Fine Particles Measurement.* New York, The Macmillan Co., 1959.

[2] Irani, R. R., and Callis, C. F.: *Particle Size Measurement, Interpretation and Application.* New York, John Wiley & Sons, Inc., 1963.

[3] Parrott, E. L.: Milling. In *The Theory and Practice of Industrial Pharmacy*, 2nd Ed., Editors, L. Lachman, H. A. Lieberman, and J. L. Kanig, Philadelphia, Lea & Febiger, 1976, pp. 466–485.

[4] It should be noted that a type of pharmaceutical preparation termed a *trituration* is a powder mixture, usually containing 10% of a potent medicinal substance in a vehicle of lactose. Triturations provide a convenient means whereby pharmacists can accurately obtain small amounts of potent drugs. For example, 50 mg of a potent drug may be obtained by weighing 500 mg of a 10% trituration of that drug.

camphor, menthol, thymol, aspirin, phenyl-salicylate, phenacetin, and other similar chemicals. To diminish contact, powder prepared from such substances is commonly mixed in the presence of an inert diluent such as light magnesium oxide or magnesium carbonate to separate physically the troublesome agents.

Trituration may be employed both to comminute and to mix powders. If comminution is especially desired, a porcelain or a Wedgwood mortar having a rough inner surface is preferred over the generally smooth working surface of the glass mortar. However, for chemicals that may stain the porcelain or Wedgwood surface, a glass mortar may be preferred. Also, if simple admixture is desired without special need for comminution, the glass mortar is usually preferred, since it cleans more readily after use. The application of firm or "heavy" trituration may have a compacting effect on a bulky fluffy powder and may be performed for this very purpose. When potent substances are to be mixed with a large amount of diluent (as in the preparation of a 10% trituration of a potent drug), a general method known as the *geometric dilution method* is employed for the purpose of ensuring the uniform distribution of potent drug. The use of this method is especially indicated in instances in which the potent and the nonpotent substances are of the same color and a visible sign of thorough mixing is lacking.[1] By this method, the potent drug is placed upon an approximately equal volume of the diluent in a mortar and the mixture is thoroughly mixed by trituration. Then a second portion of diluent equal in volume to the powder mixture in the mortar is added, and the trituration is repeated. This process is continued by adding equal volumes of diluent to that powder present in the mortar and repeating the mixing until all of the diluent is incorporated.

Powders may also be mixed by passing them through sifters like the type used in the kitchen to sift flour. This process of *sifting* generally results in a light fluffy product. This process is not generally considered acceptable for the incorporation of potent drugs into a diluent base.

Another method of mixing powders is that of *tumbling* the powder enclosed in a large container which rotates generally by a motorized process. Special *powder blenders* have been devised and mix powders by a tumbling motion (Fig. 6-2). Mixing by this process is thorough, although time-consuming. Such blenders are widely employed in industry, as are large volume powder mixers which have motorized blades to blend the powder contained in a large mixing vessel (Fig. 6-3).

Use and Packaging of Powders

Depending upon their intended use, powders are packaged and dispensed by pharmacists in two main ways, as *bulk powders* or as *divided powders*.

BULK POWDERS. After preparation of the powder mixture, a pharmacist may dispense the powder in a bulk container for either internal or external use. Among the powders commonly dispensed in this manner are (a) antacid and laxative powders, which the patient generally takes by mixing the directed amount of powder (usually a teaspoon or so) in a portion of water or other beverage and swallowing; (b) douche powders, generally dissolved in warm water by the patient for vaginal use; (c) medicated or nonmedicated powders for external application, usually dispensed in sifter cans for convenient application to the skin; (d) dentifrices or dental cleansing powders, used in dental hygiene; and (e) denture powders, some used as dentifrices and others as adhesives to hold the dentures in place.

---

[1] Some pharmacists add about 0.1% of a dry certified pharmaceutical dye or colorant to the powders and feel assured of thorough mixing when the dye is thoroughly distributed throughout the powder mixture upon visual inspection.

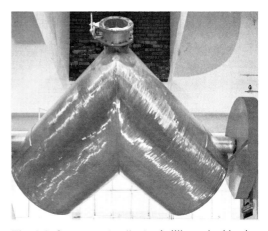

Fig. 6-2. *Large rotating "twin shell" powder blender. (Courtesy of Abbott Laboratories)*

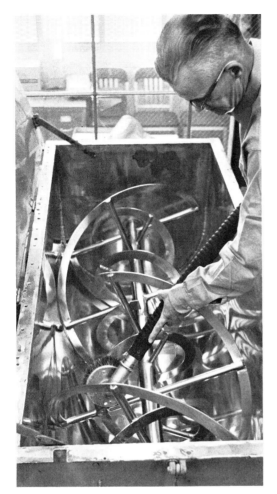

Fig. 6-3. *The meticulous cleaning of a ribbon mixer used to blend powders preparative to granulation and tablet compression. (Courtesy of Eli Lilly and Company)*

Depending upon the intended use of the powder, it may be supplied to the patient in a perforated or sifter-type can or container for external dusting, in an aerosol container for spraying onto the skin, or in a wide-mouthed jar which permits the entrance of a spoon and the easy removal of a spoonful of powder. Glass jars are generally preferred over pasteboard containers for the packaging of powders which are hydroscopic or deliquescent, or have volatile ingredients, since glass containers are much less likely to permit the entrance of moisture into the container or to permit the escape of volatile components to the atmosphere. Some glass containers are of amber or green glass to protect the light-sensitive components of the powder from decomposition. Naturally, all powders should be stored in tightly closed containers.

Dispensing powdered drugs in bulk amounts is generally limited to nonpotent substances. Powders containing potent substances or those that should be administered in controlled dosage are usually supplied to the patient in divided amounts. Powders supplied to the patient in either bulk or in divided portions that are intended for external use should bear an EXTERNAL USE ONLY or a similar label.

DIVIDED POWDERS. (Latin, *chartulae* (pl.); abbrev: *charts*.) After the powder has been properly mixed (using the geometric dilution method for potent substances), it may be divided into individual units based upon the dose to be administered or the amount to be used at a single time. Each divided portion of powder may be placed on a small piece of paper, which is then folded so as to enclose the medication.

Depending upon the potency of the drug substance, the pharmacist decides whether to weigh each portion of powder separately before enfolding in a paper or to approximate each portion by using the so-called *block-and-divide method*. By this method, used only for nonpotent drugs, the pharmacist places the entire amount of prepared powder on a flat surface such as a porcelain or glass plate or pill tile or a large sheet of paper on the prescription counter and with a large spatula forms a rectangular or square-shaped block of powder having a uniform depth. Then, using the spatula and sharp vision, he partially cuts into the powder vertically and horizontally to delineate the appropriate number of smaller, uniform blocks, each representing a dose or unit of medication. Each of the smaller blocks is then separated from the main block with the spatula and transferred to a powder paper and wrapped.

The powder papers may be of any convenient size to hold the amount of powder issued, but the most popular sizes are commercially available and include $2\frac{3}{4} \times 3\frac{3}{4}$ inches, $3 \times 4\frac{1}{2}$ inches, $3\frac{3}{4} \times 5$ inches, and $4\frac{1}{2} \times 6$ inches. The papers may be (1) simple bond paper, white or colored; (2) vegetable parchment, a thin, semi-opaque paper having limited moisture-resistant qualities; (3) glassine, a glazed, transparent paper, also having limited moisture-resistant qualities; and (4) waxed paper, a transparent, waterproof paper. The selection of the type of paper is based primarily on the nature of the powder. If the powder contains hygroscopic or deliquescent materials, a waterproof or a waxed paper should be used. In practice, such powders are double-wrapped in waxed paper, and then for aesthetic appeal they are finally wrapped in bond paper. Glassine and vegetable parchment papers may be used when only a limited barrier against moisture is necessary. Powders containing volatile components should be wrapped in waxed or in glassine papers. Powders containing neither volatile components nor ingredients adversely affected by air or moisture are usually wrapped in white bond paper.

A certain degree of expertise is required in the folding of a powder paper, and the student should practice until he becomes proficient at preparing neat and uniform papers. Basically the steps in the folding of a powder paper are as follows:

1. Place the paper flat on a hard surface and fold toward you a uniform flap of about $\frac{1}{2}$ inch of the long side of the paper. To ensure uniformity of all of the papers, this step should be performed on all the required papers concurrently, using the first folded paper as the guide (Fig. 6-4A).
2. With the flap of each paper away from you and pointing upward, place the weighed or divided amount of powder in the center of each paper.
3. Being careful not to disturb the powder excessively, bring the lower edge of the paper upward, and place it proximate to the crease of the flap (Fig. 6-4B).
4. Grasp the flap, press it down upon the tucked-in bottom edge of the paper and fold again toward you an amount of paper equal to the size of the original flap ($\frac{1}{2}$ inch) (Fig. 6-4C).
5. Pick the paper up with the flap upward and facing you, being careful not to disturb the position of the powder, and place the partially folded paper over the open powder box (to serve as the container) so that the ends of the paper extend equally beyond the sides (lengthwise) of the open container. Then, press the sides of the box slightly inward and the ends of the paper gently downward along the sides of the box to form a crease on each end of the paper. Lift the paper from the box and fold the ends of the paper along each crease sharply so that the powder cannot escape (Fig. 6-4D).
6. The folded papers are then each placed in the box so that the double-folded flaps are at

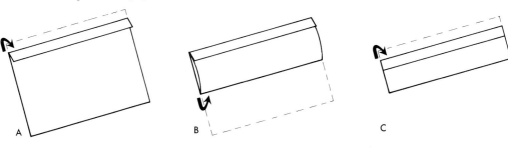

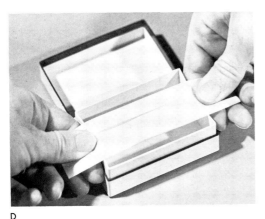

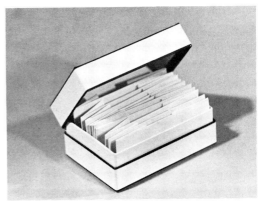

Fig. 6-4. *Steps in the folding of powder papers.*

the top, facing the operator, and the ends are folded away from the operator (Fig. 6-4E).

Papers folded properly should fit snugly in the box, have uniform folds, and should be of uniform length and height. There should be no powder in the folds, and none should be capable of escape with moderate agitation. Powder boxes, which are generally pasteboard and of the hinged type, should close easily without coming in contact with the tops of the papers. The label for the powders may be placed on the container, but some pharmacists affix a label of directions to each individual paper.

For convenience and uniformity of appearance, some pharmacists use commercially available cellophane or plastic envelopes to enclose individual doses or units of powders rather than folding individual papers. These envelopes are usually moisture resistant, and their use results in handsome and efficacious products.

Although divided powders have generally come into disuse because of more convenient and readily available unit doses of tablets and capsules, it is not unusual to find being dispensed in a pharmacy an occasional divided powder containing antacid medication or a premeasured amount of powder for use in preparing a vaginal douche solution. Further, a number of commercial preparations for the relief of pain, as Stanback Analgesic Powders and B. C. Headache Powders, are packaged in unit-dose packets.

Official Powdered Vegetable Drugs

Five vegetable drug powders are official:

Powdered Belladonna Extract, NF
Powdered Digitalis, NF
Powdered Ipecac, USP
Powdered Opium, USP
Powdered Rauwolfia Serpentina, NF

Each of these powders is official for the purpose of providing standards for these materials which are utilized in the preparation of corresponding dosage forms. Powdered belladonna extract, powdered digitalis, and powdered rauwolfia serpentina are each used in the preparation of tablets of these medicinal substances. Powdered ipecac is utilized in the preparation of ipecac syrup and powdered opium in the preparation of paregoric. In addition to the above,

Powdered Cellulose, NF is official and is utilized as a pharmaceutic aid particularly as a tablet diluent, adsorbant, and suspending agent.

Official Powders

There is presently no official powder preparation which is intended for oral administration. In fact, there are only three official powders, each of which is employed topically as indicated below.

Absorbable Dusting Powder, USP—employed as a surgeon's glove lubricant.
Compound Iodochlorhydroxyquin Powder, NF—used by vaginal insufflation as an antitrichomonal.
Methylbenzethonium Chloride Powder, NF—local anti-infective used chiefly for diaper rash in infants and chafing.

Preparations for localized application are covered more fully in subsequent chapters.

Granules

As indicated earlier, granules are prepared agglomerates of smaller particles. They are generally irregularly shaped and behave as single larger particles. They are usually in the 4- to 12-sieve size range although granules of various mesh sizes may be prepared depending upon their application.

Generally, granules are prepared by moistening the desired powder or blended powder mixture and passing the moistened mass through a screen of the mesh size that will produce the desired size granules. The larger particles thus formed are then dried by air or under heat (as the nature of the drug will allow), while they are occasionally moved about on the drying trays to prevent the adhesion of the granules. Granules may also be prepared without the use of moisture by passing compressed masses of powdered material through a granulating machine.

Granules flow well compared to powders. For the purpose of comparison, mentally visualize the pouring characteristics of granulated sugar and powdered sugar. Because of their flow properties, granulations are usually made when powder mixtures are intended to be compressed into tablets. The flow characteristics allow the material to flow freely from the hopper or feeding container into the tableting presses. This will be discussed later in this chapter in greater detail.

Granules are generally more stable physically and chemically than are the corresponding powders from which they were prepared. Granules are less likely to cake or harden upon standing than are powders. Because their surface area is less than that of powders, granules are usually more stable to the effects of the atmosphere. Since granules are more easily "wetted" by a solvent than are certain powders which tend to float on the solvent's surface, granules are frequently preferred for the making of solutions.

A number of commercial products containing antibiotic drugs which are unstable in aqueous solution are prepared as granules for reconstitution by the pharmacist with purified water just prior to dispensing. The granules are so prepared to contain not only the medicinal agent, but the colorants, flavorants, and any other desired pharmaceutic ingredient. Upon reconstitution, the resultant liquid (solution or suspension) has all of the desired medicinal and pharmaceutic features of a liquid pharmaceutical.

Other types of granular products are prepared and sold commercially including a number which are packaged in bulk and utilized as laxatives. One example of this type of product is Senokot Granules (Purdue Frederick), which are cocoa-flavored granules containing standardized senna concentrate. The granules are measured by the teaspoon and usually mixed with water upon administration. Effervescent products as Bromo Seltzer (Warner Lambert) represent another popular type of granulated product. Granulations of effervescent products may be compressed into tablet form. Alka Seltzer (Miles) is an example of a product of this type. Effervescent granules and tablets are placed in a portion of water and taken as the effervescence subsides. Effervescent granulated salts are discussed more fully below.

Effervescent Granulated Salts

Effervescent salts are granules or coarse to very coarse powders containing a medicinal agent in a dry mixture usually composed of sodium bicarbonate, citric acid, and tartaric acid. When added to water, the acids and base react to liberate carbon dioxide, resulting in effervescence. The resulting carbonated solution masks the usually saline or otherwise undesirable taste of the medicinal agent present. By using granules or coarse particles of the mixed powders rather than the ordinary smaller sized particles of these substances, the rate of solution of the substances is decreased upon addition to water, and the otherwise violent reaction and rapid, uncontrollable effervescence is eliminated. Such violent effervescence would likely overflow the glass of water to which it was added with subsequent loss of solution and little residual carbonation of the solution.

Methods of Preparation

Effervescent salts are prepared by two general methods: (1) the *wet method*, and (2) the *dry* or *fusion* method. Irrespective of the method used, the initial step is the determination of the proper formula for the preparation that will result in effective effervescence, efficient utilization of the acids and base present, a stable granulation, and a pleasant tasting and efficacious product.

Effervescent salts are usually prepared from a combination of citric and tartaric acids rather than from a single acid because the use of either acid alone presents difficulties. When tartaric acid is the sole acid, the resulting granules lose their firmness readily and crumble. Citric acid alone results in a sticky mixture difficult to granulate. Granulation is due to the presence of one molecule of water of crystallization in each molecule of citric acid, a feature that is taken advantage of and utilized in the preparation of granules by the fusion method using the combination of acids and sodium bicarbonate. Although the proportion of acids may be varied, so long as the total acidity is maintained and the bicarbonate completely neutralized, a general guideline of usual proportions of these materials can be shown from the formula of the only remaining official effervescent salt, Effervescent Sodium Phosphate, NF. The formula for this preparation is as follows:

Dried Sodium Phosphate, dried
    and powdered . . . . 200 g
Sodium Bicarbonate, in dry
    powder. . . . . 477 g
Tartaric Acid, in dry powder . . . . 252 g
Citric Acid, uneffloresced crystals. . . . 162 g
           To make about   1000 g

From this formula it can be observed that of the effervescence-producing agents, about 53% of the mixture is sodium bicarbonate, 28% is tartaric acid, and about 19% is citric acid. The reactions between citric and sodium bicarbonate (1) and tartaric acid and sodium bicarbonate (2) may be shown as follows:

(1) $H_3C_6H_5O_7 \cdot H_2O$ + $3NaHCO_3$ →
  citric acid   sodium bicarbonate

     $Na_3C_6H_5O_7$ + $4H_2O$ + $3CO_2$
      sodium citrate   water   carbon dioxide

(2) $H_2C_4H_4O_6$ + $2NaHCO_3$ →
  tartaric acid   sodium bicarbonate

     $Na_2C_4H_4O_6$ + $2H_2O$ + $2CO_2$
      sodium tartrate   water   carbon dioxide

It should be noted that it requires 3 molecules of sodium bicarbonate to neutralize 1 molecule of citric acid (1) and 2 molecules of sodium bicarbonate to neutralize 1 molecule of tartaric acid (2). In preparing a pharmaceutical formula of an effervescent salt from these components, one can determine the precise amounts of reactants to employ. For instance, using the official formula for Effervescent Sodium Phosphate, NF, one can calculate from information of the above reactions and the molecular weights of the three reactants the amount of sodium bicarbonate required to neutralize 252 g of tartaric acid and 162 g of uneffloresced citric acid:

(1) For the amount of sodium bicarbonate required to neutralize 162 g of citric acid:

$$\frac{162 \text{ g citric acid}}{210.13 \text{ g m.w. citric acid}}$$

$$= \frac{x \text{ g sodium bicarbonate}}{252.03 \text{ g m.w. sodium bicarbonate}}$$
$$(84.01) \text{ times } 3 \text{ (molecules)}$$

x = *194.3 g of sodium bicarbonate*

(2) For the amount of sodium bicarbonate required to neutralize 252 g of tartaric acid:

$$\frac{252 \text{ g tartaric acid}}{150.09 \text{ g m.w. tartaric acid}}$$

$$= \frac{x \text{ g sodium bicarbonate}}{168.02 \text{ g m.w. sodium bicarbonate}}$$
$$(84.01) \text{ times } 2 \text{ (molecules)}$$

x = *282.1 g of sodium bicarbonate*

Total: 194.3 + 282.1

    = *476.4 g of sodium bicarbonate*

The amount of medicinal agent in effervescent preparations is determined by the intended dose of the medication. Generally the dose of the drug is contained in a teaspoonful or two of the dry effervescent salt. After the formula has been determined, the powders are uniformly mixed, being certain that the powders are dry to avoid premature chemical reaction. Then the granules are prepared.

FUSION METHOD. In the fusion method, the one molecule of water present in each molecule of citric acid acts as the binding agent for the powder mixture. Just before mixing the powders, the citric acid crystals are powdered and then mixed with the other powders (previously passed through a number 60 sieve) to ensure uniformity of the mixture. The sieves and the mixing equipment should be made of stainless steel or other material resistant to the effect of the acids. The mixing of the powders is performed as rapidly as is practical, preferably in an environment of low humidity to avoid the absorption of moisture from the air by the chemicals and a premature chemical reaction. After mixing, the powder is placed on a plate or glass or a suitable dish in an oven (or other suitable source of heat) previously heated to between 93° and 104°. During the heating process, an acid-resistant spatula is used to turn the powder. The heat causes the release of the water of crystallization from the citric acid, which in turn dissolves a portion of the powder mixture, setting of the chemical reaction and the consequent release of some carbon dioxide. This causes the softened mass of powder to become somewhat spongy, and when of the proper consistency (as bread dough), it is removed from the oven and rubbed through an acid-resistant sieve to produce granules of the desired size. A No. 4 sieve may be used to produce large granules, a No. 8 sieve to produce medium size granules, and a No. 10 sieve to prepare small granules. When all of the mass has passed through the sieve, the granules are immediately dried at a temperature not exceeding 54° and immediately transferred to containers which are then promptly and tightly sealed.

The fusion method is used in the preparation of most commercial effervescent powders and in the preparation of the official Effervescent Sodium Phosphate, NF.

WET METHOD. The wet method differs from the fusion method in that the source of binding

agent is not necessarily the water of crystallization from the citric acid but may be water
added to the nonsolvent (such as alcohol),
which is employed as the moistening agent, to
form the pliable mass of material for granulation. In this method all of the powders may be
anhydrous so long as water is added to the
moistening liquid. Just enough liquid is added
(in portions) to prepare a mass of proper consistency; then the granules are prepared and
dried in the same manner as described above.

Official Effervescent Salt

Effervescent Sodium Phosphate, NF

The formula and the method of preparation
of this product is described above (fusion
method).

The preparation is used as a cathartic and
has a usual dose of 10 g. About 2 teaspoonfuls of
the granules are added to a glass of water, and
the mixture is swallowed as the effervescence
subsides. Each 10 g of the granules contain 2 g
of exsiccated sodium phosphate, the usual dose
of this agent, which is the active component of
the effervescent salt.

Capsules

Capsules may be defined as solid dosage
forms in which one or more medicinal and/or
inert substances are enclosed within a small
shell or container generally prepared from a
suitable form of gelatin. Depending upon their
formulation, the gelatin capsule shells may be
hard or soft. The majority of capsules dispensed
are intended to be swallowed whole by the patient for the benefit of the medication contained
therein.[1] However, a capsule may be prescribed

for insertion into the rectum for drug release
and absorption from that site, or the contents of
a capsule may be removed from the gelatin shell
and employed as a premeasured medicinal powder, the capsule shell being used to contain a
dose of the medicinal substance.

Hard Gelatin Capsules

Hard gelatin capsules are the type used by
the community pharmacist in the extemporaneous compounding of prescriptions and by
pharmaceutical manufacturers in the preparation of the majority of their capsule products.
The basic empty capsule shells are made from a
mixture of gelatin, sugar, and water and are
clear, colorless, and essentially tasteless. Gelatin, USP, is a product obtained by the partial
hydrolysis of collagen obtained from the skin,
white connective tissue, and bones of animals.
It is found in commerce in the form of a fine
powder, a coarse powder, shreds, flakes, or
sheets.

Gelatin is stable in air when dry but is subject to microbic decomposition when it becomes
moist or when it is maintained in aqueous solution. For this reason, soft gelatin capsules,
which contain more moisture than the hard
capsules, may be prepared with a preservative
agent added to prevent the growth of fungi in
the capsule shells. Normally, hard gelatin capsules contain between 9 and 12% of moisture.
However, if stored in an environment of high
humidity, additional moisture is absorbed by
the capsules, and they may become distorted
and lose their otherwise rigid shape. On the
other hand, in an environment of extreme
dryness, some of the moisture normally present
in the gelatin capsules may be lost, and the
capsules may become brittle and may crumble
when handled.

Since moisture may be absorbed or released
by gelatin capsules, depending upon the environmental conditions, it follows that little physical protection is afforded hygroscopic or deliquescent materials enclosed within a capsule
when stored in an area of high humidity. It is
not unusual to find capsules of such moisture-

---

[1] Dosage units, such as tablets and capsules, containing therapeutically inert materials or drug materials unrelated to the disease or condition being treated
are termed *placebos*. A placebo is deliberately prescribed by a physician for its nonspecific psychologic or
psychophysiologic effect on a patient's symptom or
illness without the patient's knowledge. Actually, a
placebo may include not only oral dosage forms, but
parenteral medication, topical preparations, inhalants,
and other types of pharmaceutical preparations as well
as mechanical, surgical, or other therapeutic techniques. A placebo may or may not actually result in a
placebo effect, and the effect may be favorable or
unfavorable to the patient and his physician. A phar-

macist may issue a placebo for a specific drug by replacing the contents of a capsule with an inert or
inappropriate (to the symptom) substance. Or, he may
receive and fill a prescription for a drug product, generally of only mild action, prescribed (in this instance)
not for a medical but for a placebo effect.

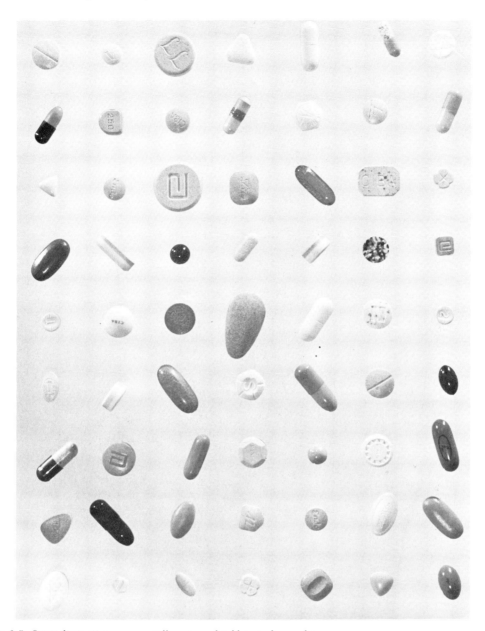

Fig. 6-5. *Some distinctive commercially prepared tablets and capsules.*

affected materials packaged in containers along with a packet of a desiccant material as a precaution against the capsules absorbing atmospheric moisture. With or without such desiccant materials, capsules should be generally stored in areas of low humidity.

Although gelatin is insoluble in cold water, it does soften through the absorption of up to ten times its weight of the water. Some patients prefer to swallow a capsule wetted with water

or saliva, since the capsule softens and slides down the throat more readily than does a dry capsule. Gelatin is soluble in hot water, and in warm gastric fluid a gelatin capsule rapidly releases its contents. Gelatin, being a protein, is digested and absorbed by the body as a nutrient.

Hard gelatin capsule shells are manufactured in two sections, the capsule body and a shorter cap. The two parts overlap when joined, with the cap fitting snugly over the open end of

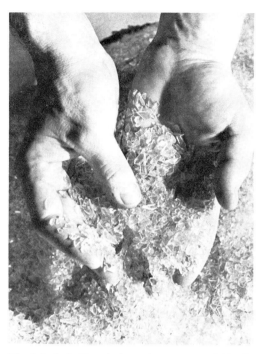

Fig. 6-6. *Pork skin gelatin used as raw material in the manufacture of gelatin capsules. (Courtesy of Smith, Kline & French Laboratories)*

the capsule body. The shells are produced by the mechanical dipping of pins or pegs of the desired shape and diameter into a reservoir of the melted gelatin mixture, maintained at a constant temperature to achieve the desired degree of fluidity. The pegs, made of manganese bronze, are affixed to plates, each capable of holding up to about 500 pegs. Each plate is mechanically lowered to the gelatin bath, the pegs being submerged to the desired depth and for the desired period of time to achieve the proper length and thickness of coating. Then the plate and the pegs are slowly lifted from the gelatin bath, and the gelatin on the pegs is gently dried by a flow of temperature and humidity controlled air. When dried, each capsule part is trimmed mechanically to the proper length and removed from the pegs, and the capsule bodies and caps are joined together. It is important that the thickness of the gelatin walls be strictly controlled so that the capsule body and cap fit snugly to prevent disengagement. Naturally, the pegs on which the caps are formed are slightly larger in diameter than the pegs on which the bodies are formed, since the caps overlap the bodies. In production, there is a continuous dipping, drying, removing, and

joining of capsules as many peg-containing plates are rotated in and out of the gelatin bath.

Several methods of making capsules distinctive are available to the pharmaceutical manufacturer. One way is to color the gelatin used in the preparation of the capsules. The compendia permit the use of certified colorants to dye the gelatin. These colorants may be used to prepare capsule bodies and caps having the same or different colors. By combining the various capsule parts, beautiful, transparent, and distinctive capsules may be prepared.

Opaque capsules may also be prepared to make a pharmaceutical product distinctive. These capsules are formed by adding an insoluble substance such as titantium dioxide to the gelatin mixture. Colored, opaque capsules may be prepared by using both a colorant and the opaque-producing substance.

A manufacturer may also alter the usually rounded shape of the capsule-making pegs to produce capsule shells of distinctive shapes. By tapering the end of the body-producing peg while leaving the cap-making peg rounded, one manufacturer prepares capsules easily differentiated from those of other manufacturers.[1] Another firm produces capsules with the ends of both the bodies and caps highly tapered, but not pointed.[2] Still another manufacturer makes distinctive and tamperproof and leakproof capsules by sealing the joint between the two capsule parts with a colored band of gelatin.[3] Removal of the band through tampering is evident, as the bands cannot be returned to place without a great deal of trouble and resealing with gelatin. As indicated previously in this text capsules may be imprinted with monograms of the manufacturer, the strength of the drug in the capsule, a code designation for product identification, or some other symbol making the product unique and distinguishable from other manufacturers' products.

Capsule Sizes

Empty gelatin capsules are manufactured in various sizes, varying both in length and in diameter. The size selected is determined by the amount of material to be encapsulated and the relative capacities of the capsule shells.

[1] Eli Lilly's *Pulvules.*
[2] Smith, Kline & French's *Spansule* capsules.
[3] Parke, Davis's *Kapseals.*

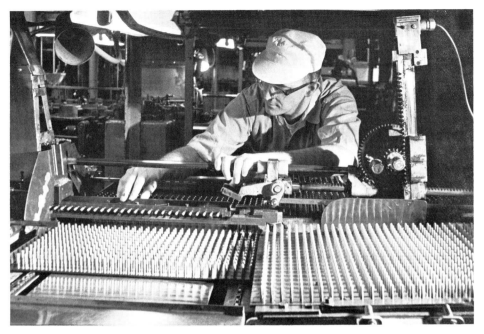

Fig. 6-7. *Body of capsules and their caps are shown as they move through automated capsule-making machine. Each machine is capable of producing 30,000 capsules per hour. It takes a 40-minute cycle to produce a capsule. (Courtesy of Smith, Kline & French Laboratories)*

Since the density and compressibility of a powder or a powder mixture will largely determine to what extent it may be packed into a capsule shell and since these are individual features of the materials themselves, there are no strict rules for predicting the proper capsule size for a given powder or formulation. However, comparison may be made with powders of well-known features (Table 6-2), and an initial judgment made as to the approximate capsule size to hold a specific amount of material, but the final decision is largely the result of trial. For human use, empty capsules ranging in size from 000, the largest, to 5, the smallest, are commercially available, plain or colored.[1] Larger capsules are available for veterinary use.

In addition to the advantages of solid dosage forms presented at the outset of this chapter, hard gelatin capsules permit a wide prescribing

latitude by the physician in that the pharmacist may extemporaneously prepare capsules containing a single chemical substance or a combination of drugs at the precise dosage level considered appropriate for the individual patient. This degree of flexibility is an advantage that capsules have as a dosage form over tablets, which cannot be prepared easily in the community pharmacy.

Preparation of Filled Hard Gelatin Capsules

The preparation of filled hard gelatin capsules may be divided into the following steps:

1. Developing and preparing the formulation and the selecting of the size capsule.
2. Filling the capsule shells with the medicinal and nonmedicinal agents.
3. Cleaning and polishing the filled capsules.

Capsule Formulation and Selection of Capsule Size

Generally speaking, hard gelatin capsules are used to encapsulate between about 65 mg and 1 g of powdered material, including drug and

[1] It is possible for pharmacists to color small numbers of plain empty gelatin capsules by placing the separated capsules in a small volume of 70% alcohol containing the desired dye (food colorings used in baking may be used), allowing the capsules to be submerged in the solution for a minute or so, decanting the solution, and drying the capsules on a paper towel. Excessive water in the dye solution or excessive exposure to the solution may result in the distortion of the capsules.

Table 6-2. APPROXIMATE CAPACITY OF EMPTY GELATIN CAPSULES*

Drug Substance	Capsule Size								
	000	00	0	1	2	3	4	5	
Quinine Sulfate	10	6	5	$3\frac{1}{2}$	3	2	$1\frac{1}{2}$	1	grains
Sodium Bicarbonate	22	15	11	8	6	5	4	2	grains
Aspirin	16	10	8	5	4	3	$2\frac{1}{2}$	$1\frac{1}{2}$	grains
Bismuth Subnitrate	28	20	14	10	8	6	4	2	grains

*Amount may vary according to the degree of pressure used in filling the capsules.

any diluent required. As indicated in Table 6-2, the smallest capsule, a No. 5 capsule, is usually capable of holding at least 1 gr or 65 mg of powders of the type used in medicine. In order to fill completely a capsule of even the smallest size, a minimum of 65 mg of material is generally required. If the dose of the drug or the amount of drug to be placed in a single capsule is inadequate to fill the volume of the capsule, a diluent is necessary to add the proper degree of bulk to the drug to produce the proper fill. When the amount of drug to be administered in a single capsule is large enough to fill a capsule completely, a diluent may not be required. Lactose is a common diluent used in capsule filling.

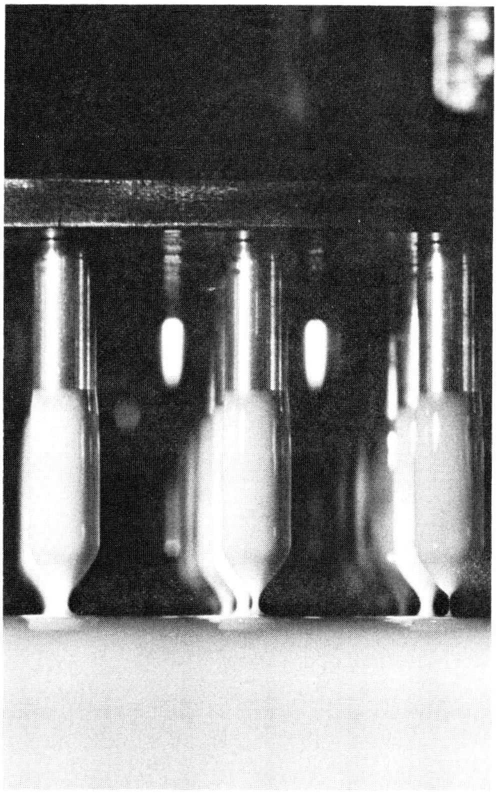

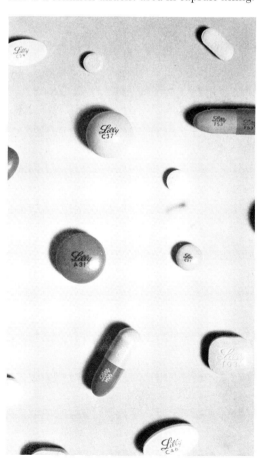

Fig. 6-8. *Capsules being dipped for coloring on automated capsule-making equipment. (Courtesy of Smith, Kline & French Laboratories)*

Fig. 6-9. *Examples of tablets and capsules marked with a letter-number code to facilitate identification. (Courtesy of Eli Lilly and Company)*

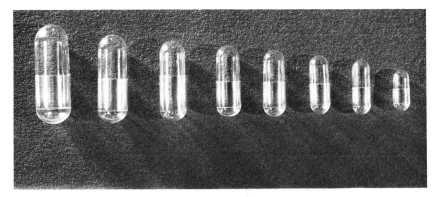

Fig. 6-10. *Actual sizes of hard gelatin capsules. From left to right, sizes 000, 00, 0, 1, 2, 3, 4, and 5.*

In many instances the amount of drug placed in a single capsule falls within the usual dosage range of that drug, a single capsule being taken as a dose of that particular medication. In other instances, especially when the amount of drug representing a usual dose is too large to place in a single capsule, two or more capsules may be required to provide the desired dose of that particular drug. For many medicinal agents, the initial or first dose may be larger than the subsequent doses, in which case more capsules may be required when drug therapy is initiated than when it is continued. In all instances, the amount of drug to be present in a single capsule is first determined, and the amount of diluent or inert materials, if any, is determined subsequently on the basis of its being needed to add bulk to the formulation, to separate chemically incompatible components of the formulation, or as a lubricant to facilitate the flow of the powder when an automatic capsule filling machine is utilized.

Magnesium stearate is a commonly used lubricant in capsule and tablet making to facilitate the flow of the drug-fill into the tableting or encapsulating machinery. Although small amounts of magnesium stearate are generally used (frequently less than 1%), the waterproofing characteristics of this insoluble material can pose a problem to the penetration of the solid dosage form by the gastrointestinal fluids intended to dissolve it. This obstacle to water and fluid penetration can delay the dissolution of the drug and its absorption. The practice of adding surfactants in capsule and tablet formulations to facilitate the wetting of the drug substance by the bathing gastrointestinal fluids is a widely followed procedure in industry. The advantage of adding a wetting agent to capsule formulations of lithium carbonate to enhance dissolution was recently demonstrated.[1] Even in instances in which magnesium stearate or some other water-insoluble lubricant is not used in capsule formulation, when the gelatin shell of a capsule dissolves, liquid must displace the air that surrounds the dry powder within the capsule and penetrate the drug before the capsule fill can be dispersed and dissolved. Powders of poorly soluble drugs have a tendency to float on the surface of the fluid and agglomerate to further minimize air-liquid contact and if wetting does not occur readily, dissolution is delayed.

Whether it be the presence of a lubricant, surfactant, or some other pharmaceutic excipient, formulation can influence the bioavailability of a drug substance and can account for differences in drug effects which may be encountered between two capsule products of the same medicinal substance.

Eutectic mixtures of drugs, or mixtures that tend to liquefy, may require a diluent or absorbant such as magnesium carbonate, kaolin, or light magnesium oxide to separate physically the interacting agents and to absorb any liquefied material. Generally, when such materials are used for this purpose, approximately 120 mg of diluent are used for each capsule. Drugs that are chemically incompatible with other drugs of the formulation may be physically separated by the same means. Another

[1] Caldwell, H. C.: Dissolution of Lithium and Magnesium from Lithium Carbonate Capsules Containing Magnesium Stearate, *J. Pharm. Sci., 63*:770–773, 1974.

method for separating drugs within a capsule is to place one of the interfering substances in a small capsule that is then placed within a larger capsule containing the other formulative components. Instead of the smaller capsule, compressed tablets may be used for this purpose.

The use of tablets within capsules is also quite common in the extemporaneous filling of a small number of capsules, each to contain a very small quantity of a potent drug. In these instances, many pharmacists insert a small tablet of the desired strength of the potent drug in each capsule, filling the remaining capsule space with the specified amounts of other required less potent and more conveniently weighed drugs and/or with an inert diluent as is necessary.

Certain salts such as sodium bromide and sodium iodide, which are extremely soluble and may be irritating to the gastric mucosa when released from the capsule, are not generally prepared in capsule form, since their rapid release and rapid dissolution in the stomach might result in highly concentrated solutions that may prove irritating and distressful to the patient. Such salts may be best administered in solution and taken with a glass of water to diminish their concentration.

Solid substances to be placed in a capsule must be thoroughly mixed before the capsules may be filled. Generally, granular materials are first powdered, since the powder form of a drug is usually more conveniently packed into capsules than is granular material. Also, two or more powders may be more uniformly mixed if their powder size and density are approximately the same.

Capsules of gelatin are unsuitable for the encapsulation of aqueous liquids, since water softens the gelatin to produce distortion of the capsules. Naturally, this would prompt the loss of the liquid contents of the capsules. However, some liquids such as fixed or volatile oils that do not interfere with the stability of the gelatin shells may be placed in gelatin capsules which then may be sealed to ensure the retention of the liquid. The pharmacist usually places the liquid in the body of the capsule with a calibrated medicine dropper, being careful not to get any of the liquid on the outside of the capsule. Then a small camel's hair brush is used to coat the inner surface of the cap with water or with a warm gelatin solution, and the cap is carefully placed onto the capsule body with a twisting motion to ensure distribution of the

sealing liquid. In large scale production, liquids are placed in soft gelatin capsules which are sealed during their manufacture. Soft capsules will be discussed later in this chapter.

Rather than placing a liquid in a capsule as such, it may be desirable in certain instances to absorb a small amount of liquid by mixing it with an absorbent, inert powder. The powder may then be placed in capsules in the usual manner. If the liquid is volatile, it may be necessary to seal the capsules. Viscous liquids frequently form a plastic-like mass when mixed with an absorbent powder. Such a mass may be placed on a glass or porcelain plate and rolled into a pencil shape with a spatula. The rolled mass may then be cut with the edge of the spatula or with a razor blade into the appropriate number of units, corresponding to the number of capsules to be prepared, and the individual units may be further rolled if necessary for uniform placement into the capsule shells. It should be remembered that upon release from the capsule within the gastrointestinal tract, drugs incorporated into a plastic mass will likely be more slowly distributed for absorption than drug substances not so incorporated.

AMOUNT OF FORMULA PREPARED. On a small or large industrial scale, the amount of formula prepared is that amount (drugs and diluents) necessary to fill the desired number of capsules. On an industrial scale this may mean many thousands of capsules. In the community pharmacy an individual prescription may call for the extemporaneous preparation of only six or a dozen capsules. Any slight loss in fill material during the preparation of the (powder) mixture or during the capsule-filling process will not materially affect the preparation of an industrial batch, but on a small scale, as in the filling of a prescription, a slight loss of fill material will likely result in an inadequate amount of powder for the last capsule. To ensure enough fill for the last capsule in the extemporaneous compounding of small numbers of capsules, the community pharmacist generally calculates for the preparation of one more capsule than is required. This procedure may not be followed for capsules containing a controlled substance, since the amount of drug used and that called for in the prescription must strictly coincide.

SELECTION OF CAPSULE SIZE. The selection of the capsule size is best done during the development of the formulation, since the amount of any inert materials to be employed is dependent upon the size or capacity of the capsule to be selected. When the formulation of medicinal materials does not require diluent to increase the bulk, the capsule size may be selected after the development and preparation of the formulation. As indicated earlier, for drugs having large doses the amount of medication in a capsule may not necessarily correspond to a full dose of that medication. Smaller capsules may be required in instances in which the drug is to be taken by youngsters or by elderly patients, and more than a single capsule may be required to provide the dose of the drug. In instances in which there is a specific need for a small capsule, the capsule size may be selected first, and the formulation may be based on that capsule size. Depending upon the particular situation and requirements of the intended patient, the capsule size may be determined by the formulation, or the formulation may be altered by the capsule size.

A properly filled capsule should have its body filled with the drug mixture and its cap fully extended down the body so as to enclose the powder in the body. The cap is not used to hold powder but to retain it, and a capsule size should be selected to meet this requirement.

Filling the Capsule Shells

In filling a small number of capsules in the pharmacy, the pharmacist generally uses the "punch" method. In this method the pharmacist takes the precise number of empty capsules to be filled from his stock container. By counting out the capsules as the initial step rather than taking a capsule from stock as each one is filled, the pharmacist guards against filling an erroneous number of capsules and avoids contaminating the stock container of empty capsules with drug particles that may cling to his fingertips. The powder to be encapsulated is placed on a sheet of clean paper or a glass or porcelain plate and with a spatula is formed into a cake having a depth of approximately one-fourth to one-third the length of the capsule body. Then the empty capsule body is held between the thumb and forefinger and "punched" vertically into the powder cake repeatedly until filled. Some pharmacists wear surgical gloves or rubber finger cots to avoid handling the capsules with bare fingers. Since the amount of powder packed into a capsule depends upon the degree of compression, the pharmacist should

punch each capsule in the same manner and after capping weigh it to ensure equal and accurate filling. When nonpotent materials are being placed in capsules, the first filled capsule should be weighed (using an empty capsule of the same size on the opposite balance pan to counter the weight of the shell) to assist in the determination of the proper capsule size and degree of compression to be used in filling, and then other capsules should be weighed periodically to check the uniformity of this operation. When potent drugs are being used, each capsule should be weighed after filling to ensure accuracy. Such weighings protect against the uneven filling of capsules and the premature exhaustion or lack of total utilization of the powder mixture. After the body of a capsule has been filled and the cap has been placed on the body, the body is squeezed gently to distribute some powder to the cap end of the capsule to give the product a full appearance. Some pharmacists place a small portion of powder in the cap before placing it on the body. Care must be exercised not to overfill a capsule so that it contains too much powder volume for the capsule and the cap does not fit completely down on the body.

Granular material that does not lend itself well to the "punch" method of filling capsules may be poured into each capsule individually from the powder paper on which it was first weighed. Liquids, as indicated earlier, may be instilled in capsules by means of a medicine dropper.

Pharmacies that prepare capsules on a regular or somewhat extensive basis may use hand-operated capsule machines. These machines are available in capacities of 24, 96, 100, and 144 capsules. When efficiently operated, they can produce from about 2000 capsules per working day for the smallest machine up to 2000 capsules per hour for the largest (Fig. 6-11).

Machines developed for industrial use can automatically remove the caps from empty capsules, fill the capsules, replace the caps, and clean the outside of the capsules at a rate of up to 90,000 capsules per working day per unit. Most industrial capsule-filling machines are designed to fill the body of the empty capsule with powder and scrape off the excess at the level of fill before capping. Therefore the formulation for each industrially produced capsule must be such that the filled body contains the amount of powder in which the right amount of drug and diluent are present. Periodic checks are made

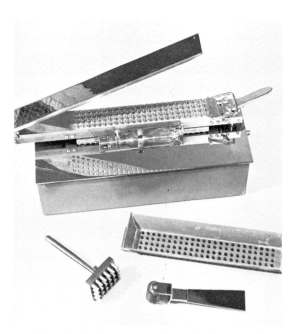

Fig. 6-11. *Hand-operated capsule-filling machine. The model shown fills 96 capsules per operation and is made to obtain an hourly production of 1000 capsules. Shown with the basic machine are the tray used to hold the fill over the empty capsules, the spreader and roller used to distribute the fill material in the tray and permit it to enter the capsules uniformly, and the packer used to compact the fill in the capsules.*

along the production line by taking capsules from production and weighing them for total powder and assaying them for active ingredient.

The USP and the NF have a weight variation requirement that must be met for official capsules. The tests that establish limits as to weight variation are as follows:

Weigh 20 intact capsules individually, and determine the average weight. The requirements are met if each of the individual weights is within the limits of 90 and 110% of the average weight.

If not all of the capsules fall within the aforementioned limits, weigh the 20 capsules individually, taking care to preserve the identity of each capsule, and remove the contents of each capsule with the aid of a small brush or pledget of cotton. Weigh the emptied shells individually, and calculate for each capsule the net weight of its contents by subtracting the weight of the shell from the respective gross weight. Determine the average net content from the sum of the individual net weights. Then determine the differ-

ence between each individual net content and the average net content: the requirements are met if (a) not more than 2 of the differences are greater than 10% of the average net content and (b) in no case is the difference greater than 25%.

If more than 2 but not more than 6 capsules deviate from the average between 10 and 25% determine the net contents of an additional 40 capsules, and determine the average content of the entire 60 capsules. Determine the 60 deviations from the new average: the requirements are met if (a) in not more than 6 of the 60 capsules does the difference exceed 10% of the average net content and (b) in no case does the difference exceed 25%.

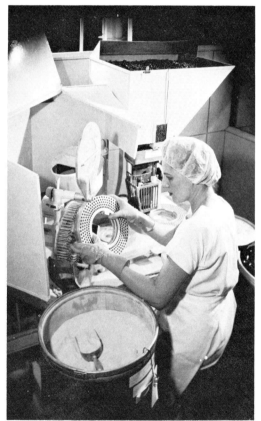

Fig. 6-12. *Filling of capsules is a semiautomatic operation. Capsules are automatically seated in holes in the metal form which is then separated to open the capsules. The form containing the bottom halves of the capsules is then filled with the dry therapeutic agent. The top section of the form is replaced, and the two halves of the capsules are automatically joined as they are ejected. (Courtesy of Parke, Davis & Company)*

Cleaning and Polishing Capsules

Capsules prepared on a small scale or on a large scale may have small amounts of the powder formulation adhering to the outside of the capsules. This powder, which may be bitter or otherwise unpalatable, should be removed before packaging or dispensing in order to improve the appearance of the capsules and to preserve their quality of being tasteless on administration. On a small scale, capsules may be cleaned individually or in small numbers by rubbing them with a clean gauze or cloth. On a large scale, many capsule-filling machines are affixed with a cleaning vacuum that removes any extraneous material from the capsules as they exit the capsule-filling equipment. Capsules may also be cleaned on a small or large scale by rotating them in a container with sucrose or sodium chloride. Capsules may be given a shine or polished by rolling or rubbing them on a cloth containing a slight amount of mineral oil or a wax. Figure 6-13 shows an industrial method of cleaning and polishing hard filled capsules using the Accela-Cota apparatus.

Soft Gelatin Capsules

Soft gelatin capsules are prepared from shells of gelatin to which glycerin or a polyhydric alcohol such as sorbitol has been added to render the gelatin elastic or plastic-like. These capsules, which may be oblong, elliptical, or spherical in shape, may be employed to contain liquids, suspensions, pasty materials, or dry powders.[1] Soft gelatin capsules are usually prepared, filled, and sealed in a continuous operation using specialized equipment. Empty soft gelatin capsules may be prepared and hermetically sealed (to prevent the walls from collapsing and adhering to one another) for filling at a later time, but this is not usually performed.

Soft gelatin capsules are useful when it is desirable to seal the medication within the capsule. The capsules are especially important to contain liquid drugs or drug solutions. Also, volatile drug substances or drug materials especially susceptible to deterioration in the presence of air may be better suited to a soft gelatin capsule than to the hard gelatin capsules.

Soft gelatin capsules are handsome and are easily swallowed by the patient. However, they are not easily prepared except on a large scale and then only with specialized equipment.

Preparation of Soft Gelatin Capsules

Soft gelatin capsules may be prepared by the plate process, using a set of molds to form the capsules, or by the more efficient and productive die processes (rotary or reciprocating). By the plate process, a warm sheet of gelatin (plain or colored) is placed on the bottom plate of the mold, and the liquid medication is evenly poured on it. Then a second sheet of the prepared gelatin is carefully laid in place on top of the medication, and the top plate of the mold is put in place. The entire mold is then subjected to a press where pressure is applied to form, fill, and seal the capsules simultaneously. The capsules are then removed and washed with a solvent harmless to the capsules. Highly automated machines have been developed for the preparation of soft capsules by the plate process and are in use today in industry.

However, most industrially produced soft capsules are probably prepared by the rotary die process, a method developed in 1933 by Robert P. Scherer. By this method, liquid gelatin flowing from an overhead tank is formed into two continuous ribbons by the rotary die machine and brought together between twin rotating

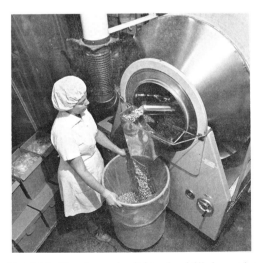

Fig. 6-13. *Cleaning and polishing hard filled capsules using the Accela-Cota apparatus. (Courtesy of Eli Lilly and Company)*

[1] Soft gelatin capsules which contain liquids and are shaped elliptical or round are commonly called "pearls." Many commercial pearls contain oleaginous vitamin preparations.

dies (Figs. 6-14 and 6-15). At the same time, metered fill material is injected between the ribbons precisely at the moment that the dies form pockets of the gelatin ribbons. These pockets of fill-containing gelatin are then sealed by pressure and heat, the capsules then being severed from the ribbon by the same process. The soft gelatin capsules may be manufactured in a number of shapes, including round, oval, oblong, tube-shape, and others. They may also be prepared of single or two-tone color, the latter resulting from the employment of two different colored ribbons of gelatin to form the sides of the capsule. A modern adaption of this method, the Accogel Capsule Machine developed by Lederle Laboratories, permits the enclosure of

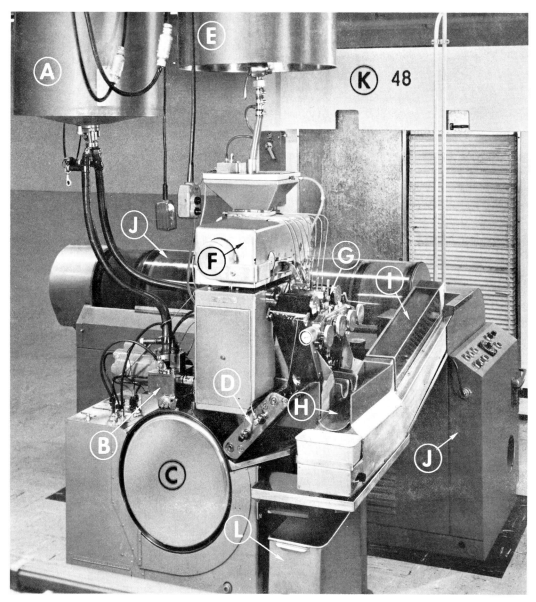

Fig. 6-14. *Rotary die process equipment.* A, *Gelatin tank;* B, *spreader box;* C, *gelatin ribbon casting drum;* D, *mineral oil lubricant bath;* E, *medicine tank;* F, *filling pump;* G, *encapsulating mechanism;* H, *capsule conveyor;* I, *capsule washer;* J, *infrared dryer;* K, *capsule drying tunnel;* L, *gelatin net receiver.* (*Courtesy of R. P. Scherer Corporation*)

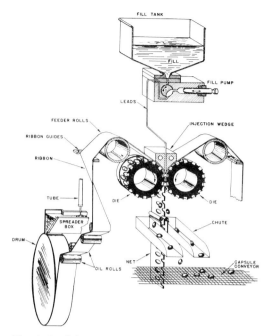

Fig. 6-15. *Schematic drawing of rotary die process. (Courtesy of R. P. Scherer Corporation)*

dry powder or liquids in soft gelatin capsules. In addition, through the use of an adaptor, the machine is capable of enclosing preformed tablets in a gelatin film.

The reciprocating die process is similar to the rotary process in that ribbons of gelatin are formed and used to encapsulate the fill, but it differs in the actual encapsulating process. The gelatin ribbons are fed between a set of vertical dies that continually open and close to form rows of pockets in the gelatin ribbons. These pockets are filled with the medication and are sealed, shaped, and cut out of the film as they progress through the machinery. As the capsules are cut from the ribbons, they fall into refrigerated tanks which prevent the capsules from adhering to one another and from getting dull.

Application of Soft Gelatin Capsules

Soft gelatin capsules may be used to contain a variety of liquid and dry fills. Liquids which may be encapsulated into soft gelatin capsules include:[1]

[1]Stanley, J. P.: Capsules, in *The Theory and Practice of Industrial Pharmacy*, by L. Lachman, H. A. Lieberman, and J. L. Kanig, Philadelphia, Lea & Febiger, 1976, pp. 404–420.

1. Water immiscible, volatile and non-volatile liquids such as vegetable and aromatic oils, aromatic and aliphatic hydrocarbons, chlorinated hydrocarbons, ethers, esters, alcohols, and organic acids.
2. Water miscible, non-volatile liquids such as polyethylene glycols, and non-ionic surface active agents as polysorbate 80.
3. Water miscible and relatively non-volatile compounds, as propylene glycol and isopropyl alcohol, depending upon factors as concentration used and packaging conditions.

Liquids which can easily migrate through the capsule shell cannot be encapsulated into soft gelatin capsules. These materials include: water, above 5%, and low molecular weight water soluble and volatile organic compounds such as alcohols, ketones, acids, amines, and esters.

Solids may be encapsulated into soft gelatin capsules as solutions in one of the suitable liquid solvents, as suspensions, or as dry powders, granules, or pelletized materials.

Among the drugs commercially prepared in soft gelatin capsules are: clofibrate (Atromid-S, Ayerst), etchlorvynol (Placidyl, Abbott), demeclocycline HCl (Declomycin, Lederle), chlorotrianisene (TACE, Merrell), chloral hydrate (Somnos, Merck, Sharp & Dohme), vitamin A, and vitamin E.

Inspecting, Counting, Packaging, and Storing Capsules

Whether capsules are produced on a small or a large scale, they are required to pass not only tests of potency and uniformity but also a visual inspection to ensure that there are no flaws in the appearance of the capsules. All capsules produced by the same method should be uniformly colored, uniformly filled, and uniformly shaped. As the pharmacist extemporaneously compounds a prescription for capsules in the community pharmacy, he must take care to prepare uniform capsules. On a large scale, however, the highly productive automatic capsule machines are capable of producing great numbers of capsules simultaneously, and these must be inspected visually as they roll off the capsule machine onto a conveyor belt. As they move past the inspectors, capsules that are visibly defective as well as those suspected of being

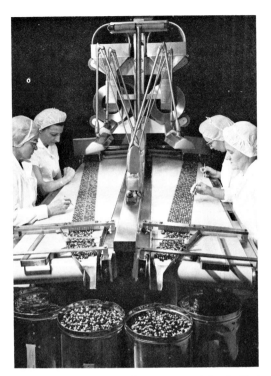

Fig. 6-16. *Cleaning and inspection of hard filled capsules. (Courtesy of The Upjohn Company)*

less than perfect are picked out. If the number of capsules removed is excessively high, some production default in the capsule-producing mechanism of the machines is suspected and checked out by machinists.

In the pharmacy, capsules that have been extemporaneously compounded or those taken from a stock package of prefabricated capsules are usually counted by hand, using specially designed counting trays to facilitate the procedure and to ensure the hygienic transfer of the capsules into the final container. One of these trays, the Abbott counting tray, is depicted in Figure 6-17. In using this tray, the pharmacist pours a supply of capsules or tablets from the bulk source onto the clean tray, and using the spatula he counts the desired number of capsules or tablets, sweeping them into the trough as he counts. When the correct number is in the trough, the pharmacist closes the trough cover, picks up the tray, returns the uncounted dosage units to the bulk container by means of the lip at the back of the tray, places the prescription contained at the opening of the trough, and carefully transfers the capsules or tablets into the container. By this method, the capsules or

tablets remain untouched by the pharmacist. To prevent contamination of tablets and capsules, the tray must be wiped clean after each counting, as powder tends to get on the tray, especially when uncoated tablets are counted.

On a larger scale, as occurs in the hospital pharmacy setting, small automatic counting and container-filling apparatus is becoming increasingly popular and useful. Some of these counting machines are shown in Figures 6-18 and 6-19.

On an industrial scale, solid dosage forms may be counted by means of large counting trays. The operator pours the dosage units on a tray containing the desired number of perforations, rotates tray until each perforation is filled with a capsule or tablet, allows the excess to slide off the tray, and then transfers the counted number from the perforations into the container. This method has largely been replaced by highly automated counting devices that both count and transfer the desired number of dosage units into the containers. Machines have been developed to count and fill a dozen or more containers simultaneously, capping and moving the filled bottles along the production line where they can again be inspected, labeled, and final packaged. One of these machines is shown in Figure 6-20.

Capsules are usually packaged in glass or in plastic containers, some containing packets of a desiccant to prevent the absorption of excessive moisture by the capsules. Soft capsules have a greater tendency than do hard capsules to soften and adhere to one another, and they must be maintained in a cool, dry place. In fact, all capsules remain stable longer if maintained tightly sealed in a cool place of low humidity.

The unit dose and strip packaging of solid dosage forms, particularly by pharmacies which service nursing homes and hospitals, provides sanitary handling of the medications, ease of identification, and security in accountability for medications. Typical small scale strip packaging equipment and commercial unit-dose packages of capsules and tablets are presented in Figures 6-21 and 6-22 respectively.

Official Capsules

There are nearly a hundred officially recognized medications in capsule form, representing a wide range of therapeutic categories. Exam-

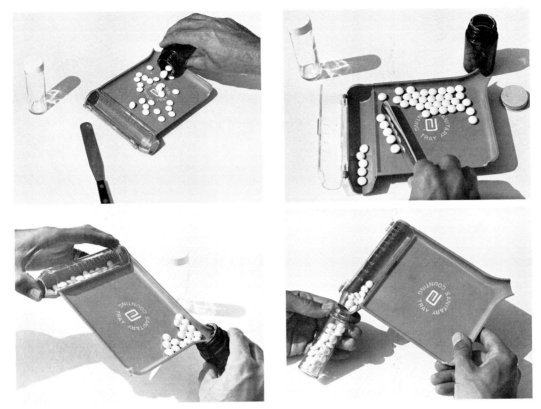

Fig. 6-17. *Steps in the counting of solid dosage units with the Abbott Sanitary Counting Tray: (1) placing units from stock package onto tray, (2) counting and transferring units to trough, (3) returning excess units to stock container, and (4) placing counted units into prescription container.*

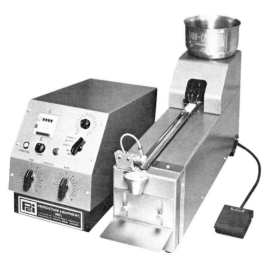

Fig. 6-18. *Mini-Counter II, small automatic tablet and capsule counting and filling apparatus. (Courtesy of Production Equipment Co.)*

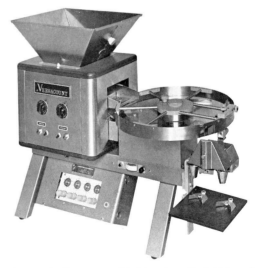

Fig. 6-19. *Versacount Model automatic tablet and capsule counting and filling apparatus. (Courtesy of Production Equipment Co.)*

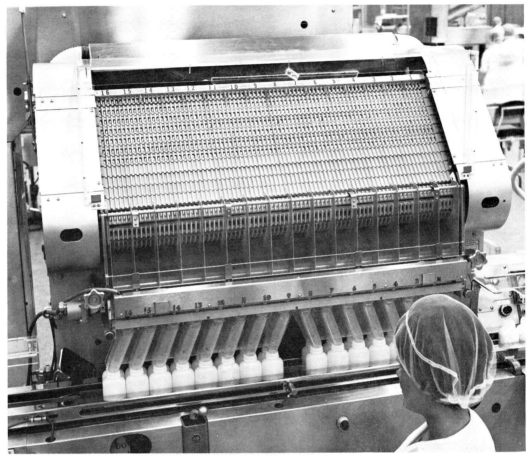

Fig. 6-20. *Large Merrill filling machine that fills 16 bottles with 200 tablets each at one time. A flipper gate in the upper manifold directs the tablets into one row of bottles while the other filled row is evacuated and a new row of bottles moves into place. (Courtesy of The Upjohn Company)*

ples of these are presented in Table 6-3. All but three of the officially recognized capsules contain a single therapeutic component. The exceptions are Decavitamin Capsules, USP, a multivitamin preparation, Oleovitamin A and D Capsules, NF, and Ephedrine Sulfate and Phenobarbital Capsules, NF. This is evidence of the current trend in medical practice toward the prescribing and utilization of single-drug products. Through the use of single-drug products the physician is better able to determine the effect that a particular drug is having on the course of an illness, and to adjust the dose, or change medications if that is indicated. This is not to say that combination-drug products do not exist or that they are not popular. Indeed, there is a vast array of such products on the market, but the majority of them are for the over-the-counter market in which the patient selects the product, usually for the relief of a minor ailment or symptom complex.

Tablets

Tablets are solid dosage forms of medicinal substances usually prepared with the aid of suitable pharmaceutical adjuncts. Different tablets may vary in size, shape, weight, hardness, thickness, disintegration characteristics, and in other aspects, depending upon the intended use of the tablets and their method of manufacture. The majority of tablets are used in the oral administration of drugs, and many of these tablets are prepared with colorants, flavorants, and coatings of various types. Other tablets such as those intended to be administered sublingually, bucally, or vaginally or those used for the preparation of pharmaceutical or medicinal solutions may not contain the same adjuncts or be prepared to possess the same types of features as tablets for oral administration. Many of the advantages of tablets for the oral administration of drugs have already been presented at the outset of this chapter and previously in Chapter 3.

Tablets are prepared by two general methods, compression and molding. Although these two methods will be discussed in detail later in this chapter, it should be briefly stated at this point that compressed tablets are manufactured with tablet machines capable of exerting great pressure in compacting the powdered or granulated tableting material through the use of various shaped punches and dies. The tablet presses are heavy equipment of various capacities selected for use on the basis of the type of tablets to be manufactured and the production rate desired. Molded tablets are prepared by hand or by tablet machinery by forcing dampened tablet material into a mold from which the formed tablet is then ejected and allowed to dry.

Types of Tablets

The various types of tablets are described as follows, with the abbreviations for the tablet types in parentheses.

COMPRESSED TABLETS (C.T.). Compressed tablets, prepared by single compression, occur in various shapes and sizes and usually contain in addition to the medicinal substance(s), a number of pharmaceutical adjuncts including (a) *diluents* or *fillers*, which add the necessary bulk to a formulation to prepare tablets of the desired size; (b) *binders* or *adhesives*, which promote the adhesion of the particles of the formulation, enabling a granulation to be prepared and the maintenance of the integrity of the final tablet;

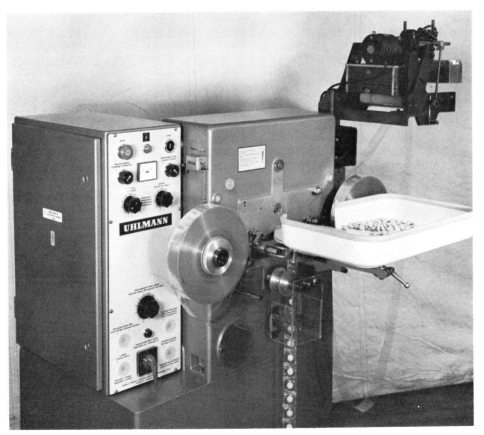

Fig. 6-21. *A strip packager for the unit dose dispensing of solid dosage forms. Drug information is imprinted on each individual package unit. The model shown has a fully automatic cutoff from 1 to 24 dosage units and is especially suited to unit-dose packaging and dispensing in hospitals, dispensaries, nursing homes, and clinics. (Courtesy of Lakso Company, Inc.)*

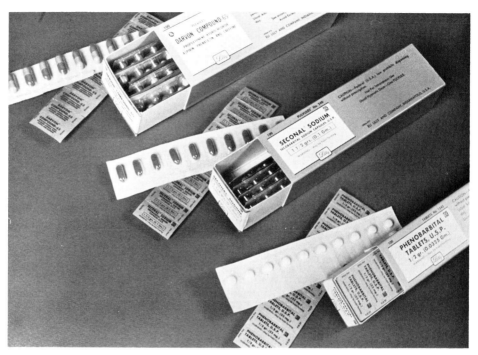

Fig. 6-22. *Example of unit-dose packaging of tablets and capsules. The drug name and other information are imprinted on the backing portion of each unit. (Courtesy of Eli Lilly and Company)*

(c) *disintegrators* or *disintegrating agents*, which promote the breakup of the tablets after administration to smaller particles for more ready drug availability; (d) *lubricants* or *lubricating agents*, which enhance the flow of the tableting material into the tablet dies, prevent the sticking of this material to the punches and dies, and produce tablets having a sheen; and (e) miscellaneous adjuncts such as colorants and flavorants. After compression, some compressed tablets may be coated with various materials as described later. Most compressed tablets are employed for the oral administration of drugs, but some may be used for the sublingual, buccal, or vaginal administration of drugs. Naturally, the types of pharmaceutical adjuncts in a tablet formulation will vary greatly depending upon the intended use of the tablet.

MULTIPLE COMPRESSED TABLETS (M.C.T.). Multiple compressed tablets are prepared by subjection to more than a single compression. The result may be a multiple-layered tablet or a tablet-within-a-tablet, the inner tablet being the *core* and the outer portion being the *shell* (Fig. 6-24). Layered tablets are prepared by the initial compaction of a portion of fill material in a die and the addition of one or more portions of fill material to the same die, each additional fill being compressed to form a two- or three-layered tablet, depending upon the number of separate fills. Usually each portion of fill material contains a different medicinal agent separated from the others for reasons of incompatibility or simply for the unique appearance of a multiple-layered tablet. Generally each portion of fill is colored differently to prepare a multiple-colored as well as a multiple-layered tablet. In the preparation of tablets having another compressed tablet as the inner core, special machines are required to place the preformed tablet precisely within the die for the second compression and the new fill material around the core tablet. The outer material is also usually medicated, the intention being to separate incompatible drugs or to prepare a timed-release type of tablet, with the outer shell providing the drug for immediate release and the inner core, the drug for sustained or delayed release.

SUGAR-COATED TABLETS (S.C.T.). Compressed tablets may be coated with a colored or an uncolored sugar. The coating is water-soluble and is quickly dissolved after swallowing. It serves the varied purposes of protecting the drug from the air and humidity and providing a taste or a

Table 6-3. EXAMPLES OF SOME OFFICIAL CAPSULES

Official Capsule	Some Representative Commercial Products*	Capsule Strengths Usually Available	Category
Amobarbital Sodium Capsules, USP	Amytal Sodium Pulvules (Lilly)	65 and 200 mg	Hypnotic; sedative
Ampicillin Capsules, USP	Amcill Capsules (Parke Davis); Polycillin Capsules (Bristol); Omnipen Capsules (Wyeth)	250 and 500 mg	Antibacterial
Aspirin Capsules, NF	· · ·	300 mg	Analgesic
Cephalexin Capsules, USP	Keflex Pulvules (Lilly)	250 and 500 mg	Antibacterial
Chloral Hydrate Capsules, USP	Felsules Capsules (Fellows); Noctec Capsules (Squibb)	250, 500, and 1000 mg	Hypnotic; sedative
Chloramphenicol Capsules, USP	Chloromycetin Kapseals (Parke Davis)	50, 100, and 250 mg	Antibacterial; antirickettsial
Chlorotrianisene Capsules, NF	TACE Capsules (Merrell-National)	12, 24, 72 mg	Estrogen
Chlordiazepoxide HCl Capsules, USP	Librium Capsules (Roche)	5, 10, and 25 mg	Sedative
Clofibrate Capsules, USP	Atromid S Capsules (Ayerst)	500 mg	Antihyperlipidemic
Chlortetracycline HCl Capsules, NF	Aureomycin HCl Capsules (Lederle)	50, 100, and 250 mg	Antibacterial; antiprotozoan
Demeclocycline HCl Capsules, NF	Declomycin HCl Capsules (Lederle)	75, 150, and 300 mg	Antibacterial
Dioctyl Sodium Sulfosuccinate Capsules, USP	Colace Capsules (Mead Johnson); Doxinate Capsules (Hoechst-Roussel)	50, 60, 100, 240, 250 and 300 mg	Stool softener
Diphenhydramine HCl Capsules, USP	Benadryl HCl Kapseals (Parke Davis)	25 and 50 mg	Antihistaminic
Ephedrine Sulfate Capsules, USP	· · ·	25 and 50 mg	Adrenergic (bronchodilator)
Erythromycin Estolate Capsules, NF	Ilosone Pulvules (Lilly)	125 and 250 mg	Antibacterial
Griseofulvin Capsules, USP	Grisactin Capsules (Ayerst)	125 and 250 mg	Antifungal
Levodopa Capsules, USP	Dopar Capsules (Eaton); Larodopa Capsules (Roche)	100, 125, 250, and 500 mg	Antiparkinsonian
Lithium Carbonate Capsules, USP	Eskalith Capsules (Smith Kline & French); Lithonate Capsules (Rowell)	300 mg	Antidepressant
Pentobarbital Sodium, USP	Nembutal Sodium Capsules (Abbott)	30, 50, and 100 mg	Hypnotic; sedative
Propoxyphene HCl Capsules, USP	Darvon Pulvules (Lilly); Dolene Capsules (Lederle)	32 and 65 mg	Analgesic
Quinine Sulfate Capsules, USP	· · ·	130, 200, and 325 mg	Antimalarial
Secobarbital Sodium Capsules, USP	Seconal Sodium Pulvules (Lilly)	30, 50, and 100 mg	Hypnotic; sedative
Tetrachloroethylene Capsules, USP	· · ·	0.2, 0.5, 1, 2.5, and 5 ml	Anthelmintic
Tetracycline HCl Capsules, USP	Achromycin V Capsules (Lederle); Panmycin HCl Capsules (Upjohn); Sumycin HCl Capsules (Squibb)	100, 125, 250, and 500 mg	Antibacterial; antiamebic; antirickettsial

Table 6-3. EXAMPLES OF SOME OFFICIAL CAPSULES (*Cont.*)

Official Capsule	Some Representative Commercial Products*	Capsule Strengths Usually Available	Category
Trimethadione Capsules, USP	Tridione Capsules (Abbott)	300 mg	Anticonvulsant
Vitamin A Capsules, USP	Aquasol A Capsules (USV Pharmaceutical)	1.5, 7.5, and 15 mg (5000, 25,000 and 50,000 units)	Anti-xerophthalmic

* The brand name products listed are intended to be representative, not inclusive. A number of the capsules presented are also commercially available under their nonproprietary (generic) names.

small barrier to objectional tasting or smelling drugs. Further, it enhances the appearance of many compressed tablets. Disadvantages to sugar-coating tablets are the time and expertise required by the process and the increase in the size and weight of the compressed tablets. Coated tablets may be 50% larger and heavier than the original uncoated tablets.

CHOCOLATE-COLORED TABLETS (C.C.T.). Chocolate-colored tablets are mainly of historic importance, since chocolate was once used to coat and color compressed tablets. Today chocolate has been replaced by other colorants such as iron oxides which are used to simulate the chocolate color.

FILM-COATED TABLETS (F.C.T.). Film-coated tablets are compressed tablets coated with a thin layer of a water-insoluble polymeric substance capable of forming a film over the tablet. The film is generally colored and has the advantage over sugar-coatings in that it is more durable, less bulky, and less time-consuming to apply. The coating ruptures in the gastrointestinal tract.

ENTERIC-COATED TABLETS (E.C.T.). Enteric-coated tablets are tablets with a coating which resists dissolution or disruption in the stomach but not in the intestines, thereby allowing for tablet transit through the stomach in favor of tablet disintegration and drug absorption from the intestines. This technique is employed in instances in which the drug substance is destroyed by gastric acid, is irritating to the gastric mucosa, or when by-pass of the stomach enhances drug absorption from the intestines to a significant extent.

BUCCAL OR SUBLINGUAL TABLETS. Buccal or sublingual tablets are generally flat, oval tablets intended to be dissolved in the buccal pouch (*buccal tablets*) or beneath the tongue (*sublingual tablets*) for absorption through the oral mucosa. They are useful in providing for the absorption of drugs that are destroyed by the gastric juice and/or poorly absorbed from the gastrointestinal tract. Although few drugs are absorbed from the oral cavity, some important ones to note are nitroglycerin and many steroid

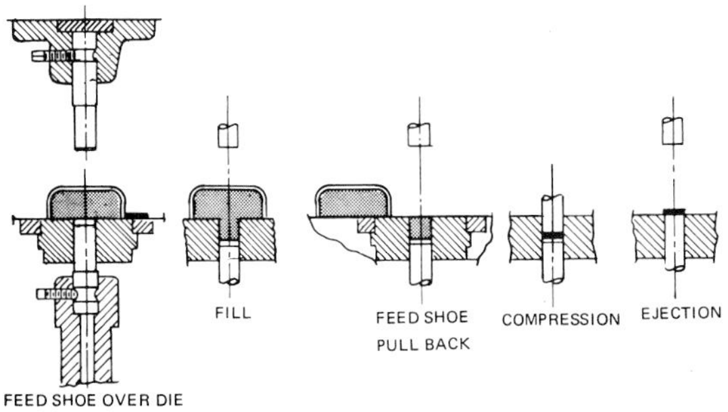

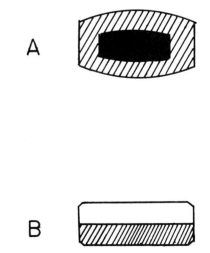

Fig. 6-23. *Steps in the compression of a tablet on a single punch press. (Courtesy of Cherry-Burrell Corporation)*

FILL   FEED SHOE PULL BACK   COMPRESSION   EJECTION

FEED SHOE OVER DIE

Fig. 6-24. *Diagram of multiple-compressed tablets. A, having a core of one drug and a shell of another, and B, a multiple-layered tablet of two drugs.*

hormones. Tablets intended for buccal administration (as progesterone tablets) are prepared to erode or to dissolve slowly, while those for sublingual use (as nitroglycerin tablets) dissolve very promptly to give rapid drug effects.

CHEWABLE TABLETS. Chewable tablets, which have a smooth, rapid disintegration when chewed or allowed to dissolve in the mouth, yield a creamy base of a specially flavored and colored mannitol. The tablets are especially useful in tablet formulations for children and are commonly employed in the preparation of multiple vitamin tablets. They find other uses in the administration of antacids and antibiotics. These tablets are prepared by compression.

EFFERVESCENT TABLETS. Effervescent tablets are prepared by compressing granular effervescent salts or other materials having the capacity to release gas when in contact with water. Commercially, alkalinizing-analgesic tablets and saccharin tablets are frequently made to effervesce to encourage fast disintegration and solution when added to water or an aqueous beverage.

DISPENSING TABLETS (D.T.). Dispensing tablets might better be termed *compounding tablets*, since they are used by the pharmacist in compounding and are never dispensed as such to the patient. The tablets contain relatively large amounts of highly potent drug substances and are prepared as a convenience to the pharmacist, enabling him to obtain quickly accurately measured amounts of potent drugs. He may use the tablets in preparing other solid or liquid dosage forms. The diluent or base of the tablets is usually water-soluble to permit the preparation of clear aqueous solutions. Dispensing tablets may be prepared by either molding or compression. Disintegrating agents, water-insoluble lubricants, colorants, flavorants, and coatings are not used in the preparation of dispensing tablets. Primarily because of the potential hazard in the inadvertent dispensing of these tablets to patients, very few, if any, dispensing tablets are used today. Nowadays, the pharmacist more commonly employs commercially prepared compressed tablets or tablet triturates in the compounding of prescriptions calling for a drug substance unavailable in bulk, but available in these dosage forms.

TABLET TRITURATES (T.T.). Tablet triturates are small, usually cylindrical, molded (M.T.T.) or compressed tablets (C.T.T.) containing small amounts of usually potent drugs. Most tablet triturates are produced industrially by compression but they may also be prepared by molding for small-scale production, since the molds are more easily used and considerably less expensive than tablet presses. Tablet triturates must be readily and completely soluble in water; thus when these tablets are prepared by compression, a minimal amount of pressure is exerted. A combination of sucrose and lactose is usually the diluent, and any water-insoluble material is avoided in the formulation. Some tablet triturates are used for the oral administration of drugs and some for sublingual use (as nitroglycerin tablets). Many pharmacists employ tablet triturates in compounding procedures in the preparation of other solid or liquid dosage forms. For instance, the tablets may be easily inserted into capsules to provide accurate amounts of potent drug substances. They may also be used by pharmacists to fortify liquid preparations, as prescribed, by dissolving the appropriate number of tablets in a small portion of water and then bringing the preparation to the required volume with the liquid medication being fortified.

HYPODERMIC TABLETS (H.T.). Hypodermic tablets are tablet triturates for use by the physician in his extemporaneous preparation of parenteral solutions. The physician dissolves the required number of tablets in a suitable vehicle, attains sterility of the preparation, and performs the injection. The tablets were originally intended as a convenience to the physician, since he could carry in his medicine bag a variety of lightweight hypodermic tablets and a suitable vehicle and prepare corresponding injections of the desired strength and volume according to the needs of the individual patient. However, the difficulty in achieving sterility and the recent availability of a number of drugs in injectable form, some in disposable syringes, have diminished the utility of hypodermic tablets. They are prepared by molding or by soft compression without the intent of achieving sterility, but with a high degree of sanitation.

TIMED-RELEASE TABLETS. Sustained-release and delayed-action dosage forms will be discussed later in this chapter.

Compressed Tablets

Characteristics and Quality

The physical features of compressed tablets are well known to even the layman. Some tablets are round, others oblong, and still others triangular. Some are thick; others are thin. Some tablets have larger diameters than others. Some tablets are flat; others have varying degrees of convexity. Some are *scored* or grooved in halves or in quadrants to permit the fairly accurate breaking of the tablet for the administration of a partial amount or for easier administration of smaller pieces of the tablet. Some tablets are engraved with a symbol of the manufacturer to denote the company, the product, or both. Tablets are produced in different colors to make them further distinctive.

Tablet diameters and shapes are determined by the die and punches used for the compression of the tablet. The less concave the punches, the more flat the resulting tablets; conversely, the more concave the punches, the more convex the resulting tablets. Punches having raised impressions will produce recessed impressions on the tablets; punches having recessed etchings will produce tablets having raised impression or monograms. Monograms may be placed on one or on both sides of a tablet, depending upon whether monogram-producing lower and/or upper punches are used. Scored tablets are generally grooved on a single side.

The thickness of a tablet is determined by the amount of fill permitted to enter the die and the amount of pressure applied during compression.

In addition to these apparent features of tablets, pharmacists are aware that tablets must meet other physical specifications that are generally unknown to the layman. These include tablet weight, tablet thickness, tablet hardness, tablet disintegration, and for some tablets, drug dissolution. These factors must be controlled within the production of a batch of tablets as well as from production batch to production batch in order to guarantee not only the outward appearance of the product but also its therapeutic efficacy.

TABLET WEIGHT. The amount of fill placed in the die of a tablet press will determine the weight of the resulting tablet. The volume of fill (granulation or powder) permitted to enter the dies must be adjusted with the first few tablets produced to yield tablets of the desired weight. Adjustment is necessary, since tablet formulations are based on the weight of the tablets to be prepared. For example, if a tablet is to contain 20 mg of a drug substance and if 10,000 tablets are to be produced, 200 g of that drug are employed in the formula. After the addition of the pharmaceutical additives such as the diluent, disintegrant, lubricant, and binder, the formulation may weigh 2000 g, which means that each tablet must weigh 200 mg in order for 20 mg of drug to be present. Thus, the depth of fill in the tablet die must be adjusted to hold a volume of granulation weighing 200 mg.[1] Once the fill is properly set, production may start.

The USP and the NF have weight variation standards to which the official tablets must conform. The official test, which refers to uncoated tablets, is as follows:

> Weigh individually 20 whole tablets, and calculate the average weight; the weights of not more than 2 of the tablets differ from the average weight by no more than the percentage listed and no tablet differs by more than double that percentage.

A control of quality is necessary during production, and periodic checks are made of tablet

[1] It should be apparent that when reference is made to a "20-mg tablet," the reference is to the amount of drug contained in the tablet and not to the actual weight of the tablet. Tablets such as aspirin tablets which generally have small amounts of pharmaceutical adjuncts present may actually weigh only slightly more than the amount of active ingredient present. Generally tablets made from drugs with large doses have proportionately less diluent present than do tablets made from drugs with small doses, and there is a closer relationship between drug present and tablet weight for the former type of drug than for the latter.

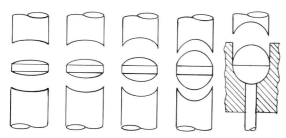

Fig. 6-25. *Contours of the punches determine the shape of the tablets. From left to right, flat face, shallow cup, standard cup, deep cup, and modified ball. (Courtesy of Cherry-Burrell Corporation)*

Weight Variation Tolerances for Uncoated Tablets

Average Weight of Tablet, mg	Percentage Difference
130 or less	10
From 130 through 324	7.5
More than 324	5

weights, since a great expense would be incurred if the tablets were found *after* production not to meet the specifications. During production, there is time to determine the cause of the poor quality and to make the necessary adjustments.

Naturally, the size of tablets produced depends not only on the volume and weight of the fill but also on the diameter of the die and upon the pressure applied to the fill on compaction.

TABLET THICKNESS. As indicated above, the thickness desired in a tablet must be coordinated with the volume of fill issued to the die, the diameter of the die, and the pressure applied to the fill by the punches. In order to produce tablets of uniform thickness during production and between productions for the same formulation, care must be exercised to employ the same volume of fill and the same pressure. Tablets of the same product which vary in size not only might alarm the patient but also might cause problems in packaging. Tablets are measured with a caliper during production to make certain of consistent thickness. It should be pointed out that since pressure applied affects not only the thickness of the tablet but also its hardness and since the latter factor is probably the more important of the two, the thickness of a tablet is varied more by the size of the die and the fill permitted than by the pressure. Pressure adjustments are made primarily to control the softness or the hardness of the tablets.

TABLET HARDNESS. It is not unusual for a tablet press to exert as little as 3000 and as much as 40,000 pounds of force in the production of tablets. Generally speaking, the greater the pressure applied, the harder the tablets, although the characteristics of the granulation also determine the hardness of the tablet. Certain tablets, such as lozenges and

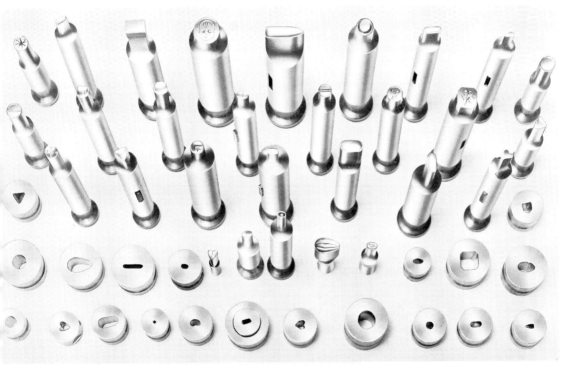

Fig. 6-26. *Various Stokes punches and dies for the production of distinctive tablets. (Courtesy of Stokes Equipment Division, Pennwalt Chemicals Corporation)*

buccal tablets that are intended to dissolve slowly, are intentionally made hard; other tablets, such as compressed tablet triturates that are intended to dissolve rapidly, are made soft. In general, tablets should be sufficiently hard to resist breaking during packaging, shipment, and normal handling and yet soft enough to dissolve or disintegrate properly after administered or to be broken between the fingers when a part of a tablet is to be taken.

A number of tablet hardness testers in use today measure the degree of force (in kilograms, pounds, or in arbitrary units) that is required to break a tablet. In the industry, a force of about 4 kilograms is considered to be the minimum permitted for a satisfactory tablet. Hardness determinations are made during production to determine the need for pressure adjustments on the tablet presses.

Another means of determining the hardness of tablets is through the use of a *friabilator*. This apparatus determines the tablet's *friability*, (that is, its tendency to crumble) by allowing the tablet to roll and fall within a rotating tumbling apparatus. The tablets are weighed before and after a specified number of rotations, and the loss in weight is determined. Resistance to loss of weight indicates the tablet's ability to withstand abrasion in handling, packaging, and shipment.

TABLET DISINTEGRATION. In order for the medicinal component of a tablet to become fully available for absorption from the gastrointestinal tract, the tablet must first disintegrate and discharge the drug to the body fluids for dissolution. This is not to say that a tablet which disintegrates will guarantee the absorption of the medicinal component. As pointed out in Chapter 3, a drug must first be in solution to be absorbed, and unless the drug becomes solubilized in the gastrointestinal tract, it cannot be absorbed, irrespective of the disintegration performance of the dosage form which merely acts as the delivery system. Tablet disintegration is also important for those tablets bearing medicinal agents (such as antacids and anti-diarrheals) that are not intended to be absorbed but rather to act locally within the gastrointestinal tract. In these instances, tablet disintegration provides to the environment a great number of tablet and drug particles with a greater surface area for its localized activity within the body.

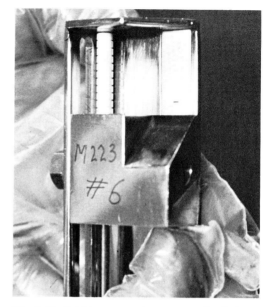

Fig. 6-27. *Tablet gauge used to measure the thickness of tablets. (Courtesy of Eli Lilly and Company)*

The USP and the NF tablets must pass the official Tablet Disintegration Test, which is conducted *in vitro* with a special testing apparatus (Fig. 6-30). Briefly, the apparatus consists of a basket-rack assembly containing 6 open-ended glass tubes held vertically upon a 10-mesh stainless steel wire screen. During testing, a tablet is placed in each of the six tubes of the basket and through the use of a mechanical device, the basket is raised and lowered in the immersion fluid at a frequency of between 28 and 32 cycles per minute, the wire screen always being maintained below the level of the fluid. For uncoated tablets, buccal tablets, and sublingual tablets, water maintained at about 37° serves as the immersion fluid unless another fluid is specified in the individual monograph. Buccal tablets must disintegrate within 4 hours, and the sublingual and other uncoated tablets within the limits of the official monograph, usually 30 minutes but varying from about 2 minutes for Nitroglycerin Tablets, USP, to an hour or longer for other tablets. For these tests, disintegration is defined as "that state in which any residue of the tablet, except fragments of insoluble coating, remaining on the screen is a soft mass having no palpably firm core." For plain coated tablets, initial soaking in water at room temperature for 5 minutes is permitted to remove any water-soluble external coating. Then the tablets are immersed in simu-

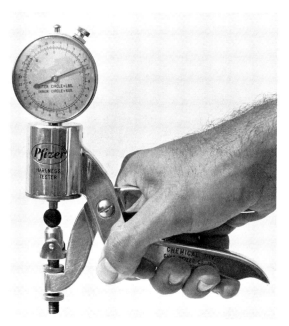

Fig. 6-28. *Pfizer tablet hardness tester. (Courtesy of Pfizer Laboratories)*

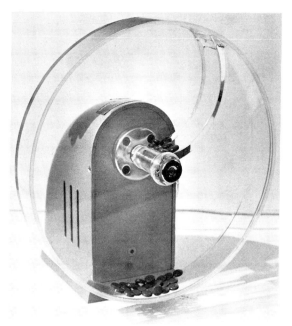

Fig. 6-29. *Erweka tablet testing apparatus for rolling and impact durability. Tablets are weighed and placed in the plexiglass drum in which a curved baffle is mounted. When the motor is activated by setting the timer, the tablets roll and drop. If the free fall within the drum results in the breakage or excessive abrasion of the tablets, they are considered not suited to withstand shipment without being damaged. The motor makes 20 rpm. After the tablets have been tested, they are removed and weighed again. The difference in weight within a given time indicates the rate of abrasion. (Courtesy of Chemical and Pharmaceutical Industry Co., Inc.)*

lated gastric fluid at 37° for 30 minutes, and if they fail to disintegrate, they are subjected to the test using simulated intestinal fluid also at 37° for the prescribed period according to the individual monograph. Enteric-coated tablets are similarly tested, except that the tablets are permitted to be tested in the gastric fluid for one hour after which no sign of dissolution or disintegration must be seen. They are then actively immersed in the simulated intestinal fluid for an individually designated length of time during which the tablets should have disintegrated. In each of the above cases, if 1 or 2 of the 6 tablets fail to disintegrate completely, tests are repeated on 12 additional tablets, and not less than 16 of the total of 18 tablets tested must disintegrate completely to meet the standard.[1]

TABLET DISSOLUTION. The official compendia contain a test for tablet and capsule dissolution for use when stated in the individual drug monographs. The test affords an objective means of determining the dissolution characteristics of a drug present in a solid dosage form. Since drug absorption and physiologic availability are largely dependent upon having the drug in the dissolved state, simple dissolution character-

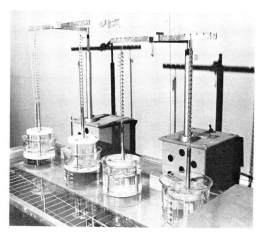

Fig. 6-30. *Tablet disintegration testing apparatus. (Courtesy of Eli Lilly and Co.)*

[1] The USP or the NF should be consulted for the full details of the apparatus and the testing procedure.

istics are an important property of a satisfactory drug product.

Briefly, the apparatus for testing the dissolution characteristics of a capsule or tablet dosage form consists of (1) a variable speed stirrer motor, (2) a cylindrical stainless steel basket to be affixed to the end of the stirrer shaft, (3) a 1000-ml vessel of glass or other inert, transparent material, fitted with a cover having a center port for the shaft of the stirrer, and three additional ports, two for the removal of samples, and one for the placement of a thermometer, and (4) a suitable water bath to maintain the temperature of the dissolution medium in the vessel (Fig. 6-31). In each test, usually 900 ml of the dissolution medium (as stated in the individual monograph) is placed in the vessel and allowed to come to 37° ±0.5°. Then, the basket containing the single tablet or capsule to be tested is immersed in the medium to a point 2 cm from the bottom of the vessel and rotated at the speed specified in the monograph. At specified intervals, samples of the medium are withdrawn for chemical analysis of the proportion of drug dissolved. The test is repeated on 5 additional dosage units and all 6 tablets or capsules must meet the monographic requirement for rate of dissolution. If they do not, the test is repeated on 6 additional dosage units and not less than 10 of the 12 total units must conform to the requirements.

With the increased emphasis on dissolution

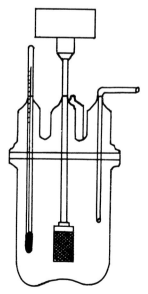

Fig. 6-31. *Dissolution test apparatus.*

testing and the determination of the bioavailability of drugs from solid dosage forms has come the introduction of sophisticated systems for the testing and analysis of tablet dissolution. One of these systems is shown in Figure 6-32.

Certain drug products have demonstrated either *biologic* or *clinical in*equivalency with their *chemically*-equivalent products in clinical practice, and thus particular emphasis has been placed on establishing standards for products of these chemical substances. Among the official tablets and capsules for which there is presently an official drug dissolution requirement are the following:

Acetohexamide Tablets, USP
Digoxin Tablets, USP
Hydrochlorothiazide Tablets, USP
Indomethacin Capsules, NF
Meprobamate Tablets, USP
Methylprednisolone Tablets, NF
Nitrofurantoin Tablets, USP
Phenylbutazone Tablets, USP
Prednisolone Tablets, USP
Prednisone Tablets, USP
Sulfisoxazole Tablets, USP
Sulfamethoxazole Tablets, NF
Theophylline, Ephedrine HCl, and Phenobarbital Tablets, NF
Tolbutamide Tablets, USP

CONTENT UNIFORMITY TEST. The principle of requiring a demonstration of uniformity of the content of the active ingredient(s) in solid dosage forms from a given container or batch was introduced in the USP XVII and the NF XII, with a small number of the monographs for tablets having a *Content Uniformity* test as part of the official requirement. This requirement has been greatly extended since that time, and now the test is included in all monographs for tablets in which (1) the active ingredient is present in relatively low quantities—usually 50 mg or less of any strength available—and (2) test procedures and similar considerations indicate that it is feasible to apply the specification. The test is also applied to other dosage forms—such as capsules and sterile solids—when considered desirable. In brief, the test involves the individual *assay* of a specified number of dosage units to determine the homogeneity of their preparation.

It should be mentioned that the *Content Uniformity* test would be impractical were it

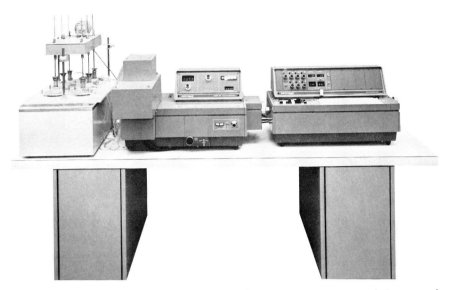

Fig. 6-32. *Beckman Model 25-7 dissolution system. A spectrophotometric system accommodating seven channels of analysis. Six dosage forms and a blank may be tested at one time. The constant temperature water bath is seen on the far left with six tablet basket assemblies in operation simultaneously. Using a multi-channel pump, solution from each of the six test vessels may be continuously sampled to a series of flow cells for UV or colorimetric analysis. (Courtesy of Beckman Instruments, Inc.)*

not for techniques of automated analyses, and the official compendia, in recognizing this fact, make the necessary provisions. The *Content Uniformity* test should not be confused with the *Weight Variation* test, which provides limits for the permissible variations in the *weights* (not active ingredient content) of individual dosage units. The test for *Weight Variation* is still a monographic requirement for those tablets and capsules that contain greater than 50 mg of active constituent and are therefore not generally subjected to the *Content Uniformity* test.

Methods of Preparation

The three current methods for the preparation of compressed tablets are the *wet granulation method*, the *dry granulation method*, and *direct compression*.

Wet Granulation

Wet granulation is undoubtedly the most widely employed method for the production of compressed tablets. Although the process is time consuming, the rewards are great in that the product resulting is generally a pharmaceutically acceptable one. The steps required in the preparation of tablets by this method may be separated as follows: (1) weighing and blending the ingredients, (2) preparing the granulation, (3) screening the damp mass, (4) drying, (5) dry screening, (6) lubrication, and (7) tableting by compression.

WEIGHING AND BLENDING. The active ingredient and any diluent and disintegrating agent required in the tablet formulation are weighed in amounts required for the preparation of the number of tablets to be produced and are mixed thoroughly, generally in a motor-driven powder mixer. Among the diluents used are lactose, kaolin, mannitol, starch, powdered sugar, and calcium phosphate. The selection of the diluent is based partly on the experience of the manufacturer in the preparation of other tablets and also on its cost and compatibility with the other formulative ingredients. For example, calcium salts must not be employed as fillers in the preparation of tablets or capsules of tetracycline antibiotics, since the calcium interferes with the absorption of these drugs from the gastrointestinal tract.

Disintegrating agents include corn and potato starches, starch derivatives as sodium starch glycolate, cellulose derivatives as sodium carboxymethylcellulose, cation-exchange resins, and other materials that swell or expand on exposure to moisture and effect the rupture or breakup of the tablet after it enters the gastro-

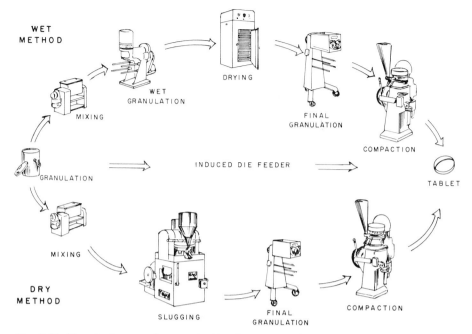

Fig. 6-33. *Steps in the manufacture of tablets by wet granulation, dry granulation, and direct compression with induced die feeder. (Courtesy of Cherry-Burrell Corporation)*

intestinal tract. Results of water-sorption studies show that the disintegrants with the highest water uptake are generally the most effective in most tablet systems.[1] Sodium starch glycollate and the cation exchange resins were shown to be particularly effective in the taking up of moisture. In studies of the mechanism of starch as a tablet disintegrant, it has been observed that the rupture of tablet surfaces occurs where agglomerates of starch grains were found and that tablet break-up probably results from the hydration of the hydroxy groups of the starch molecules causing them to move apart.[2] When starch is employed, 5% is usually suitable to promote disintegration, but up to about 15% may be used to promote more rapid tablet disintegration. The total amount of disintegrant is not always added to the drug-diluent mixture, but a portion (sometimes half of that used) is reserved for later addition, with the lubricant, to the prepared granulation of the drug. This process results in a double disintegration of the tablet—the first from that portion of the disintegrant added last and effecting the breakup of the tablets into small pieces or chunks of tablet and the second disintegration from the initial addition of disintegrant and breaking up the pieces of tablet into fine particles.

Care must be exercised to achieve thorough mixing of the components to insure proper dosage administration as well as the uniform disintegration of all of the tablets produced. Sometimes the blended powders are passed through a sifter or a screen of appropriate fineness to eliminate clumps or compacts of powder.

PREPARING THE GRANULATION. For the powder mixture to flow evenly and freely from the hopper (the funnel-like container holding the drug and guiding its flow into the machine for tableting) into the dies, filling the latter evenly and fully at each occurrence, it is usually necessary to convert the powder mixture to free-flowing granules called the *granulation*. This is accomplished by adding a liquid binder or an adhesive to the powder mixture, passing the wetted mass through a screen of the desired mesh size, drying the granulation, and then passing through a second screen of smaller mesh to reduce further the size of the granules. The binding agent present in the tablets also contributes to the adhesion of the granules to one another, maintaining the integrity of the

[1] Khan, K. A., and Rhodes, C. T.: Water-Sorption Properties of Tablet Disintegrants, *J. Pharm. Sci.*, 64:447, 1975.

[2] Lowenthal, W., and Wood, J. H.: Mechanism of Action of Starch as a Tablet Disintegrant VI: Location and Structure of Starch in Tablets, *J. Pharm. Sci.*, 62:287, 1973.

tablet after compression. Among the binding agents used are a 10 to 20% aqueous preparation of corn starch, a 25 to 50% solution of glucose, molasses, various natural gums (as acacia), cellulose derivatives (as methylcellulose, carboxymethylcellulose and microcrystalline cellulose), gelatins, and povidone. If the drug substance is adversely affected by an aqueous binder, the binding agents may be nonaqueous or may be added dry. In general, the binding action is more effective when the adhesive is mixed with the powders in liquid form. The amount of binding agent used is part of the operator's art and is dependent upon the other formulative ingredients. However, an amount that will render the drug mixture moist enough so that the powder is compactible by squeezing in the hand is usually sufficient. Care must be exercised not to overwet or underwet the powder. Overwetting usually results in granules that are too hard for proper tableting; underwetting usually results in the preparation of tablets that are too soft and tend to crumble. If desired, a suitable colorant or flavorant may be added to the binding agent to prepare a colored or flavored granulation.

SCREENING THE DAMP MASS. Generally the wet granulation is pressed through a No. 6- or 8-mesh screen. This may be done by hand or by special granulation equipment, some of which prepares the granulation by extrusion through perforations in the apparatus. After all of the material has been converted into granules, the granulation is spread evenly on large pieces of paper in shallow trays and dried.

DRYING THE GRANULATION. In most instances, the granules are dried in special drying cabinets that have circulating air systems and are thermostatically controlled. Among the newer methods of drying in use today is *fluidization* conducted in *fluid bed driers* (Fig. 6-36). In this method the granules are dried by being suspended and agitated by a stream of warm air. If the effectiveness of the binder is dependent upon the presence of minute amounts of moisture, the granulation is not completely dried. However, an excessive amount of moisture remaining in a granulation is frequently the cause of ruptures occurring to coatings later placed on the compressed tablets.

Granulation may also be accomplished by mechanical granulating equipment, including by fluidized layer spray granulation. In this

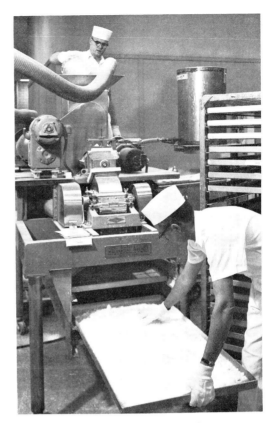

Fig. 6-34. *Fitzpatrick malaxating machine, a continuous wet granulator that combines dry material and granulating excipient and discharges the wet granulation for spreading on a drying tray. Tray of wet granulation is then placed on truck for drying. (Courtesy of The Upjohn Company)*

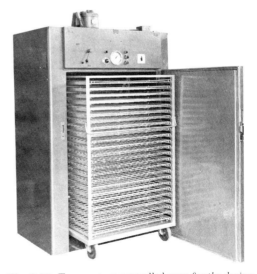

Fig. 6-35. *Temperature-controlled oven for the drying of wet granulation preparative to tablet compression. (Courtesy of Stokes Equipment Division, Pennwalt Corporation)*

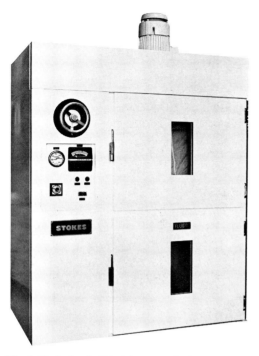

Fig. 6-36. *Stokes fluid bed dryer in which heated air is passed at controlled high velocity through the material to be dried, converting it into a fluidized bed and surrounding each individual particle with a stream of drying air. Because of the efficient mass heat transfer involved, materials previously requiring a 16-hour or longer drying cycle may be dried in less than 45 minutes, depending upon air-steam velocity, drying temperature and the physical properties of the material being processed. (Courtesy of Pennwalt Corporation)*

process, the powder mixture to be granulated is converted to a solution or suspension and spray dried in a fluidized bed to achieve uniform and free flowing granules.

DRY SCREENING. After drying, the granules are passed through a screen of a smaller mesh than that used to prepare the original granulation. The degree to which the granules are reduced depends upon the size of the punches to be used and the tablets to be produced. The proper selection is based on experience; however, in general, the smaller the tablet to be produced, the smaller are the granules used to produce it. Screens from 12- to 20-mesh size are generally used for this purpose. Sizing of the granules is necessary so that the small die cavity for the production of small tablets may be completely filled by the flowing granulation. The voids or air spaces left by a large granulation in a small die cavity would likely result in the production of tablets of varying evenness.

LUBRICATION. After dry screening, a dry lubricant is generally added to the granulation. So that each granule is covered with lubricant, it may be dusted over the spread-out granulation through a fine mesh screen. Among the more commonly used lubricants are talc, magnesium stearate, and calcium stearate, but many other agents are occasionally employed. The quantity of lubricant used varies from one tableting operation to another and may range from a low of about 0.1% of the weight of the granulation to as much as 5%. Lubricants contribute to the preparation of compressed tablets in several ways; they improve the flow of the granulation in the hopper to the die cavity, they prevent the adhesion of the tablet formulation to the punches and dies during compression, they reduce friction between the tablet and the die wall during the tablet's ejection from the tablet machine, and they give a sheen to the finished tablet.

TABLETING. There are a number of types of tablet presses or tableting machines, each varying in its productivity but similar in its basic operation. That operation is the compression of the tablet granulation within a steel die cavity by the pressure exerted by the movement of two steel punches, a lower punch and an upper punch.

There are single-punch tablet machines, some hand operated and some motor driven, which are capable of producing a single tablet upon completion of each up and down movement of the set of punches. As the lower punch drops, the feed shoe filled with granulation (from the hopper) is positioned over the die cavity which then fills. The feed shoe then retracts, scraping the excessive granulation from the stage and leveling the layer of granulation in the die cavity. The upper punch lowers and compresses the material in the die cavity to form the tablet. The upper punch then retracts, and the lower punch rises to the precise level of the stage, lifting the tablet to be ejected from the stage by the feed shoe which moves over the die cavity once again to repeat the process (Fig. 6-23). The tablet is ejected into a barrel or other suitable container. The first few tablets collected, as well as some tablets prepared during the course of production, are examined for weight variation, hardness, thickness, and disintegration, and the necessary adjustments are made in the volume of fill or the pressure of compression to prepare tablets of the desired quality.

Ordinary rotary tablet machines and high speed rotary tablet machines equipped with multiple punches and dies can greatly out-produce the single punch machines through the continuous, rotating movement of the punches and continuous tablet compression. In contrast to the single punch tablet machines generally having a capacity of about 100 tablets per minute, a single rotary press with 16 stations (16 sets of punches and dies) may produce up to 1150 tablets per minute. Double rotary tablet presses with 27, 33, 37, 41, or 49 sets of punches and dies are capable of producing 2 tablets for each die for each complete revolution of the die head because of having two tableting mechanisms. Some of these machines can produce 5000 and more tablets per minute of operation. For such high speed production, induced die feeders are required (Fig. 6-40). These induced feeders force granulation into the dies by the rotary action of an agitator. This feeding is much more rapid than standard gravity feeding and is necessary for the fast production rates achieved with these tableting machines.

As indicated earlier, tablet machines have been developed to form multiple-layered tablets by the multiple feed and multiple compression of fill material within a single die. Also, a layer of material can be compressed onto a tablet core placed strategically and automatically in the die by a special feed apparatus using a special tableting machine.

Dry Granulation

In the dry granulation method the granulation is formed not by moistening or adding a binding agent to the powdered drug mixture but by compacting large masses of the mixture and

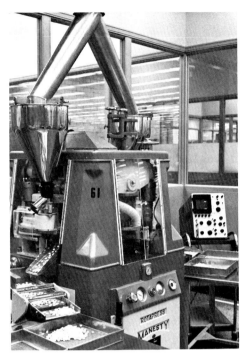

Fig. 6-38. *Manesty Rotapress rotary compression machine making compressed tablets. Tablets leaving the machine run over a tablet duster to screen where they are inspected. Material to be compressed is being fed from overhead hopper through yoke to each of the two compressing machine hoppers. Hardness of tablet is monitored electronically by oscilloscope at the right. (Courtesy of The Upjohn Company)*

subsequently breaking up and sizing these pieces into smaller granules. By this method, either the active ingredient or the diluent must have cohesive properties in order for the large masses to be formed. This method is especially applicable to materials that cannot be prepared by the wet granulation method due to their sensitivity to moisture or to the elevated temperatures required for drying.

After weighing and mixing the ingredients in the same manner as in the wet granulation method, the powder is "slugged" or compressed into large flat tablets of about 1 inch in diameter. It is possible to do this because the flow of the powder into the slugging machine is facilitated by the large cavity and the tablets need not be of exact size or weight. The slugs must be hard enough to be broken up without producing an excessive amount of powder. The slugs are broken up by hand or by a mill and passed through a screen of desired mesh for sizing. Lubricant is added in the usual manner, and tablets are prepared by compression. Aspirin,

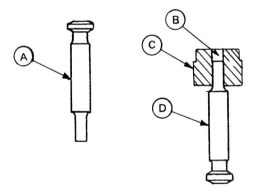

Fig. 6-37. *Punch and die set: (A) upper punch, (B) die cavity, (C) die, and (D) lower punch. (Courtesy of Cherry-Burrell Corporation)*

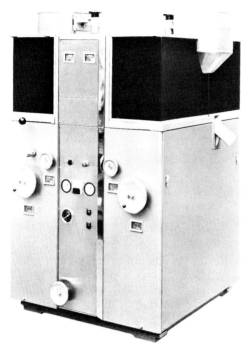

Fig. 6-39. *New Stokes Ultra Press, a double-sided rotary press capable of producing over 10,000 tablets per minute. (Courtesy of Stokes Equipment Division, Pennwalt Corporation)*

which is hydrolyzed on exposure to moisture, is commonly prepared into tablets after slugging. Instead of the slugging method, compaction mills may be used to increase the density of a powder by pressing it between high-pressure rollers. The densified material is then broken up,

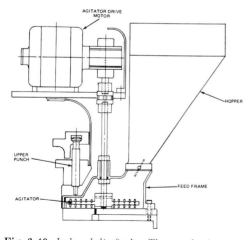

Fig. 6-40. *Induced die feeder. The standard gravity-fed open feed frame can be replaced with an induced die feeder. Using this accessory, granulation is forced into the die by the rotary action of the agitator. (Courtesy of Cherry-Burrell Corporation)*

sized, and lubricated, and tablets are prepared by compression in the usual manner.

Direct Compression

Some granular chemicals like potassium chloride, potassium iodide, ammonium chloride, and methenamine possess free flowing as well as cohesive properties that enable them to be compressed directly in a tablet machine without need of either wet or dry granulation. In past years the number of medicinal substances that could be tableted without prior granulation was quite small. Today the use of spray-dried diluents rather than plain powdered diluents imparts to certain tablet formulations the required qualities for tablet production by direct compression, and a number of additional products may now be produced in this manner. In addition, the forced or induced feeders which have been developed permit the preparation of certain additional tablets by direct compression because the deaerating action of the feeder on light, bulky powders makes them more dense and permits them to flow evenly and completely into the die cavities under moderate pressure. This deaeration also eliminates air entrapment within the die as the tablets are compressed, thereby reducing a major cause of *capping* or splitting of tablets upon compression.[1]

Tablet Coating

Since the reasons for coating tablets and the different types of coatings (i.e., enteric, sugar, film) have already been mentioned, this section will be limited to the general methods involved in the application of these coatings.

Sugarcoating Tablets

The sugarcoating of tablets may be divided into the following steps: (1) waterproofing and

---

[1]The capping or splitting of tablets may be caused by a number of factors and is not limited to tablets prepared by direct compression. For instance punches that are not immaculately clean and perfectly smooth may result in capped tablets as may dies that are old or imperfect. Too much pressure on compression can cause capping as can a granulation which is too soft. Generally there is a portion of "fines" or a fine powder which results when the dry granulation is sized and generally amounts to 10 to 20% of the weight of the granulation and are necessary to properly fill the die cavity. However, an excess of these fines can also lead to capping.

sealing (if needed), (2) subcoating, (3) smoothing and final rounding, (4) finishing and coloring (if desired), and (5) polishing. Generally the entire coating process is conducted in a series of mechanically operated coating pans, which are acorn-shaped vessels of galvanized iron, stainless steel, or copper partially open in the front and with diameters ranging from about 1 to 4 feet and therefore of various capacities. The smaller pans are used for experimental, developmental, and pilot plant operations; the larger pans, for industrial production. The pans are fixed and operate at about a 40° angle, which permits the tablets to remain inside the pan during its revolutions yet also permits the operator to observe and handle the tablets from the open end of the pan. During each of the operations involved in the coating of tablets, the pan is rotated by a motor at moderate speeds, allowing the tablets to tumble and roll about in the pan and make contact with each other and with the coating solutions. As they rotate, the coating solution is gently poured or sprayed on the tablets in portions, and warm air is introduced into the pan to hasten the drying of each coat so that the tablets do not stick to one another and so that the entire process may be hastened, since the tablets require many coats of material and each subsequent coat may be applied only after the previous coat has dried. Tablets intended to be coated are generally compressed tablets that have been prepared to be highly convex and have as thin an edge as possible to permit the coatings to form rounded rather than angular edges.

WATERPROOFING AND SEALING COATS. For tablets containing components that may absorb moisture or be adversely affected on contact with moisture, a waterproofing layer or coating of a material such as shellac is placed on the compressed tablets before the subcoating application. The shellac or other waterproofing agent is applied in solution (usually alcoholic) form and is gently poured on the compressed tablets rotating in the coating pans or is sprayed on as a fine spray. Warm air is blown into the pan during the coating to hasten the drying and to prevent tablets from sticking together. A second coat of the waterproofing substance may be added to the tablets after the first coat has dried to ensure against moisture penetration into the compressed tablets.

SUBCOATING. After the waterproofing or sealing coats (if they are necessary) have been applied, the tablets are given about 3 to 5 subcoats of a sugar-based syrup for the purpose of rounding the tablets and bonding the sugar coating to the compressed tablet. In applying the subcoating, a heavy syrup generally containing gelatin and sometimes acacia is added to the tablets as they roll in the coating pan. When the tablets are partially dry they are sprinkled with a dusting powder, which is usually a mixture of powdered sugar and starch but may also contain talc, acacia, or precipitated chalk. Warm air is applied to the rolling tablets, and when they are dry, the subcoating process is repeated and repeated again until the tablets are of the desired shape and size. At this point, the tablets are usually removed from the coating pan, the excess powder is shaken off the tablets by gently jostling them on a cloth screen, and the coating pan is then washed to remove extraneous coating material.

	PAN SIZE	CAPACITY (APPROX.) GALS.		PAN SIZE	CAPACITY (APPROX.) GALS.
	8	.22		8	.37
	9	.28		9	.48
	10	.4		10	.67
	12	.7		12	1.15
	14	1.1		14	1.8
	16	1.6		16	2.7
	18	2.47		18	4.15
	20	3.28		20	5.5
	24	5.5		24	9.2
	28	8.7		28	14.6
	30	10.9		30	18.25
GALVANIZED	32	13.	STAINLESS	32	21.8
COATING &	36	19.6	STEEL	36	33.
POLISHING	38	22.75	COATING &	38	38.25
PANS	40	26.25		40	44.
	42	30.5	POLISHING PANS	42	51.25

Fig. 6-41. *Sizes and shapes of usual coating and polishing pans. The size of the tablets and the size of the batch to be coated or polished determine the diameter of the pan. (Courtesy of Cherry-Burrell Corporation)*

SMOOTHING AND FINAL ROUNDING. After the tablets have been subcoated to the desired shape (roundness), 5 to 10 additional coatings of a very thick syrup are applied to the rolling tablets for the purpose of completing the rounding of the tablets and smoothing the coatings. This syrup may be composed of a sucrose-based simple syrup, or it may have additional components like starch and calcium carbonate. As the syrup is applied, the operator moves his hand through the rolling tablets to distribute the syrup and to prevent the sticking of the tablets to one another. A dusting powder may or may not be used between syrup applications, but warm air is generally applied to hasten the drying time of each coat. If the coating is to be colored, the

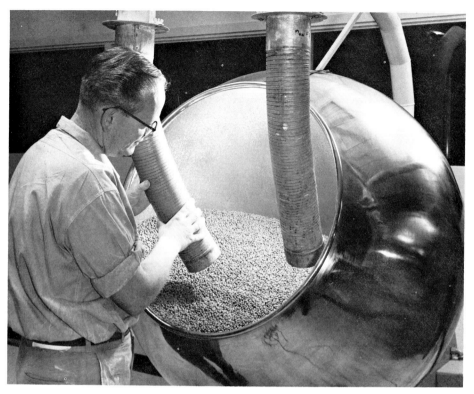

Fig. 6-42. *Tablet coating, showing the warm air supply and the exhaust. (Courtesy of Wyeth Laboratories)*

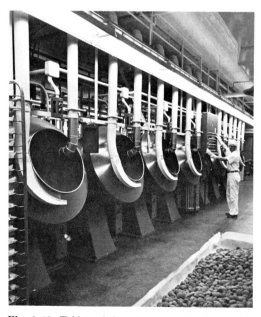

Fig. 6-43. *Tablet polishing in canvas-lined pans. Air and exhaust ducts to facilitate drying are automatically operated from central board. Similar pans without canvas linings are used in coating operations. (Courtesy of Eli Lilly and Company)*

suitable dye may be added to the syrup during this step of the coating process as well as during the next step.

FINISHING AND COLORING. To attain final smoothness and the appropriate color to the tablets, several coats of a thin syrup containing the desired colorant (if any) are applied. This step is usually performed in a clean pan, free from previous coating materials.

A recent innovation in tablet coating equipment is the Accela-Cota coating pan shown in Figure 6-44. This system provides for the automated spraying of coating material into the pan with a simultaneous flow of air being drawn across the revolving bed of tablets. The result is a more uniform tablet coating and a decrease in the time of the coating operation. The tablets may be coated with this procedure using film coatings, a cellulose acetate phthalate, or sugar-based coatings.

Tablets, coated by any of the methods, may then be passed through special imprinting machines to impart any distinctive symbol or identification code on the tablets (Fig. 6-45).

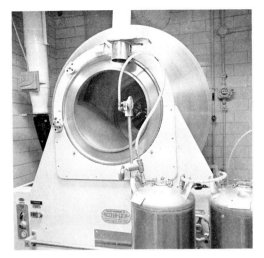

Fig. 6-44. *Tablet coating by spray technique using the Accela-Cota equipment. (Courtesy of Eli Lilly and Company)*

POLISHING. Coated tablets may be polished in special drum-shaped pans made by stretching a cloth fabric over a metal frame or in ordinary coating pans lined with canvas. The fabric or the canvas may be impregnated with a wax such as carnauba wax with or without the addition of beeswax and the tablets polished as they roll about in the pan. Or, the wax may be dissolved in a nonaqueous solvent such as acetone or petroleum benzin and sprayed on the rolling tablets in small amounts. After each coat has dried, the addition of a small amount of talc to the tumbling tablets contributes to their high luster. Two or three coats of wax may be applied, depending upon the desired gloss. Another method of polishing tablets simply involves placing pieces of wax in the polishing pan along with the tablets and permitting the tablets to tumble over the wax until the desired sheen is attained.

Film Coating Tablets

As one can ascertain from the previous discussion of sugarcoating, the process is not only tedious and time-consuming, requiring the expertise of a highly skilled technician, but it also results in the preparation of coated tablets that may be twice the size and weight of the original uncoated compressed tablets. These factors are important to a manufacturer in his consideration of the expense of both packaging materials and shipping. From a patient's point of view,

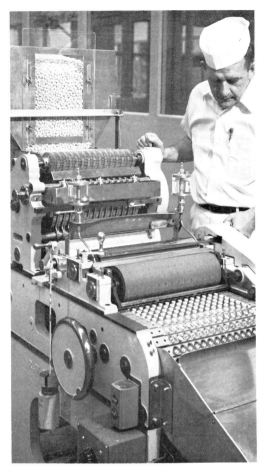

Fig. 6-45. *Branding of coated compressed tablets on a Hartnett branding machine. (Courtesy of The Upjohn Company)*

large tablets are not as convenient to swallow as are small tablets. Also, the coatings of tablets by the application of the sugar coating may vary slightly from batch to batch and within the batch. The film-coating process, which places a thin, skin-tight coating of a plastic-like material over the compressed tablet, was developed to produce coated tablets having essentially the same weight, shape, and size as the originally compressed tablet. The coating is thin enough to reveal any depressed or raised monograms punched into the tablet by the tablet punches. In addition, film-coated tablets are far more resistant to destruction by abrasion than are sugar-coated tablets, and like sugar-coated tablets, the coating may be colored to make the tablets attractive and distinctive.

Film-coating solutions generally contain the

following types of materials to provide the desired coating to the tablets:[1]

(1) A *film former* capable of producing smooth, thin films reproducible under conventional coating conditions and applicable to a variety of tablet shapes. Example: cellulose acetate phthalate.
(2) An *alloying substance* providing water solubility or permeability to the film to insure penetration by body fluids and therapeutic availability of the drug. Example: polyethylene glycol.
(3) A *plasticizer* to produce flexibility and elasticity of the coating and thus provide durability. Example: castor oil.
(4) A *surfactant* to enhance spreadability of the film during application. Example: polyoxyethylene sorbitan derivatives.
(5) *Opaquants* and *colorants* to make the appearance of the coated tablets handsome and distinctive. Examples: Opaquant, titanium dioxide; colorant, F.D. & C. or D. & C. dyes.
(6) *Sweeteners, flavors,* and *aromas* to enhance the acceptability of the tablet to the patient. Examples: sweeteners, cyclamate-saccharin; flavors and aromas, vanillin.
(7) A *glossant* to provide luster to the tablets without a separate polishing operation. Example: beeswax.
(8) A *volatile solvent* to allow the spread of the other components over the tablets while allowing rapid evaporation to permit an effective yet speedy operation. Example: alcohol-acetone mixture.

Tablets are film coated by the application or spraying of the film-coating solution upon the tablets in ordinary coating pans. The volatility of the solvent enables the film to adhere quickly to the surface of the tablets.

Enteric Coating

The purpose of enteric coating for solid dosage forms has been previously discussed. Since the pH within the various depths of the gastrointestinal tract may vary between patients and within a given patient at different times, it is generally considered preferable to base the design of an enteric coating upon the length of time required for disintegration or drug release rather than on specific environmental conditions of the intestine. However, enteric preparations may be based on one factor or the other, or on both. If the tablet is coated to various thicknesses with certain coating materials that are not immediately dissolved by the gastric fluid, the tablet may be prevented from disintegrating until it has time to reach the intestinal tract. Among the materials used in enteric coatings are phenyl salicylate (salol), a combination of 45 parts of n-butyl stearate, 30 parts of carnauba wax, and 25 parts of stearic acid, and cellulose acetate phthalate. These materials may be applied on a large industrial scale by the usual coating methods, or they may be applied to a few capsules, pills, or tablets extemporaneously by the pharmacist. The application of salol to dosage forms by the practicing pharmacist is a difficult procedure and often results in only partially coated tablets. The use of the mixture of n-butyl stearate, carnauba wax, and stearic acid frequently meets with better success. In coating solid dosage forms with this combination of substances, the three ingredients are melted together at 75° and maintained in the molten state while a dosage unit, held with tweezers, is dipped at least half way into the mixture and withdrawn, touching it slightly to the edge of the container to remove excess coating. When dry, the other half of the dosage unit is similarly coated, so as to overlap the first coat slightly. The process is repeated two or more times to ensure complete coating. All three of the components of the coating resist the gastric fluid, and all but the carnauba wax are hydrolyzed in the intestine. In a similar manner, solid dosage units may be extemporaneously coated with a 10% solution of cellulose acetate phthalate in acetone, placed in a small vessel. Three coatings are usually applied. In the intestine the cellulose acetate phthalate is disintegrated by the esterases and also by ions that combine with the carboxyl groups of the molecules of the coating material to produce a soluble compound which erodes and reveals the compressed tablet for intestinal disintegration.

Air Suspension Coating

This process, also known as the Wurster process after its developer, may be employed for the rapid coating of granules, powders, or tablets. The items to be coated are fed into a verti-

[1] From Gross, H. M., and Endicott, C. J.: Transformation to Filmcoating, *Drug Cosmetic Ind.*, 86:170, 1960.

cal cylinder and are supported by a column of air that enters from the bottom of the cylinder. Within the air stream, the solids rotate both vertically and horizontally. As the coating solution enters the system, it is rapidly placed on the suspended, rotating solids, with rounding coats being applied in less than an hour with the assistance of warm air blasts released in the chamber.

Compression Coating

In a manner similar to the preparation of multiple compressed tablets having an inner core and an outer shell of drug material, core tablets may be sugarcoated by compression. The coating material in the form of a granulation or a powder is compressed onto a tablet core of drug with a special tablet press. This method eliminates the time-consuming and tedious operation previously described in this section. Compression coating is an anhydrous operation and thus may be safely employed in the coating of tablets having a drug that is sensitive to moisture. The resulting coat is more uniform than the usual sugar coating applied using pans, and less of a coating is required. Resulting tablets are lighter and smaller and are therefore easier to swallow and less expensive to package and ship.

Chewable Tablets

Chewable tablets are tablets which are intended to disintegrate smoothly in the mouth at a moderate rate, either with or without actual chewing. Characteristically, chewable tablets have a smooth texture upon disintegration, are pleasant tasting, and leave no bitter or unpleasant aftertaste. Mannitol, a white cyrstalline hexahydric alcohol, which possesses many of the characteristics desired for the excipient in chewable tablets, is widely employed for this purpose. Mannitol is said to be about 70% as sweet as sucrose with a cool taste and mouth-feel, the latter resulting from its negative heat of solution and a moderate solubility in water. Mannitol's nonhygroscopicity also makes it an ideal excipient for the preparation of chewable tablets containing moisture-sensitive drugs. Chewable tablets are prepared by wet granulation and compression, using minimum degrees of tablet hardness. In many chewable tablet formulations, mannitol may account for 50% or more of the weight of the formulation. Some-

times, other sweetening agents, as sorbitol, lactose, dextrose and glucose, may be substituted for part or all of the mannitol. Lubricants and binders which do not detract from the texture or desired hardness of the tablet are used in formulating chewable tablets. To enhance the appeal of the tablets, colorants and tart or fruity flavorants are commonly employed. Among the types of products prepared into chewable tablets are antacids and vitamins, aspirin, and antibiotic preparations intended for children.

Molded Tablets

As indicated at the beginning of this section, molded tablets include tablet triturates, hypodermic tablets, and dispensing tablets although each of these tablet types may also be prepared by soft compression with a tablet press. It should be recalled that these tablets must be completely and rapidly soluble in water. Tablets prepared by molding are generally softer than tablets prepared by compression because less pressure is applied during compaction, and as a result they are usually more rapidly soluble. The types of tablets described in this section are characteristically small and contain small amounts of potent drugs. Tablet triturates and hypodermic tablets generally do not weigh more than 65 mg or so, including the diluent. Dispensing tablets, which are prepared to contain a multiple of the usual dose of the potent drug generally do not weigh more than 200 or 300 mg, including the diluent.

Preparation of Molded Tablet Triturates

THE MOLD. The mold used in the preparation of molded tablets is usually made of hard rubber, metal, or a hard plastic composition, and it consists of two parts, the upper part, or the *die* portion, and the lower part containing squat, flat punches. The die portion is simply a plate of the thickness of the desired tablets and generally having from 50 to 200 uniformly drilled and spaced circular holes. The lower part of the mold contains punches corresponding in number, position, and diameter with the holes of the die. When the two parts of the mold are joined, the punches fit precisely in the holes of the upper plate. When the die is filled with the material to be tableted and the die is placed upon the lower portion of the mold, the punches gently lift the fill material from the holes to rest openly on the flat punches for drying. In assembling the two parts of the mold, the pharmacist must make certain that the upper plate is right side up and facing in the proper direction in order that the punches may be properly directed and fit snugly in the holes. To assist the pharmacist, the mold manufacturers generally make the two parts of the mold each with one slightly rounded end and one squared end which are each placed in the same direction when the two parts are joined. The upper plate also usually bears a number which corresponds to the number of the bottom of the mold to identify the two parts as a unit. In positioning the upper plate, the number usually faces upwards for the proper fit on the punches.

PREPARING THE TABLET FORMULATION FOR MOLDING. The base for tablet triturates is generally a mixture of finely powdered lactose alone or in combination with an amount of powdered sucrose varying from about 5 to 20% of the base. The addition of sucrose results in the production of tablets that are less brittle than when lactose alone is employed. The greater the proportion of sucrose added, the harder will be the resulting tablet triturates. To the base is added the amount of drug substance required to prepare the desired number of tablets of the desired drug strength. It should be pointed out that the medicinal agent is generally added to the base by geometric dilution, since the drug is generally a potent substance.

The molding of the tablets is effected by the solvent action of a liquid *excipient* used to moisten the powder mixture preparative to molding. The excipient is usually a mixture of alcohol and water in equal proportions. The water portion of the excipient exerts the solvent action on a portion of the base, effecting the binding action on drying. The alcoholic portion of the excipient speeds the drying process. If a large proportion of the powder formulation is very rapidly soluble in water, it is usually desirable to use an excipient of a greater alcoholic content than the mixture described above. Care must also be exercised in selecting the proper excipient with respect to chemical interaction or drug destruction (as from hydrolysis) due to an interaction between a part of the excipient and the drug. For drugs adversely affected by alcohol, the alcoholic content of the excipient must therefore be reduced or eliminated. Similarly, for drugs adversely affected by water, an excipient of greater than usual alcoholic strength may be preferred.

The amount of excipient used to dampen the powder mixture is largely determined by experience, but it may be said that the powder mixture should be damp but not wet. The particles

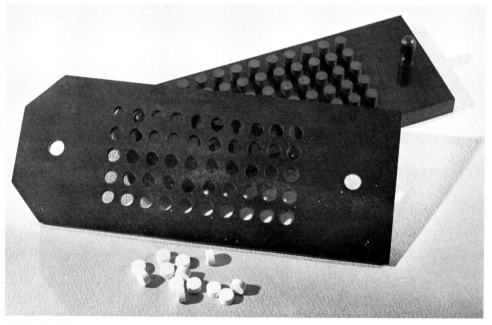

Fig. 6-46. *A tablet triturate mold.*

of powder should have the tendency to cling together when pressed slightly between the fingers.

The moistened powder is added to the mold by placing the upper part of the mold flatly on a glass or porcelain plate and forcing the moistened material into the openings of the mold by a rubbing motion with a steel spatula. The spatula should be moved so that the fill in each opening is complete and flat with the surface. The underside of the mold should be inspected to make certain that the fill is complete on that side also. It is permissible to work both sides with the spatula until the mold is evenly and completely filled. After the mold has been filled, it is placed upon the lower punch of the mold, and the tablets are ejected for drying.

STANDARDIZING THE MOLD. Since the upper plate of the mold is capable of holding different weights of materials depending upon the densities of the materials, each mold must be "standardized" by the pharmacist in terms of weight for each formulation that is molded into tablets. It is advisable for him to maintain a record of such standardizations for each mold so that they need not be repeated the next time the same formula is prepared into tablets. Although several methods for standardizing the mold have been presented, perhaps the most efficient in terms of preparing the proper amount to fill completely all of the perforations with the proper amount of drug and base is the following method:

1. Weigh the proper amount of medicinal substance for the preparation of the desired number of tablets which corresponds to the number of openings in the mold.
2. Mix the medicinal substance with an amount of base known to be insufficient to fill the mold completely.
3. Moisten the mixture and place it in the openings as far as it will go, spending little time trying to achieve uniform distribution.
4. Moisten an additional amount of base (with no medicinal agent present) and use this to finish filling the mold, being careful not to remove any of the medicated base from the openings.
5. Punch out the tablets, remove them from the punches, and remix thoroughly to obtain a uniform distribution of the medicinal substance.

6. Refill the mold with the thoroughly blended mixture and punch out the tablets and allow them to dry.

The final weight of the dry tablets should be taken and recorded as the standard weight for that mold for that particular formulation. On the next occasion that formulation is prepared, the identical mold and same formula may be employed. This of course assumes that the same degree of manual pressure is used in each occasion in packing the mold.

Preparation of Hypodermic Tablets

Hypodermic tablets are prepared in the same general manner as tablet triturates with the following exceptions. Since hypodermic tablets are intended to be used as the source of drug for injection, the tablets are prepared under rigid aseptic conditions (even though the tablets are not sterilized nor claimed to be sterile) so that an efficacious injection may be prepared by the physician. They are prepared in dust-free environments. Lactose that has been specially recrystallized is used as the base to ensure rapid and complete solution of the hypodermic tablets. It is the physician's responsibility to handle the tablets aseptically and to sterilize the final solution after preparation. As mentioned earlier, the claim of convenience for hypodermic tablets is becoming less vocal, with unit-dose parenteral preparations in disposable syringes becoming more and more prevalent.

Naturally, neither tablet triturates nor hypodermic tablets are coated. Examples of hypodermic tablets presently commercially available include those of atropine sulfate and codeine sulfate.

Preparation of Dispensing Tablets

Dispensing tablets are prepared either by molding in the same manner as tablet triturates using molds having larger perforations than the tablet triturate molds or by soft compression.

Timed-Release Forms

Some solid dosage forms are designed to release their medication to the body for absorption rapidly and completely; other products may be designed to release the drug slowly for more prolonged drug release and sustained drug action. The latter type of dosage form is commonly referred to by a designation such as a *sustained-action, prolonged-action, sustained-release, prolonged-release, timed-release, extended-action,* or *extended-release* tablet or capsule. Some tablets or capsules may contain two or more full doses of medication and are designed to release each subsequent dosage of medication in its full amount after the previous dose has been absorbed and is being metabolized and excreted. Such dosage forms enable the patient to be maintained on the drug for longer than usual periods following the administration of a single dosage unit. These types of products are usually termed *repeat-action* tablets or capsules. Many of these specialized types of dosage forms are protected by patents and have been given trademark names that help to identify both the manufacturer and the type of pharmaceutical product.[1]

Sustained-Action Forms

Most sustained-action dosage forms are designed so that the administration of a single dosage unit provides the immediate release of an amount of drug that promptly produces the desired therapeutic effect and gradual and continual release of other amounts of drug to maintain this level of effect over an extended period, usually 8 to 12 hours. The advantage of this type of dosage form is the production of even blood levels of the drug without the necessity of the repeated administration of dosage units.

In this type of dosage form, the design must be based primarily on the particular qualities of each individual drug, especially as reflected in its biological performance. What may be an effective type of dosage form design for one drug simply is ineffective in promoting the sustained release of another drug because of the peculiar physical, chemical, and biological qualities of each individual drug substance. In order to maintain the constant level of drug in the system, the drug must be released from the dosage form at a rate that will replace the amount of drug being metabolized and excreted from the body. For each drug, this is a highly individualized quality. In general, the drugs best suited

for incorporation into a sustained release product are those having a fairly rapid rate of absorption and excretion, those having relatively small doses, drugs that are uniformly absorbed from the gastrointestinal tract, and those drugs used in the treatment of chronic rather than acute conditions.[1]

The reasons for these desired qualities for sustained-action forms may be briefly explained as follows. Drugs with slow rates of absorption and excretion are usually inherently long-acting, and their preparation into sustained-action type dosage forms is not necessary. Drugs given in large doses are not suitable for the preparation of the sustained-action product because the individual dosage unit needed to maintain the constant therapeutic blood level of the drug would likely have to be too large for the patient to swallow. Drugs absorbed at different rates as they pass along the gastrointestinal tract are not good candidates for sustained-release products, since their drug release and therefore drug absorption will fluctuate, depending upon the position of the drug in the gastrointestinal tract and its rate of movement within the tract. Drugs for acute conditions generally require more physician control of the dosage than that provided by sustained-release products.

Although there are a variety of types of sustained-release products, they may be grouped into five main categories according to the pharmaceutical mechanism by which they provide sustained release: (1) specially coated beads or granules or microencapsulated drug, (2) embedding drug in a slowly eroding matrix, (3) embedding drug in inert plastic matrix from which it is leached, (4) formation of slowly dissolving chemical complexes of the drug, and (5) use of ion exchange resins. A brief explanation of these methods follows.

COATED BEADS OR GRANULES OR MICRO-ENCAPSULATED DRUG. In this method a solution of the drug substance in a non-aqueous solvent such as a mixture of acetone and alcohol is coated onto small inert beads made of a combination of sugar and starch. In instances in which the dose of the drug is large, the starting granules of material may be composed of the drug itself. Then with some of the beads or granules remaining uncoated and intended to

---

[1] A number of lists of these names are available. One such list may be found in the following reference: Winek, C. I.: Dosage Form Names & Product Identification. Amer. J. Hosp. Pharm., 22:82–89, 1965.

[1] This and the following discussion adapted in part from Shangraw, R. F.: Timed Release Pharmaceuticals. Hosp. Pharm. 2:No. 10, 19–27, 1967.

provide the immediately released dose of drug when taken, coats of a lipid material like beeswax or a cellulosic material like ethylcellulose are applied to the remainder (about two-thirds to three-fourths) of the granules, with some granules receiving a few coats and others many coats. Then the beads or granules of different thicknesses of coatings are blended in the desired proportions to achieve the proper blend. The coating material may be colored with a dye material so that the beads of different coating thicknesses will be darker in color and distinguishable from those having fewer coats and being lighter in color. When properly blended, the granules may be placed in capsules or tableted. The variation in the thickness of the coats and in the type of material used in the coating is reflected in the speed with which the body fluids are capable of penetrating the coating and in dissolving the drug. Naturally, the thicker the coat, the more resistant to penetration and the more delayed will be the drug release. The presence of drug granules of various coating thicknesses therefore produces the sustained drug release and action. Examples of these types of dosage forms include: *Spansules* (Smith Kline & French), *Medules* (Upjohn), *Tempules* (Armour), and *Sequels* (Lederle). The Spansule capsule and the rupturing of one of the coated pellets is shown in Figure 6-47.

Microencapsulation is a process by which solids, liquids or even gases may be encapsulated into microscopic size particles through the formation of thin coatings of "wall" material around the substance being encapsulated. The process had its early origin in the late 1930's as a "clean" substitute for carbon paper and carbon ribbons as sought by the business machines industry. The ultimate development in the 1950's of reproduction paper and ribbons which contained dyes in tiny gelatin capsules released upon impact by a typewriter key or the pressure of a pen or pencil was the stimulus for the development of a host of microencapsuled materials, including drugs. Gelatin is a common wall forming material but synthetic polymers as polyvinyl alcohol, ethylcellulose, or polyvinyl chloride have been used. The typical encapsulation process usually begins with the dissolving of the prospective wall material, say gelatin, in water. The material to be encapsulated is added and the two-phase mixture thoroughly stirred. With the material to be encapsulated broken up to the desired particle size, a solution of a second material is added, usually acacia. This additive material is chosen to have the ability to concentrate the gelatin (polymer) into tiny liquid droplets. These droplets (coacervate) then form a film or coat around the particles of the substance to be encapsulated as a consequence of the extremely low interfacial tension of the gelatin. The next step is the removal of the residual water or solvent in the wall material so that a continuous, tight, film coating remains on the particle. The final dry microcapsules are free-flowing, discrete particles of coated material. Of the total particle weight, the wall material usually represents between 2 and 20%. By varying the wall thickness of microencapsulated drug particles, their dissolution rates may be altered accordingly and sustained release obtained. An example of a drug commercially available in microencapsulated dosage form is aspirin as *Measurin* (Breon Laboratories).

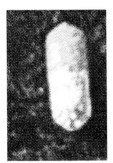 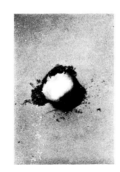 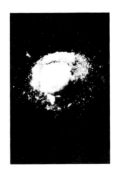 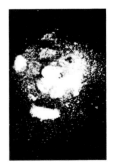

Fig. 6-47. *The* Spansule *capsule showing the hard gelatin capsule containing hundreds of tiny pellets for sustained drug release and the rupturing of one of the pellets as occurs in the gastric fluid. (Courtesy of Smith Kline & French)*

EMBEDDING DRUG IN SLOWLY ERODING MATRIX. By this process, the portion of the drug intended to have sustained action is combined with lipid or cellulosic material processed into granules that can be placed into capsules or tableted. When these granules are combined with granules of drug prepared without the special lipid or cellulosic excipient, the untreated portion provides the immediate drug effect, and the treated portion the prolonged effect. The treated granules slowly erode in the body fluids. The types of materials used in the preparation of the granules may be varied to achieve different rates of erosion. Examples of dosage forms of this type include: *Lontabs* (Ciba), *Space-Tabs* (Sandoz), *Endurets* (Geigy), *Dosespan* (Merrell) and *Ten-Tabs* (National).

Two-layered tablets may be prepared from the granules, with one layer containing the untreated drug for immediate release and the other layer having the drug for sustained release. Three-layered tablets may be similarly prepared, with both outer layers containing the drug for immediate release. Some commercial tablets are prepared with an inner core containing the sustained release portion of drug and an outer shell completely enclosing the core and containing the drug portion for immediate release. Tablets prepared from the type of material described in the next method may be similarly constructed.

EMBEDDING DRUG IN INERT PLASTIC MATRIX. By this method, the drug in granulated with an inert plastic material such as polyethylene, polyvinyl acetate, or polymethacrylate, and the granulation is compressed into tablets. The drug is slowly released from the inert plastic matrix by leaching by the body fluids. The compression of the tablet creates the matrix or plastic form that retains its shape during the leaching of the drug and through its elimination from the alimentary tract. The initially released drug is present on the surfaces of the tablet or is only superficially embedded. The primary example of a dosage form of this type is the *Gradumet* (Abbott).

COMPLEX FORMATION. Certain drug substances when chemically combined with certain other chemical agents form chemical complexes that may be only slowly soluble in body fluids, depending upon the pH of the environment. This slow dissolution rate is effective in providing the sustained action of the drug. One such type of complex is composed of tannic acid with any one of a number of amine-containing drug molecules. The addition of certain buffering agents to the formulation can further alter the rate of dissolution and enhance the sustained release of the drug. An example of a dosage form of this type is *Durabond* (Mallinckrodt).

It should be remembered that certain drug substances that are only slowly soluble in body fluids without special complexation or other treatment are inherently long acting.

ION-EXCHANGE RESINS. A solution of the cationic drug is passed through a column containing the ion-exchange resin, to which it complexes by the replacement of hydrogen atoms. The resin-drug complex is then washed and may be tableted, encapsulated, or suspended in an aqueous vehicle. The release of the drug is dependent upon the pH and the electrolyte concentration in the gastrointestinal tract. Generally, release is greater in the acidity of the stomach than the less acidic small intestine. Examples of drug products of this type include *Biphetamine* capsules (resin complexes of amphetamine and dextroamphetamine) and *Ionamin* capsules (phentermine resin) both by Pennwalt.

Repeat Action Forms

Some specialized tablets are prepared so that an initial dose of the drug is released from the tablet shell and a second dose from an inner core of the tablet, which is separated from the outer shell by a slowly permeable barrier coating. Generally the barrier coating is penetrated and drug from the inner core is exposed to the body fluids some 4 to 6 hours after the swallowing of the tablet. Such a tablet permits the release of two doses of drug from a single tablet, eliminating the need for more frequent drug administration. Examples of this type of dosage form include *Repetabs* (Schering) and *Chronotabs* (White). As for the sustained-action type of dosage forms, the repeat-action forms are best suited for those drugs having low dosage and employed in chronic conditions and for drugs having regular absorption patterns with fairly rapid rates of absorption and excretion.

Delayed Action Forms

The release of a drug from a dosage form may be intentionally delayed until it reaches the intestinal environment for any of several reasons. Among these may be the fact that the drug is destroyed by the gastric juices, or it may be excessively irritating to the lining of the stomach or a nauseating drug, or it may be better absorbed from the intestines than from the stomach. Capsules and tablets coated so as to remain intact in the stomach but yield their ingredients in the intestines are said to be *enteric coated*. The coating may be composed of a material that is pH dependent and breaks down in the less acidic environment of the intestine, or the coating may erode due to moisture and on a time basis coinciding with the time required for the tablet or capsule to reach the intestines. Other coatings may deteriorate due to the hydrolysis-catalyzing action of certain intestinal enzymes. Among the many agents used to enteric coat tablets and capsules are fats, fatty acids, waxes and mixtures of these, shellac, and cellulose acetate phthalate. Phenyl salicylate (salol) and beeswax are commonly used by the pharmacist in his extemporaneous enteric coating of capsules. In this effort, the pharmacist carefully applies a coating of one of these materials around a capsule by dipping it in a melted portion of the material contained in a small beaker. An even application of the enteric coating is a challenge to the pharmacist but a necessity for an effective product.

Testing Timed-Release Tablets and Capsules

A procedure for assay and the necessary apparatus to conduct the tests for the determination of release of drug from timed-release preparations are described in the *National Formulary*. The tests are conducted *in vitro*, that is, in glass and not within an animal body (*in vivo*), so that the relationship between the results of the assay and the release of the drug within the body is not necessarily a direct one. In fact, the NF Cautions:

> This *in vitro* method is not designed to assure or measure safety or effectiveness, both of which must be determined through comprehensive *in vivo* studies and clinical evaluation. From the *in vivo* test data and clinical evaluation, however, suitable *in vitro* release limits may be established.

The test method presented by the NF is intended to serve as a guide and is not intended to set a standard for any official preparation.

Basically, the test involves the exposure of the timed-release tablets or capsules to extracting fluids of various pH values, prepared by mixing various proportions of simulated gastric fluid with simulated intestinal fluid.[1] The tablets or capsules are rotated at a given rate in bottles containing the fluids and submerged in a water bath at 37°. At periods corresponding to 1, 2, 3.5, 5, and 7 hours of rotation time, assays are performed on the tablet or capsule residues (or the filtered extracts) to determine the rate and the amount of drug released from the dosage units.

Pharmaceutic Factors Affecting the Bioavailability of Drugs from Solid Dosage Forms

Differences in the bioavailability of drugs from different types of dosage forms, as tablets, suspensions, solutions are easily understood and attributed to the basic differences in the physical state in which the drug is present in the dosage form (as a solution or as solid particles) and the consequent differences in its dissolution rate and its resultant absorption. Differences which exist in the bioavailability of a drug substance when present in the *same* type of dosage form, but from different manufacturers may not be as clear or as easily understood. However, the differences generally are the result of the following: (1) differences in the physical or chemical quality of the starting materials, both therapeutic and pharmaceutic, (2) differences in the pharmaceutical adjuncts employed and in the methods of dosage form manufacture, including on-line quality control procedures, and (3) differences in the packaging, storage, and age of the fabricated dosage form.

Quality of Starting Materials

As discussed previously in Chapter 3, many therapeutic and pharmaceutical materials ex-

---

[1] The formulas for these two fluids are given in the USP as follows: *Simulated Gastric Fluid:* Sodium Chloride, 2.0 g, Pepsin, 3.2 g, Hydrochloric Acid, 7.0 ml, and sufficient water to make 1000 ml. The pH of the solution is about 1.2.

Simulated Intestinal Fluid: Monobasic Potassium Phosphate, 6.8 g, Pancreatin, 10 g, plus water and enough 0.2 N Sodium Hydroxide to prepare 1000 ml of solution having a pH of about 7.5.

hibit differences in their dissolution characteristics depending upon their physical form, as amorphous or crystalline, small or large particle size, etc. It is well known, for example, that different absorption rates occur from poorly soluble drugs, as griseofulvin, depending upon the drug particle size present in the dosage form. Thus, different drug products manufactured from such a drug, but with varying particle size would be expected to exhibit different dissolution rates and thus different rates of absorption. Manufacturers must be consistent in utilizing starting materials of identical physical and chemical standards in the production of each batch of their products, or variations could occur batch-to-batch. The importance of chemical purity of the substances used not only relates to the therapeutic advantages of such pure materials, but also to the pharmaceutic advantages of minimizing the risk of product instability due to impurities and the possible occurrence of interactions between the impurity and other formulative components or packaging materials.

Formulation and Methods of Manufacture

In the manufacture of a solid dosage form of a given therapeutic agent, different manufacturers utilize different formulations. The differences may be the amount or type of binder, filler, disintegrant, lubricant, colorant or flavorant used. Such variations in tablet or capsule formulation may result in vast differences in drug bioavailability between chemical equivalents of competing products. The different pharmaceutical adjuncts used may produce differences in the hardness of a tablet granulation, for instance, resulting in differences in tablet disintegration and in drug dissolution. The type and amount of disintegrating agent employed in a tablet formulation materially affect the ability and rate of disintegration and thus the availability for dissolution of the drug substance. As noted previously, the type of lubricant used and the amount employed could have a bearing on the wetting of the therapeutic agent present in a tablet or capsule and on its subsequent rate of dissolution and availability for absorption. Certainly tablets with different types of coatings would also be expected to have different release rates for the drug contents.

The method of manufacture of a tablet or capsule can have a profound influence on the release of its medication. Whether the granulation was prepared by the wet or dry granulation method, by hand screening or by granulating machine, can result in granules of different dissolution characteristics. Also, the size of the granules can affect their rate of dissolution; the larger the granule, the slower its dissolution rate. The compression force applied in the manufacture of compressed tablets is another factor that can lead to variation in drug bioavailability between products. Hard tablets may be generally expected to release their medication slower than softer tablets due to the reduction in the porosity of the tablet and the decreased penetrability by the gastrointestinal fluids. The hard packing of material into capsules can similarly affect the release of the contents following rupture of the capsule shell by the gastric fluids.

The quality of the final product is only as good as the materials, methods of manufacture, and quality control that went into its production. Thus, the control of the various processes that comprise the methods of manufacture of dosage forms is essential to the production of a product of consistent high quality. On-line quality control of these methods and of the materials during the various stages of production is the best means of assuring a quality product. This means, for example, the determination of the uniformity of the powder mixture before granulation, the quality of the granules before tableting, and the testing of tablet size, content uniformity, hardness, disintegration and drug dissolution features of the produced tablets *during* the course of batch production and not only at the end. By utilizing good process control techniques, not only is the good quality of the product assured, wastefulness is reduced by the ability to halt production and implement corrections at any point at which production standards are not being met.

Packaging, Storage, and Aging of Dosage Forms

To ensure the maintenance of the original quality of a dosage form, it must be packaged in materials and containers that will protect it from any deteriorating effects of moisture, air, light, etc. Differences in the packaging of pharmaceutical products could result in differences in their chemical and/or physical stability and thus produce differences in their therapeutic effectiveness. In most instances of dispensing, the pharmacist is well advised to use a similar type of container as provided by the manufacturer of the product and the patient advised to maintain the drug in the container dispensed. Proper storage conditions as recommended for the particular drug should be maintained by the pharmacist and patient and expiration dates observed. The pharmacist should be aware also that the hardness of certain tablets may change upon aging usually resulting in a decrease in the disintegration and dissolution rates of the product. The increase in tablet hardness can frequently be attributed to the increased adhesion of the binding agent and other formulative components within the tablet. Examples of increased tablet hardening with age have been reported for a number of drugs including aluminum hydroxide, sodium salicylate and phenylbutazone.[1] Certain tablets containing volatile drugs, as nitroglycerin, may experience the migration of the drug between tablets in the container thereby resulting in a lack of uniformity among the tablets.[2] Further, packing materials, as cotton and rayon, in contact with nitroglycerin tablets may absorb varying amounts of nitroglycerin rendering the tablets sub-potent.[3]

In 1972, the Food and Drug Administration issued a number of regulations covering the packaging, labeling, and dispensing of nitroglycerin products. These regulations include:

1. All nitroglycerin tablets must be packaged in glass containers with tightly fitting metal screw caps.
2. No more than 100 tablets may be packaged in each container.
3. Nitroglycerin tablets must be dispensed in their original containers and bear the label—"Warning: To prevent loss of potency, keep these tablets in the original container. Close tightly immediately after use."
4. All nitroglycerin tablets should be stored at controlled room temperatures of between 59° and 86°F.

[1]Barrett, D. and Fell, J. T.: Effect of Aging on Physical Properties of Phenylbutazone Tablets, *J. Pharm. Sci.*, 64:335, 1975.
[2]Page, D. P., *et al.*: Stability Study of Nitroglycerin Sublingual Tablets, *J. Pharm. Sci.*, 64, 140, 1975.
[3]Fusari, S. A.: Nitroglycerin Sublingual Tablets I: Stability of Conventional Tablets, *J. Pharm. Sci.*, 62, 122, 1973.

Implementation of these regulations contributed to the maintenance of better content uniformity standards for nitroglycerin tablets than had been achieved previously. However, since nitroglycerin is a volatile liquid at room temperature, some nitroglycerin is lost to the atmosphere when the containers are opened and particularly if they are not closed tightly. In a further effort to reduce the loss of nitroglycerin from tablets and to prevent the migration of the substance from tablet to tablet, pharmaceutical manufacturers of these tablets have recently been developing "stabilized" nitroglycerin tablets. The main method used is to include a small amount of a nonvolatile substance in the formulation which has the effect of reducing the vapor pressure of the nitroglycerin and thus its tendency to escape from the tablet. One such marketed product is *Nitrostat* by Parke-Davis which contains polyethylene glycol as the stabilizer.

Packaging and Storing Tablets

Tablets are best stored in tight containers and in places of low humidity protected from extremes in temperature. Tablets that are especially prone to decomposition by moisture may be copackaged with a desiccant. Tablets that are adversely affected by light are packaged in light-resistant containers. With a few exceptions, tablets that are properly stored will be stable for several years or more.

Official Tablets

There are almost four hundred tablets which are official in the USP and NF. Examples of these are presented in Table 6-4.

Other Solid Dosage Forms
for Oral Administration

Pills

Pills are small, round solid dosage forms containing a medicinal agent and intended to be administered orally. Although the manufacture and administration of pills was at one time quite prevalent, today pills have largely been replaced by compressed tablets and capsules. Pills may be prepared extemporaneously by the pharmacist

Table 6-4. EXAMPLES OF SOME OFFICIAL TABLETS

Official Tablet*	Some Representative Commercial Products**	Tablet Strengths Usually Available	Category and Comments
Acetaminophen	Tylenol (McNeil); Tempra (Mead Johnson)	120, 325 and 500 mg	Analgesic and anti-pyretic
Acetazolamide	Diamox (Lederle)	125 and 250 mg	Carbonic anhydrase inhibitor used in secretion control (diuretic)
Allopurinol	Zyloprim (Burroughs Wellcome)	100 and 300 mg	Xanthine-oxidase inhibitor used primarily in the treatment of gout
Dried Aluminum Hydroxide Gel	Amphojel (Wyeth)	300, 500, and 600 mg	Antacid
Aminophylline	—	100 and 200 mg	Smooth muscle relaxant; plain or enteric coated tablets
Amitriptyline HCl	Elavil HCl (Merck, Sharp & Dohme)	10, 25, and 50 mg	Antidepressant
Ascorbic Acid	Cevalin (Lilly)	50, 100, 250 and 500 mg	Antiscorbutic vitamin (vitamin C)
Aspirin	—	65, 81, 162, 325, 500 and 650 mg	Analgesic; some tablets enteric-coated, some chewable, some sustained release.
Atropine Sulfate	—	0.3, 0.4, and 0.6 mg	Anticholinergic; tablets usually compressed or molded tablet triturates.
Bisacodyl	Dulcolax (Geigy)	5 mg	Cathartic; enteric coated tablets.
Chlorambucil	Leukeran (Burroughs Wellcome)	2 mg	Antineoplastic
Chlorothiazide	Diuril (Merck Sharp & Dohme)	250 and 500 mg	Diuretic; antihypertensive
Chlorpheniramine Maleate	Chlor-Trimeton Maleate (Schering)	2, 4, 8, and 12 mg	Antihistaminic; some tablets sustained-release
Chlorpromazine Hydrochloride	Thorazine (Smith, Kline & French)	10, 25, 50, 100, and 200 mg	Tranquilizer
Chlorpropamide	Diabinese (Pfizer)	100 and 250 mg	Antidiabetic
Codeine Phosphate	—	15, 30, and 60 mg	Antitussive; narcotic analgesic
Colchicine	—	0.5 and 0.6 mg	Suppressant for gout
Cortisone Acetate	—	5, 10, and 25 mg	Adrenocortical steroid (anti-inflammatory)
Dexamethasone	Decadron (Merck Sharp & Dohme); Deronil (Schering)	0.25, 0.5, 0.75, 1.5 and 4.0 mg	Adrenocortical steroid (anti-inflammatory)
Dextroamphetamine Sulfate	Dexedrine Sulfate (Smith, Kline & French)	5 and 10 mg	Central stimulant

*Tablets presented are official in the USP XIX.

**The products listed are examples and not a complete listing; many of the tablets are available under their nonproprietary names. The word *Tablet* has been omitted for each product to conserve space.

Table 6-4. EXAMPLES OF SOME OFFICIAL TABLETS (*Cont.*)

Official Tablet*	Some Representative Commercial Products**	Tablet Strengths Usually Available	Category and Comments
Diazepam	Valium (Roche)	2, 5, and 10 mg	Tranquilizer (Minor)
Diethylstilbestrol	—	0.1, 0.25, 0.5, 1, 5, 25, 50 and 100 mg	Estrogen
Digitoxin	Crystodigin (Lilly); Purodigin (Wyeth)	0.05, 0.1, 0.15 and 0.2 mg	Cardiotonic
Digoxin	Lanoxin (Burroughs Wellcome)	0.25 and 0.5 mg	Cardiotonic
Dimenhydrinate	Dramamine (Searle)	50 mg	Antinauseant
Diphenoxylate HCl and Atropine Sulfate	Lomotil (Searle)	2.5 mg diphenoxylate and 25 mcg atropine sulfate	Antidiarrheal
Ephedrine Sulfate	—	25 and 30 mg	Sympathomimetic
Ergotamine Tartrate	Gynergen (Sandoz)	1 and 2 mg	Specific analgesic
Ethinyl Estradiol	Estinyl (Schering); Lynoral (Organon)	10, 20, 50 and 500 mg	Estrogen
Ferrous Sulfate	Feosol (Smith, Kline & French); Fero-Gradumet Filmtab (Abbott)	200 and 300 mg	Hematinic
Furosemide	Lasix (Hoescht)	20 and 40 mg	Diuretic
Griseofulvin	Fulvicin U/F (Schering); Grifulvin V (McNeil)	125, 250, and 500 mg	Antifungal. Official tablets are of microcrystalline griseofulvin.
Guanethidine Sulfate	Ismelin (Ciba)	10 and 25 mg	Antihypertensive
Hydrochlorothiazide	Esidrix (Ciba); Hydro-Diuril (Merck, Sharp & Dohme); Oretic (Abbott)	25 and 50 mg	Diuretic; antihypertensive
Imipramine Hydrochloride	Tofranil (Geigy)	10, 25, and 50 mg	Antidepressant
Isoniazid	Nydrazid (Squibb)	50, 100, and 300 mg	Antibacterial (tuberculostatic)
Isoproterenol Hydrochloride	Isuprel (Winthrop)	10 and 15 mg	Adrenergic (bronchodilator) sublingual tablets; disintegration time, 3 minutes
Levodopa	Dopar (Eaton); Larodopa (Roche)	100, 250, and 500 mg	Antiparkinsonian
Meclizine Hydrochloride	Bonine (Pfizer)	12.5 and 25 mg	Antinauseant. Commercial product is a chewable tablet.
Meperidine Hydrochloride	Demerol (Winthrop)	50 and 100 mg	Narcotic analgesic
Meprobamate	Equanil (Wyeth); Miltown (Wallace)	200, 400 and 600 mg	Sedative
Methotrexate	As methotrexate (Lederle)	2.5 mg	Antineoplastic
Methyldopa	Aldomet (Merck, Sharp & Dohme)	250 and 500 mg	Antihypertensive
Metronidazole	Flagyl (Searle)	250 mg	Antiamebic; Antitrichomonal
Methylphenidate Hydrochloride	Ritalin Hydrochloride (Ciba)	5, 10, and 20 mg	Central stimulant

Table 6-4. EXAMPLES OF SOME OFFICIAL TABLETS (*Cont.*)

Official Tablet*	Some Representative Commercial Products**	Tablet Strengths Usually Available	Category and Comments
Methyltestosterone	Metandren (Ciba); Oreton Methyl (Schering)	5, 10, and 25 mg	Androgen
Nitrofurantoin	Furadantin (Eaton)	50 and 100 mg	Antibacterial (Urinary)
Nitroglycerin	—	150, 300, 400 and 600 mg	Anti-anginal sublingual tablets (T.T.s); disintegration time, 2 min.; dispense in original glass container to retain potency.
Norgestryl and Ethinyl Estradiol	Estradiol Ovral (Wyeth)	Norgestryl: 500 μg; and Ethinyl estradiol: 50 μg	Oral contraceptive
Phenobarbital	Luminal (Winthrop)	15, 30, 60, and 100 mg	Hypnotic; sedative anticonvulsant
Phenylbutazone	Butazolidin (Geigy)	100 mg	Antiarthritic; anti-inflammatory
Piperazine Citrate	Antepar Citrate (Burroughs Wellcome)	500 mg	Anthelmintic
Potassium Penicillin G	Pentids (Squibb)	100,000, 250,000, 400,000, 500,000 and 800,000 units	Antibacterial
Penicillin V Potassium	Compocillin-VK Filmtabs (Abbott); Pen Vee K (Wyeth); V-Cillin K (Lilly)	125, 250, and 500 mg (200,000, 400,000 and 800,000 units)	Antibacterial
Potassium Permanganate	—	60, 120, and 300 mg	Local anti-infective (oxidant); to prepare external solutions
Prednisolone	Delta-Cortef (Upjohn)	1, 2.5, and 5 mg	Adrenocortical steroid (anti-inflammatory)
Prednisone	Delta-Dome (Dome); Deltasone (Upjohn); Meticorten (Schering)	1, 2.5, 5, 10, 20, and 25 mg	Adrenocortical steroid (anti-inflammatory)
Pyrvinium Pamoate	Povan (Parke, Davis)	50 mg	Anthelmintic (intestinal pinworms). Tablet is to be swallowed whole, without chewing.
Quinine Sulfate	—	120, 200, and 300 mg	Antimalarial
Reserpine	Rau-Sed (Squibb); Serpasil (Ciba)	0.1, 0.25, 0.5, 1, 2, 4, and 5 mg	Antihypertensive
Sodium Warfarin	Coumadin Sodium (Endo); Panwarfin (Abbott)	2, 2.5, 5, 7.5, 10, and 25 mg	Anticoagulant
Sulfisoxazole	Gantrisin (Roche)	500 mg	Antibacterial
Thyroid	—	15, 30, 60, 100, 125, 150, 200, 250, and 500 mg	Thyroid hormones
Tolbutamide	Orinase (Upjohn)	500 mg	Antidiabetic
Tripelennamine Hydrochloride	Pyribenzamine Hydrochloride (Ciba)	25 and 50 mg	Antihistaminic
Trisulfapyrimidines	Terfonyl (Squibb)	250 or 500 mg (83 or 167 mg ea. of sulfadiazine, sulfamerazine, and sulfamethazine)	Antibacterial

with simple pharmaceutical equipment, or they may be prepared on a large industrial scale with highly specialized pill-making equipment. Basically, pills are prepared by mixing the powdered drug substance with a powdered diluent to provide bulkiness and a liquid excipient, which alone or together with the powdered diluent provides cohesiveness of the powders. The plastic-like mass which results is then shaped by hand or by machine into the characteristic round pill. Typical powder diluents used are tragacanth and starch, and typical liquid excipients are liquid glucose, and acacia mucilage. Pills may be left uncoated or coated with a sugar or enteric coating as desired. A common procedure for the extemporaneous preparation of pills on a small-scale may be found in the previous edition of this text.

Official Pills

At the present time, there is only one official pill, Hexylresorcinol Pills, NF, which are prepared by a special patented process to enclose the medication in a gelatin coating that is sufficiently tough to resist breaking even by chewing.

Hexylresorcinol Pills, NF

Hexylresorcinol is a chemical agent that is extremely irritating to the respiratory tract and to the skin. For this reason the official pills, which are taken for the anthelmintic (intestinal roundworms and trematodes) effect of hexylresorcinol, are coated with a rupture-resistant coating that is dispersible in the digestive tract. The NF describes a test for the "rupture resistance" of the pills as well as a test for their disintegration. The latter test requires that the pills disintegrate in simulated gastric fluid according to the usual test procedure within a period of 4 hours.

Hexylresorcinol pills usually contain 100 and 200 mg of hexylresorcinol. The usual dose (adult) of hexylresorcinol is 1 g.

Lozenges

Lozenges are disk-shaped, solid dosage forms containing a medicinal agent and generally a flavoring substance and intended to be slowly dissolved in the oral cavity for localized effects. Lozenges are frequently called *troches* and less frequently referred to as *pastilles*. Many of the commercially available lozenges have a hard candy as the base or a base of sugar and an adhesive substance such as a mucilage or gum.

Commercially, lozenges may be made by compression, using a tablet machine and large, flat punches. The machine is operated at a high degree of compression to produce lozenges that are harder than ordinary tablets so that they slowly dissolve or disintegrate in the mouth. Medicinal substances that are heat stable may be prepared into a hard, sugar candy lozenge by candy-making machines that process a warm, highly concentrated, flavored syrup as the base and form the lozenges by molding and drying.

Official Lozenges

At present, there is only one official lozenge, Cetylpyridinium Chloride Lozenges, NF. Lozenges sold commercially under the name of Cepacol Throat Lozenges (Merrell-National) contain a 1:1500 concentration of cetylpyridinium chloride and 0.3% of benzyl alcohol, a local anesthetic, in a flavored hard candy base. Cetylpyridinium chloride is a quaternary ammonium compound which exerts surface activity against microorganisms. The lozenge is utilized primarily to stimulate salivation thereby providing soothing relief of dryness and minor irritation of the throat.

Solid Dosage Forms for Other than the Oral Route of Administration

There are a few solid dosage forms which are used by routes of administration other than oral. For instance, dosage forms called *pellets* or *inserts* are implanted under the skin by special injectors or by surgical incision for the purpose of providing for the continuous release of medication. Such implants provide the patient with an economical means of obtaining long-lasting effects (up to several months following implantation) and obviate the need for frequent injections or oral dosage administration. Hormonal substances are most frequently administered in this manner. Another solid dosage form called *vaginal tablets* or *inserts* are specially formulated and shaped tablets intended to be placed in the vagina by special inserters, where the medication is released, generally for localized effects. Still another example of a solid dosage form intended for use by means other than swallowing is a specially prepared capsule containing a micronized powder intended to be released from the capsule and inhaled deep into the lungs through the use of a special inhaler-device. These dosage forms will be discussed in subsequent chapters devoted to injections, vaginal preparations, and inhalations, respectively.

Selected Reading

Bakan, J. A. and Sloan, F. D.: Microencapsulation of Drugs. *Drug and Cosmetic Industry*, *110*:34, 1972.

Carver, L. D.: Particle Size Analysis. *Industrial Research*, 40–43, (Aug.) 1971.

Conine, J. W. and Hadley, H. R.: Preparation of Small Solid Pharmaceutical Spheres. *Drug & Cosmetic Industry*, *106*:38, 1970.

Cook, C. H., Jr., and Webber, M. G.: An Extemporaneous Method of Preparing Enteric Coated Capsules. *Amer. J. Hosp. Pharm.*, 22:95–99, 1965.

Daoust, R. G. and Lynch, M. J.: Mannitol in Chewable Tablets. *Drug and Cosmetic Industry*, 93:25, 1963.

Fusari, S. A.: Nitroglycerin Sublingual Tablets I: Stability of Conventional Tablets. *J. Pharm. Sci.*, 62:122–129, 1973.

Gross, H. M. and Endicott, C. J.: Transformation to Filmcoating. *Drug and Cosmetic Ind.*, 86:170, 1960.

Kahn, K. A. and Rhodes, C. T.: Water-Sorption Properties of Tablet Disintegrants. *J. Pharm. Sci.*, 64:447–451, 1975.

Lachman, L.: Physical and Chemical Stability Testing of Tablet Dosage Forms. *J. Pharm. Sci.*, 54:1519–1526, 1965.

Lazarus, J. and Cooper, J.: Absorption Testing and Clinical Evaluation of Oral Prolonged-Action Drugs. *J. Pharm. Sci.*, 50:715–732, 1961.

Lloyd, P. J., Yeung, P. C. M., and Freshwater, D. C.: The Mixing and Blending of Powders. *J. Soc. Cosmetic Chemists*, 21:205–220, 1970.

Lowenthal, W. and Wood, J. H.: Mechanism of Action of Starch as a Tablet Disintegrant VI. Location and Structure of Starch in Tablets. *J. Pharm. Sci.*, 62:287–293, 1973.

Luzzi, L.: Microencapsulation. *J. Pharm. Sci.*, 59:1367–1375, 1970.

Mendes, R. W.: Tablet Binders. *Drug and Cosmetic Industry*, *103*:46, 1968.

Milosovich, G.: Direct Compression of Tablets. *Drug and Cosmetic Industry*, 92:557, 1963.

Morrison, A. B. and Campbell, J. A.: Tablet Disintegration and Physiologic Availability of Drugs. *J. Pharm. Sci.*, 54:1–8, 1965.

Newton, J. M. and Rowley, G.: On the Release of Drugs from Hard Gelatin Capsules. *J. Pharm. Pharmacol*, 22:163S–168S, 1970.

Page, D. P., *et al.*: Stability Study of Nitroglycerin Sublingual Tablets. *J. Pharm. Sci.*, 64:140–147, 1975.

Paikoff, M. and Drumm, G.: Method for Evaluating Dissolution Characteristics of Capsules. *J. Pharm. Sci.*, 54:1693–1694, 1965.

Seidler, W. M. K. and Rowe, R. J.: Influence of Certain Factors on the Coating of a Medicinal Agent on Core Tablet. *J. Pharm. Sci.*, 57:1007–1010, 1968.

Shangraw, R. F.: Timed-Release Pharmaceuticals. *Hosp. Pharm.*, 2:No. 10, 19–27, 1967.

Shangraw, R. F. and Contractor, A. M.: New Developments in the Manufacture and Packaging of Nitroglycerin Tablets. *J. Am. Pharm. Assoc.*, *NS12*:633–636, 1972.

Sinotte, L. P.: Tableting Controls. *Drug and Cosmetic Industry*, *105*:47, 1969.

Srivastava, L. K. and Maney, P. V.: Development and Testing of Enteric Coatings. *Mfg. Chem. Aerosol News*, 36:55–58, 1965.

Stempel, E.: Patents for Prolonged Action Dosage Forms, Part I. *Drug Cosmetic Ind.*, *98*:No. 1, 44, 1966; Part II. *ibid.*, *98*:No. 2, 36, 1966.

Sutaria, R. H.: The Art and Science of Tablet Coating. *Manufacturing Chemist and Aerosol News*, 39:37–42, 1968.

Swintosky, J. V.: Design of Oral Sustained-Action Dosage Forms. *Drug Cosmetic Ind.*, 87:464, 1960.

Williams, J. C.: *Powder Technology*, 2:13–20, 1968.

Chapter 7

Tinctures, Fluidextracts, Extracts, and Other Pharmaceuticals Prepared by Extraction

CERTAIN PHARMACEUTICAL preparations are prepared by the process of *extraction*—that is, by the withdrawal of desired constituents from crude drugs through the use of selected solvents in which the desired constituents are soluble. Crude drugs may be defined as either vegetable or animal drugs that have undergone no other processes than collection and drying. Since each crude drug contains a number of constituents that may be soluble in a given solvent, the products of extraction, termed *extractives*, do not contain just a single constituent but rather varying numbers of constituents, depending upon the drug used and the conditions of the extraction. The general purpose of extraction as applied to the preparation of tinctures, fluidextracts, extracts, and other similar prepara-

tions is therefore not the separation and isolation of single pure plant or animal substances; it is the separation from the crude drug of all of its pharmacologically active constituents to make from them more concentrated and more palatable preparations in an effort to eliminate the need for taking bulky, distasteful crude drugs.

Today, as in the past, plants, rather than animals, represent the most used sources of crude drugs to be subjected to extractive procedures. In fact, no presently official tincture, fluidextract, or extract is prepared from an animal source. The most recently official animal preparation of this type was Cantharides Tincture, official in the NF X. It was prepared by extracting the dried insect, *Cantharis vesicatoria*, in a solvent mixture of glacial acetic acid and alcohol, the final product being used as an irritant and vesicant.

Both plant and animal tissues are composed of heterogeneous mixtures of constituents, some of which are pharmacologically active and therefore considered desirable and others that are pharmacologically inactive and considered inert. If an inert substance interferes with the stability of either the active constituent or of the final extractive or in some way makes the preparation discolored, unsightly, or unpalatable, steps would be taken either to prevent its extraction or to remove it from the extractive after its extraction. Among the varied plant constituents are sugars, starches, mucilages, proteins, albumins, pectins, cellulose, gums, inorganic salts, fixed and volatile oils, resins, tannins, coloring materials, and a number of very active constituents such as alkaloids and glycosides. Unfortunately, the solvents generally suitable for extraction dissolve not only the active components but some of the inactive ones as well. The solvent systems must be selected on the basis of their capacity to dissolve the maximum amount of active constituents and the minimum amount of those considered undesirable. A great deal of experimentation has been conducted to determine the most suitable solvents for use in each of the official products prepared by extraction, and the monographs for these products reflect the conclusions of the research by the solvents recommended.

Many vegetable drugs contain more than a single active constituent. Fortunately in many instances the active constituents of a plant drug are of the same general chemical type and have similar solubility characteristics and can be extracted simultaneously with a single solvent or a single solvent-mixture. And, since the active agents from a given plant generally provide the same type of pharmacologic effects, there is no need to isolate them, but rather it is desirable to extract them all, for in this way the extractive reflects most closely the total pharmacologic activity of the crude plant source. The process of extraction concentrates the active constituents of a crude drug and removes from it the extraneous matter. In drug extraction, the solvent or solvent-mixture is referred to as the *menstruum*, and the drug residue, which is exhausted of active constituents, is termed the *marc*.

Preparing the Crude Drug for Extraction

Most crude drugs are dried soon after collection to reduce any enzymatic activity that could result in the destruction of the active constituents, to prevent the growth of bacteria, mold, and yeasts, and to facilitate packaging, storage, and shipping of the bulky material. Before a plant drug is dried, the active constituents are generally present within the cells in aqueous solution or in colloidal suspension. After drying, the active constituents have been divested of their aqueous vehicle and occur within the dried cells as crystalline or amorphous substances. If the dried, intact drug were placed in an appropriate solvent, in time some of the active constituents would likely dissolve in the solvent, entering the cell by osmosis, and some small amount would likely be released to the extracellular solvent through broken tissues. However, the active constituents would be much more readily and completely extracted if the cell wall barriers were removed and the soluble constituents exposed to the bathing action of the menstruum. In the process of extraction, the dried crude drugs are generally ground or comminuted into a powder to break the majority of the cell walls. The powder must not be comminuted so fine as to allow it to compress too tightly during the extraction process and prevent total exposure to the menstruum. Experimentation with the individual drugs and with the solvents used to extract them has resulted in monographic requirements as to the proper powder size to be used during the process of extraction of a particular drug.

The Menstruum

The selection of the menstruum to use in the extraction of a crude drug is based primarily upon the relative solubility in it of the active constituents and the inactive and undesirable constituents and also upon the type of pharmaceutical product desired—for example, aqueous, hydroalcoholic, or alcoholic. Although water and alcohol and, to a lesser extent, glycerin are probably the most frequently employed solvents in drug extraction, acetic acid and organic solvents like ether may be used for special purposes.

Because of its ready availability, cheapness, and good solvent action for many plant constituents, water is considered to be a useful menstruum in drug extraction, particularly when used in combination with other solvents. However, as a sole solvent it has many disadvantages and is used alone only infrequently. For one thing, most active plant constituents are complex organic chemical compounds that are less soluble in water than in alcohol. Although water has a great solvent action on such plant constituents as sugars, gums, starches, coloring principles, and tannins, most of these are not particularly desirable components of an extracted preparation. Water also tends to extract plant principles which upon standing in the extractive later separate leaving an undesired residue. Finally, unless preserved, aqueous preparations serve as excellent growth media for molds, yeasts, and bacteria. When water alone is employed as the menstruum, alcohol is frequently added to the extractive or to the final preparation as an antimicrobial preservative. To counteract certain of its shortcomings as a menstruum, other solvents are frequently added to water to increase its utility. Acidified water, by making water-soluble salts of alkaloidal bases, is useful in increasing the aqueous extraction of these important and highly potent active constituents. Occasionally an alkalinized aqueous menstruum may be required to extract a substance from a crude drug. Hydroalcoholic mixtures are perhaps the most versatile and most widely employed menstruums. They combine the solvent effects of both water and alcohol, and the complete miscibility of these two agents permits a flexible combining of the two agents to form solvent mixtures most suited to the extraction of the active principles from a particular drug. A hydroalcoholic menstruum generally provides inherent protection against microbial contamination and helps to prevent the separation of extracted material on standing. Alcohol is used alone as a menstruum only when necessary because it is more expensive than hydroalcoholic mixtures.

Glycerin, a good solvent for many plant substances, is occasionally employed as a cosolvent with water or alcoholic menstruums because of its ability to dissolve, help extract, and then prevent the precipitation of inert material from the extractive upon standing. It is especially useful in this regard in preventing the separation of tannin and tannin oxidation products in extractives. Also, since glycerin has preservative action, depending upon its concentration in the final product, it may contribute to the stability of a pharmaceutical extractive. Being nonvolatile, glycerin used during extraction remains in the final extractive and should not be used in instances in which this may be undesirable.

Other solvents may be employed in drug extraction as may be required to prepare a potent and therapeutically efficacious extractive. Frequently an organic solvent such as ether or chloroform may be employed as the menstruum in a preliminary extraction of a crude drug to remove fats and waxy coats on the tissues in order to facilitate a subsequent extraction with an aqueous or other menstruum.

Methods of Extraction

The principal methods of drug extraction are (1) maceration, (2) percolation, (3) digestion, (4) infusion, and (5) decoction. Of the five methods, the first two are the most important in contemporary pharmacy. For a given crude drug, the most efficient method of extraction is established primarily by experimentation. Generally speaking, the method of extraction finally selected for a given drug depends on several factors: (a) the nature of the crude drug and its adaptability to each of the various extraction methods, (b) the interest of the pharmacist in obtaining complete or near-complete extraction of the drug, and (c) the skill of the operator and the relative importance of his time and the cost of the operation compared with the value of obtaining drug exhaustion. The nature of the crude drug is a primary factor to be considered in selecting the method of extraction. Certain

drugs simply do not lend themselves to the process of percolation, which demands that they be capable of being ground to a uniform powder and packed firmly and evenly, but not too compactly, in the percolation apparatus. Other drugs, although packable in a percolator, may yield their active constituents so readily to a solvent that they simply need to be soaked in it to provide a satisfactory extractive. They may be extracted by maceration rather than by percolation. Generally speaking, the process of percolation requires a greater skill on the part of the operator than does maceration, and of the two processes, percolation is perhaps more expensive to conduct, since it requires specialized equipment and a great deal of the operator's time.

Most frequently a combination of maceration and percolation is actually employed in the extraction of a crude drug. The drug is macerated first to soften the plant tissues and to dissolve much of the active constituents, and the percolation process is then conducted to achieve the separation of the extractive from the marc.

Maceration

The term "maceration" comes from the Latin *macerare*, meaning "to soak." It is a process in which the properly comminuted drug is permitted to soak in the menstruum until the cellular structure is softened and penetrated by the menstruum and the soluble constituents are dissolved.

In the maceration process, the drug to be extracted is generally placed in a wide-mouth bottle or jar with the prescribed menstruum, the vessel is stoppered tightly, and the contents are agitated repeatedly over a period usually ranging from 2 to 14 days. The agitation permits the repeated flow of fresh solvent over the entire surface area of the comminuted drug. An alternative to this repeated shaking is to place the drug in a porous cloth bag that is tied and suspended in the upper portion of the menstruum, much the same as a tea bag is suspended in water in the preparation of a cup of tea. As the soluble constituents dissolve in the menstruum, they tend to settle to the bottom because of an increase in the specific gravity of the liquid due to its added weight. Fresh menstruum then comes to the top and the process continues in a cyclic manner. Occasional dipping of the drug bag may facilitate the speed of the extraction. The extractive is separated from the marc by expressing the bag of drug and washing it with additional fresh menstruum, the washings being added to the extractive. If the maceration is performed with an unbagged drug, the marc may be removed by straining and/or filtration, with the marc being washed free of extractive by the additional passage of menstruum through the strainer or filter into the total extractive.

One maceration of a given drug does not usually result in the total extraction of the soluble constituents because a portion of these constituents invariably remains in the liquid with the marc, even after attempts at expression. Repeated macerations with fresh menstruum can produce total extraction and separation; however, this is time consuming and expensive in terms of time and solvent, especially if alcohol is employed in the extractions. In most instances, the official preparations prepared by extraction employ the more efficient method of percolation whenever total extraction is desired. However, for drugs containing little or no cellular material, such as benzoin, aloe, tolu, and styrax, which dissolve almost completely in the menstruum, maceration is the method of choice, since percolation is neither suitable nor necessary to extract these drugs. Presently there are four official tinctures for which the prescribed method of extraction is maceration, officially called "Process M." They are Compound Benzoin, Sweet Orange Peel, Compound Cardamom, and Tolu Balsam tinctures. In addition, the preparation of many other tinctures and fluidextracts that are extracted by percolation also utilize a preliminary maceration period within the percolation apparatus to soak the drug free of the active constituents.

Maceration is most usually conducted at a temperature of between 15° to 20° and, according to the USP for a period of "3 days or until the soluble matter is dissolved."

Percolation

The term *percolation*, from the Latin *per*, meaning "through," and *colare*, meaning "to strain," may be described generally as a process in which a comminuted drug is extracted of its soluble constituents by the slow passage of a suitable solvent through a column of the drug. The drug is packed in a special extraction apparatus termed a *percolator*, with the extractive

collected called the *percolate*. Most drug extractions are performed by percolation.

In the process of percolation the flow of the menstruum over the drug column is generally downward to the exit orifice, impelled by the force of gravity as well as the weight of the column of liquid. In certain specialized and more sophisticated percolation apparatus, additional pressure on the column is exerted with positive air pressure at the inlet and suction at the outlet or exit. Other equipment utilizes continuous columns of drug so that pressures alternately force the menstruum downward in one drug column and upward in the next, the process being repeated for as long as the series of columns is arranged. However, the usual percolation apparatus, particularly that utilized for small-scale extractions, permits the normal downward flow of menstruum through a single drug column, unassisted by added air pressure or by suction.

Percolators for drug extraction vary greatly as to their shape, capacities, composition, and, most important, their utility. Percolators employed in the large-scale industrial preparation of extractives are generally made of stainless steel or are glass-lined large metal vessels that vary greatly in size and in operation. Percolators used to extract leaves, for instance, may be 6 to 8 feet in diameter and 12 to 18 feet high (Fig. 7-1). Percolators employed to extract other vegetable parts like seeds that are greater in density than leaves and would pack too tightly in percolators of such large dimensions are extracted in much smaller percolators. Some special industrial percolators are designed to percolate with hot menstruums; in others pressure is utilized to force the menstruum through the drug columns.

Percolation on a small scale generally involves the use of glass percolators of various shapes for extraction of small amounts (perhaps up to 1000 g) of crude drug. If percolation with a hot menstruum is desirable, metallic percolators (copper or copper lined with tin) are required. The shape of percolators in common laboratory and small-scale use are generally (a) cylindrical, with little if any taper except for the lower orifice; (b) cylindrical-like, but with a definite taper downward; and (c) conical, or funnel-shaped (Fig. 7-2). Each type has a special utility in drug extraction.

The cylindrical percolator, if narrow and elongated rather than stubby, is particularly

cle is more repeatedly exposed to passing solvent. The menstruum, which makes contact with drug over a long flow-pattern becomes highly concentrated in solute, and if the rate of flow of percolate is adjusted to slower than usual, the menstruum just entering the column remains highly efficient in solubilizing and retaining the soluble constituents. The percolate collected is therefore richer in active constituents than would be a percolate collected after having made a more rapid pass over a shorter column of drug. This is an important aspect in the preparation of fluidextracts, which are highly concentrated by definition,[1] and are best

[1] Fluidextracts are liquid preparations of which each ml contains the therapeutic constituents of 1 g of the standard drug which it represents.

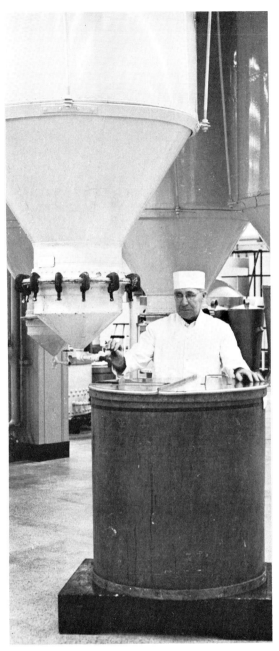

Fig. 7-1. *Large industrial percolators used in extracting crude drugs to make fluidextracts, tinctures, and powdered extracts. (Courtesy of the Upjohn Company)*

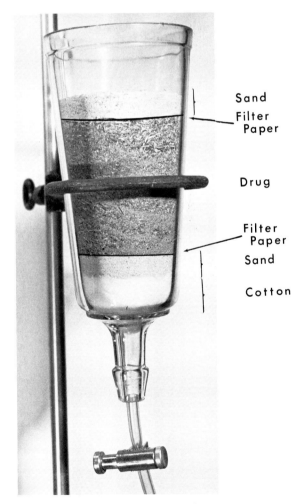

Sand
Filter Paper

Drug

Filter Paper
Sand

Cotton

Fig. 7-2. *A packed laboratory percolator.*

suited to the complete extraction of drugs with a minimal expenditure of menstruum. By the passage of the menstruum over the drug contained in a high, narrow column (rather than in a lower, wider column obtained if a different-shaped percolator were used), each drug parti-

prepared with a minimal amount of menstruum, since any extra menstruum must ultimately be removed from the final preparation, generally by evaporation. However, when the nature of the soluble substances is such that their extraction and retention in the menstruum of a drug column produce a viscosity that hinders the movement of the liquid in the column, a wider column of drug would be preferred, and a wider percolator and perhaps a faster collection rate of percolate would be desired. In preparing tinctures by extraction, a wider cylindrical or a tapered percolator would do nicely, since both the volume of percolate collected in preparing a tincture and the quantity of menstruum to be used is greatly in excess of that generally required to exhaust the drug. A funnel-shaped percolator is probably used least frequently. It is useful for the percolation of drugs that swell a great deal during the maceration process, since the large upper surface permits the expansion of the drug column with little risk of a too tightly packed column or breakage of a glass percolator.

The drug and the type of product being prepared both greatly influence the type of percolator to employ. As a general rule, the size (not shape) of the percolator should be selected on the basis of the quantity of drug to be extracted, with the rule of thumb being that about two thirds of the percolator should be filled after proper drug packing. The remaining space is required for a column head of menstruum to prevent the drying out of the column (which could cause the formation of channels in the drug column) and to provide pressure to force the menstruum through the drug column.

Whichever percolator is selected, the process involves the same general principles. The passage of the solvent through the drug column exercises its solvent power on successive layers or portions of drug, taking with it as it moves downward an ever increasing concentration of dissolved solute. Each successive portion of menstruum passing over a drug particle continues the extraction process and replaces any menstruum that may have entered the cellular structures or may have adhered to the drug particle. As this process continues, there is less and less solute remaining to be dissolved, and each successive portion of percolate collected is less and less concentrated with solute. This process is commonly observed in the different intensities of color seen in each of the consecutively collected portions of percolate due to a large initial extraction of the plant's soluble coloring principles followed by progressively diminished amounts.

Several distinct operations are required in the extraction of drugs by percolation:

1. Preparation of the dried crude drug for percolation
   a. Powdering
   b. Moistening
2. Packing the percolator
3. Period of maceration
4. Percolation and collection of percolate
5. Adjustment of concentration of percolate as required.

Preparation of the Dried Crude Drug for Percolation

As indicated earlier, the crude vegetable drug, freed of all extraneous matter, is dried after collection and properly stored so that its potency remains at a high level. Before percolation, the drug must be subdivided into small particles so that a large surface area of the cellular parts is created for maximum exposure to the solvent action of the menstruum. Many factors contribute to the degree of comminution desired in preparing a crude drug for percolation. These factors include such things as the adaptability of the drug's various potential powder sizes to packing in a percolator, the ease of solubility of the desired plant constituents in the selected menstruum, the amount of time one is willing to expend in order to exhaust the drug of active constituents, and the desired relationship between the amount of menstruum to be used and the amount of drug to be extracted. Naturally, if the desired constituent is very readily soluble in the menstruum, a coarse powder will suffice in contrast to a fine powder that may be required of drugs in which the active constituents are more tenaciously held by the nonsoluble plant parts. If there is a limitation on the volume of menstruum (as in the preparation of a fluidextract), a fine powder, which will be apt to release the constituents more readily than a coarse powder of the same drug, will conserve the menstruum. The same general rule applies to the conservation of the operator's time. The disadvantage to fine powders is their capability of packing too tightly, which may result in delayed passage of the menstruum through the drug column, and may in some cases prevent percolation altogether by plugging the column. Uniformity of powder size is of the utmost importance, as an uneven powder size would result in uneven packing of the percolator and an irregular passage of menstruum through the column. Generally, a drug to be extracted with an alcoholic menstruum needs to be powdered finer than if water were used because alcohol tends to harden plant tissues, making them less responsive to solvent-penetration than does water, which actually softens tissues and renders them more easily penetrable.

After reducing the crude drug to a powder of the proper size, the material is moistened with a portion of the intended menstruum. This is generally done in a beaker, dish, or other large container that permits the drug to absorb the liquid and swell. The swelling obtained outside of the percolator averts the plugging and column distortion that might result if the drug were packed dry and moistened within the percolator.

The amount of menstruum used to moisten the drug should be adequate to encourage total swelling of the powdered drug but not an amount that will yield extractive into the beaker or mixing dish. The menstruum should be added to the powdered drug in small portions, blending the two components thoroughly after each addition. The mixing may be done entirely in the mixing vessel with a stirring rod, or it may be performed by rubbing the moistened drug between the hands. Whatever the method, the drug should be made uniformly damp but not wet. The amount of menstruum required to accomplish this varies greatly, depending upon the nature of the drug, the fineness of the powder, and the type of menstruum. For many powdered drugs, a half milliliter of menstruum for each gram of drug accomplishes the purpose, but there is no hard and fast rule for this task. It is part of the art of pharmacy to determine the proper degree of moistness for each drug and for each percolation on an individual basis. After the drug has been moistened, a 15-minute period is generally sufficient to allow maximum swelling. After swelling, the moistened drug may be packed in the percolator.

Packing the Percolator

Proper packing of the percolator is extremely important. If it is packed unevenly with some places tighter than others or with empty spaces or channels, the menstruum in its downward course will seek the route of least resistance, and the extraction will not be as efficient as it should. The first step in packing a percolator is to open the lower orifice (usually by adjusting the glass stopcock or clamp on rubber tubing) so that the air in the column will have an exit and will not remain entrapped in the column to disrupt the wetting of the drug during the maceration period or the percolation process later. During percolation, entrapped air, which would have a tendency to rise to the top of the column, could disrupt the uniformity of the drug column and result in channeling. For small scale percolation, a pledget of cotton large enough to cover the orifice is inserted into the base of the percolator. It must be packed loosely enough to allow the percolate to pass freely and firm enough to prevent crude drug particles from reaching the orifice. Its purpose is primarily to prevent clogging of the orifice and to filter off any solid particles that may be flowing with the menstruum. Care must be exercised not to pack the cotton too tightly so that it becomes an impregnable plug that hinders the flow and collection of the percolate. Generally, the cotton is held in place by a thin layer of washed sand, which acts as a filter and as a leveling layer upon which the drug column may be firmly and uniformly packed. The moistened drug is placed in the percolator in portions, each portion being positioned, leveled, and firmly pressed down by a device such as a cylindrical plug of wood or a cork attached to a stirring rod. Each successive layer of drug must be carefully packed to avoid interspaces between the layers. These are usually prevented by packing the layers successively harder. After all of the drug has been packed, the column should be inspected to detect any sign of unevenness. The uniform column is held in place by a filter paper shaped to the dimension of the inner circumference of the percolator, and on top of that is a layer of sand, washed pebbles, or a porous glass or porcelain plate. This prevents disturbance of the drug column as the menstruum is poured on top of the column to initiate the period of maceration within the percolator.

With the lower orifice still open, menstruum is slowly added to the top of the percolator. As the menstruum descends, the operator can follow its flow (if a glass percolator is used) and notice the evenness and rate of the descent. If the column was packed properly, the menstruum descends the column slowly and evenly. The addition of menstruum is continued until the first portion reaches the cotton and a few drops of percolate reach the lower orifice. At that point the orifice is closed, and sufficient menstruum is added to the percolator to provide a definite layer above the surface of the column. The drug is then permitted to macerate.

Period of Maceration

The length of the period of maceration varies with the individual character of the drug-menstruum mixture. The period should be sufficient to permit the menstruum to enter all of the crevices of the drug structures and dissolve much of the soluble constituents. Naturally the greater the length of exposure, the greater the chance of complete extraction. However, an optimum time must be determined for each drug-menstruum combination to avoid premature percolation or unnecessary waste of time waiting for the soluble constituents to be dissolved in the menstruum. The maceration period may require several hours or several days for optimum extraction.

Care must be observed during the period of maceration to make certain that a layer of menstruum remains above the drug column and any portion lost through evaporation is replaced with a fresh portion. This precaution is particularly applicable to a volatile menstruum and to procedures requiring an unusually lengthy period of maceration. The constant presence of the menstruum above the drug column is necessary to prevent the drug from becoming dry and disrupted. A cover may be placed atop the percolator to prevent the evaporation of menstruum during the maceration period.

Percolation and Collection of Percolate

After the proper maceration period, the lower orifice is opened, and percolate is collected at the prescribed rate while maintaining the layer of fresh solvent above the drug column. The speed of the percolation flow is important if thorough and efficient extraction is to be achieved. If the rate is too rapid, the fresh solvent entering the drug column may not be given adequate opportunity to extract the soluble constituents of the drug particles it contacts. If the rate is too slow, efficiency will be lost; if the solute-solvent extraction ratio is high, the extractive may become too viscous to pass easily through the cotton pledget at the orifice. The

rates of flow are indicated in the monographs for each of the official preparations prepared by percolation, and they are described as follows for the extraction of 1000 g of drug:

> "percolate slowly"—a rate not exceeding 1 ml of percolate per minute
> "percolate at a moderate rate"—rate of 1 to 3 ml per minute
> "percolate rapidly"—rate of 3 to 5 ml per minute.

The rates of flow may be increased for larger amounts of drugs and decreased for smaller amounts to achieve comparable efficiency.

Most commonly, one menstruum is employed for the moistening, maceration, and percolation of a drug. However, in certain instances one menstruum may be employed during one stage of the process and another during another stage for the purpose of increasing the yield or the ease of the extraction.

Adjustment of Concentration of Percolate

The percolation is generally continued until the desired volume of product has been collected or until the drug is shown by the appropriate test to be exhausted of the desired constituents. These tests may involve such things as the absence of color in the last portion of collected percolate, the absence of a bitter taste, or the absence of alkaloids as determined qualitatively with an alkaloidal reagent, the tests depending upon the nature of the constituent being extracted.

For some extractives, particularly those obtained from potent drugs, an assay of the potency of the near-final product is undertaken for the purpose of adjusting the final strength of the extractive. As is required, either additional menstruum is added to dilute the extractive or solvent is removed (usually by evaporation) to concentrate the extractive to meet the desired potency.

Decoction, Infusion, and Digestion

Although decoction, digestion, and infusion are not prescribed methods of extraction for any preparations presently official, they are each employed on occasion in the chemical and pharmaceutical industries.

Decoction

Decoction is a process of boiling vegetable substances with water to extract the soluble principles. Generally an amount of cold water equal to the intended volume of the finished product is added to a drug in a suitable vessel, and the mixture is stirred and then boiled for approximately 15 minutes. After cooling, the marc is expressed of liquid extractive and the latter is strained if necessary and made to volume with additional water.

Obviously, the process may be employed only in instances in which the desired constituents are both water soluble and heat stable. Since sugars and albuminous and mucilaginous matter are usually coextracted with the desired constituents, decoctions do not keep well and tend to support the growth of microorganisms. Therefore, only freshly prepared decoctions must be used.

Infusion

Infusion is a process in which vegetable drugs, generally coarsely comminuted, are extracted of their water-soluble constituents by steeping or drenching them in water, the resulting products being termed *infusions*. Generally infusions are prepared by first macerating the drug with cold water for a period of about 15 minutes. An amount of water equal to the weight of the drug may be used. This is followed by the addition of boiling water, in an amount equal to about 90% of the intended volume of the finished infusion, and the vessel is covered tightly. The mixture is permitted to remain in this condition until cool, usually about 30 minutes, after which time it is strained, and sufficient water is added through the strainer to make the product to the desired volume. Infusions are subject to the same instabilities as decoctions and thus must also be freshly prepared upon request. The drugs best suited to the process of infusion are those that are light in structure rather than dense and those in which the desired constituents are easily water soluble. The drugs are coarsely ground, since finely powdered drugs would not permit the ease of separation of the marc by straining.

Digestion

Digestion is a form of maceration in which gentle heat is applied to the drug-menstruum mixture and maintained throughout the extraction to increase the solvent powers of the menstruum. It differs from the processes of decoction and infusion in that the period of maceration is extended and the temperature maintained is lower, usually between 40 and 60°. If the menstruum is volatile at the temperatures used, it is generally recovered through the use of a reflux condenser affixed to the digestion vessel. Naturally, the drug must be stable at the temperatures employed for the process to be effectively conducted.

Tinctures

Tinctures are defined by the USP as "alcoholic or hydroalcoholic solutions prepared from vegetable materials or from chemical substances."

The official tinctures vary widely in their method of preparation, the strength of their active ingredient, their alcoholic content, and their intended use in medicine or pharmacy. When they are prepared from chemical substances (e.g., iodine, nitromersol, etc.) tinctures are prepared by simple solution of the chemical agent in the solvent and their concentrations vary widely depending upon the optimum concentration determined for the particular chemical agent with regard to its therapeutic application. When tinctures are prepared from crude vegetable drugs, they are termed "compound" if they are prepared by extracting more than a single drug (e.g., compound cardamom tincture, which contains the extractive from cardamom seed, cinnamon powder, and caraway powder). There is no set strength for compound tinctures; they vary with the particular preparation. However, for tinctures prepared from single vegetable drugs (e.g., belladonna tincture), the amounts of crude drug used to prepare each 100 ml of tincture is generally as follows:

> Potent drug (e.g., Belladonna Leaf), 10 g
> Nonpotent drug (e.g., Tolu Balsam), 20 g
> Undried fresh fruit peel (e.g., Sweet Orange Peel), 50 g

Depending upon the amount of soluble active constituents in a given drug, the actual concentration of active constituents will vary between tinctures prepared from different drugs, even though the amount of starting material may have been the same.

The variation in the concentration of active

constituents present in the official tinctures may be demonstrated by pointing out that Belladonna Tincture, USP, which is prepared by percolating belladonna leaf, contains between 0.027 and 0.033% of active constituents (the alkaloids of the leaf) in contrast to Tolu Balsam Tincture, NF, which contains in each 100 ml nearly all of the 20 g of solid starting material exposed to alcohol in the process of maceration.

Tinctures generally are considered to be stable preparations. The extremes of alcohol content among the official tinctures are Green Soap Tincture, NF, with between 28 and 32% alcohol and Tolu Balsam Tincture, NF, with between 77 and 83% alcohol. The high alcoholic content protects against microbial growth, and unless some of the alcoholic solvent is lost through evaporation permitted by an untight closure, the solvent system is generally sufficient to maintain the solution of the dissolved solute.

The specified alcoholic content present in the various tinctures is generally fairly critical in maintaining the integrity of the solution. Similarly, a hydroalcoholic tincture has the desired balance of alcohol and water to effect and maintain the solution of the desired solute. Thus, tinctures cannot generally be mixed successfully with liquids too diverse in solvent character without the likelihood of either increasing the instability of the product or actually inducing the precipitation of the solute. For example, tolu balsam tincture, prepared with alcohol as the sole menstruum, has dissolved in it alcohol-soluble principles that are immediately expelled from solution upon the addition of water.

Because of the alcoholic content of tinctures and its essential presence in the original proportion, tinctures must be tightly stoppered and not exposed to excessive temperatures. Also, because many of the constituents found in tinctures undergo a photochemical change upon exposure to light, many tinctures must be stored in light-resistant containers and protected from sunlight.

The Preparation
of Tinctures by
Maceration

Most drugs prepared into tinctures by maceration either contain a large proportion of soluble constituents or are incapable of being packed uniformly in a percolator and are thus not suited to the percolation process.

According to the USP and the NF, a general method of maceration may be employed when the official monograph presents no specific method for preparing a tincture by maceration. The general method recommended is essentially the same in the two compendia and is designated as "Process M," for maceration. The method of the USP, which is applicable for the preparation of 1000 ml of tincture, is as follows:

> Process M—Macerate the drug with 750 ml of the prescribed solvent or solvent mixture in a container that can be closed, and put in a warm place. Agitate it frequently during 3 days or until the soluble matter is dissolved. Transfer the mixture to a filter, and when most of the liquid has drained away, wash the residue on the filter with a sufficient quantity of the prescribed solvent or solvent mixture, combining the filtrates, to produce 1000 ml of tincture, and mix.

Tinctures prepared by maceration are identified in Table 7-1.

Tinctures prepared by solution generally have as their main ingredient agents as iodine, nitromersol, and thimerosol, as indicated in Table 7-1. The preparation of tinctures by solution involves the dissolution of the chemical agent in the solvents employed, generally varying proportions of alcohol and water. Occasionally some solubilizing agent is added to enhance or facilitate the dissolution process. Some tinctures, as paregoric, are combinations of vegetable extractive (opium extractive in the case of paregoric) with additional agents added, and thus are prepared by a combination of methods as percolation and solution.

Official Tinctures

As shown in Table 7-1, there are very few official tinctures compared with other dosage forms. For the purpose of this discussion, they may be conveniently separated into those which are medicated and taken orally, those which are nonmedicated and used as pharmaceutic aids in flavoring other preparations, and those which are employed topically.

Table 7-1. OFFICIAL TINCTURES AND FLUIDEXTRACTS

Preparation	Method of Preparation	Use and Comments
Tinctures		
Belladonna Tincture, USP	Percolation	Anticholinergic with a usual oral dose of 0.6 to 1 ml three or four times a day. See text for additional discussion.
Paregoric, USP (Camphorated Opium Tincture)	Maceration/Solution	Antiperistaltic with a usual dose of 5 to 10 ml one to four times a day. See text for additional discussion.
Compound Benzoin Tincture, USP	Maceration	Topical protectant. See text and Chapter 10 for additional discussion.
Green Soap Tincture, NF	Solution	Topical detergent. See Chapter 10 for additional discussion.
Benzethonium Chloride Tincture, USP	Solution	
Iodine Tincture, USP	Solution	
Nitromersol Tincture, NF [Metaphen Tincture (Abbott)]	Solution	Topical anti-infectives. See Chapter 10 for additional discussion.
Thimerosal Tincture, NF [Merthiolate Tincture (Lilly)]	Solution	
Compound Cardamom Tincture, NF	Maceration	
Sweet Orange Peel Tincture, NF	Maceration	Flavoring tinctures. See text for additional discussion.
Tolu Balsam Tincture, NF	Maceration	
Vanilla Tincture, NF	Maceration/Percolation	
Fluidextracts		
Aromatic Cascara Fluidextract, USP	Maceration/Percolation	Cathartic with a usual dose of 5 ml. See text for additional discussion.
Cascara Sagrada Fluidextract, NF	Process D percolation	Cathartic with a usual dose of 1 ml. See text for additional discussion.
Senna Fluidextract, NF	Process A percolation	Cathartic with a usual dose of 2 ml. See text for additional discussion.
Eriodictyon Fluidextract, NF	Process A percolation	Flavoring fluidextracts. See text for additional discussion.
Glycyrrhiza Fluidextract, NF	Percolation	

Medicated Tinctures Taken Orally

Medicated tinctures taken orally are becoming a thing of the past. For one thing, they are bad-tasting. A person requiring oral medication nowadays would prefer to take a tablet or capsule or a pleasant tasting elixir or syrup. Secondly, physicians prefer to prescribe single drugs and not preparations of plant extractives which contain many plant constituents, both active and inactive. Thirdly, since tinctures generally have a rather high alcoholic content, many physicians and patients alike prefer other forms of medication.

The only presently official medicated tinctures which are employed orally are Belladonna Tincture, USP and Paregoric, USP formerly official as Camphorated Opium Tincture. Some aspects of these two preparations are presented below.

Belladonna Tincture, USP

Belladonna tincture is prepared by percolation, as modified for assayed tinctures, using 10 g of belladonna leaf for each 100 ml of tincture and a mixture of 3 volumes of alcohol and 1 volume of water as the menstruum. The extractive is adjusted to contain for each 100 ml, 30 mg of the alkaloids of belladonna leaf, the principal alkaloid being atropine. The highly alcoholic menstruum is effective in extracting both the alkaloids of belladonna and chlorophyll, thereby producing an attractive green product. Prior to the USP XI, the menstruum employed was half alcohol and half water, which was effective in extracting the alkaloids but resulted in a displeasing brown-green tincture because of excessive extraction of water-soluble brown coloring matter. The disadvantage of the present tincture is that the high alcoholic content occasionally results in the separation of some alcohol-soluble resinous material from the tincture when it is mixed with a preparation having a low alcoholic content.

The tincture is employed as an anticholinergic primarily to overcome intestinal spasm and to check secretions. The usual dose is 0.6 ml, three times a day, generally diluted with water. Because of the small dose, the tincture is generally dispensed to the patient by the pharmacist in a dropper bottle calibrated to deliver the dose by either a specified number of drops or by a marked level on the dropper itself. The tincture is preserved in tight, light-resistant containers and is maintained away from excessive heat and direct sunlight.

Paregoric, USP

Paregoric is made by macerating powdered opium, anise oil, benzoic acid, and camphor in diluted alcohol containing a small volume of glycerin. During the maceration period of 5 days, the mixture is occasionally agitated to ensure total extraction of the alkaloids of opium and the solution of the other agents. After maceration, the mixture is filtered, a portion of diluted alcohol is passed through the filter, and the filtrate is assayed for the morphine content. The filtrate is then adjusted so that it contains 0.04% of anhydrous morphine (40 mg per 100 ml), about 0.4% each of anise oil, camphor, and benzoic acid, 4% of glycerin, and about 45% alcohol.

Paregoric is officially categorized as an antiperistaltic and as such is commonly used to relieve the peristalsis accompanying diarrhea. It is also frequently used as an antitussive and as an anodyne to relieve menstrual cramps and abdominal pain. The usual dose is 5 ml, one to four times a day. It is a narcotic preparation and is subject to the laws governing narcotics under federal and state requirements. It is best stored in tight, light-resistant containers away from direct sunlight and excessive heat.

The Preparation of Tinctures by Percolation

Tinctures prepared by percolation may be prepared by the general method of percolation, termed "Process P," in the official compendia, unless otherwise indicated in the individual monograph. The general methods presented in the NF and the USP are essentially the same, and the USP method is as follows:

Process P—Carefully mix the ground drug or mixture of drugs with a sufficient quantity of the prescribed solvent or solvent mixture to render it evenly and distinctly damp, allow it to stand for 15 minutes, transfer it to a suitable percolator, and pack the drug firmly. Pour on enough of the prescribed solvent or solvent mixture to saturate the drug, cover the top of the percolator, and when the liquid is about to drip from the percolator, close the lower orifice and allow the drug to macerate for 24 hours or for the time specified in the monograph. If no assay is directed, allow the percolation to proceed slowly, or at the specified rate, gradually adding sufficient solvent or solvent mixture to produce 1000 ml of tincture, and mix. If an assay is directed, collect only 950 ml of percolate, mix this, and assay a portion of it as directed. Dilute the remainder with such quantity of the prescribed solvent or solvent mixture as calculation from the assay indicates is necessary to produce a tincture that conforms to the prescribed standard, and mix.

Tinctures prepared by percolation are identified in Table 7-1.

The Preparation of Tinctures by Solution

Flavoring Tinctures

The four flavoring tinctures presented in Table 7-1 are employed pharmaceutically in the flavoring of other types of preparations, generally syrups. Each of these tinctures has an alcoholic concentration above 40% to maintain the flavoring principles in solution. Occasionally the addition of these tinctures to an aqueous preparation will result in the separation of some of the principles from solution, and filtration is necessary to remove the separated portion.

Tinctures Employed Topically

The tinctures employed topically are presented in Table 7-1, and with the exception of Compound Benzoin Tincture, USP, are prepared by solution. The majority of these tinctures are applied to the skin for the anti-infective activity of their main chemical component. Since all of these tinctures contain greater than 45% alcohol, they sting when placed on the broken skin. Many of the agents represented in these tinctures, as iodine, nitromersol, and thimerosol, are also available in aqueous solution and may be preferred to the tincture. However, the tinctures because of their alcoholic content can provide additional antisepsis effect. Further discussion of dermatologic preparations will be presented in Chapter 10.

Fluidextracts

Fluidextracts are defined by the USP and the NF as "liquid preparations of vegetable drugs, containing alcohol as a solvent or as a preservative, or both, and so made that each ml contains the therapeutic constituents of 1 g of the standard drug that it represents." Because they contain alcohol and are highly concentrated, fluidextracts are sometimes referred to as "100% tinctures." Fluidextracts of potent drugs are ten times as concentrated or potent as the corresponding tincture. For example, although 100 g of belladonna leaf are extracted to prepare each 1000 ml of belladonna tincture, the preparation of each 1000 ml of belladonna fluidextract would require the extraction of 1000 g of belladonna leaf. The usual dose of the tincture is 0.6 ml; the dose of the ten times more potent fluidextract would be one-tenth of that, or 0.06 ml.

Because of their concentrated nature, many fluidextracts are considered too potent to be safely taken in self-administration by the patient and their use *per se* is steadily diminishing in medical practice. Also, many fluidextracts are simply too bitter tasting or otherwise un-palatable to be accepted by the patient. Therefore, most fluidextracts today are either modified by the addition of flavoring or sweetening agents before use, or are used pharmaceutically as the drug source component of other liquid dosage forms, such as syrups.

The Preparation of Fluidextracts

All official fluidextracts are prepared by percolation, the menstruum used in each case being prescribed in the individual monograph. The selection of the menstruum is based primarily on achieving a complete but economical extraction of the active constituents from a plant drug while keeping to a minimum the extraction of inactive materials. These inactive materials frequently have a tendency to deposit from solution upon standing, and although this does not generally affect the potency or therapeutic efficacy of the product, it does render it unsightly and pharmaceutically unattractive. To avoid this occurrence on the pharmacist's shelves, the manufacturer of a fluidextract generally permits a period of aging before final packaging to allow any insoluble material to settle out so that it may be removed by filtration before distribution. Because the menstruum is selected for its ability to dissolve extract and keep in solution the active constituents of a plant drug, the sediment rarely involves a desired constituent. Should a sediment be found by a pharmacist at the bottom of a bottle of a fluidextract, he can, if he wishes, decant the supernatant liquid, filter it if necessary, and be reasonably confident of the therapeutic efficacy of the clarified fluidextract.

Usually a narrow, cylindrical percolator is employed in the preparation of fluidextracts, since, as explained earlier, this type of percolator is most efficient in extracting a concentrated product. Concentration is important, since any excess of percolate collected over the intended final volume of product must be reduced in volume by evaporation to maintain the standard of potency for fluidextracts (i.e., 1 g of drug = 1 ml of fluidextract). The least amount of menstruum required to exhaust a drug is beneficial in terms of time, effort, and conservation of solvent. A cone-shaped percolator may be used in the preparation of fluidextracts if the drug is known to swell considerably and the chance of causing a blockage within the drug column of a cylindrical percolator is considered likely. For each fluidextract, the period of maceration and the rate of percolation are stated in the monograph.

Three general methods are presently given by the NF for the preparation of fluidextracts and are designated as Processes A, B, and C. They are briefly outlined as follows.

Process A

Process A involves the exhaustive percolation of a drug with an alcoholic or hydroalcoholic menstruum. The essential feature of the process is the setting aside or the "reserving" of the first 85% of the percolate (the first 850 ml collected in the preparation of 1 liter of fluidextract). The percolation process is continued with the collection of "weak percolate" until the drug is exhausted of desired constituents. Generally, more than 1000 ml of total percolate must be collected by Process A in the extraction of each 1000 g of drug, and by reserving the concentrated first portion of percolate, only the second and weaker portion needs be reduced in volume to achieve the proper amount of product. The weak percolate is subjected to the minimum required temperature to facilitate evaporation of solvent. When the extractive is concentrated to a soft, pliable mass, it is dissolved in the reserve percolate, and the fluidextract is adjusted with the proper hydroalcoholic diluent to bring the preparation to the required volume and concentration of drug and alcohol. The lowest possible temperature is used to avoid as far as is possible the destruction of any active components that may be unstable at high temperature. The use of vacuum distillation generally is effective in the rapid removal of solvent at a relatively low temperature.

Process B

Process B is used in the preparation of fluidextracts, with boiling water as the menstruum and alcohol generally added to the concentrated percolate as a preservative. A heat-resistant glass or metallic percolator must be used in this process.

Obviously this process is suited to those drugs whose active constituents are water solu-

ble and are not destroyed by heat. The drug is exhausted of constituents and the aqueous percolate is subjected to evaporation by a water bath or vacuum still to prepare the specified volume of product. *All* of the percolate is subjected to heat, and no reserve percolate is set aside because aqueous extractions of vegetable drugs are usually albuminous in their content and as such are especially subject to growth of molds and bacteria. Heating the entire percolate destroys organisms present and preserves the percolate until such time as the alcohol is added. To prevent loss through volatilization, the alcohol must not be added until the percolate is cooled. The product is permitted to stand for several days or longer in a stoppered container to permit any insoluble material to settle. It is then clarified by decantation and filtration and made to volume with water and alcohol to achieve the proper total volume and alcohol concentration (usually between 15 and 25%).

Process C

Process C, which is intended to facilitate total drug extraction by collecting 1000 ml of percolate from each 1000 g of drug, uses long narrow columns of drug and percolation under pressure. A single cylindrical percolator may be used if total drug extraction is ensured with the collection of 1000 ml of percolate, or a series of such percolators joined together may be employed when necessary. By the latter method, the columns of drug are set up vertically and parallel to one another and are joined together by U-shaped tubes also packed with drug. The menstruum is added to the first vertical tube and forced by pressure through the system of vertical tubes and connecting U-tubes. The percolate, which is highly concentrated at first, is collected from the last tube of the series, and after collection of the desired volume, the drug is usually exhausted of active constituents. The advantage to the method is the elimination of the need to concentrate the percolate through the use of heat. Process C may be used as a substitute for Process A. The major disadvantage of the process is the time consumed in packing, setting up, and cleaning the narrow tubes of drug. The collection of percolate is generally made at a rate half that specified for the percolation of the drug by another process.

Most fluidextracts should be stored in tight,

light-resistant containers away from excessive heat and direct sunlight.

There are five officially recognized fluidextracts. Two of them, Glycyrrhiza Fluidextract, NF and Eriodictyon Fluidextract, NF, are employed as flavoring agents largely in the preparation of the corresponding syrups. Both glycyrrhiza and eriodictyon are effective in masking the bitter or salty taste of drugs. The remaining three official fluidextracts are used as cathartics and are described briefly below.

Cascara Sagrada Fluidextract, NF

Cascara sagrada fluidextract is prepared by Process B, using boiling water as the menstruum and about 20% alcohol for preservation and stabilization.

The water-soluble principles of cascara sagrada are active cathartics, and the fluidextract owes its value to these agents. The preparation has a dose of about 1 ml. However, since it is so intensely bitter, due to the nature of the extractive, the more palatable and less concentrated Aromatic Cascara Sagrada Fluidextract, USP, having a dose of 5 ml is usually preferred.

Aromatic Cascara Sagrada Fluidextract, USP

Aromatic cascara sagrada fluidextract is prepared by Process B, with magnesium oxide being mixed with the drug prior to percolation for the purpose of neutralizing and thereby partially preventing the extraction of some of the bitter principles of the cascara. This procedure and the addition to the percolate of several flavoring oils, saccharin, and pure glycyrrhiza extract for a licorice flavor and sweetness make this fluidextract more palatable than the plain, untreated fluidextract of the NF. About 20% of alcohol is used to solubilize the oils and to act as a preservative.

Because some of the irritating bitter but cathartic principles are not extracted, this treated fluidextract is less active than the plain preparation previously mentioned and must be taken in larger amounts, usually 5 ml.

Senna Fluidextract, NF

Senna fluidextract is prepared by Process A, using a hydroalcoholic menstruum composed of 2 volumes of water for each volume of alcohol. This highly aqueous menstruum reduces the extraction of some of the undesired resinous material present in the powdered senna leaf. The fluidextract is used mainly in the preparation of Senna Syrup, NF, although the fluidextract may be used alone as a cathartic. The dose of the fluidextract is 2 ml. Senna contains emodin and other bitter and griping principles, and its action as a cathartic is considered harsh. The syrup is generally preferred over the fluidextract because it is more palatable and the coriander oil in the syrup is thought to reduce the griping caused by the senna principles.

Extracts

Extracts as defined by the USP are "concentrated preparations of vegetable or animal drugs obtained by removal of the active constituents of the respective drugs with suitable menstrua, evaporation of all or nearly all of the solvent, and adjustment of the residual masses or powders to the prescribed standards." Extracts are potent preparations, usually between two and six times as potent on a weight basis as the crude drug used as the starting material. They contain the active constituents of the crude drug, a great portion of the inactive constituents and structural components of the crude drug having been removed. Their function is to provide in small amounts and in convenient, stable physical form the medicinal activity and character of the more bulky plants that they represent. As such, they are useful in the compounding of prescriptions or in product formulation.

In the manufacture of most extracts, percolation is employed to remove the active constituents from the drug, with the percolates generally being reduced in volume by evaporation of the solvent by distillation under reduced pressure, the latter being used to reduce the degree of heat and protect the drug substances against thermal decomposition. When thermolabile drugs are involved in the process, the temperature is generally maintained below 60° during the entire period of concentrating the percolate. The extent of the removal of the solvent determines the final physical character of the extract. Extracts are made into three forms: (a) *semiliquid extracts* or those of a syrupy consistency prepared without the intent of removing all or even most of the menstruum, (b) *pilular* or *solid extracts* of a plastic consistency prepared with nearly all of the menstruum removed, and (c) *powdered extracts* prepared to be dry by the removal of all of the menstruum insofar as is feasible or practical. Pilular and powdered extracts differ only by the slight amount of remaining solvent in the former preparation, and for all practical purposes are interchangeable from a therapeutic standpoint, but each has its pharmaceutical advantage because of its physical form. For instance, the pilular extract is preferred in compounding a plastic dosage form such as an ointment or paste or one in which a pliable material facilitates compounding, whereas the powdered form is preferable in the compounding of such dosage forms as powders, capsules, and tablets.

In the preparation of extracts, the selection of the menstruum is based on the same primary requirements as in the preparation of fluid-extracts and tinctures—that is, the ability of the solvent to dissolve the great bulk of the desired constituents and the minimal amount of undesired constituents. Alcoholic, hydro-alcoholic, and aqueous menstruums all are employed from time to time, depending upon the nature of the drug and its active constituents.

Generally speaking, if a powdered extract is to be prepared from a drug containing alcohol-soluble active constituents, a menstruum of alcohol would be preferred over a hydro-alcoholic menstruum for reasons other than the required solubility of the active constituents in alcohol. In preparing a powdered extract, it is necessary to remove all of the menstruum, and since alcohol has a greater volatility than a hydroalcoholic menstruum, it would be removed more readily and at a lower temperature. Also, an alcoholic menstruum keeps to a minimum the extraction of undesired water-soluble constituents of plants, such a gums and mucilages. When alcohol is used in the large-scale industrial preparation of an extract, the cost of the process may be lowered considerably if upon evaporation of that solvent, the alcohol is recovered by distilling and condensing it. However, in small-scale preparation in the pharmacy or laboratory, the small amounts of alcohol used are generally left unrecovered after evaporation from the percolate.

In preparing a pilular extract, it is not the intent to render the product dry, and therefore

an aqueous or hydroalcoholic menstruum is of no great disadvantage. When a hydroalcoholic menstruum is used, the alcohol is evaporated more readily because of its greater volatility than the water, and a portion of the water is permitted to remain in the final extract to give it its characteristic pliable, plastic character.

Although extracts considered to be non-potent are not required to be assayed for potency, those considered to be potent must be assayed after preparation, and their strength must be adjusted to the proper standard. In most instances in which an assay is required, the extract has excessive potency and requires dilution to achieve the proper concentration of active constituents. Most usually, liquid glucose is employed as the diluent for pilular extracts, and starch dried at 100° is the diluent for powdered extracts. However, other diluents may be employed so long as they do not interfere in any way with the potency or therapeutic efficacy of the product. Among the other useful diluents for pilular extracts are malt extract and/or glycerin or glucose. Alternate diluents for powdered extracts are powdered sucrose, lactose, powdered glycyrrhiza, magnesium carbonate, magnesium oxide, calcium phosphate, and the finely powdered marc remaining after the extraction of the crude drug. It should be noted that the alkaline reaction of certain of the diluents such as magnesium oxide and magnesium carbonate in the presence of moisture negates their usefulness as diluents for extracts containing active constituents destroyed by the alkalinity. Hence, these agents are not used for such extracts as belladonna extract, the alkaloids of which are hydrolyzed and rendered impotent by the alkaline substances.

The official compendia permit the diluent of a powdered extract to be colored with chlorophyll to make it green or with caramel to make it brown or with a combination of the two agents to produce a color corresponding with the natural color of the undiluted extract so that after dilution it does not look "pale" or impotent. For a powdered extract, the powdered marc used as a diluent accomplishes the same purpose.

Powdered extracts prepared from drugs that contain a large proportion of inactive oily or fatty material generally are treated to remove this material in order to obtain a stable and satisfactory product. Such material may be removed from a powdered extract, before assay if one is required, by repeated washing with solvent hexane, the washed extract being dried and any adjustments to proper strength being made in the usual manner. Another method involves the repeated washing of the undried, pilular extract with hot acidified water, cooling the mixture and skimming the oily or fatty material off the top of the water layer. If each of these methods is unsatisfactory, another suitable method may be employed.

Packaging and Storage of Extracts

Pilular extracts must be packaged in containers such as wide-mouthed jars or metallic or plastic tubes that permit their easy removal. The containers must close tightly to prevent the loss of moisture from a pilular extract, which would result in its becoming hard and unsuitable for use. On the other hand, powdered extracts must be protected from the entrance of moisture into the container. Upon exposure to moisture, powdered extracts may become caked and lose their utility in the preparation of other pharmaceutical dosage forms.

Generally stated, most pharmaceutical extracts are best stored in tight, light-resistant containers preferably at a temperature not above 30°.

Official Extracts

Belladonna Extract, NF

Belladonna extract is official in both pilular and powdered forms, each type being required to contain an average of 1.25 g of the alkaloids of belladonna for each 100 g of extract. The extract is approximately four times as concentrated in active ingredients as is the fluidextract (about 300 mg of alkaloids in each 100 ml) or the crude drug (about 350 mg per 100 g) and about forty times as concentrated as the corresponding tincture (about 30 mg of alkaloids in each 100 ml). Because of its concentration with respect to the crude drug, belladonna extract is frequently referred to as a ''400%'' extract, meaning it is four times as potent as the original material. The dose of the extract is thus propor-

tionately lower, 15 mg being the usual dose for its anticholinergic action to reduce secretions in the treatment of colds or to control gastrointestinal spasma or irritation. The pilular extract is used in some proprietary antihemorrhoidal suppositories for its anodyne effects.

Cascara Sagrada Extract, NF

Cascara sagrada extract is a powdered extract prepared with boiling water as the menstruum and starch as the diluent and adjusted to represent in each g the potency of 3 g of the dried bark of cascara sagrada.

The extract may be used as a concentrated powdered source of cascara sagrada in the manufacture of other dosage forms, especially capsules and tablets, for use as cathartics. The usual dose of the extract is 300 mg.

Pure Glycyrrhiza Extract, USP

Pure Glycyrrhiza Extract, USP, is a pilular extract prepared by the percolation of glycyrrhiza, in granular powder, with boiling water until the drug is exhausted. Diluted ammonia solution is added to the percolate to convert the glycoside glycyrrhizin to the ammoniated compound, which is more soluble and sweeter than the glycyrrhizin itself. After nearly complete evaporation of the solvent, the residue is a black, pilular mass with the sweet, licorice taste characteristic of the ammoniated glycyrrhizin.

The extract is employed as a flavor to mask bitter tasting drugs, most notably in Aromatic Cascara Sagrada Fluidextract, USP, to mask the bitterness of cascara sagrada.

Trichinella Extract, USP

This is an aqueous extract of the killed, washed, defatted and powdered larvae of *Trichinella spiralis*, usually obtained from inoculated rodents. It is employed by intradermal injection as a diagnostic aid for trichinosis.

Resins and Oleoresins

In addition to the synthetic resins used in pharmacy, as the ion-exchange resins, there are *natural resins* and *prepared resins* and also *natural oleoresins* and *prepared oleoresins,* and a distinction must be made between them. The natural resins and oleoresins are plant materials that make themselves available for collection by their natural exudation from the plant material. The prepared resins and oleoresins are obtained by exhausting a drug of these materials through the use of a proper solvent or solvent mixture.

Resins

Resins may be defined as solid or semisolid exudations from plants or from insects feeding on plants. As indicated above, they may reveal themselves naturally, or they may be obtained by extraction. Chemically resins are usually the oxidized terpines of the volatile oils of plants and, like their precursors, are insoluble in water, but unlike the volatile oils they generally do not possess an appealing, fragrant odor. The formerly official Mastic, NF XI, is an example of a natural resin.

Prepared resins are obtained by percolating to exhaustion the crude drug having the resin as its active constituent, using an alcoholic menstruum. The percolate obtained is then poured into a large volume of water, causing the separation of the water-insoluble resin which then may be collected as a precipitate, washed with additional water, and dried. Ipomea Resin and Jalap Resin, both formerly official in the NF XI, are examples of prepared resins obtained in this manner. Resins may also be prepared from natural oleoresins by using heat to drive off the volatile oil, leaving the resin as the residue. Rosin, NF XIII, is prepared in this manner from turpentine, an oleoresin.

These natural products should be distinguished from the various synthetic resins, which are polymeric substances generally prepared by either condensation or addition from many different chemical substances.

Resins are best stored in well-closed containers.

Official Resin

Podophyllum Resin, USP

Podophyllum resin is a powdered mixture of resins removed from the dried rhizome and roots of *Podophyllum peltatum* by percolation with alcohol and subsequent precipitation of the resins from the percolate upon its addition to water acidified with 1.0% of hydrochloric acid. The acidified water results in a more complete precipitation of the resins than does water alone. Podophyllum is required to contain not less than 5% resin, and since the drug is exhausted by percolation, this amount of resin is usually recovered from the percolate.

The resin is officially categorized as a caustic for certain papillomas and is used for this purpose generally as a 25% dispersion of the resin in compound benzoin tincture or as a solution in alcohol. In addition, the resin is considered to be among the most drastic of the hydrogogue cathartics. However, because of its unpredictable and highly irritant action, it is gradually coming into disuse in human preparations but finds some acceptance in veterinary products. The USP cautions that the resin is "highly irritating to the eye and to mucous membranes in general"; therefore, it should be handled with appropriate caution.

The resin occurs as a light brown to greenish yellow, amorphous powder that turns darker when exposed to light or to temperatures exceeding 25°. It must be stored in tight, light-resistant containers, and exposure to excessive heat must be avoided.

Oleoresins

Natural oleoresins, as their name indicates, are mixtures of volatile oils and resin. They are generally obtained by incising the trunks of the trees in which they are found. Turpentine, NF XI, is an example of a natural oleoresin. Prepared oleoresins may contain components other than the volatile oil and resin, since they are prepared by percolating drugs with a solvent such as alcohol, acetone, or ether which is capable of dissolving and extracting plant constituents other than the oleoresin. The percolate is concentrated by the evaporation of the solvent by distillation, and the residue contains the oleoresin. The relative proportion of volatile oil to resin varies greatly among the oleoresins, with some containing much larger proportions of resin than others. Oleoresins are stored in tight containers. The most recently official prepared oleoresin was Ginger Oleoresin, NF XIII, used as a flavoring agent.

Selected Reading

Brochmann-Hanssen, E.: Studies on the Effects of Surface-Active Agents on the Extraction of Crude Drugs. J. Amer. Pharm. Ass., Sci. Ed., 43:27–31, 1954.

Davis, H.: Extraction. In *Bentley's Text-Book of Pharmaceutics*, 6th ed. London, Bailliere, Tindall and Cox, 1954, pp. 272–307.

Ovadia, M. E., and Skauen, D. M.: Effects of Ultrasonic Waves on the Extraction of Alkaloids. J. Pharm. Sci., 54:1013–1016, 1965.

Riebling, P. W. and Walker, G. C.: Extraction and Extractives. In *Remington's Pharmaceutical Sciences*, 15th ed., Easton, Pa., Mack Publishing Co., 1975, pp. 1509–1522.

Svoboda, G. H.: Methodology of Selective Extraction and Gradient pH Extraction Techniques. Lloydia, 27:299–301, 1964.

Chapter 8

Injections, Biological Products, and Sterile Fluids

C ONSIDERED IN this chapter are important pharmaceutical dosage forms that have the common characteristic of being prepared to be sterile; that is, free from contaminating microorganisms. Among these sterile dosage forms are the various small- and large-volume injectable preparations, irrigation fluids intended to bathe body wounds or surgical openings, dialysis solutions, and biological preparations as vaccines, toxoids, antitoxins, blood replenishment products, etc. Sterility in these preparations is of utmost importance since they are placed in direct contact with the internal body fluids or tissues where infection can easily arise. Ophthalmic preparations which are also prepared to be sterile will be discussed separately in Chapter 11.

Injections

Injections may be broadly defined as sterile, pyrogen-free preparations intended to be administered parenterally. The term *parenteral* as commonly used refers to the injectable routes of administration as well as to the various preparations administered by injection. The word has its derivation from the Greek words *para*

and *enteron*, meaning outside of the intestine, and denotes routes of administration other than the oral route. *Pyrogens* are fever-producing organic substances arising from microbial contamination and are responsible for many of the febrile reactions which occur in patients following intravenous injection. Pyrogens and the determination of their presence in parenteral preparations will be discussed later in this chapter. In general, the parenteral routes of administration are undertaken when rapid drug action is desired, as in emergency situations, when the patient is uncooperative, unconscious, or unable to accept or tolerate medication by the oral route, or when the drug itself is ineffective by other routes. With the exception of insulin injections, which are commonly self-administered by diabetic patients, most injections are administered by the physician or his agent in the course of medical treatment. Thus injections are employed mostly in the hospital and clinic and less frequently in the home; consequently, the pharmacist generally supplies most injectable preparations directly to the physician or his agent rather than to the patient as with most other types of medication.

Interesting historical accounts of the origin and development of injection therapy may be found in the references cited below.[1,2]

Parenteral Routes of Administration

Drugs may be injected into almost any organ or area of the body, including the joints (*intra-articular*), a joint-fluid area (*intrasynovial*), the spinal column (*intraspinal*), into spinal fluid (*intrathecal*), arteries (*intra-arterial*), and in an emergency, even into the heart (*intracardiac*). However, most commonly injections are performed into a vein (*intravenous, I.V.*), into a muscle (*intramuscular, I.M.*), into the skin (*intradermal, I.D., intracutaneous*), or under the skin (*subcutaneous, S.C., Sub-Q, S.Q., hypodermic, "Hypo."*).

---

[1]Van Itallie, P. H.: The Rugged Beginnings of Injection Therapy, *Pulse of Pharmacy* (Wyeth Laboratories), *19*:3–17, 1965.
[2]Griffenhagen, G. B.: The History of Parenteral Medication, *Bulletin Parenteral Drug Assoc.*, *16*:12, 1962.

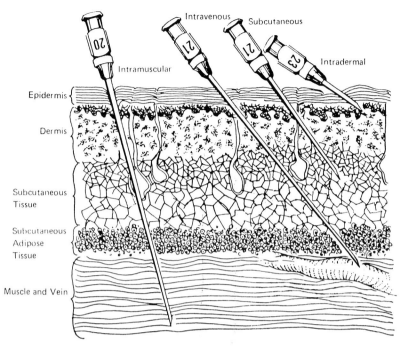

Fig. 8-1. *Routes of parenteral administration. Numbers on needles indicate size or gauge of needle based on outside diameter of needle shaft. (Turco, S. and King, R. E.,* Sterile Dosage Forms: Their Preparation and Clinical Applications. *Courtesy of Lea & Febiger, 1974.)*

Intravenous Route

The intravenous injection of drugs had its scientific origin in 1656 in the experiments of Sir Christopher Wren, architect of St. Paul's Cathedral and amateur physiologist. Using a bladder and quill for a syringe and needle, he injected wine, ale, opium, and other substances into the veins of dogs and studied their effects. Intravenous medication was first given to man by Johann Daniel Major of Kiel in 1662, but was abandoned for a period because of the occurrence of thrombosis and embolism in the patients so treated. The invention of the hypodermic syringe toward the middle of the 19th century created new interest in intravenous techniques and toward the turn of the century, intravenous administration of solutions of sodium chloride and glucose became popular. Today, the intravenous administration of drugs is a common occurrence in the hospital, although there are still recognized dangers associated with the practice. Thrombus and embolus formation are still induced by intravenous needles and catheters, and the recently recognized generation of particulate matter in parenteral solutions poses new concerns for those involved in the development, administration, and use of intravenous solutions.

Drugs administered intravenously provide rapid action compared to other routes of administration and because drug absorption is not a factor, optimum blood levels may be achieved with the accuracy and immediacy not possible by other routes. In emergency situations, the intravenous administration of a drug may be a life-saving procedure because of the placement of the drug directly into the circulation and the prompt action which ensues. On the negative side, once a drug is administered intravenously, it cannot be retrieved. In instances of an adverse reaction to the drug, for instance, the drug cannot be easily removed from the circulation as it could, for example, by vomiting following the oral administration of the same drug.

Although most superficial veins are suitable for venipuncture, the veins of the antecubital area (situated in front of the elbow) are usually selected for direct intravenous injection. The veins in this location are large, superficial, and easy to see and enter. Most clinicians insert the needle with the bevel facing upward, at the most acute angle possible with the vein, to ensure that the direction of flow of the injectable is that of the flow of the blood. Strict aseptic precautions must be taken at all times to avoid risk of infection. Not only are the injectable solutions sterile, the syringes and needles employed must also be sterilized and the point of entrance must be cleansed to reduce the chance of carrying bacteria from the skin into the blood via the needle.

Both small and large volumes of drug solutions may be administered intravenously. The use of 500-ml containers of solutions for intravenous infusion is commonplace in the hospital. These solutions containing such agents as nutrients, blood extenders, electrolytes, amino acids, antibiotics and other therapeutic agents are generally administered through an indwelling needle or catheter by continuous drip. The drip or flow rates may be adjusted by the clinician according to the needs of the patient. Generally, flow rates of 2 to 3 ml per minute are employed. For intravenous infusion, the needle or catheter is generally placed in the prominent veins of the forearm or leg and taped firmly to the patient so that it will not slip from place during infusion. The main hazard of intravenous infusion is the possibility of thrombus formation induced by the touching of the wall of the vein by the catheter or needle. Thrombi are more likely to occur when the infusion solution is of an irritating nature to the biologic tissues. A *thrombus* is a blood clot formed within the blood vessel (or heart) due usually to a slowing of the circulation or to an alteration of the blood or vessel wall. Once such a clot circulates, it becomes an *embolus*, carried by the blood stream until it lodges in a blood vessel, obstructing it, and resulting in a blockage or occlusion referred to as an *embolism*. Such an obstruction may be a critical hazard to the patient, depending upon the site and severity of the obstruction.

Drugs administered intravenously must be in aqueous solution; they must mix with the circulating blood and not precipitate from solution. Such an event could lead to thrombus formation and the subsequent blockage of blood passage. For similar reasons, suspensions of drugs may not be safely administered intravenously. It is also the reason for the growing concern when particulate matter (insoluble particles) is found to be present in solutions intended for intravenous administration.

Naturally, the intravenous route is utilized in the administration of blood transfusions and it also serves as the point of exit in the removal of blood from patients for diagnostic work and for obtaining blood from donors.

Intramuscular Route

Intramuscular injections of drugs provide drug effects that are less rapid, but generally of greater duration than that obtained from intravenous administration. Aqueous or oleaginous solutions or suspensions of drug substances may be administered intramuscularly. Depending upon the type of preparation employed, the absorption rates may vary widely. Generally it would be expected that drugs from solutions would be more rapidly absorbed than from suspensions and that drugs in aqueous preparations would be more rapidly absorbed than when in oleaginous preparations. The type of preparation employed is based on the properties of the drug itself and on the therapeutic goals desired.

Intramuscular injections are performed deep into the skeletal muscles. The point of injection should be as far as possible from major nerves and blood vessels. Injuries to patients from intramuscular injection usually are related to the point where the needle entered and where the medication was deposited. Such injuries include paralysis resulting from neural damage, abscesses, cysts, embolism, hematoma, sloughing of the skin, and scar formation.

In adults, the upper outer quadrant of the gluteus maximus is the most frequently used site for intramuscular injection. In infants, the gluteal area is small and composed primarily of fat, not muscle. What muscle there is is poorly developed. An injection in this area might range dangerously close to the sciatic nerve, especially if the child is resisting the injection and squirming or fighting. Thus, in infants and young children, the deltoid muscles of the upper arm or the midlateral muscles of the thigh are preferred. An injection given in the upper or lower portion of the deltoid would be well away from the radial nerve. The deltoid may also be used in adults, but the pain is more noticeable here than in the gluteal area. If a series of injections are to be given, the injection site is usually varied. To be certain that a blood vessel has not been entered, the clinician may aspirate slightly on the syringe following insertion of the needle to observe if blood enters the syringe. Usually, the volume of medication which may be conveniently administered by the intramuscular route is limited; generally a maximum of 5 ml is administered intramuscularly in the gluteal region and 2 ml in the deltoid of the arm.

Intradermal Route

A number of substances may be effectively injected into the corium, the more vascular layer of the skin just beneath the epidermis. These substances include various agents for diagnostic determinations, desensitization, or immunization. The usual site for intradermal injection is the anterior surface of the forearm. A short ($\frac{3}{8}$ in.) and narrow gauge (23- to 26-gauge) needle is usually employed. The needle is inserted horizontally into the skin with the bevel facing upward. The injection is made when the bevel just disappears into the corium. Usually only about 0.1 ml volumes may be administered in this manner.

Subcutaneous Route

The subcutaneous route may be utilized for the injection of small amounts of medication. The injection of a drug beneath the surface of the skin is usually made in the loose interstitial tissues of the arm, forearm, thigh, or buttocks. The site of injection is usually changed when injections are frequently given. Prior to injection, the skin at the injection site should be thoroughly cleansed. The volume of a subcutaneous injection is seldom greater than 2 ml. Thus a 2-ml syringe is generally employed with a $\frac{1}{2}$ or $\frac{3}{4}$ inch needle of 22- to 26-gauge. Upon insertion, if blood appears in the syringe a new site should be selected.

Drugs which are irritating or those which are present in thick suspension form may produce induration, sloughing, or abscess formation and may be painful to the patient. Such preparations should be considered not suitable for subcutaneous injection.

Official Types of Injections

According to the USP and the NF, injections are separated into five distinct types, generally defined as follows:

(1) Medicaments or solutions, or emulsions suitable for injection, bearing titles of the form, "_____ *Injection*." (Ex: Insulin Injection, USP)

(2) Dry solids or liquid concentrates containing no buffers, diluents, or other added substances, and which, upon the addition of suitable solvents, yield solutions conforming in all aspects to the requirements for Injections, and which are distinguished by titles of the form, "*Sterile* _____" (Ex: Sterile Procaine Hydrochloride, USP)

(3) Preparations as those described in (2) except that they contain one or more buffers, diluents, or other added substances, and which are distinguished by titles of the form, "_____ *for Injection*" (Ex: Glucagon for Injection, USP)

(4) Solids which are suspended in a suitable fluid medium and which are not to be injected intravenously or into the spinal canal, distinguished by titles of the form, "*Sterile* _____ *Suspension.*" (Ex: Sterile Hydrocortisone Acetate Suspension, USP)

(5) Dry solids, which, upon the addition of suitable vehicles, yield preparations ·conforming in all respects to the requirements for Sterile Suspensions, and which are distinguished by titles of the form, "*Sterile* _____ *for Suspension.*"

The form into which a given drug is prepared for parenteral use by the manufacturer depends upon the nature of the drug itself, with respect to its physical and chemical characteristics, and also upon certain therapeutic considerations. Generally, if a drug is unstable in solution, it may be prepared as a dry powder intended for reconstitution with the proper solvent at the time of its administration, or it may be prepared as a suspension of the drug particles in a vehicle in which the drug is insoluble. If the drug is unstable in the presence of water, that solvent may be replaced in part or totally by a solvent in which the drug is stable. If the drug is insoluble in water, an injection may be prepared as an aqueous suspension or as a solution of the drug in a suitable nonaqueous solvent, such as a vegetable oil. If an aqueous solution is desired, a water-soluble salt form of the insoluble drug is frequently prepared to satisfy the required solubility characteristics. Therapeutically, only aqueous or blood-miscible solutions may be injected directly into the blood stream, since blood-immiscible liquids, as oleaginous injections, would interrupt the normal flow of blood within the circulatory system. Suspensions of drugs will also interfere with blood flow within the circulatory system and perhaps block the smaller blood vessels, and their use is generally restricted to other than intravenous administration. As indicated previously, the onset and duration of action of a drug may be somewhat controlled by the chemical form of the drug used, the physical state of the injection (solution or suspension), and the vehicle employed. Drugs that are very soluble in body fluids generally have the most rapid absorption and onset of action. Thus drugs in aqueous solution have a more rapid onset of action than do drugs in oleaginous solution. Drugs in aqueous suspension are also more rapid acting than drugs in oleaginous suspension due to the greater miscibility of the aqueous preparation with the body fluids after injection and the subsequent more rapid contact of the drug particles with the body fluids. Oftentimes more prolonged drug action is desired to reduce the necessity of frequently repeated injections. These long-acting types of injections are commonly referred to as "respository" or "depot" types of preparations.

The solutions and suspensions of drugs intended for injection are prepared in the same general manner as was discussed previously in this text for oral solutions (Chapter 4) and oral suspensions (Chapter 5), with the following differences:

1. Solvents or vehicles used must meet special purity and other standards assuring their safety by injection.
2. The use of added substances, as buffers, stabilizers, and antimicrobial preservatives, fall under specific guidelines of use and are restricted in certain parenteral products. The use of coloring agents is strictly prohibited.
3. Parenteral products are always sterilized and meet sterility standards and must be pyrogen-free.
4. Parenteral solutions must be free of particulate matter.
5. Parenteral products must be prepared in environmentally controlled areas, under strict sanitation standards, and by personnel specially trained and clothed to maintain the sanitation standards.
6. Parenteral products are packaged in special hermetic containers of specific and high quality. Special quality control procedures are utilized to ensure their hermetic seal and sterile condition.
7. Each container of an injection is filled to a volume in slight excess of the labeled "size" or volume to be withdrawn. This excess permits the ease of withdrawal and administration of the labeled volumes.
8. There are compendial restrictions over the volume of injection permitted in multiple-dose containers and also a limitation over the types of containers (single-dose or multiple-dose) which may be used for certain injections.
9. Specific compendial labeling regulations apply to injections.
10. Sterile powders intended for solution or suspension immediately prior to injection are frequently packaged as lyophilized or freeze-dried powders to permit ease of solution or suspension upon the addition of the solvent or vehicle.

Solvents and Vehicles for Injections

The most frequently used solvent in the large scale manufacture of injections is *Water for Injection, USP*. This water is purified by distillation or by reverse osmosis and meets the same standards for the presence of total solids as does *Purified Water, USP*, not more than 1 mg per 100 ml. Water for Injection, USP may not contain added substances. Although water for injection is not required to be sterile, it must be pyrogen-free. The water is intended to be used in the manufacture of injectable products which are to be sterilized after their preparation. Water for injection should be stored in tight containers at temperatures below or above the range in which microbial growth occurs.[1]

[1] For each species of bacteria there is a temperature at which it is in every way most active (optimum-growth temperature) and temperatures above (maximum-growth temperature) or below (minimum-growth temperature) which the organism is inactive. At temperatures below the minimum-growth temperature, bacteria cease to develop, but most species are not killed by cold. Bacteriologists successfully keep many cultures alive in the ordinary refrigerator (2–15°C) for several days or weeks. Indeed, many organisms will survive for weeks frozen in ice and will grow normally again when the ice melts. High temperatures are much more injurious to microorganisms than are cold temperatures. If any bacterium is heated above its maximum-growth temperature to a sufficient degree and for sufficient length of time, it will be killed. Although thermal death temperature may range between 30°C for cold-loving organisms and 90° for heat-loving organisms, nearly all nonsporeforming bacteria when exposed in aqueous media to temperatures of 60 to 75°C are killed within 30 minutes. (Burdon, K. L., and Williams, R. P.: *Microbiology*, 5th ed. New York, The Macmillan Co., 1964, pp. 145–158.)

Water for injection is intended to be used within 24 hours following its collection. Naturally, the water should be collected in sterile and pyrogen-free containers. The containers are usually glass or glass-lined.

Sodium chloride (0.9%) is added to water for injection to render it isotonic, and this is permitted by the compendia so long as it is not interdicted in the specific monograph for the injection to be prepared. Similarly, Sodium Chloride Injection, USP and Ringer's Injection, USP may be used as vehicles for the preparation of parenteral products.

Sterile Water for Injection, USP is water for injection which has been sterilized and packaged in single-dose containers of not greater than 1-liter size. As water for injection, it must be pyrogen-free and may not contain an antimicrobial agent or other added substance. This water may contain a slightly greater amount of total solids than water for injection due to the leaching of solids from the glass-lined tanks during the sterilization process. This water is intended to be used as a solvent, vehicle or diluent for already-sterilized and packaged injectable medications. In use, the water is aseptically added to the vial of medication to prepare the desired injection. For instance, a suitable injection may be prepared from the dry powder, Sterile Ampicillin Sodium, USP, by the aseptic addition of sterile water for injection.

Bacteriostatic Water for Injection, USP is sterile water for injection containing one or more suitable antimicrobial agents. It is packaged in prefilled syringes or in vials containing not more than 30 ml of the water. The container label must state the name and proportion of the antimicrobial agent(s) present. The water is employed as a sterile vehicle in the preparation of small volumes of injectable preparations. Because of the presence of antimicrobial agents the water must only be used in parenterals that are administered in small volumes. Its use in parenterals administered in large volume is restricted due to the excessive and perhaps toxic amounts of the antimicrobial agents which would be injected along with the medication. Generally, if volumes of greater than 5 ml of solvent are required, sterile water for injection rather than bacteriostatic water for injection is preferred. In using bacteriostatic water for injection, due regard must also be given to the chemical compatibility of the bacteriostatic agent(s) present with the particular medicinal agent being dissolved or suspended.

Although an aqueous vehicle is generally preferred for an injection, its use may be precluded in a formulation due to the limited water solubility of a medicinal substance or its susceptibility to hydrolysis. When such physical or chemical factors limit the use of a wholly aqueous vehicle, the pharmaceutical formulator must turn to one or more nonaqueous vehicles. The selected agent must be nonirritating, nontoxic in the amounts administered, and nonsensitizing. Like water, it must not exert a pharmacologic activity of its own, nor may it adversely affect the activity of the medicinal agent. In addition, the physical and chemical properties of the solvent must be considered, evaluated, and determined to be suitable for the task at hand before it may be employed. Among the many considerations are the solvent's stability at various pH levels, its viscosity, which must be such as to allow ease of injection, its fluidity, which must be maintained over a fairly wide temperature range, its boiling point, which should be sufficiently high to permit heat sterilization, its miscibility with body fluids, its flammability, and its constant purity or ease of purification and standardization. There is no single solvent that is free of limitations, and thus the cross-consideration and the assessment of each solvent's advantages and disadvantages help the formulator determine the most appropriate solvent for use in a given preparation. Among the nonaqueous solvents presently employed in parenteral products are fixed vegetable oils, glycerin, polyethylene glycols, propylene glycol, alcohol, and a number of lesser used agents as ethyl oleate, isopropyl myristate, and dimethylacetamide.[1] These and other nonaqueous vehicles may be used provided they are safe in the amounts administered and do not interfere with the therapeutic efficacy of the preparation or with its response to prescribed assays and tests.

The USP and the NF set restrictions on the fixed vegetable oils which may be employed in parenteral products. For one thing, they must remain clear when cooled to 10° to ensure the stability and clarity of the injectable product upon storage under refrigeration. The oils must not contain mineral oil or paraffin, as these materials are not absorbed by body tissues. The fluidity of a vegetable oil generally depends upon the proportion of unsaturated fatty acids,

[1] A review of nonaqueous solvents in parenteral products was prepared by Spiegel, A. J., and Noseworthy, M. M.: *J. Pharm. Sci.*, 52:917, 1963.

such as oleic acid, to saturated acids, such as stearic acid. Oils to be employed in injections must meet officially stated requirements of iodine number and saponification number.

Although the toxicities of vegetable oils are generally considered to be relatively low, some patients exhibit allergic reactions to specific oils. Thus, when vegetable oils are employed in parenteral products, the label must state the specific oil present. The most commonly used fixed oils in injections are corn oil, cottonseed oil, peanut oil, and sesame oil. Castor oil and olive oil have been used on occasion. In all cases, the oil must be free of any odor or taste suggesting rancidity.

By the selective employment of solvent or vehicle, a pharmacist can prepare injectable preparations as solutions or suspensions of a medicinal substance in either an aqueous or nonaqueous vehicle. Again, the immiscibility of unemulsified fixed oils with the blood precludes their use in intravenous injections. For the most part, oleaginous injections are administered intramuscularly. Some examples of official injections employing oil as the vehicle are presented in Table 8-1.

Added Substances

The USP and the NF permit the addition of suitable substances to the official preparations intended for injection for the purpose of increasing their stability or usefulness, provided the substances are not interdicted in the individual monographs and are harmless in the amounts administered and do not interfere with the therapeutic efficacy of the preparation or with specified assays and tests. Many of these added substances are antibacterial preservatives, buffers, solubilizers, antioxidants, and other pharmaceutical adjuncts. Agents employed solely for their coloring effect are strictly prohibited in parenteral products.

The compendia direct that one or more suitable substances to prevent the growth of microorganisms must be added to parenteral products that are packaged in multiple-dose containers, regardless of the method of sterilization employed, unless otherwise directed in the individual monograph or unless the injection's active ingredients are themselves bacteriostatic. Such substances are used in concentrations that prevent the growth of or kill microorganisms in

Table 8-1. EXAMPLES OF SOME OFFICIAL INJECTIONS IN OIL*

Injection	Category
Desoxycorticosterone Acetate Injection, USP	Adrenocortical steroid
Diethylstilbestrol Injection, USP	Estrogen
Dimercaprol Injection, USP†	Antidote to arsenic, gold and mercury poisoning
Sterile Epinephrine Oil Suspension, USP	Adrenergic (bronchodilator)
Estradiol Benzoate Injection, NF	Estrogen
Estradiol Cypionate Injection, USP	Estrogen
Estradiol Dipropionate Injection, NF	Estrogen
Estradiol Valerate Injection, USP	Estrogen
Estrone Injection, NF	Estrogen
Menadione Injection, NF	Prothrombogenic
Sterile Procaine Penicillin G with Aluminum Stearate Suspension, USP‡	Antibacterial
Sterile Propyliodone Oil Suspension, USP§	Radiopaque medium (bronchographic)
Testosterone Cypionate Injection, USP	Androgen
Testosterone Enanthate Injection, USP	Androgen
Testosterone Propionate Injection, USP	Androgen

*In instances other than those indicated by footnote, the oil to be used is described by the USP and NF as any "suitable oil" and is left to the discretion of the manufacturer.

†In a mixture of benzyl benzoate and vegetable oil.

‡In refined peanut or sesame oil.

§In peanut oil.

the preparations. Because many of the usual preservative agents are toxic when given in excessive amounts or irritating when administered parenterally, special care must be exercised in the selection of the appropriate preservative agents. For the following preservatives, the indicated maximum limits prevail for use in a parenteral product unless otherwise directed: for agents containing mercury and the cationic, surface-active compounds, 0.01%; for agents like chlorobutanol, cresol, and phenol, 0.5%; for sulfur dioxide as an antioxidant, or for an equivalent amount of the sulfite, bisulfite, or metabisulfite of potassium or sodium, 0.2%. It should be recognized that it is not the percentage concentration of the added substance that is hazardous (unless it is unusually high) but rather the total amount of the preservative that is received by the patient at one time. Thus, the USP and NF caution that special care in the choice and use of preservative agents should be taken when the amount of preparation to be administered exceeds 5 ml in volume. When antimicrobial preservatives or antioxidants are used in a parenteral product, it is a requirement that they be identified and the amounts present be plainly declared on the label of the container. Many parenteral products are given in large volumes of 1000 ml or more—for example, Dextrose Injection, USP, and Dextrose and Sodium Chloride Injection, USP. The use of antimicrobial preservatives in these and other large volume parenterals is strictly prohibited, lest an extremely large dose of preservative agent be administered to the patient along with the nutrient or therapeutic solution. On the other hand, many small volume parenterals, as Insulin Injection, USP, have as a monographic requirement, a designated amount of a specified preservative.

In addition to the stabilizing effect of the additives, the air within an injectable product is frequently replaced with an inert gas, such as nitrogen, to enhance the stability of the product by preventing chemical reaction between the oxygen in the air and the drug.

Methods of Sterilization

The term *sterilization*, as applied to pharmaceutical preparations, means the complete destruction of all living organisms and their spores of their complete removal from the preparation. The USP outlines five methods for the sterilization of pharmaceutical products:[1]

1. Steam sterilization
2. Dry-heat sterilization
3. Sterilization by filtration
4. Gas sterilization
5. Sterilization by ionizing radiation

The method used in attaining sterility in a pharmaceutical preparation is determined largely by the nature of the preparation and its ingredients. However, regardless of the method used, the resulting product must pass a test for sterility as proof of the effectiveness of the method and the performance of the equipment and the personnel.

In the following discussion, it is not the intent to reproduce the precise details of each of the methods of sterilization in the USP but rather to point out the general features of each of the methods and to show their utility.

Steam Sterilization

Steam sterilization is generally conducted in an autoclave (or in a pressure cooker on a small scale as in a community pharmacy) and employs steam under pressure. It is recognized as the method of choice in most cases where the product is capable of withstanding such treatment.

Most pharmaceutical products are adversely affected by heat and cannot be heated safely to the temperature required for dry-heat sterilization (about 170°C). When moisture is present, bacteria are coagulated and destroyed at a considerably lower temperature than when moisture is absent. In fact, bacterial cells with a large percentage of water are generally killed rather easily. Spores, which contain a relatively low percentage of water, are comparatively difficult to destroy. The mechanism of microbial destruction in moist heat is thought to be by denaturation and coagulation of some of the organism's essential protein. It is the presence of the hot moisture within the microbial cell that permits destruction at relatively low temperature. Death by dry heat is thought to be by the dehydration of the microbial cell followed by a slow burning or oxidative process. Since it is not possible to raise the temperature of steam

[1] *United States Pharmacopeia* XIX, pp. 709–714, 1975.

above 100° under atmospheric conditions, pressure is employed to achieve higher temperatures. It should be recognized that the temperature, not the pressure, is destructive to the microorganisms and that the application of pressure is solely for the purpose of increasing the temperature of the system. Time is another important factor in the destruction of microorganisms by heat. Most modern autoclaves have gauges to indicate to the operator the internal conditions of temperature and pressure and a timing device to permit the desired exposure time for the load. The usual steam pressures, the temperatures obtainable under these pressures, and the approximate length of time required for sterilization after the system reaches the indicated temperatures are as follows:

10 pounds pressure (115.5°), for 30 minutes
15 pounds pressure (121.5°), for 20 minutes
20 pound pressure (126.5°), for 15 minutes.

As can be seen, the greater the pressure applied, the higher the temperature obtainable and the less the time required for sterilization.

The temperature at which most autoclaves are routinely operated is usually 121°, as measured at the steam discharge line running from the autoclave. It should be understood that the temperature attained in the chamber of the autoclave must also be reached by the interior of the load being sterilized, and this temperature must be maintained for an adequate time. The penetration time of the moist heat into the load may vary with the nature of the load, and the exposure time must be adjusted to account for this latent period. For example, a solution packaged in a thin-walled 50-ml ampule may reach a temperature of 121° in from 6 to 8 minutes after that temperature is registered in the steam discharge line, whereas 20 minutes or longer may be required to reach that temperature within a solution packaged in a completely filled thick-walled 1000-ml glass bottle. An estimate of these latent periods must be added to the total time in order to ensure adequate exposure times. Since this sterilization process depends upon the presence of moisture and an elevated temperature, air is removed from the chamber as the sterilization process is begun, since a combination of air and steam yields a lower temperature than does steam alone under the same condition of pressure. For instance, at 15 pounds pressure the temperature of saturated

steam is 121.5°, but a mixture of equal parts of air and steam will reach only about 112°.

In general, this method of sterilization is applicable to pharmaceutical preparations and materials that can withstand the required temperatures and are penetrated by, but not adversely affected by, moisture. In sterilizing aqueous solutions by this method, the moisture is already present, and all that is required is the elevation of the temperature of the solution for the prescribed period of time. Thus solutions packaged in sealed containers, as ampules, are readily sterilized by this method. The method is also applicable to bulk solutions, glassware, surgical dressings, and instruments. It is not useful in the sterilization of oils, fats, oleaginous preparations, and other preparations not penetrated by the moisture or the sterilization of exposed powders that may be damaged by the condensed moisture.

Dry-Heat Sterilization

Dry-heat sterilization is usually carried out in sterilizing ovens designed specifically for this purpose. The ovens may be heated either by gas or electricity and are generally thermostatically controlled.

Since dry heat is less effective in killing microorganisms than is moist heat, higher temperatures and longer periods of exposure are required. These must be determined individually for each product with consideration to the size and type of product and the container and its heat distribution characteristics. In general, individual units to be sterilized should be as small as possible, and the sterilizer should be loaded in such a manner as to permit free circulation of heated air throughout the chamber. Dry-heat sterilization is usually conducted at temperatures of 160° to 170° for periods of 1 to 4 hours. Higher temperatures permit shorter exposure times for a given article; conversely, lower temperatures require longer exposure times. For example, if a particular chemical agent melts or decomposes at 170°, but is unaffected at 140°, the lower temperature would be employed in its sterilization, and the exposure time would be increased over that required to sterilize another chemical that may be safely heated to 170°.

Dry-heat sterilization is generally employed for substances that are not effectively sterilized by moist heat. Such substances include fixed oils, glycerin, various petroleum products such as petrolatum, liquid petrolatum (mineral oil), and paraffin and various heat-stable powders such as zinc oxide. Dry-heat sterilization is also an effective method for the sterilization of glassware and surgical instruments. Dry-heat sterilization is the method of choice when dry apparatus or dry containers are required, as in the handling or packaging of dry chemicals or nonaqueous solutions.

Sterilization by Filtration

Sterilization by filtration, which depends upon the physical removal of microorganisms by adsorption on the filter medium or by a sieving mechanism, is used for the sterilization of heat-sensitive solutions. Medicinal preparations sterilized by this method are required to contain a bacteriostatic agent unless otherwise directed.

The available bacterial filters include (1) test-tube shaped filters called "filter candles" which are made of compressed infusorial earth (Berkefeld and Mandler filters); (2) filter candles made of unglazed porcelain (Pasteur-Chamberland, Doulton, and Selas filters); (3) disks of compressed asbestos fastened in a special holder in the filtration apparatus (Seitz, and Swinney filters); (4) glass Buchner-type funnel with a fused fritted glass holder (Millipore). In practice, the filter, its accessories, and the receiving vessel must all be rendered sterile by suitable means; then the solution to be sterilized is passed through the filter as rapidly as possible (using positive pressure at the non-sterile end of the system or suction at the receiving end, if necessary) and collected in the sterile receiving vessel. This method of sterilization demands rigid adherence to aseptic technique. The apparatus must be thoroughly inspected prior to its use for cracks or breaks that may render it ineffective as a bacterial filter.

The commercially available filters are produced with a variety of pore-size specifications. It would be well to mention briefly one type of these modern filters, the Millipore filters.[1] Millipore filters are thin plastic membranes of cellulosic esters with millions of pores per square inch of filter surface. The pores are made to be extremely uniform in size and occupy approximately 80% of the filter membrane's volume, the remaining 20% being the solid filter material. This high degree of porosity permits flow rates much in excess of other filters having the same particle-retention capability. Millipore filters are made from a variety of polymers to provide membrane characteristics required for the filtration of almost any liquid or gas system. Also, the filters are made of various pore sizes to meet the selective filtration requirements of the operator. They are available in pore sizes from 14 to 0.01 microns. For comparative purposes, the period that ended the last sentence is approximately 500 microns in size. The size of the smallest particle visible to the naked eye is about 40 microns, a red blood cell is about 6.5

[1] Millipore Filter Corporation, Bedford, Massachusetts.

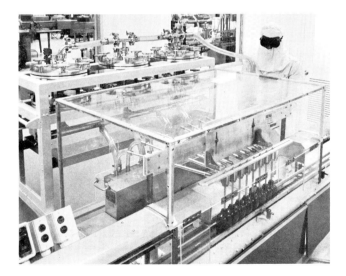

Fig. 8-2. *Sterilization by filtration. An eight-head bottle-filling machine using three large sterilizing filters for sterile filling of bottles in large scale pharmaceutical production. (Courtesy of Millipore Corporation.)*

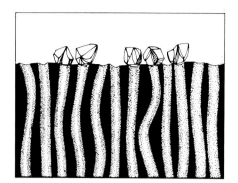

Fig. 8-3. *Membrane filters act as microporous screens which retain on their surface all particles and microorganisms larger than the rated pore size. (Courtesy of Millipore Corporation.)*

microns, the smallest bacteria, about 0.2 micron, and a polio virus, about 0.01 micron.

Although the pore size of a bacterial filter is of prime importance in the removal of microorganisms from a liquid, there are other factors such as the electrical charge on the filter and that of the microorganism, the pH of the solution, the temperature, and the pressure or vacuum applied to the system.

The major advantages of bacterial filtration include its speed in the filtration of small quantities of solution, its ability to sterilize effectively thermolabile materials, the relatively inexpensive equipment required, and the complete removal of living and dead microorganisms as well as other particulate matter from the solution. The disadvantages are less numerous and apply mainly to certain filters which have a tendency to absorb some active ingredients from the solution being filtered (infusorial earth) and to impart an alkalinity to the solution being filtered (asbestos filters). These disadvantages have largely been obviated through the use of the membrane filters. One serious disadvantage to the use of bacterial filters is the possibility of a flaw in the construction of the filter and thus some uncertainty of sterility, a circumstance not true of methods involving dry- or moist-heat sterilization in which the procedures are just about guaranteed to give effective sterilization. Also, filtration of large volumes of liquids would require more time, particularly if the liquid were viscous, than would, say, steam sterilization. In essence, the bacterial filters are useful when heat cannot be used and also for small volumes of liquids.

Bacterial filters may be used conveniently and economically in the community pharmacy

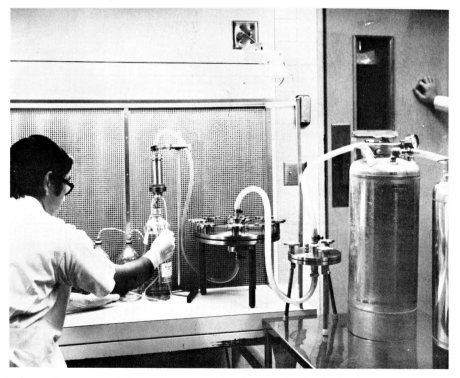

Fig. 8-4. *Hyperalimentation solutions being prepared in a laminar flow hood using Millipore sterilizing filtration in the hospital pharmacy. (Courtesy of Millipore Corporation.)*

to filter extemporaneously prepared solutions (as ophthalmic solutions) that are required to be sterile. By this method, it would matter little if the liquid were thermolabile or thermostable, since heat is not employed in any case.

Gas Sterilization

Some heat-sensitive and moisture-sensitive materials can be sterilized much better by exposure to ethylene oxide or propylene oxide gas than by other means. These gases are highly flammable when mixed with air but can be employed safely when properly diluted with an inert gas such as carbon dioxide or a suitable fluorinated hydrocarbon. Such mixtures are commercially available.

Sterilization by this process requires specialized equipment resembling autoclaves, and many combination steam autoclaves-ethylene oxide sterilizers are commercially available. Greater precautions are required for this method of sterilization than for some of the others, since the variables—for instance, time, temperature, gas concentration, and humidity—are not as firmly quantitated as those of dry-heat and steam sterilization. In general, sterilization with gas is enhanced, and the exposure time required is reduced, by increasing the relative humidity of the system (to about 60%) and by increasing the exposure temperature (to between 50 and 60°C). If the material being sterilized cannot tolerate either the moisture or the elevated temperature, exposure time will have to be increased. Generally, sterilization with ethylene oxide gas requires from 4 to 16 hours of exposure. Ethylene oxide is thought to function as a sterilizing agent by its interference with the metabolism of the bacterial cell.

The great penetrating qualities of ethylene oxide gas make it a useful sterilizing agent in certain special applications, as in the sterilization of medical and surgical supplies and appliances such as catheters, needles, and plastic disposable syringes in their final plastic packaging just prior to shipment. The gas is also used to sterilize certain heat-labile enzyme preparations, certain antibiotics, and other drugs, with tests being performed to assure of the absence of chemical reaction or other deleterious effects on the drug substance.

Sterilization by Ionizing Radiation

Techniques are available for the sterilization of some types of pharmaceuticals by gamma rays and by cathode rays, but the application of such techniques is limited because of the highly specialized equipment required and the effects of irradiation on products and their containers.

The exact mechanism by which irradiation sterilizes a drug or preparation is still subject to investigation. One of the proposed theories involves an alteration of the chemicals within or supporting the microorganism to form deleterious new chemicals capable of destroying the cell. Another theory proposes that vital structures of the cell, such as the chromosomal nucleoprotein, are disoriented or destroyed. It is probably a combination of irradiation effects that causes the cellular destruction, which is complete and irreversible.

Sterility Tests

Regardless of the method of sterilization employed, pharmaceutical preparations required to be sterile must undergo sterility tests to confirm the absence of microorganisms. Both the USP and NF have outlined the required procedures, and these detailed methods should be referred to whenever the tests are performed. The compendia direct that the sterility tests should be conducted by personnel having had expert training and experience in rigid aseptic techniques.

Pyrogens and Pyrogen Testing

As indicated earlier, *pyrogens* are fever-producing organic substances arising from microbial contamination and responsible for many of the febrile reactions which occur in patients following injection. Pyrogenic materials may be the dead microorganisms themselves. Pyrogenic materials are water-soluble complex polysaccharides. Because they are water-soluble, they may remain in water even after sterilization by autoclaving or by bacterial filtration.

Manufacturers of water for injection may employ any suitable method for the removal of pyrogens from their product. Because pyrogens are organic substances, one of the more common means of facilitating their removal is by oxidizing them to easily eliminated gases or to nonvolatile solids, both of which are easily separated from water by fractional distillation. Potassium permanganate is usually employed as the oxidizing agent, with its efficiency being increased by the addition of a small amount of barium hydroxide serving to impart alkalinity to the solution and to make nonvolatile barium salts of any acidic compounds that may be present. These two reagents are added to water that has previously been distilled several times, and the distillation process is repeated with the chemical-free distillate being collected under strict aseptic conditions. When properly conducted, this method results in a highly purified, sterile, and pyrogen-free water. However, in each instance the official pyrogen test must be performed for assurance of the absence of these fever-producing materials.

PYROGEN TEST. The USP Pyrogen Test utilizes healthy rabbits that have been properly maintained in terms of environment and diet prior to performance of the test. Normal, or "control" temperatures are taken for each animal to be used in the test. These temperatures are used as the base for the determination of any temperature increase resulting from the injection of a test solution. In a given test, rabbits are used whose temperatures do not differ by more than one degree from each other and whose body temperatures are considered to be unelevated. The actual procedure of the test is as follows:[1]

Render the syringes, needles, and glassware free from pyrogens by heating at 250° for not less than 30 minutes or by other suitable method. Warm the product to be tested to approximately 37°.

Inject into an ear vein of each of three rabbits 10 ml of the product per kg of body weight within 40 minutes subsequent to the control temperature reading. Record the temperature at 1, 2, and 3 hours subsequent to the injection.

If no rabbit shows an individual rise in temperature at 0.6° or more above its respective control temperature, and if the sum of the three temperature rises does not exceed 1.4°, the material under examination meets the requirements for the absence of pyrogens. If any rabbits show a temperature rise of 0.6° or more, or if the sum of the temperature rises exceeds 1.4°, repeat the test using five other rabbits. If not more than three of the eight rabbits show individual rises in temperature of 0.6° or more, and if the sum of the eight temperature rises does not exceed

[1]Adapted from *The United States Pharmacopeia*, XIX, 1975, p. 613.

3.7°, the material under examination meets the requirements for the absence of pyrogens.

The Preparation of Parenteral Products

Once the formulation for a particular parenteral product is determined, including the selection of the proper solvents or vehicles and additives, the production pharmacist must follow rigid aseptic procedures in preparing the injectable products. In most manufacturing plants the area in which parenteral products are made is maintained bacteria-free through the use of ultraviolet lights, a filtered air supply, sterile manufacturing equipment, such as flasks, connecting tubes, and filters, and sterilized work clothing worn by the personnel in the area.

In the preparation of parenteral solutions, the required ingredients are dissolved according to good pharmaceutical practice either in water for injection, in one of the alternate solvents, or in a combination of solvents. The solutions are then usually filtered until sparkling clear through either sintered glass, porcelain, hard filter paper, or most commonly through a membrane-type filter. After filtration, the solution is transferred as rapidly as possible and with the least possible exposure into the final containers. The product is then sterilized, preferably by autoclaving, and samples of the finished product are tested for sterility and pyrogens. In instances in which sterilization by autoclaving is impractical due to the nature of the ingredients, the individual components of the preparation that are heat or moisture labile may be sterilized by other appropriate means and added aseptically to the sterilized solvent or to a sterile solution of all of the other components sterilizable by autoclaving.

Suspensions of drugs intended for parenteral use may be prepared by reducing the drug to a very fine powder with a ball mill, micronizer, colloid mill, or other appropriate equipment and then suspending the material in a liquid in which it is insoluble. It is frequently necessary to sterilize separately the individual components of a suspension before combining them, as frequently the integrity of a suspension is destroyed by autoclaving. Autoclaving of a parenteral suspension may alter the viscosity of the

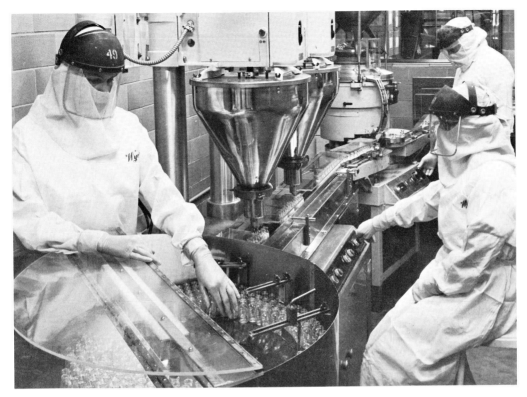

Fig. 8-5. *Sterile filling of vials. (Courtesy of Wyeth Laboratories.)*

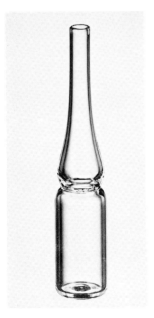

Fig. 8-6. *Ampule, before filling and sealing (Courtesy of Owens Illinois.)*

product, thereby affecting the suspending ability of the vehicle, or change the particle size of the suspended particles, thereby altering both the pharmaceutic and the therapeutic characteristics of the preparation. If a suspension remains unaltered by autoclaving, this method is generally employed to sterilize the final product. Since parenterally administered emulsions, which are dispersions or suspensions of a liquid throughout another liquid, are generally destroyed by autoclaving, an alternate method of sterilization must be employed for this type of injectable.

Some injections are packaged as dry solids rather than in conjunction with a solvent or vehicle due to the instability of the therapeutic agent in the presence of the liquid component. These dry powdered drugs are packaged as the sterilized powder in the final containers to be reconstituted with the proper liquid prior to use, generally to form a solution or less frequently a suspension. The method of sterilization of the powder may be dry heat or another method that is appropriate for the particular drug involved. Examples of sterile drugs pre-

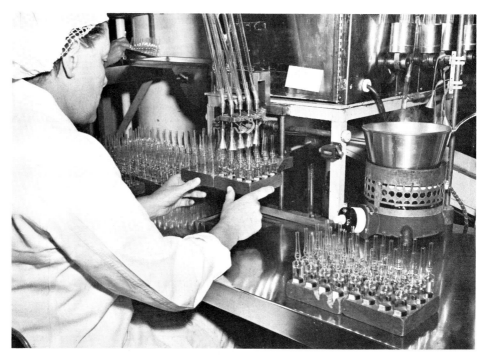

Fig. 8-7. *Ampul filling. (Courtesy of Abbott Laboratories.)*

pared and packaged *without* the presence of pharmaceutical additives as buffers, preservatives, stabilizers, tonicity agents, and other substances include:

Sterile Amobarbital Sodium, USP
Sterile Ampicillin Sodium, USP
Sterile Chlordiazepoxide Hydrochloride, USP
Sterile Phenobarbital Sodium, USP
Sterile Phenytoin Sodium, USP

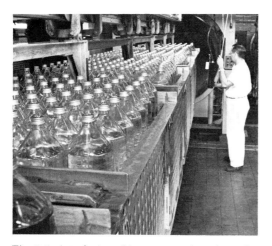

Fig. 8-8. *Autoclaving of intravenous electrolyte solutions. (Courtesy of Abbott Laboratories.)*

Sterile Polymyxin B Sulfate, USP
Sterile Secobarbital Sodium, USP
Sterile Streptomycin Sulfate, USP
Sterile Urea, USP
Sterile Vancomycin Hydrochloride, USP
Sterile Vinblastine Sulfate, USP
Sterile Viomycin Sulfate, USP

Those sterile drugs formulated *with* pharmaceutical additives and intended to be reconstituted prior to injection include the following:

Amphotericin B for Injection, USP
Corticotropin for Injection, USP
Dactinomycin for Injection, USP
Erythromycin Lactobionate for Injection, USP
Hydrocortisone Sodium Succinate for Injection, USP
Methohexital Sodium for Injection, USP
Nafcillin Sodium for Injection, USP
Oxacillin Sodium for Injection
Oxytetracycline Hydrochloride for Injection, USP
Penicillin G Potassium for Injection, USP
Prednisolone Sodium Succinate for Injection, USP
Streptomycin Sodium for Injection, USP
Tetracycline Hydrochloride for Injection, USP
Thiopental Sodium for Injection, USP

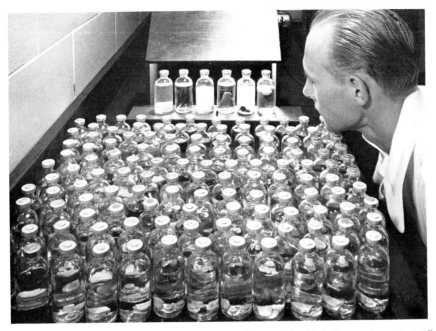

Fig. 8-9. *Testing compatibility of rubber closures with the solution with which they are in contact. (Courtesy of Abbott Laboratories.)*

In certain instances, a liquid is packaged along with the dry powder for use at the time of reconstitution. This liquid is sterile and may contain some of the desired pharmaceutical additives as the buffering agents. More frequently, the solvent or vehicle is not provided along with the dry product, but the labeling on the injection generally lists suitable solvents. Sodium chloride injection or sterile water for injection are perhaps the most frequently employed solvents used to reconstitute dry-packaged injections. The dry powders are packaged in containers large enough to permit proper shaking with the liquid component when the latter is aseptically injected through the container's rubber or plastic closure during its reconstitution. To facilitate the dissolving process, the dry powder is prevented from caking upon standing by the appropriate means, including its preparation by lyophilization.[1] Powders so treated form a honeycomb, lattice structure that is rapidly penetrated by the liquid, and solution is rapidly effected because of the large surface area of powder exposed.

[1] Lyophilization, a process also known as "freeze drying," involves the removal of water from products in the frozen state at extremely low pressures. The process is generally used to dry products that are thermolabile and would be destroyed or otherwise adversely affected by heat-drying.

Packaging, Labeling, and Storage of Injections

Containers for injections, including the closures, must not interact physically or chemically with the preparation so as to alter its strength or efficacy. If the container is made of glass, it must be clear and colorless or of a light amber color to permit the inspection of its contents. The type of glass suitable and preferred for each parenteral preparation is usually stated in the individual monograph. Injections are placed either in single-dose containers or in multiple-dose containers. By definition:

Single-dose Container—A single-dose container is a hermetic container holding a quantity of sterile drug intended for parenteral administration as a single dose, and which when opened cannot be re-sealed with assurance that sterility has been maintained.

Multiple-dose Container—A multiple-dose container is a hermetic container that permits withdrawal of successive portions of the contents without changing the strength, quality, or purity of the remaining portion.

Single-dose containers, commonly called ampuls, are sealed by fusion of the glass container under aseptic conditions. The glass con-

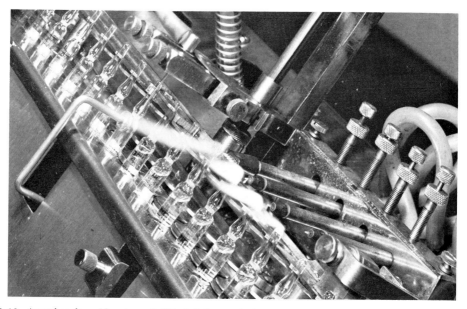

Fig. 8-10. *Ampul sealing. (Courtesy of Abbott Laboratories.)*

tainer is made so as to have a neck portion that may be easily separated from the body of the container without fragmentation of the glass. After opening, the contents of the ampul may be drawn into a syringe with a hypodermic needle. Once opened, the ampul cannot be resealed, and any unused portion may not be retained and used at a later time, since the contents would have questionable sterility. The types of glass for parenteral product containers have already been pointed out in Chapter 2, and the student should recall that Types I, II, and III are suitable for parenteral products, with Type I being the most resistant to chemical deterioration. The type of glass to be used as the container for a particular injection is indicated in the individual monograph for that preparation.

One of the prime requisites of solutions for parenteral administration is clarity. They should be sparkling clear and free of all particu-

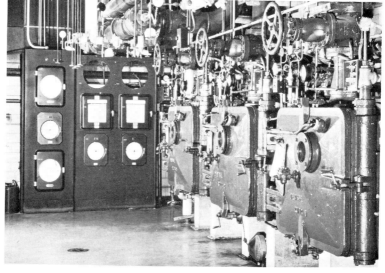

Fig. 8-11. *Antibiotic lyophilizers. (Courtesy of Abbott Laboratories.)*

late matter, that is, all of the mobile, undissolved substances which are unintentionally present. Included are such contaminants as dust, cloth fibers, glass fragments, material leached from the glass or plastic containers or seals, and any other material which may find its way into the product during its manufacture or administration, or develop during storage.

In order to prevent the entrance of unwanted particles into parenteral products, a number of precautions must be taken during the manufacture, storage, and use of the products. During manufacture, for instance, the parenteral solution is usually final filtered before being placed into the parenteral containers. The containers are carefully selected to be chemically resistant to the solution being added and of the highest available quality to minimize the chances of container components being leached into the solution. It has been recognized for some time, that some of the particulate matter found in parenteral products is generated from leached material from the glass or plastic containers. Once the container is selected for use, it must be carefully cleaned to be free of all extraneous matter. During container-filling, extreme care must be exercized to prevent the entrance of air-borne dust, lint or other contaminants into the container. The provision of filtered and directed air flow in production areas is useful in reducing the likelihood of contamination. Laminar flow hoods have been developed which allow for the draft-free flow of clean, filtered air over the work area. These hoods are commonly found in the hospital setting for both the manufacture and the incorporation of additives into parenteral and ophthalmic products. The personnel involved in the manufacture of parenterals must be made acutely aware of the importance of cleanliness and aseptic techniques. They are provided uniforms made of monofilament fabrics that do not shed lint. They wear face hoods, caps, gloves and disposable shoe covers to prevent contamination.

After the containers are filled and hermetically sealed, they are visually inspected for particulate matter. Usually an inspector passes the filled container past a light source with a black background to observe for mobile particles. Particles of approximately 50 microns in size may be detected in this manner. Reflective particles, such as fragments of glass, may be visualized in smaller size, about 25 microns in size. Other methods are used to detect particulate matter

smaller than that which may be detected by the unaided eye including microscopic examinations as well as the use of sophisticated equipment as the Coulter Counter which electronically counts particles present in a sample presented to it. Once past the inspection following production the product may be labeled. Prior to its use, however, the pharmacist should inspect each parenteral solution dispensed for evidence of particulate matter.

Although the total significance of injecting or infusing parenteral solutions containing particulate matter into a patient has not been ascertained, it is apparent that particulate matter has the potential of inducing thrombi and vessel blockage and depending upon the chemical composition of the particles the additional potential for introducing into the patient chemical agents which are undesired and possibly toxic.

In formulating a single-dose parenteral product, the pharmacist must consider not only the physicochemical aspects of the drug, but also the intended therapeutic use of the product itself. Some single-dose preparations are prepared to be administered rapidly in small volumes, but other preparations are allowed to drip slowly into the circulatory system over a period of hours. Most small-volume parenterals are formulated so that a convenient amount of solution, say 0.5 to 2 ml, contains the usual dose of the drug although larger volumes of more diluted solutions are frequently administered intravenously and intramuscularly. Generally, several strengths of injections of a given drug are marketed to permit a wider dosage selection by the physician without being wasteful of the drug as would be the case if he administered only part of a given single-dose parenteral solution. The large-volume, single-dose preparations generally are those solutions used to expand the blood volume or to replenish nutrients or electrolytes and are given by slow intravenous drip. However, in no instance may a single-dose container permit the withdrawal and administration of greater than 1000 ml. In addition, a pharmacopeial requirement is that preparations intended for intraspinal, intracisternal, or peridural administration must be packaged only in single-dose containers as a precaution against contamination.

Frequently in the hospital, a physician may order an additional agent to be placed in a large-volume parenteral solution for infusion. In these instances, the person filling such an

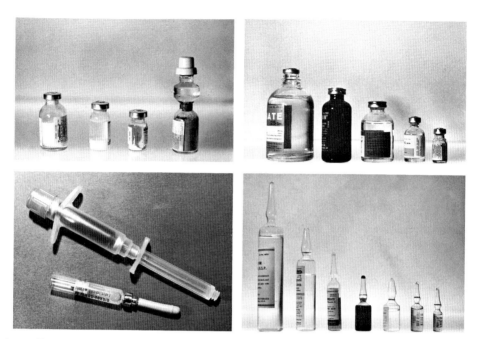

Fig. 8-12. *Examples of packaging of injectable products. A. Multiple-dose vials of suspensions and dry powders for reconstitution. B. Vials of solutions, including one of light-protective glass. C. Unit dose, disposable syringes. D. Various size ampuls.*

order must be certain that aseptic conditions are employed and that the additive is compatible with the contents of the original large volume parenteral solution. Care must also be exercized not to introduce particulate matter into the solution. Many pharmaceutical companies have developed special devices for the aseptic transfer of pharmaceutical additives to large volume parenterals. An ordinary sterile needle and syringe, preferably affixed with a filtering device, may be effectively employed to transfer solutions from one parenteral product to another.

Multiple-dose containers are affixed with rubber or plastic closures to permit the penetration of a hypodermic needle without the removal or destruction of the closure. Upon withdrawing the needle from the container, the closure reseals and protects the contents from airborne contamination. The needle may be inserted to withdraw a portion of the prepared liquid injection, or it may be used to introduce a solvent or vehicle to a dry powder intended for injection. In either instance, the sterility of the injection may be maintained so long as the needle itself is sterile at the time of entry into the container. It should be recalled that unless otherwise indicated in the monograph, multiple-dose injectables are required to contain added antibacterial preservatives. Also, unless

otherwise specified, multiple-dose containers are not permitted to be of greater than 30-ml capacity[1] to limit the number of penetrations

[1] Package-size limitations as stated for single-dose and multiple-dose containers do not apply to injections labeled for veterinary use.

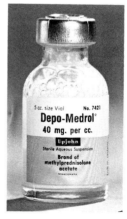

Fig. 8-13. *A typical vial used for sterile injectable products. It is made from Type I (borosilicate) glass. The rubber closure has been specially selected as regards compatibility with the product, desirable physical characteristics, etc. The overseal holds the closure in place and provides a means for ready access to the contents of the vial. (Courtesy of the Upjohn Company.)*

made into the closure and thus protect against loss of sterility. The limited volume also guards against an excessive amount of antibacterial preservative being inadvertently coadministered with the drug when unusually large doses of an injection are required, in which case a non-preserved single-dose preparation is advisable. The usual multiple-dose container contains about ten usual doses of the injection, but quantity may vary greatly with the individual preparation and manufacturer.

Because it is impossible in practice to transfer the entire volume of a single-dose container or the last dose in a multiple-dose container into a hypodermic syringe, the compendia permit a slight excess in volume of the contents of ampuls and vials over the labeled "size" or volume of the package. Table 8-2 presents the recommended "overages" permitted by the USP and NF to allow the withdrawal and administration of the labeled volumes.

The labels on containers of parenteral products must state: (1) the name of the preparation; (2) for a liquid preparation, the percentage content of drug or the amount of drug present in a specified volume, or for a dry preparation, the amount of active ingredient present and the volume of liquid to be added to the dry preparation to prepare a solution or suspension; (3) the route of administration; (4) a statement of storage conditions and an expiration date; (5) the name of the manufacturer or distributor; (6) the manufacturing lot number, which when referred to indicates all manufacturing processes for that preparation. Injections for veterinary use are labeled to that effect. Preparations intended to be used as irrigation fluids should meet the requirements for injections, except those relating to volume present in the containers, and should bear a statement indicating that the

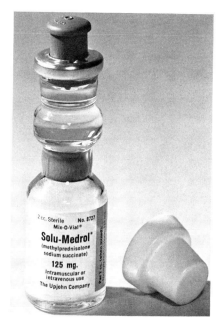

Fig. 8-14. *The Mix-O-Vial shown above is a combination vial containing dry ingredients in the bottom compartment and a liquid diluent in the top compartment, separated by a specially formulated center seal. The bottom compartment can either be liquid filled, frozen and dried to make a lyophilized product, or it may be powder filled. The top diluent contains a preservative and may or may not contain one or more active ingredients.*

To use the vial, the dust cover is removed (as shown above), pressure is applied with the thumb to the top plunger which dislodges the center seal and the vial is shaken until the solution is effected. The top of the plunger is then swabbed with a disinfectant; the syringe needle inserted through the target circle on the plunger and the contents of the vial withdrawn into the syringe.

The Mix-O-Vial offers stability of product (until it is activated), convenience, fast operation and safety as regards the right drug with the proper diluent in the correct proportions. (Courtesy of The Upjohn Company.)

Table 8-2. RECOMMENDED OVERAGES FOR OFFICIAL PARENTERAL PRODUCTS

Labeled Size	Excess Volume for Mobile Liquids	Excess Volume for Viscous Liquids
0.5 ml	0.10 ml	0.12 ml
1.0 ml	0.10 ml	0.15 ml
2.0 ml	0.15 ml	0.25 ml
5.0 ml	0.30 ml	0.50 ml
10.0 ml	0.50 ml	0.75 ml
20.0 ml	0.60 ml	0.90 ml
30.0 ml	0.80 ml	1.20 ml
50.0 ml or more	2%	3%

solution is not intended to be injected. All containers appropriately labeled should allow a sufficient area of the container to remain free of label for its full length or circumference to permit inspection of the contents. Any injection whose visual inspection reveals particulate matter other than normally suspended material should be discarded.

Each individual monograph for the official injections states the type of container (single-dose and/or multiple-dose) permitted for the injection, the type of glass preferred for the container, exemptions, if any, to usual pack-

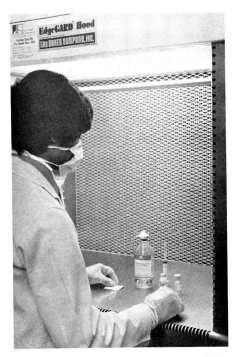

Fig. 8-15. *Pharmacist preparing a parenteral admixture in a laminar flow hood.*

age-size limitations, and any special storage instructions. Most injections prepared from chemically pure medicinal agents are stable at room temperature and may be stored without special concern or conditions. However, most biological products—insulin injection and the various vaccines, toxoids, toxins, and related products—are usually stored under refrigeration. Reference should be made to the individual monograph to find the proper storage temperature for a particular injection.

Official Injections

There are about 300 official injections, with hundreds of nonofficial injections also on the market. Tables 8-4 and 8-5 present examples of some of the most widely used injections with certain official injections of especial interest being discussed more fully in the following pages.

Small Volume Parenterals

Table 8-4 presents some of the most commonly employed injections given in small volume. Some of these injections are solutions and others suspensions. The injections are given for

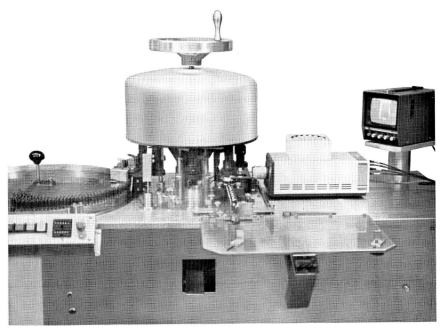

Fig. 8-16. *The AUTOSKAN automatic inspection machine which detects the presence of particulate matter in injectables with a television camera and electronics, and automatically rejects them from the production line. (Courtesy of Lakso Company, Inc.)*

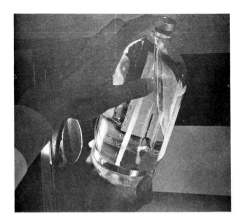

Fig. 8-17. *Examining a large volume parenteral fluid for particulate matter prior to use in the hospital.*

the therapeutic benefit of the medicinal agent present. For many of these agents, the drug is also available in dosage forms for oral administration. The injectable form is utilized commonly in emergency situations or those in which rapid drug effects are desired, in instances in which the patient is unwilling or unable to take medication orally, in instances in which there is uncertainty as to the completeness of drug absorption by other routes of administration and such assurance of total drug availability is desired by the physician.

Among the most used of the small volume injections are the various insulin preparations described below. Insulin, the active principle of the pancreas, enables the diabetic patient to utilize carbohydrates and fats in a comparatively satisfactory manner. Insulin promotes the oxidation of glucose, lowers the blood sugar level, and regulates the formation of sugar from noncarbohydrate sources. Thus, insulin, which is effectively administered only by injection, is used in the treatment of *diabetes mellitus*, in instances in which the condition cannot be controlled satisfactorily by dietary regulation alone or by oral hypoglycemic drugs. Insulin may also be used to improve the appetite and increase the weight in selected cases of nondiabetic malnutrition and is frequently added to intravenous infusions.

Insulin Injection, USP

Insulin Injection, USP is a sterile acidified aqueous solution of insulin. Commercially, the solution is prepared from beef or pork pancreas or both. The source must be stated on the labeling. The first insulin developed for clinical use was an amorphous insulin. This type has since been replaced by a more purified crystalline insulin composed of zinc-insulin crystals which produces a clear aqueous solution. Until recently, insulin injection ("regular insulin") has been produced at a pH of 2.8 to 3.5. This was necessary, because particles formed in the vial when the pH was increased above the acid range. However, recent changes in the manufacturing methods resulting in the production of insulin of greater purity has allowed for the preparation of insulin injection having a neutral pH. The neutralized product has been shown to exhibit greater stability than the acidic product. The USP requires the word "neutral" to appear on the label of insulin injection prepared from neutral solution.

Insulin Injection is prepared to contain 40, 80, 100, or 500 USP Insulin Units in each ml. The first three strengths are packaged in 10-ml multiple-dose vials and latter strength in 20-ml vials. The labeling must state the potency, in USP Insulin Units in each ml, and the

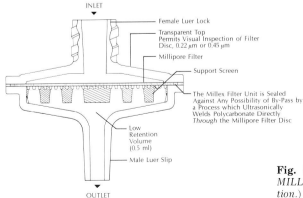

INLET
▼

Female Luer Lock

Transparent Top
Permits Visual Inspection of Filter
Disc, 0.22 μm or 0.45 μm

Millipore Filter

Support Screen

The Millex Filter Unit is Sealed
Against Any Possibility of By-Pass by
a Process which Ultrasonically
Welds Polycarbonate Directly
Through the Millipore Filter Disc

Low
Retention
Volume
(0.5 ml)

Male Luer Slip

▼
OUTLET

Fig. 8-18. *Cutaway showing composition of the MILLEX filter unit. (Courtesy of Millipore Corporation.)*

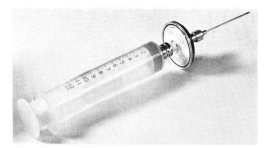

Fig. 8-19. *Luer-Lock syringe adapted with a MILLEX Filter Unit and hypodermic needle. (Courtesy of Millipore Corporation.)*

expiration date, which must not be later than 24 months after the date of distribution from the manufacturer's storage. As an added precaution against the inadvertent use of the incorrect strength of insulin by the patient during self-administration of the drug, the package

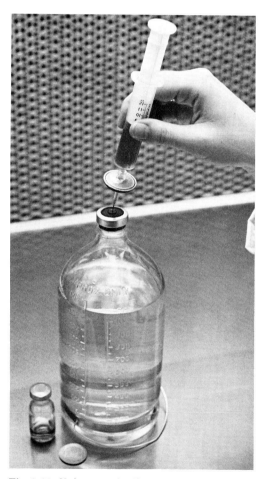

Fig. 8-20. *Utilization of a filter syringe for the aseptic addition of an additive to a large volume parenteral solution. (Courtesy of Millipore Corporation.)*

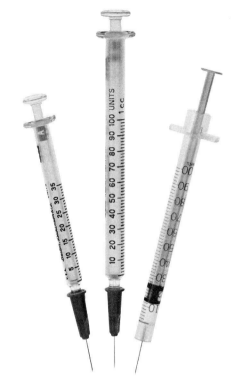

Fig. 8-21. *Examples of insulin syringes calibrated in Units. (Courtesy of Becton, Dickinson and Company.)*

colors vary, depending upon the strength of the insulin. For instance, all insulins (of the various types) containing 40 units per ml, have red in their package design, all 80 units per ml insulins have green, 100 units per ml have orange, and the 500 units per ml preparation has brown with diagonal white stripes.

Insulin injection is a colorless to straw-colored solution, depending upon its concentration; that containing 500 Units per ml is straw-colored. It is substantially free from turbidity. A small amount of glycerin (1.4 to 1.8%) is added for stability and 0.1 to 0.25% of either phenol or cresol is added for preservation. Insulin remains stable if stored in a cold place, preferably the refrigerator. Freezing should be avoided, as this reduces potency.

The various insulin preparations differ as to their rapidity of action (onset of action) after injection, their peak of action, and their duration of action (Table 8-3). Insulin injection, being a solution, is categorized as a prompt-acting insulin preparation. Insulin preparations that are suspensions are slower acting. Only insulin injection may be administered intravenously (in an emergency); all others, as well as

Table 8-3. APPROXIMATE ONSET OF ACTION, PEAK OF ACTION, AND DURATION OF ACTION OF THE OFFICIAL INSULIN PREPARATIONS

Preparation	Physical Form	Time, in hours, required for action		
		Onset	Peak	Duration
Insulin Injection	Solution	Rapid ($\cong$1 hr)	2–3	5–7
Prompt Insulin Zinc Suspension	Suspension	″ ″	4–8	12–16
Globin Zinc Insulin Injection	Solution	Intermediate ($\cong$1–2 hrs)	6–12	18–24
Isophane Insulin Suspension	Suspension	″ ″	10–12	24–28
Insulin Zinc Suspension	Suspension	″ ″	10–12	24–28
Extended Insulin Zinc Suspension	Suspension	Prolonged ($\cong$2–6 hrs)	12–16	36–more
Protamine Zinc Insulin Suspension	Suspension	″ ″	16–24	36–more

insulin injection, are normally given subcutaneously, usually ½ to 2 hours before a meal so that its physiological effects will parallel the absorption of glucose. The dosage is individually determined, and the usual dosage range, as stated by the USP is 5 to 100 USP Units. The insulin injection containing 500 units per ml is employed in insulin coma therapy and in cases of insulin resistance requiring very large doses.

Commercial Product: Regular Iletin (Lilly)

Globin Zinc Insulin Injection, NF

Globin Zinc Insulin Injection, USP, is a sterile solution modified by the addition of zinc chloride and globin. The globin is obtained from globin hydrochloride prepared from beef blood. The injection is an almost colorless liquid, substantially free from turbidity and insoluble matter. About 1.5% glycerin and either 0.15 to 0.20% cresol or from 0.20 to 0.26% phenol are added for stability and preservation. The injection's label bears an expiration date of not more than 18 months after the immediate container was filled. Injections are available containing either 40, 80, or 100 USP Insulin Units per ml of injection, packaged in 10-ml vials. The injection is best stored in a refrigerator avoiding freezing.

Globin zinc insulin is an intermediate-acting insulin preparation, having a duration of action between that produced by short-acting regular

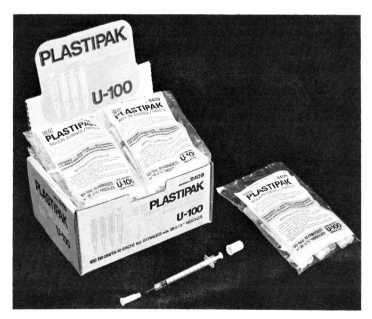

Fig. 8-22. *Example of packaging of disposable sterile insulin syringes and needles. (Courtesy of Becton, Dickinson and Company.)*

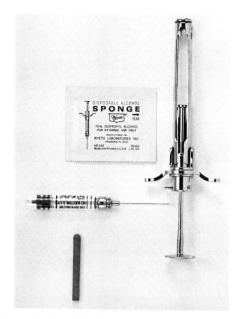

Fig. 8-23. *The TUBEX closed injection system, which delivers accurately measured doses with each sterile, prefilled cartridge-needle unit. (Courtesy of Wyeth Laboratories.)*

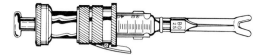

Fig. 8-24. *Diagram of the BUSHER Automatic Injector, utilized by patients who find it difficult to administer medication by self-injection. (Courtesy of Becton, Dickinson Company.)*

insulin injection and the long-acting insulin preparations.

The dose of the injection, subcutaneously, is individualized to the needs of the diabetic patient, with the usual dosage range being 10 to 80 USP units.

Isophane Insulin Suspension, USP

Isophane Insulin Suspension, USP, is a sterile suspension, in an aqueous vehicle buffered with dibasic sodium phosphate to between pH 7.1 and 7.4, of insulin prepared from zinc-insulin crystals modified by the addition of protamine so that the solid phase of the suspension consists of crystals composed of insulin, zinc, and protamine. Protamine is prepared from the sperm or the mature testes of fish belonging to

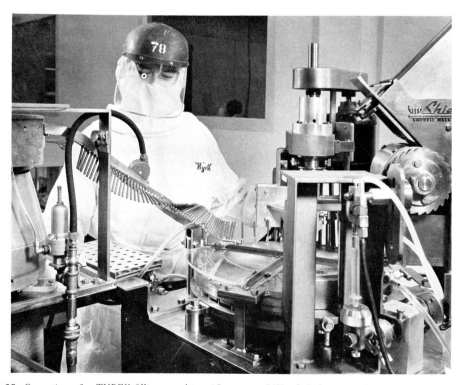

Fig. 8-25. *Operation of a TUBEX filling machine. (Courtesy of Wyeth Laboratories.)*

the genus *Oncorhynchus* and others. As mentioned earlier during the discussion of the aqueous insulin solutions, suspensions of insulin with a pH on the alkaline side are inherently of a longer duration of action than those preparations that are solutions. Insulin is most insoluble at pH 7.2.

The rod-shaped crystals of isophane insulin suspension should be approximately 30 microns in length and the suspension free from large aggregates of crystals following moderate agitation. This is necessary in order for the insulin suspension to pass freely within the needle used in injection and for the absorption of the drug from the site of injection to be consistent from one manufactured batch of injection to another. When a portion of the suspension is examined microscopically, the suspended matter is largely crystalline with only traces of amorphous material. The official injection is required to contain glycerin and phenol for stability and preservation. The specified expiration date occurring in the labeling is 18 months after the immediate container was filled by the manufacturer. The suspension is packaged in multiple-dose containers having not less than 10 ml of injection. Each ml of the injection contains either 40 or 80 Units of insulin per ml of suspension as stated on the package. The suspension is best stored in a refrigerator, but freezing must be avoided.

As indicated earlier, isophane insulin suspension is an intermediate-acting insulin preparation administered as required mainly as hormonal replacement in diabetes mellitus. The usual dosage range subcutaneously is 10 to 80 USP Units.

Commercial Product: NPH[1] Iletin (Lilly)

Insulin Zinc Suspension, USP

Insulin for Insulin Zinc Suspension, USP, is modified by the addition of zinc chloride so that the suspended particles consist of a mixture of crystalline and amorphous insulin in a ratio of approximately 7 parts of crystals to 3 parts of amorphous material. The sterile suspension is

[1] The "NPH" stands for "Neutral Protamine Hagedorn," since the preparation is about neutral (pH about 7.2), contains protamine, and was developed by Hagedorn. The term "isophane" is based on the Greek: *iso* and *phane,* meaning "equal" and "appearance" and refers to the equivalent balance between the protamine and insulin.

in an aqueous vehicle buffered to pH 7.2 to 7.5 with sodium acetate. In treating insulin with zinc chloride, it is possible to obtain both crystalline and amorphous zinc insulin. The amorphous form has the most prompt hypoglycemic effect, since the particles are the smallest and are absorbed into the system more rapidly after subcutaneous injection than are the zinc insulin crystals. Also, the larger the crystals the less prompt and the longer-acting will be the insulin suspension. By combining the crystalline and amorphous forms into one preparation, an intermediate-acting suspension is obtained. As noted in Table 8-3, the time-activity of insulin zinc suspension is essentially the same as that for isophane insulin suspension. The advantage of the former is that no additional foreign protein (other than the insulin) is present, such as protamine, which may produce local sensitivity reactions. Also, it may be combined as desired with either of the following two suspensions to produce an insulin preparation having the time-activity characteristics that most closely meet the desires and requirements of the individual patient. Suspensions available contain 40, 80, and 100 USP Insulin Units per ml packaged in 10-ml vials. The individual crystalline and amorphous particles may be seen microscopically, with the crystals being predominantly between 10 to 40 microns in maximum dimension and the amorphous particles no greater than 2 microns in maximum dimension.

In addition to the sodium acetate as a buffer, the suspension contains about 0.7% sodium chloride for tonicity and 0.10% methylparaben for preservation. The expiration date of the suspension is 24 months after the immediate container was filled. The suspension must be stored in a refrigerator with freezing being avoided. As with all such preparations, the dose depends upon the individual needs of the patient, but generally ranges between 10 and 80 USP Units.

Commercial Product: Lente Iletin (Lilly)

Extended Insulin Zinc Suspension, USP

Extended insulin zinc suspension is a sterile suspension of zinc insulin crystals in an aqueous medium buffered to between pH 7.2 and 7.5 with sodium acetate. Present also are 0.7% sodium chloride for tonicity and 0.1% methylparaben for preservation. Because the suspended matter is composed solely of zinc

Table 8-4. EXAMPLES OF SOME INJECTIONS USUALLY PACKAGED AND ADMINISTERED IN SMALL VOLUME

Injection	Physical Form	Category and Comments
Aminophylline Injection, USP	solution	Smooth muscle relaxant; usually administered I.V. as a bronchodilator in treating asthma, emphysema, congestive heart failure and other conditions.
Caffeine and Sodium Benzoate Injection, USP	solution	Administered I.M. or SubQ. as a central stimulant in treating emergency cardiac and respiratory failure.
Sterile Cortisone Acetate Suspension, USP	suspension	Adrenocortical steroid administered I.M. for rheumatoid, allergic, and other conditions.
Repository Corticotropin Injection, USP	viscous liquid	Adrenocorticotropic hormone with prolonged activity (24–72 hours) following SubQ. or I.M. injection due to presence of gelatin in the formulation.
Digoxin Injection, USP	solution	Cardiotonic given I.M. or I.V. with highly individualized and monitored dosage.
Ergotamine Tartrate Injection, USP	solution	Analgesic agent specific in migraine, given I.M. or SubQ.
Fluorescein Sodium Injection, USP	solution	Diagnostic aid given I.V. in determination of circulation time.
Histamine Phosphate Injection, USP	solution	Diagnostic aid given SubQ. in the testing of gastric secretion capacity.
Heparin Sodium Injection, USP	solution	Anticoagulant administered I.V. or SubQ. as indicated by prothrombin time determination.
Iron Dextran Injection, USP	colloidal solution	Hematinic administered I.M. or I.V. in cases of iron deficiency anemia.
Isoproterenol HCl Injection, USP	solution	Adrenergic (bronchodilator) given I.M., SubQ., or I.V.
Lidocaine HCl Injection, USP	solution	Cardiac depressant given I.V. as an antiarrhythmic; also as a local anesthetic, epidurally, by infiltration, and in peripheral nerve block.
Meperidine HCl Injection, USP	solution	Narcotic analgesic given I.M. or SubQ.
Morphine Sulfate Injection, USP	solution	Narcotic analgesic.
Oxytocin Injection, USP	solution	Oxytocic, given I.M. or I.V. obstetrically for the therapeutic induction of labor.
Sterile Penicillin G Benzathine Suspension, USP	suspension	Antibacterial given I.M. with blood levels lasting one to four weeks following single injections, depending upon the dose.
Pentobarbital Sodium Injection, USP	solution	Hypnotic-sedative, given I.M. or I.V.
Phytonadione Injection, USP	dispersion	Vitamin K (prothrombogenic) employed in hemorrhagic situations. An aqueous emulsion of phytonadione, a viscous liquid.
Procaine HCl Injection, USP	solution	Local anesthetic given by epidural, infiltration, peripheral nerve block, and spinal.
Scopolamine HBr Injection, USP	solution	Anticholinergic used in conjunction with depressants in preanesthesia, to control delirium tremens, and to prevent motion sickness.
Streptomycin Sulfate Injection, USP	viscous liquid	Antibacterial administered I.M. as a tuberculostatic.

insulin crystals, which are slowly absorbed, this preparation is classified as a long-acting insulin preparation. Because of the compatibility between the preparations, this suspension may be mixed with either insulin zinc suspension or prompt insulin zinc suspension to achieve the proper time-activity requirements of an individual patient. The usual dosage range is 10 to 80 USP Units. The suspension is commercially available in 10-ml vials providing either 40, 80, or 100 USP Insulin Units per ml. The suspension must be stored in a refrigerator with freezing being avoided. Under proper storage conditions, the expiration date of the injection is not later than 24 months after the immediate container was filled.

Commercial Preparation: Ultralente Iletin (Lilly)

Prompt Insulin Zinc Suspension, USP

The sterile suspension of insulin in Prompt Insulin Zinc Suspension, USP, is modified by the addition of zinc chloride so that the solid phase of the suspension is amorphous. The maximum dimension of the shapeless particles of zinc insulin must not exceed 2 microns. The suspension is available in 40, 80, or 100 USP Insulin Units per ml in vials of 10 ml. This preparation has the same pH and additives as extended insulin zinc suspension, and they may be mixed as desired to achieve a preparation having the desired time-activity characteristics. This is a rapid-acting insulin preparation. It must be stored in a refrigerator and not permitted to freeze. Its expiration date is not greater than 24 months after the immediate container was filled.

Commercial Product: Semilente Iletin (Lilly)

Protamine Zinc Insulin Suspension, USP

Protamine Zinc Insulin Suspension, USP, is a sterile suspension of insulin modified by the addition of zinc chloride and protamine. Because of a larger proportion of both zinc and protamine in this preparation, it has a much less prompt onset of action and a longer duration of action than does isophane insulin suspension, which also contains zinc and protamine. This suspension is stabilized and preserved with about 1.6% of glycerin and either 0.20% of cresol or 0.25% of phenol. It is packaged and stored, as are the other insulin suspensions, in 10-ml containers having either 40, 80, or 100 USP Units per ml. It has an expiration date of not later than 24 months after the immediate container was filled.

Commercial Product: Protamine, Zinc & Iletin (Lilly)

Large Volume Parenterals

Common examples of large volume parenterals in use today are presented in Table 8-5. These solutions are generally administered by intravenous infusion to replenish body fluids, electrolytes, or to provide nutrition. They are usually administered in volumes of 250 ml to liter amounts and more per day by slow intravenous drip. Because of the large volumes administered, these solutions may not contain bacteriostatic agents or other pharmaceutical additives. They are packaged in large single-dose containers.

As indicated previously, therapeutic additives as antibiotic drugs and others are frequently incorporated into large volume parenterals for coadministration to the patient. It is the responsibility of the pharmacist to be knowledgeable of the physical and chemical compatibility of the additive in the solution in which it is placed. Obviously, an incompatible combination which results in the formation of insoluble material or which affects the efficacy or potency of the therapeutic agent of the vehicle is not acceptable.

Large volume parenteral solutions are employed in *maintenance therapy* for the patient entering or recovering from surgery, or for the patient who is unconscious and unable to obtain fluids, electrolytes, and nutrition orally. The solutions may also be utilized in *replacement therapy* in patients who have suffered a heavy loss of fluids and electrolytes.

MAINTENANCE THERAPY. When a patient is being maintained on parenteral fluids for only several days, simple solutions providing adequate amounts of water, dextrose, and small amounts of sodium and potassium generally suffice. When patients are unable to take oral nutrition or fluids for slightly longer periods, say 3 to 6 days, solutions of higher caloric content may be used. In instances in which oral feeding must be deferred for periods of weeks or longer, total parenteral nutrition must be implemented to provide all of the essential nutrients to minimize tissue break-down and to

Table 8-5. EXAMPLES OF SOME INJECTIONS ADMINISTERED IN LARGE VOLUME BY INTRAVENOUS INFUSION[1]

Injection	Usual Contents	Category and Comments
Dextrose Injection, USP	2.5, 5.0, 10, 20% dextrose, and other strengths	Fluid and nutrient replenisher.
Dextrose and Sodium Chloride Injection, USP	Dextrose varying from 2.5 to 25% and sodium chloride from 0.11 to 0.9%	Fluid, nutrient, and electrolyte replenisher.
Fructose Injection, NF	10% fructose	Fluid replenisher and nutrient.
Fructose and Sodium Chloride Injection, NF	10% fructose and 0.9% sodium chloride	Fluid replenisher, nutrient, and electrolyte replenisher.
Mannitol Injection, USP	5, 10, 15, 20 and 25% mannitol	Diagnostic aid in renal function determinations; diuretic.
Mannitol and Sodium Chloride Injection, USP	5, 10, and 15% mannitol and 0.45% sodium chloride	Diuretic
Protein Hydrolysate Injection, USP	5, 7, and 10% protein hydrolysate with or without varying proportions of dextrose, alcohol, and fructose.	Fluid and nutrient replenisher.
Ringer's Injection, USP	0.86% sodium chloride, 0.03% potassium chloride, and 0.033% calcium chloride	Fluid and electrolyte replenisher.
Lactated Ringer's Injection, USP	2.7 mEq calcium, 4 mEq potassium, 130 mEq sodium and 2.45 g lactate per liter	Systemic alkalizer; fluid and electrolyte replenisher
Sodium Chloride Injection, USP	0.9% sodium chloride	Fluid and electrolyte replenisher; isotonic vehicle.

[1]These solutions are generally administered in volumes of 1 liter or more, alone, or with other drugs added.

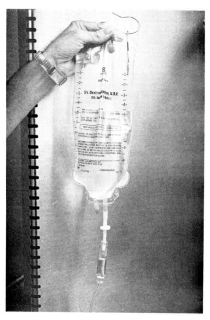

Fig. 8-26. *Intravenous solution packaged in pliable plastic.*

maintain normalcy within the body. Included in these solutions would be protein hydrolysate, carbohydrates, vitamins, minerals, electrolytes, and adequate water.

REPLACEMENT THERAPY. In instances in which there is a heavy loss of water and electrolytes, as in severe diarrhea or vomiting, greater than usual amounts of these materials may be administered initially and then maintenance therapy provided.

WATER REQUIREMENT. In normal individuals, the daily water requirement is that amount needed to replace normal and expected losses. Water is lost daily in the urine, feces, skin and from respiration. The normal daily requirement of water for adults is about 25 to 40 ml/kg of body weight, or an average of about 2,000 ml per square meter of body surface area.[1] Nomograms for the determination of body surface area from body height and weight are given in the Appendix. Children and small adults need more water per pound of body weight than do

[1]Vidt, D. G.: Use and Abuse of Intravenous Solutions, *J.A.M.A.*, 232:533, 1975.

larger adults; water requirements correlate more closely with body surface area than with weight. However, in the newborn, the volume administered in the first week or two should be about half that calculated from body surface area.

In water replacement therapy for adults, 70 ml of water per kg per day may be required in addition to the maintenance water requirements; a badly dehydrated infant may require even a greater proportion.[1] Thus, a 50-kg patient may require 3500 ml for replacement plus 2400 ml for maintenance. In order to avoid the consequences of fluid overload, especially in elderly patients, and those with renal or cardiovascular disorders, monitoring of blood pressure is desirable.

Because water administered intravenously as such may cause the osmotic hemolysis of red blood cells, and, since a patient who requires water generally requires nutrition and/or electrolytes, the parenteral administration of water is generally as a solution with dextrose or electrolytes in which the solution has sufficient tonicity (sodium chloride equivalency) to protect the red blood cells from hemolyzing.

ELECTROLYTE REQUIREMENT. Potassium, the primary intracellular cation, is particularly important for normal cardiac and smooth muscle function. The usual daily intake of potassium is about 100 mEq and the usual daily loss is about 40 mEq. Thus, any replacement therapy should include a minimum of 40 mEq plus the amount needed to replace additional losses. Sodium, the principal extracellular cation, is vital to maintain normal extracellular fluids. Average daily intake of sodium is 135 to 170 mEq (8 to 10 g of sodium chloride). The body is able to conserve sodium when this ion is lost or removed from the diet. When there is sodium loss or a deficit, the daily administration of 3 to 5 g of sodium chloride (51 to 85 mEq of sodium) should prevent a negative sodium balance.[1] Although other electrolytes and minerals as calcium, magnesium, and iron are lost from the body, they generally are not required during short-term parenteral therapy.

CALORIC REQUIREMENTS. Generally patients requiring parenteral fluids are given 5% dex-

trose to reduce the caloric deficit that usually occurs in patients undergoing maintenance or replacement therapy. The use of dextrose also minimizes ketosis and the break-down of protein. Basic caloric requirements may be estimated by body weight; in the fasting state, the average daily loss of body protein is approximately 80 g/day for a 70 kg man. Daily ingestion of at least 100 g of glucose reduces this loss by half.

PARENTERAL HYPERALIMENTATION. This is the infusion of large amounts of basic nutrients sufficient to achieve active tissue synthesis and growth. It is employed in the long-term intravenous feeding of protein solutions containing high concentrations of dextrose (approximately 20%), electrolytes, vitamins, and in some instances insulin. The large proportion of dextrose increases the caloric value of the solution, while keeping the volume required to be administered to a minimum. The solutions are administered slowly through a large vein, such as the subclavian. The use of the subclavian, which is located immediately beneath the clavicle and near to the heart, permits the rapid dilution of the concentrated hyperalimentation fluid and minimizes the risk of tissue or cellular damage due to the hypertonicity of the solution.

BLOOD REPLENISHMENT PREPARATIONS. Table 8-6 describes the official products used in the replenishment of blood, namely whole human blood, human red blood cells, normal human serum albumin, and human plasma protein fraction. In collecting human blood from donors for the purpose of preparing transfusions of the whole blood or the blood cells, care must be taken to prevent the blood from clotting. The following official solutions are used for this purpose.

Anticoagulant Acid Citrate Dextrose Solution, USP (ACD Solution)

Anticoagulant acid citrate dextrose solution is a sterile solution of citric acid, sodium citrate, and dextrose in water for injection. The solution is prepared by dissolving the ingredients, filtering the solution until clear, and then transferring the liquid to suitable containers and sterilizing. The final product must be pyrogen free. It may not contain bacteriostatic agents.

[1]Vidt, D. G.: Use and Abuse of Intravenous Solutions, J.A.M.A., 232:533, 1975.

Table 8-6. OFFICIAL PREPARATIONS FOR BLOOD REPLENISHMENT

Preparation	Description
Whole Human Blood, USP	Whole human blood is blood that has been drawn from selected human donors under rigid aseptic precautions. It contains citrate ion or heparin as an anticoagulant. The collected blood is stored at temperatures between 1° and 10°, held constant within a 2° range. The expiration date is not later than 21 days after the date of collection when citrate ion is used as the anticoagulant and not greater than 48 hours if heparin is used. The blood is usually contained in 1 unit (500 ml) volumes and administered by intravenous infusion first making certain of the compatibility of the donor's and recipient's blood.
Human Red Blood Cells, USP	This is whole human blood from which the plasma has been removed. The plasma may be removed from the cells by centrifugation within 6 days following the collection of the whole human blood. The blood cells are stored at the same temperatures as whole human blood, or they may be stored frozen at −65°. The frozen blood may be stored for as long as 3 years but must be used within 24 hours following removal from the freezing temperature and placement in 1° to 10° conditions.
Normal Human Serum Albumin, USP	This is a sterile preparation of serum albumin obtained by fractionating blood from healthy human donors. Not less than 96% of the protein must be albumin. It is a solution containing in each 100 ml, either 25 g of serum albumin osmotically equivalent to 500 ml of normal human plasma, or 5 g equivalent to 100 ml of normal human plasma. It is administered as a blood-volume supporter by intravenous infusion, generally in volumes equivalent to 25 to 75 g of albumin daily. The expiration date ranges from 3 to 10 years, depending upon the conditions of storage.
Human Plasma Protein Fraction, USP	This is a sterile solution of selected proteins derived from the blood plasma of adult human donors. It contains approximately 5 g of protein per 100 ml of which 83 to 90% is albumin, the remainder is alpha and beta globulins. It is generally administered in volumes of 250 to 500 ml (sometimes up to 1500 ml) as a blood volume supporter. Its expiration date is between 3 and 5 years, depending upon conditions of storage.

Two formulas are given in the USP for the preparation of the solution and are designated Solution A and Solution B:

	Solution A	Solution B
Citric acid	7.3 g	4.4 g
Sodium citrate (dihydrate)	22.0 g	13.2 g
Dextrose (monohydrate)	24.5 g	14.7 g
Water for injection, a sufficient quantity to make......................	1000 ml	1000 ml

Solution B contains the ingredients in approximately the same ratio as Solution A, but is only about 60% as concentrated. In practice, either 75 ml of Solution A or 125 ml of Solution B are employed in the preservation of 500 ml of whole blood. When the solution is packaged, the label must indicate the number of ml required per 100 ml of blood.

The solution prevents the coagulation of blood by virtue of the citrate ion's ability to bind the calcium ions of the blood to form a nonionizing calcium citrate complex, thereby preventing the calcium ions from participating in the clotting mechanism which is rendered ineffective by its absence. The dextrose adds sufficient tonicity to the solution to prevent the osmotic hemolysis of the erythrocytes during storage.

The solution is commercially available prepackaged in transfusion bottles that are only partially filled by the solution. For example, a 500-ml bottle containing 100 ml of Solution B would be suitable for the entry and preservation of 400 ml of whole blood. During collection, the blood-solution mixture is swirled gently and stored continuously in a refrigerator preferably between 1° and 10°C. Under these conditions blood may be stored safely for 21 days. Prior to its administration as a blood transfusion, the mixture is made uniform by gentle swirling and is then injected intravenously without warming, using sterile equipment.

Anticoagulant Citrate Phosphate Dextrose Solution, USP (CPD Solution)

This is a sterile solution of citric acid, sodium citrate, sodium biphosphate and dextrose in water for injection. It is used in the proportion of 70 ml of solution for each 500 ml of whole blood as an anticoagulant. This solution is less acid than the ACD solution (pH 5 to 6 for CPD vs. pH 4.5 to 5.5 for ACD) and this is thought to be of some advantage in preserving the red blood cell. The solution is also more nearly isotonic to the red blood cell and is considered better able to maintain the red cell membrane under physiological conditions.

Anticoagulant Heparin Solution, USP

Heparin sodium is used in the preparation of this anticoagulant solution. Heparin sodium is a mixture of active principles having the property of prolonging the clotting of blood. The substance is usually obtained from the lungs, intestinal mucosa or other suitable tissues of animals used for food by man. The potency of heparin is based on USP Heparin Units and must meet the requirements of not less than 120 such units per mg when derived from lungs and 140 such units per mg when derived from other tissues. The anticoagulant heparin solution contains 2250 Units per 30 ml, the amount of solution required to stabilize each 500 ml of whole blood.

Biologics

In pharmacy, the broad term *biologics* refers to such pharmaceutical products as vaccines, toxins, toxoids, antitoxins, immune serums, blood derivatives, certain diagnostic aids, and other related preparations. For the most part, biologics are administered by injection (a nota-

ble exception being the oral type of polio vaccine), and for this reason they are presented in this chapter.

Biologics are produced by manufacturers licensed to do so in accordance with the terms of the federal Public Health Service Act of 1944, and each product must meet the specified standards of the Bureau of Biologics of the federal Food and Drug Administration. Generally, each lot of a biologic product must pass rigid control requirements before it may be distributed for general use.

Biologics intended to be administered by injection are packaged and labeled in the same manner as other injections. In addition, however, the label of a biological product must include the manufacturer's name, address, and the *license number* granted him to manufacture the particular product.

With a few exceptions most biologics are stored in a refrigerator at between 2° and 8°, and freezing is avoided. In many instances it is not the biologic substance that is harmed by freezing, but rather the container which may be broken through the freezing and expansion of an aqueous vehicle so that some of the product is lost. The expiration date for biological products varies with the product and the storage temperatures employed. Generally, most biological products have an expiration date of a year

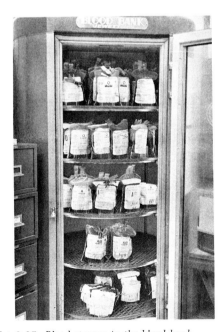

Fig. 8-27. *Blood storage in the blood bank.*

or longer after the date of manufacture or issue. Biologics must be dispensed in their original containers in order to avoid contamination and deterioration. They are sterile when packaged and are injected by aseptic techniques.

As indicated by the listings in Table 8-7, some biologics are diagnostic aids, others are prophylactic, and some are therapeutic. Although it is not within the scope of this book to undertake a discussion of immunity, some brief definitions may assist in the understanding of the use of the official products presented. Also, it is not the intent here to discuss the detailed methods of preparation for these biologics, and only brief descriptions of the products are given. If additional information is desired, the student is encouraged to read other references.[1]

IMMUNITY—The power of the body to resist and overcome infection.

NATURAL, INNATE, OR NATIVE IMMUNITY—A constitutional attribute of individuals who because of race, species specificity, endocrine balance, and other factors may be resistant to a particular toxic agent. It is something with which they are born and is not acquired through the use of biologics.

ACQUIRED IMMUNITY—A specific immunity that may be actively acquired (active immunity) or passively acquired (passive immunity).

ACTIVE IMMUNITY—Specific immunity developed in an individual in response to the introduction of antigenic substances into his body. This may occur by natural means, as by infection, in which case it is termed *naturally acquired active immunity*, or it may be developed in response to the administration of a specific vaccine or toxoid, in which case it is termed *artificially acquired active immunity*. In either case, the body builds up its own defenses in response to the antigen.

PASSIVE IMMUNITY—Immunity developed by the introduction of already formed antibodies into the body to combat the specific antigen. If the antibodies are passed to the individual naturally, as by the placental transfer of antibodies from the mother to the fetus, the term *naturally acquired passive immunity* applies. However, if the antibodies are

passed on to the individual through the injection of a specific antitoxin, the immunity is referred to as *artificially acquired passive immunity*. Passive immunity is not long-lasting.

VACCINES—Agents administered primarily for prophylactic action in the development of active immunity (acquired). Vaccines may contain living, attenuated (weakened), or killed viruses; killed rickettsia; or killed bacteria.

TOXOIDS—Toxins modified and detoxified by the use of moderate heat and chemical treatment so that the antigenic properties remain. They are employed for the development of active immunity.

TOXINS—Poisonous bacterial products that act as antigens and cause the human body to develop specific antibodies to combat their presence. Most toxins are used for diagnostic purposes to determine the susceptibility of the patient to the disease caused by the toxin-containing organism.

ANTITOXINS—Substances prepared from the blood of animals, usually horses, which have been immunized by repeated injections of specific bacterial toxins. The resulting antitoxins produce passive immunity, or they may be used for curative purposes for persons already known to be infected by the specific antigen.

ANTISERUMS—Serums prepared in the same manner as the antitoxins, except that bacteria or viruses are injected into the animal to stimulate the production of specific antibodies. The antibody-rich blood serum may be employed to produce passive immunity.

HUMAN IMMUNE SERUMS AND GLOBULINS—Serums containing the specific antibodies obtained from the blood of humans and produced as a result of having had the specific disease or having been immunized against it with a specific biologic product. They provide passive immunity.

Other Injectable Products— Pellets or Implants

Pellets or implants are sterile, small, usually cylindrical-shaped solid objects about 3.2 mm in diameter and 8 mm in length, prepared by compression and intended to be implanted subcutaneously for the purpose of providing the

---

[1] More detailed descriptions of the methods of producing the individual biologic products may be found in: Claus, E. P., Tyler, V. E. and Brady, L. R.; "Pharmacognosy," 6th Ed., Lea & Febiger, Philadelphia, 1970, Chapter 14, pp. 399–431.

Table 8-7. OFFICIAL BIOLOGICAL PRODUCTS

Biological Product	Nature of Contents	Route of Administration[1]	Use
Vaccines and Vaccine Combinations			
BCG Vaccine, NF	Dried, living culture of the bacillus Calmette-Guerin strain of *Mycobacterium tuberculosis* var. *bovis*	Intradermal	Active immunizing agent (tuberculosis)
Cholera Vaccine, USP	Suspension of killed cholera vibrios (*Vibrio comma*)	Subcutaneous or intramuscular	Active immunizing agent
Diphtheria and Tetanus Toxoids and Pertussis Vaccine, NF	Suspension of killed pertussis bacilli (*Bordetella pertussis*) in a mixture of diphtheria toxoid and tetanus toxoid	Subcutaneous or intramuscular	Active immunizing agent
Adsorbed Diphtheria and Tetanus Toxoids and Pertussis Vaccine, USP	Suspension of the precipitate obtained after treating a mixture of diphtheria and tetanus toxoids and pertussis vaccine with alum, aluminum hydroxide, or aluminum phosphate	Intramuscular	Active immunizing agent
Influenza Virus Vaccine, USP	Aqueous suspension of inactivated influenza virus prepared from extra-embryonic fluid of influenza virus-infected chick embryo. May contain an adsorbant such as calcium phosphate or protamine.	Intramuscular or subcutaneous	Active immunizing agent
Live Attenuated Measles Virus Vaccine, USP	Live measles virus grown on cultures of either chicken embryo tissue or canine renal tissue.	Subcutaneous	Active immunizing agent
Live Measles, Mumps, and Rubella Virus Vaccine, USP	Combination of viruses grown on either chicken or duck embryo tissue.	Subcutaneous	Active immunizing agent
Live Measles and Rubella Virus Vaccine, USP	Live viral vaccine with the measles virus grown on chicken embryo tissue and the rubella virus on duck embryo tissue.	Subcutaneous	Active immunizing agent
Inactivated Mumps Virus Vaccine, NF	Sterile suspension of killed mumps virus prepared in the chick extra-embryonic fluid. The virus is killed with formaldehyde solution and suspended in isotonic sodium chloride solution.	Subcutaneous	Active immunizing agent
Pertussis Vaccine, NF	Suspension of killed pertussis bacilli (*Bordetella pertussis*)	Subcutaneous	Active immunizing agent
Adsorbed Pertussis Vaccine, NF	Killed pertussis bacilli precipitated or adsorbed by the addition of alum, aluminum hydroxide, or aluminum phosphate and resuspended.	Intramuscular	Active immunizing agent
Plague Vaccine, USP	Suspension of killed plague bacilli (*Pasteurella pestis*)	Intramuscular or subcutaneous	Active immunizing agent
Poliomyelitis Vaccine, USP	Suspension of inactivated poliomyelitis virus of Types 1, 2, and 3, grown separately in primary cultures of monkey kidney tissue and combined after inactivation.	Intramuscular or subcutaneous	Active immunizing agent

Table 8-7. OFFICIAL BIOLOGICAL PRODUCTS (*Cont.*)

Biological Product	Nature of Contents	Route of Administration[1]	Use
Vaccines and Vaccine Combinations (cont.)			
Live Oral Poliovirus Vaccine, USP	A preparation of one or a combination of the three types of live, attenuated polioviruses, grown separately in primary cultures of monkey kidney tissue.	Oral	Active immunizing agent
Rabies Vaccine, USP	A preparation in liquid or dried form of killed fixed virus of rabies, obtained from brain tissue of rabbits or from duck embryo that have been infected with the virus.	Subcutaneous	Active immunizing agent
Rocky Mountain Spotted Fever Vaccine, USP	Suspension of inactivated *Rickettsia rickettsii* prepared by growing the virus on domestic fowl.	Subcutaneous	Active immunizing agent
Live Rubella Virus Vaccine, USP	Live rubella (German measles) virus grown on duck embryo or rabbit kidney tissue	Subcutaneous	Active immunizing agent
Live Rubella and Mumps Viral Vaccine, USP	Combination of rubella virus grown on cultures of duck embryo tissue and mumps virus grown on chicken embryo tissue	Subcutaneous	Active immunizing agent
Smallpox Vaccine, USP	A liquid or dried form of living virus of vaccinia that has been grown in the skin of a vaccinated bovine calf or in membranes of a chick embryo.	Percutaneous	Active immunizing agent
Typhoid Vaccine, USP	Suspension of killed typhoid bacilli (*Salmonella typhosa*)	Subcutaneous	Active immunizing agent
Typhus Vaccine, USP	Suspension of killed rickettsial organisms of a strain or strains of epidemic typhus rickettsia (*Rickettsia prowazeki*), derived from infected yolk sac membrane.	Subcutaneous	Active immunizing agent
Yellow Fever Vaccine, USP	Dried, frozen, attenuated strain of living yellow fever virus prepared by culturing the virus in the living embryo of the domestic fowl, separating, and freeze-drying.	Subcutaneous	Active immunizing agent
Toxoids			
Diphtheria Toxoid, USP	Solution of the formaldehyde-treated products of the growth of the diphtheria bacillus (*Corynebacterium diphtheriae*).	Intramuscular or subcutaneous	Active immunizing agent
Adsorbed Diphtheria Toxoid, USP	Suspension of diphtheria toxoid (as above) precipitated or adsorbed by the addition of alum, aluminum hydroxide, or aluminum phosphate.	Intramuscular or subcutaneous	Active immunizing agent

Table 8-7. OFFICIAL BIOLOGICAL PRODUCTS (*Cont.*)

Biological Product	Nature of Contents	Route of Administration[1]	Use
Toxoids (cont.)			
Diphtheria and Tetanus Toxoids, NF	Solution of mixed diphtheria toxoid and tetanus toxoid.	Intramuscular or subcutaneous	Active immunizing agent
Adsorbed Diphtheria and Tetanus Toxoids, USP	Suspension prepared by mixing adsorbed diphtheria toxoid and adsorbed tetanus toxoid.	Intramuscular or subcutaneous	Active immunizing agent
Tetanus Toxoid, USP	Solution of formaldehyde-treated products of growth of the tetanus bacillus (*Clostridium tetani*)	Subcutaneous	Active immunizing agent
Adsorbed Tetanus Toxoid, USP	Suspension of tetanus toxoid precipitated or adsorbed by the addition of alum, aluminum hydroxide, or aluminum phosphate	Intramuscular or subcutaneous	Active immunizing agent
Adsorbed Tetanus and Diphtheria Toxoids for adult use, USP	Suspension of adsorbed tetanus toxoid and adsorbed diphtheria toxoid	Intramuscular	Active immunizing agent
Antitoxins			
Botulism Antitoxin, USP	Solution of refined and concentrated proteins, chiefly globulins, containing antitoxin obtained from the blood serum or plasma of healthy horses immunized against the toxins produced by both type A and B strains of *Clostridium botulinum.*	Intramuscular or intravenous	Passive immunizing agent
Tetanus Antitoxin, USP	Solution of the refined and concentrated proteins, chiefly globulins, containihg antitoxic antibodies obtained from the blood serum or plasma of a healthy animal, usually the horse, that has been immunized against tetanus toxoid or toxin.	Intramuscular or subcutaneous (prophylactic) or intravenous (therapeutic)	Passive immunizing agent
Tetanus and Gas Gangrene Antitoxins, NF	Solution of antitoxic substances obtained from the blood of healthy animals that have been immunized against the toxins of *Clostridium tetani*, *C. perfringens*, and *C. septicum.*	Parenteral as required	Passive immunizing agent
Toxins			
Diphtheria Toxin for Schick Test, USP	Solution of the toxic products of growth of the diphtheria bacillus (*Corynebacterium diphtheriae*).	Intradermal	Diagnostic aid (dermal reactivity indicator)
Serums and Globulins			
Antirabies Serum, USP	Solution containing antiviral substances from the blood serum or plasma of a healthy animal, usually the horse, that has been immunized against rabies by means of vaccine.	Intramuscular	Passive immunizing agent

Table 8-7. OFFICIAL BIOLOGICAL PRODUCTS (*Cont.*)

Biological Product	Nature of Contents	Route of Administration[1]	Use
Serums and Globulins (cont.)			
Iodinated I 125 Serum Albumin, USP	Isotonic solution containing radio-iodinated (125_I) normal human serum albumin	Intravenous	Diagnostic aid (blood volume determination)
Iodinated I 131 Serum Albumin USP	Isotonic solution containing radio-iodinated (131_I) normal human serum albumin	Intravenous	Diagnostic aid (blood volume determination; intrathecal scanning)
Anti-A Blood Grouping Serum, USP	Agglutinates human red cells containing B-agglutinogens	. . .	Diagnostic aid (in vitro)
Anti-Rh Typing Serums, USP	Derived from human blood having specific Rh antibodies	. . .	Diagnostic aid (in vitro)
Immune Human Serum Globulin, USP	Solution of globulins containing many antibodies normally present in adult human blood. Each lot is derived from an original plasma or serum pool representing venous or placental blood from at least 1000 individuals.	Intramuscular	Passive immunizing agent (infectious hepatitis, poliomyelitis, rubella, rubeola, varicella)
Vaccinia Immune Human Globulin, USP	Sterile solution of globulins from blood plasma of human donors who have been immunized with vaccinia virus smallpox vaccine	Intramuscular	Passive immunizing agent
Pertussis Immune Human Globulin, USP	Solution of globulins derived from the blood plasma of adult human donors who have been immunized with pertussis vaccine.	Intramuscular	Passive immunizing agent
Tetanus Immune Human Globulin, USP	Solution of globulins derived from the blood plasma of adult human donors who have been immunized with tetanus toxoid.	Intramuscular	Passive immunizing agent
Miscellaneous Biological Products			
Blastomycin, NF	Liquid concentrate of the soluble growth products developed by the fungus *Blastomyces dermatitidis* when grown in the mycelial phase on a synthetic medium	Intradermal	Diagnostic aid (North American blastomycosis)
Polyvalent Crotaline Antivenin, USP	A preparation derived by drying a frozen solution of specific venom-neutralizing globulins obtained from the serum of healthy horses immunized against venoms of four species of pit vipers, *Crotalus atrox*, *C. adamanteus*, *C. terrificus*, and *Bothrops atrox*.	Intramuscular or intravenous	Passive immunizing agent

Table 8-7. Official Biological Products (*Cont.*)

Biological Product	Nature of Contents	Route of Administration[1]	Use
Miscellaneous Biological Products (cont.)			
Human Fibrinogen, USP	Fraction of normal human plasma, dried from the frozen state, which in solution has the property of being converted into insoluble fibrin when thrombin is added.	Intravenous	Coagulant (clotting factor)
Histoplasmin, USP	Liquid concentrate of the soluble growth products developed by the fungus *Histoplasma capsulatum* when grown in the mycelial phase on a synthetic medium.	Intradermal	Diagnostic aid (histoplasmosis)
Human Plasma Protein Fraction, USP	Solution of selected proteins derived from the blood plasma of adult human donors. It contains about 5% of protein, about 85% of which is albumin, the remainder alpha and beta globulins.	Intravenous	Blood-volume supporter
Trichinella Extract, USP	Aqueous extract of the killed, washed, defatted, and powdered larvae of *Trichinella spiralis*, usually obtained from inoculated rodents.	Intradermal	Diagnostic aid (trichinosis)
Tuberculin, USP	Solution of the concentrated, soluble products of growth of the tubercle bacillus, *Mycobacterium tuberculosis*. (Old Tuberculin), or, a soluble partially purified product of growth of the tubercle bacillus prepared in a special liquid medium free from protein (Purified Protein Derivative, PPD).	Intradermal	Diagnostic aid (tuberculosis)

[1] The doses to be administered and the schedule of doses vary widely with the patient, depending upon his age, exposure, previous record of immunizations, etc.

continuous release of medication over a prolonged period of time. The pellets, which are implanted under the skin (usually of the thigh or abdomen) with a special injector or by surgical incision, are used for potent hormones. Their implantation provides the patient with an economical means of obtaining long-lasting effects (up to many months after a single implantation) and obviates the need for frequent parenteral or oral hormone therapy. The implanted pellet, which may contain 100 times the amount of drug given by other routes of administration, slowly dissolves under the skin to release the drug to the tissues for absorption into the general circulation.

Pellets must not contain any binder, diluent, or excipient in order to permit total dissolution and absorption of the pellet from the site of implantation.

Official Pellets

The official pellets must meet various requirements including a test for weight variation and sterility. Pellets are aseptically packaged in tight containers, each holding one pellet.

Desoxycorticosterone Acetate Pellets, NF

Desoxycorticosterone acetate pellets usually contain 75 and 125 mg of desoxycorticosterone acetate, an adrenocortical hormone. The usual intramuscular dose of desoxycorticosterone acetate is 1 mg, and the buccal dose is 2 mg daily.

Estradiol Pellets, NF

Estradiol pellets usually contain 10 and 25 mg of the estrogen estradiol (the usual single oral or parenteral dose of estradiol is about 250 mcg).

Testosterone Pellets, NF

Testosterone pellets usually contain 75 mg of testosterone. The usual dose of testosterone is 10 mg buccally, 25 mg intramuscularly, and 300 mg by implantation. Four tablets usually are implanted for prolonged androgenic effects of the drug.

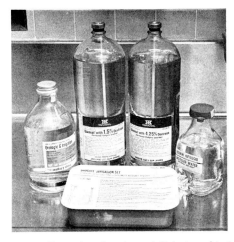

Fig. 8-28. *Examples of peritoneal dialysis and irrigation fluids.*

Irrigation and Dialysis Solutions

Solutions for irrigation of body tissues and for dialysis resemble parenteral solutions in that

Table 8-8. OFFICIAL IRRIGATION SOLUTIONS

Solution	Description
Acetic Acid Irrigation, USP	This solution is employed topically to the bladder as a 0.25% solution for irrigation. It has a pH of between 2.9 and 3.3 and is employed during urologic procedures. It is administered to wash blood and surgical debris away while maintaining suitable conditions for the tissue and permitting the surgeon an unobstructed view.
Aminoacetic Acid Irrigation, USP	This solution is employed topically to body cavities as a 1.5% solution having a pH of between 4.5 and 6.5. The solution is employed commonly in urethral surgery.
Neomycin Sulfate and Polymyxin B Sulfate Solution for Irrigation, USP	This solution is employed as a topical antibacterial in the continuous irrigation of the bladder.
Ringer's Solution, NF	This solution contains sodium chloride, potassium chloride, and calcium chloride in purified water, in the same proportions, as is present in Ringer's Injection, USP. The solution is sterile and pyrogen-free. It is used topically as an irrigation and must be labeled "not for injection."
Sodium Chloride Irrigation, USP	This solution contains 0.9% sodium chloride which is isotonic with body fluids. The solution is employed topically to wash wounds and into body cavities where absorption into the blood is not likely. The solution may also be employed rectally as an enema; for simple evacuation, 150 ml is usually employed and for colonic flush, 1500 ml may be used.
Sterile Water for Irrigation, USP	This is water for injection that has been sterilized and suitably packaged. The label must state "for irrigation only" and "not for injection." The water must not contain any antimicrobial or other added agent.

they are subject to the same stringent standards. The difference is in their use. These solutions are not injected into the vein, but employed outside of the circulatory system. Since they are generally used in large volumes, they are packaged in large volume containers, generally of the screw-cap type which permits the rapid pouring of the solution.

Irrigation Solutions

Irrigation solutions are intended to bathe or wash wounds, surgical incisions, or body tissues. Official irrigation solutions are presented in Table 8-8. In addition to the official solutions, a number of commercial products are available.

Dialysis Solutions

Dialysis may be defined as a process whereby substances may be separated from one another in solution by taking advantage of their differing diffusibility through membranes. *Peritoneal dialysis* solutions, allowed to flow into the peritoneal cavity, are used to remove toxic substances normally excreted by the kidney. In cases of poisoning or kidney failure, or in patients awaiting renal transplants, dialysis is an emergency life-saving procedure. Solutions are commercially available containing dextrose as a major source of calories, vitamins, minerals, electrolytes, and amino acids or peptides as a source of nitrogen. The solutions are made to be hypertonic (with dextrose) to plasma to avoid absorption of water from the dialysis solution into the circulation. The peritoneal cavity, containing the hypertonic fluid, acts as a semipermeable membrane and allows for the flow of undesired elements into the peritoneal dialysis fluid which is removed by peritoneal tube to collection vessels.

Hemodialysis is employed to remove toxins from the blood. In this method, the arterial blood is shunted through a polyethylene catheter through an artificial dialyzing membrane bathed in an electrolyte solution. Following the dialysis, the blood is returned to the body circulation through a vein.

There are no official dialysis solutions *per se*, however, various solutions are available commercially and the pharmacist may be called upon to provide them or to make adjustments in their composition.

Selected Reading

Anschel, J.: Solubilizing Agents for Parenteral Drugs. *Bull. Parenteral Drug Assoc.*, 20:24–27, 1966.

Ballard, B. E., and Nelson, E.: Absorption of Implanted Solid Drug. *J. Pharm. Sci.*, 51:915–924, 1962.

Best, C. H.: The History of Insulin. *Diabetes, 11*:495–503, 1962.

Carleton, F. J.: Aqueous and Nonaqueous Solvents in Parenteral Preparations. *Bull Parenteral Drug Assoc.*, 21:142–147, 1967.

Davis, N. N., Turco, S., and Sively, E.: Particulate Matter in I.V. Infusion Fluids. *Bull. Parenteral Drug Assoc.*, 24:257–270, 1970.

Diabetes Mellitus, 7th ed., Indianapolis, Eli Lilly and Company, 1973.

Dudrick, S. J. and Rhoads, J. E.: New Horizons for Intravenous Feeding. *JAMA*, 215:939–949, 1971.

Dudrick, S. J.: Rational Intravenous Therapy. *Am. J. Hosp. Pharm.*, 28:82–91, 1971.

Dwyer, J. L.: The Technology of Absolute Microfiltration. *Technical Quarterly*, 5:243–249, 1968.

Farnsworth, N. R.: Immunizing Biologicals. *Tile and Till*, 56:20–24 1970; *ibid*: 56:52–57, 1970; *ibid*: 56:62–64, 1970.

Gallelli, J. F.: Stability Studies of Drugs Used in Intravenous Solutions. *Amer. J. Hosp. Pharm.*, 24:425–433, 1967.

Geyer, R. P.: Parenteral Nutrition. *Bull. Parenteral Drug Assoc.*, 21:215–225, 1967.

Gross, M. A.: The Danger of Particulate Matter in Solutions for Intravenous Use. *Drug Intelligence*, 1:12–13, 1967.

How to Give an Intramuscular Injection, New York, Pfizer Laboratories, 1967.

Intravenous Techniques, New York, Pfizer Laboratories, 1967.

Johnson, C., Cloyd, J., and Rapp, R. P.: Parenteral Hyperalimentation. *Drug Intelligence and Clinical Pharmacy*, 9:493–499, 1975.

Lamy, P. P.: Laminar Flow Concepts, *Drug & Cosmetic Industry*, 104:51, 1969.

Latiolais, C. J., Shoup, I. K., and Thur, M. P.: Stability of Drugs after Reconstitution. *Amer. J. Hosp. Pharm.*, 24:667–691, 1967.

Lawlis, J. F.: Quality Control of Biological Products. *Bull. Parenteral Drug. Assoc.*, 18:30–32, 1964.

Lin, K. S., Anschel, J., and Swartz, C. J.: Parenteral Formulations IV: Solubility Considerations in Developing a Parenteral Dosage Form. *Bull. Parenteral Drug Assoc.*, 25:40–50, 1971.

Macke, T. J.: Preparation of Parenteral Dispersions. *J. Pharm. Sci.*, 52:694–699, 1963.

McLeod, D. C.: Single Unit Packages of Drugs Available Today: Injections in Prefilled Disposable Syringes. *Amer. J. Hosp. Pharm.*, 24:696–703, 1967.

Meyers, E. L.: Packaging and Labeling of Parenteral Products. *Bull. Parenteral Drug Assoc.*, 21:1–6, 1967.

"Parenteral Administration," Chicago, Abbott Laboratories, 1959.

Parker, E. A., Boomer, R. J., and Bell, S. C.: Parenteral Incompatibilities—Past, Present and Future. *Bull. Parenteral Drug Assoc.,* 21:197–207, 1967.

Personeus, G. R.: Pyrogen Testing of Biologicals and Small Volume Parenterals. *Bull Parenteral Drug Assoc.,* 23:201–207, 1969.

Rendell-Baker, L. and Roberts, R. B.: Safe Use of Ethylene Oxide Sterilization in Hospitals. *Anesthesia and Analgesia . . . Current Researches,* 49:919–921, 1970.

Scheindlin, S.: Stabilizers for Parenteral Drugs. *Bull. Parenteral Drug Assoc.,* 20:61–64, 1966.

Shoup, L. K.: Reconstitution of Parenterals. *Amer. J. Hosp. Pharm.,* 24:692–695, 1967.

Spiegel, A. J., and Noseworthy, M. M.: Use of Nonaqueous Solvents in Parenteral Products. *J. Pharm. Sci.,* 52:917–927, 1963.

Stokes, T. F., Sumner, E. D., and Needham, T. E.: Particulate Contamination and Stability of Three Additives in 0.9% Sodium Chloride Injection in Plastic and Glass Large-Volume Containers. *Am. J. Hosp. Pharm.* 32:821–826, 1975.

Turco, S. and King, R. E.: *Sterile Dosage Forms: Their Preparation and Clinical Applications,* Philadelphia, Lea & Febiger, 1974.

Van Itallie, P. H.: The Rugged Beginnings of Injection Therapy. *Pulse of Pharmacy,* 19:3–17, 1965.

Vidt, D. G.: Use and Abuse of Intravenous Solutions. *JAMA,* 232:533–536, 1975.

Virginia, M.: Physical Incompatibilities of Parenteral Drugs, *Hosp. Pharm.,* 2:7–13, 1967.

Wilmore, D. W. and Dudrick, S. J.: An In-Line Filter for Intravenous Solutions. *Arch Surg,* 99:462, 1969.

Chapter 9

Aerosols, Inhalations, and Sprays

Pharmaceutical Aerosols

Pharmaceutical aerosols may be defined as "pressurized dosage forms containing one or more active ingredients which upon actuation give a fine dispersion of liquid and/or solid materials in a gaseous medium." Pharmaceutical aerosols are similar to other dosage forms in that they require the same types of considerations with respect to formulation, product stability, and therapeutic efficacy. However, they differ from most other dosage forms in their dependence upon the function of the container, its valve assembly, and an added component—the propellant—for the physical delivery of the medication in proper form.

The term *pressurized package* is commonly used when referring to the aerosol container or completed product. Pressure is applied to the aerosol system through the use of one or more liquefied or gaseous propellants. Upon activation of the valve assembly of the aerosol, it is the pressure exerted by the propellant which forces the contents of the package out through the opening of the valve. The physical form in which the contents are emitted is dependent upon the formulation of the product and the type of valve employed. Aerosol products may be designed to expel their contents as a fine mist, a coarse, wet or a dry spray, a steady stream, or as a stable or a fast-breaking foam. The physical form selected for a given aerosol is based on the intended use of that product. For instance, an aerosol intended for inhalation therapy, as in the treatment of asthma or emphysema, must present particles in the form of a fine liquid mist or as finely divided solid particles if the product is to be efficacious. It has been generally accepted that particles less than 6 microns will reach the respiratory bronchioles, and those less than 2 microns will reach the alveolar ducts and alveoli.[1] However, when deposition in the trachea and the primary or secondary bronchioles is desired for localized effects, a particle range of 20 to 60 microns is indicated. In contrast, the particle size for a dermatologic spray intended for deposition on the skin would be more coarse and generally less critical to the therapeutic efficacy of the product. Some dermatologic aerosols present the medication in the form of a powder, a wet spray, a stream of liquid (usually a local anesthetic), or an ointment-like product. Other pharmaceutical aerosols include vaginal and rectal foams.

Aerosols used to provide an airborne mist are termed *space sprays*. Room disinfectants, room deodorizers, and space insecticides characterize this group of aerosols. The particle size of the released product is generally quite small, usually below 50 microns, and must be carefully controlled so that the dispersed droplets or particles remain airborne for a prolonged period of time. A one-second burst from a typical aerosol space spray will produce 120 million particles, a substantial number of which will remain suspended in the air for an hour.

Aerosols intended to carry the active ingredient to a surface are termed *surface sprays* or *surface coatings*. The dermatologic aerosols can be placed in this group. Also included are a great many non-pharmaceutical aerosol products, as personal deodorant sprays, cosmetic hair lacquers and sprays, perfume and cologne sprays, shaving lathers, toothpaste, surface pesticide sprays, paint sprays, and various household products such as spray starch, waxes, polishers, cleaners, and lubricants. A number of veterinary and pet products have been put into aerosol form as have been such food products as dessert toppings and food spreads. Physically, some of these products are sprays; others, foams; and a few, paste-like products.

[1] Mitchell, R. I.: Retention of Aerosol Particles in the Respiratory Tract. Amer. Rev. Resp. Dis., 82:627, 1960.

Advantages of the Aerosol Dosage Form

Some features of pharmaceutical aerosols that may be considered advantages over other types of dosage forms are as follows:

1. A portion of medication may be easily withdrawn from the package without contamination or exposure to the remaining material.
2. By virtue of its hermetic character, the aerosol container protects medicinal agents adversely affected by atmospheric oxygen and moisture. Being opaque, the usual aerosol container also protects drugs adversely affected by light. This protection persists during the use and the shelf-life of the product. If the product is packaged under sterile conditions, sterility may also be maintained during the shelf-life of the product.
3. Topical medication may be applied in a uniform, thin layer to the skin, without touching the affected area. This method of application reduces the irritation that usually accompanies the mechanical (fingertip) application of topical preparations. Aerosol application results in firm applications of the medication. The rapid volatilization of the propellant also provides a cooling, refreshing effect.
4. By proper formulation and valve control, the physical form and the particle size of the emitted product may be controlled which may contribute to the efficacy of a drug; e.g., the fine controlled mist of an inhalant aerosol. Through the use of metered valves, dosage may be controlled.
5. Aerosol application is a "clean" process, requiring little or no "wash-up" by the user.

The Aerosol Principle

An aerosol formulation consists of two component parts, the product concentrate and the propellant. The product concentrate is the active ingredient of the aerosol combined with the required adjuncts, such as antioxidants, surface-active agents, and solvents, to prepare a stable and efficacious product. The propellant in pharmaceutical aerosols is usually a liquefied gas or a mixture of liquefied gases which frequently serves the dual role of propellant and solvent or vehicle for the product concentrate. In certain aerosol systems, nonliquefied compressed gases, as carbon dioxide, nitrogen, and nitrous oxide, are employed as the propellant.

The liquefied gas propellants used in the preparation of aerosols are principally fluorinated hydrocarbons.[1] Some of these propellants are presented in Table 9-1. Fluorinated hydrocarbons are gases at room temperature. They may be liquefied by cooling below their boiling point or by compressing the gas at room temperature. For example, dichlorodifluoromethane ("Freon 12") gas will form a liquid when cooled to $-22°F$ or when compressed to 70 psig (pounds per square inch gauge) at $70°F$. Both of these methods for liquefying gases are employed in aerosol packaging as will be discussed later in this section.

When a liquefied gas propellant or propellant mixture is sealed within an aerosol container with the product concentrate, an equilibrium is quickly established between that portion of propellant which remains liquefied and that which vaporizes and occupies the upper portion of the aerosol container. The vapor phase exerts pressure in all directions—against the walls of the container, the valve assembly, and the surface of the liquid phase, which is composed of the liquefied gas and the product concentrate. It is this pressure which upon actuation of the aerosol valve forces the liquid phase up the dip tube and out of the orifice of the valve into the atmosphere. As the propellant meets the air, it immediately evaporates due to the drop in pressure, leaving the product concentrate as airborne liquid droplets or dry particles, depending upon the formulation (Fig. 9-1). As the liquid phase is removed from the container, equilibrium between the propellant remaining liquefied and that in the vapor state is reestablished. Thus even during expulsion of the product from the aerosol package, the pressure within remains virtually constant, and the product may be continuously released at an even rate and with the same propulsion. However, when the liquid reservoir is depleted, the pressure may not be maintained, and the gas may be expelled from the container with diminishing pressure until it is exhausted.

[1] Many of these propellants are products of the DuPont Company, marketed as "Freon" propellants or refrigerants. They are also available as "Genetrons" from the General Chemical Division, Allied Chemical Corporation, or as "Ucons" from Union Carbide Chemicals Company, Division of Union Carbide Corporation.

Table 9-1. PHYSICAL PROPERTIES OF SOME FLUORINATED HYDROCARBON PROPELLANTS

Chemical Name	Chemical Formula	Numerical Designation[a]	Vapor Pressure (psia[b]) 70°F	Boiling Point (1 ATM) °F	Liquid Density (g/ml.) 70°F
Trichloromonofluoromethane	CCl_3F	11	13.4	74.7	1.485
Dichlorodifluoromethane	CCl_2F_2	12	84.9	−21.6	1.325
Dichlorotetrafluoroethane	$CClF_2CClF_2$	114	27.6	38.4	1.468
Chloropentafluoroethane	$CClF_2CF_3$	115	117.5	−37.7	1.29
Monochlorodifluoroethane	CH_3CClF_2	142b	43.8	15.1	1.119
Difluoroethane	CH_3CHF_2	152a	76.4	−11.2	0.911
Octafluorocyclobutane	$CF_2CF_2CF_2CF_2$	C318	40.1	21.1	1.513

[a] The numerical designations for fluorinated hydrocarbon propellants have been designed within the refrigeration industry to simplify communications when referring to these agents. The numerical designations are arrived at by the following method: (1) the digit at the extreme right refers to the number of fluorine atoms in the molecule; (2) the second digit from the right represents one *greater* than the number of hydrogen atoms in the molecule; (3) the third digit from the right is one *less* than the number of carbon atoms in the molecule; if this number is zero, it is omitted and a two-digit number is used; (4) a capital letter "C" is used before a number to indicate the cyclic nature of a compound; (5) the small letters following a number are used to indicate decreasing symmetry of isomeric compounds, with the "b" indicating less symmetry than the "a," and so forth. The number of chlorine atoms in a molecule may be determined by subtracting the total number of hydrogen and fluorine atoms from the total number of atoms which may be added to the carbon chain.

[b] psia is pounds per square inch absolute, which is equal to psig + 14.7.

Aerosol Systems

The pressure of an aerosol is critical to its performance. It can be controlled by (1) the type and amount of propellant and (2) the nature and amount of material comprising the product concentrate. Thus, each formulation is unique unto itself, and a specific amount of propellant to be employed in aerosol products cannot be firmly stated. However, some general statements may be made within the context of this discussion. Space sprays generally contain a greater proportion of propellant than do aerosols intended for surface coating, and thus they are released with greater pressure, and the resultant particles are projected more violently from the valve. Space aerosols usually operate at pressures between 30 and 40 psig at 70°F and may contain as much as 85% propellant. Surface aerosols commonly contain 30 to 70% propellant with pressures between 25 and 55 psig at 70°F. Foam aerosols usually operate between 35 and 55 psig at 70°F and may contain only 6 to 10% propellant.

Foam aerosols may be considered to be emulsions, in that the liquefied propellant is partially emulsified with the product concentrate rather than being dissolved in it. Since the fluorinated hydrocarbons are nonpolar organic solvents having no affinity for water, the liquefied propellant does not dissolve in the aqueous formulation. The utilization of surfactants or emulsifiers in the formulation encourages the mixing of the two components to enhance the emulsion. Shaking of the package prior to use further mixes the propellant throughout the product concentrate. When the aerosol valve is activated, the mixture is expelled to the atmosphere where the propellant globules vaporize rapidly, leaving the active ingredient in the form of a foam.

Blends of the various liquefied gas propellants are generally used in pharmaceutical aerosols to achieve the desired vapor pressure and to provide the proper solvent features for a given product. Some propellants are eliminated from use in certain products because of their reactivity with other formulative materials, or with the proposed container or valve components. For instance, trichloromonofluoromethane tends to form free hydrochloric acid when formulated with systems containing water or ethyl alcohol, the latter a commonly used cosolvent in aerosol systems. The free hydrochloric acid not only affects the efficacy of the product, but also exerts a corrosive action on some container components.

The physiologic effect of the propellant must also be considered in formulating an aerosol to assure safety of the product in its intended use. Even though an individual propellant or propellant blend and the active ingredient of a

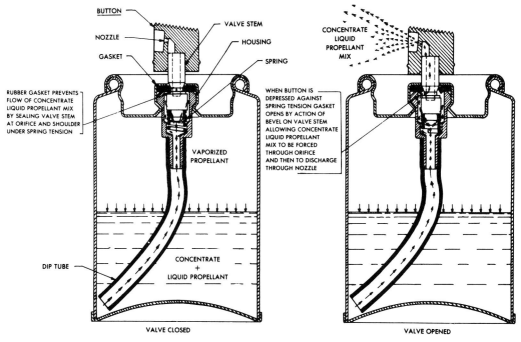

Fig. 9-1. *Cross section sketches of contents and operation of a typical two-phase aerosol system. (Courtesy of Armstrong Laboratories, Inc., Division of Aerosol Techniques, Inc.)*

formulation are nontoxic when tested individually, the use of the combination in aerosol form may have undesirable features. For instance, when an active ingredient ordinarily used in a nasal or oral spray is placed in a fine aerosol mist, it may reach deeper into the respiratory tract than desired and may result in irritation. In other instances, as with new dermatologic, vaginal, and rectal aerosol products, the influence of the aerosol form of the drug on the recipient tissue membranes must be evaluated for irritating effects and changes in the absorption of the drug from the site of application. The absorption pattern of a drug may change due to an increased rate of solubility of the fine particles usually produced in aerosol products.

Although the fluorinated hydrocarbons have a relatively low order of toxicity and are generally nonirritating, certain individuals, who may be sensitive to the propellent agent and who utilize an inhalation aerosol, may exhibit cardiotoxic effects following rapid and repeated use of the aerosol product.[1] Recent concern has also been expressed over the potential of fluorocarbon gases to reduce the ozone level of the

[1] Chiou, W. L.: Aerosol Propellants: Cardiac Toxicity and Long Biological Half-Life, *JAMA:*227:658, 1974.

earth's protective mantle thereby permitting greater exposure of the earth to harmful ultraviolet radiation.

TWO-PHASE SYSTEMS. The two-phase aerosol system is comprised of the liquid phase, containing the liquefied propellant and product concentrate, and the vapor phase (see Fig. 9-1). In this system, the product concentrate is either soluble or miscible with the liquefied propellant. Large volumes of water must be avoided, as water is immiscible with the liquefied fluorinated hydrocarbon propellants. For highly aqueous preparations, a three-phase system may be employed.

THREE-PHASE SYSTEMS. Due to the immiscibility of the liquefied propellant and a highly aqueous product concentrate, individual liquid layers of these components exist, along with the vapor phase, in a three-phase system. Since the liquefied propellant usually has a greater density than the aqueous layer, it generally is positioned at the bottom of the container with the aqueous phase floating above it. As with the two-phase system, upon activation of the valve, the pressure of the vapor phase causes the liquid phase to rise in the dip tube and be expelled from the container. To avoid expulsion of the reservoir of liquefied propellant, the dip tube must extend only within the aqueous phase and not down into the layer of liquefied propellant. The aqueous product is broken up into a spray by the mechanical action of the valve. If the container is shaken immediately prior to use, some liquefied propellant may be mixed with the aqueous phase and be expelled through the valve to facilitate the dispersion of the exited product or the production of foam, depending upon the formulation. The vapor phase within the container is replenished from the liquid propellant phase.

COMPRESSED GAS SYSTEMS. Compressed, rather than liquefied, gases may be used to prepare aerosols. The pressure of the compressed gas contained in the headspace of the aerosol container forces the product concentrate up the dip tube and out of the valve. The use of gases that are insoluble in the product concentrate, as is nitrogen, will result in the emission of a product in essentially the same form as it was placed in the container, since no gas will be emitted from the valve to induce particle dispersion or foaming. Thus, any particle size reduction on emission of the product would be a function of the type of valve employed. An advantage of nitrogen as a propellant is its inert behavior toward other formulative components and its protective influence on products subject to oxidation. Further, nitrogen is an odorless and tasteless gas and thus does not contribute adversely to the smell or taste of a product.

Other gases, such as carbon dioxide and nitrous oxide, which are slightly soluble in the liquid phase of aerosol products may be employed in instances in which their expulsion with the product concentrate is desired in order to achieve spraying or foaming.

Unlike aerosols prepared with liquefied gas propellants, there is no reservoir of liquid propellant in compressed gas filled aerosols. Thus higher gas pressures are generally required in these systems, and the pressure in these aerosols progressively diminishes as the product is used.

The Aerosol Container and Valve Assembly

The effectiveness of a pharmaceutical aerosol is dependent upon achieving the proper combination. of formulation, container, and valve assembly. The formulation must not chemically interact with the container or valve components so as to interfere with the stability of the formulation or with the integrity and operation of the container and valve assembly. The container and valve must be capable of withstanding the pressure required by the product, it must be corrosive-resistant, and the valve must contribute to the form of the product to be emitted.

CONTAINERS. Various materials have been used in the manufacture of aerosol containers, including (1) glass, uncoated or plastic coated; (2) metal, including tin-plated steel, aluminum, and stainless steel; and (3) plastics. The selection of the container for an aerosol product is based on its adaptability to production methods, compatibility with formulation components, ability to sustain the pressure intended for the product, the interest in design and aesthetic appeal on the part of the manufacturer, and the cost.

Were it not for their brittleness and danger of breakage, glass containers would be preferred for most aerosols. Glass presents fewer problems with respect to chemical compatibility with the formula than do metal containers and is not subject to corrosion. Glass is also more adaptive to creativity in design. On the negative side, glass containers must be precisely engineered to provide the maximum in pressure safety and impact resistance. Plastic coatings are commonly applied to the outer surface of glass containers to render them more resistant to accidental breakage, and in the event of breaking, the plastic coating prevents the scattering of glass fragments. When the total pressure of an aerosol system is below 25 psig and no more than 50% propellant is used, glass containers are considered quite safe. When required, the inner surface of glass containers may be coated to render them more chemically resistant to formulation materials.

At the present time, tin-plated steel containers are the most widely used metal containers for aerosols. Since the starting material used is in the form of sheets, the completed aerosol cylinders are seamed and soldered to provide a sealed unit. When required, special protective coatings are employed within the container to prevent corrosion and interaction between the container and formulation. The containers must be carefully examined prior to filling to ensure that there are no flaws in the seam or in the protective coating that would render the container weak or subject to corrosion.

Most aluminum containers are manufactured by extrusion or by other methods that make them seamless. They have the advantage over the seam type of container in that there is greater safety against leakage, incompatibility, and corrosion. Stainless steel is employed to produce containers for certain small volume aerosols in which a great deal of chemical resistance is required. The main limitation of stainless steel containers is their high cost.

Plastic containers have not met with a great deal of success or utilization in the packaging of aerosols due to their inherent problem of being permeated by the vapor within the container. Also, drug-plastic interactions, which have been found to occur, affect the release of drug from the container and reduce the efficacy of the product.

THE VALVE ASSEMBLY. The function of the valve assembly is to permit the expulsion of the contents of the can in the desired form, at the desired rate, and, in the case of metered valves, in the proper amount or dose. The materials used in the manufacture of valves must be inert toward the formulations and must be approved by the Food and Drug Administration. Among the materials used in the manufacture of the various valve parts are plastic, rubber, aluminum, and stainless steel.

The usual aerosol valve assembly is composed of the following parts (Fig. 9-2):

1. *Actuator*—The actuator is the button which the user presses to activate the valve assembly for the emission of the product. The actuator permits the easy opening and closing of the valve. It is through the orifice in the actuator that the product is discharged. The design of the inner chamber and size of the emission orifice of the actuator contribute to the physical form (mist, coarse spray, solid stream, or foam) in which the product is discharged. The combination of the type and quantity of propellant used, and the actuator design and dimensions control the particle size of the emitted product. Larger orifices (and less propellant) are used for products to be emitted as foams and solid streams than for those intended to be sprays or mists.

2. *Stem*—The stem supports the actuator and delivers the formulation in the proper form to the chamber of the actuator.

3. *Gasket*—The gasket, placed snugly with the stem, serves to prevent leakage of the formulation when the valve is in the closed position.

4. *Spring*—The spring holds the gasket in place and also is the mechanism by which the actuator retracts when pressure is released, thereby returning the valve to the closed position.

5. *Mounting cup*—The mounting cup, which is attached to the aerosol can or container, serves to hold the valve in place. Since the underside of the mounting cup is exposed to the formulation, it must receive the same consideration as the inner part of the container, with respect to meeting criteria of compatibility. If necessary, it may be coated with an inert material (as an epoxy resin or vinyl) to prevent an undesired interaction.

6. *Housing*—The housing, located directly below the mounting cup, serves as the link between the dip tube and the stem and actuator. With the stem, its orifice helps to determine the delivery rate and the form in which the product is emitted.

7. *Dip tube*—The dip tube, which extends from the housing down into the product, serves to bring the formulation from the container to

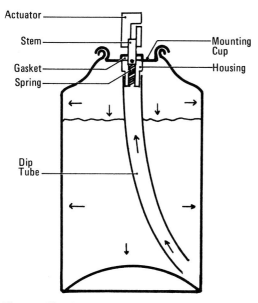

Fig. 9-2. *Sketch showing valve assembly components.*

the valve. The viscosity of the product and its intended delivery rate dictate to a large extent the inner dimensions of the dip tube and housing for a particular product.

The actuator, stem, housing, and dip tube are generally made of plastic, the mounting cup and spring of metal, and the gasket of rubber predetermined to be resistant to the formulation.

Metering valves are employed when the formulation is a potent medication, as in inhalation therapy (Fig. 9-3). In these metered valve systems, the amount of material discharged is regulated by an auxiliary valve chamber by virtue of its capacity or dimensions. A single depression of the actuator causes the evacuation of this chamber and the delivery of its contents. The integrity of the chamber is controlled by a dual valving mechanism. When the actuator valve is in the closed position, a seal is effected between the chamber and the atmosphere. However, in this position the chamber is permitted to fill with the contents of the container to which it is open. Depression of the actuator causes a simultaneous reversal of positions sealed; the chamber becomes open to the atmosphere, releasing its contents, and at the

same time becomes sealed from the contents of the container. Upon release of the actuator, the system is restored for the next dose. The NF XIV contains a test to determine quantitatively the amount of medication from a metered valve.

Most aerosol products have a protective cap or cover which fits snugly over the valve and mounting cup. This serves to protect against accidental activation of the valve and to protect the valve against contamination with dust and dirt. The cap, which is generally made of plastic or metal, also serves a decorative function.

Filling Operations

As explained earlier, fluorinated hydrocarbon gases may be liquefied by cooling below their boiling points or by compressing the gas at room temperature. These two features are utilized in the filling of aerosol containers with propellant.

COLD FILLING. In the cold method, both the product concentrate and the propellant must be cooled to temperatures of $-30°$ to $-40°F$. This temperature is necessary to liquefy the propellant gas. The cooling system may be a mixture of dry ice and acetone or a more elaborate refrigeration system. After the chilled product concentrate has been quantitatively metered into an equally cold aerosol container, the liquefied gas is added. The heavy vapors of the cold liquid propellant generally displace the air present in the container. However, in the process, some of the propellant vapors are also lost. When sufficient propellant has been added, the valve assembly is immediately inserted and crimped into place. Because of the low temperatures required, aqueous systems cannot be filled by this process, since the water turns to ice. For nonaqueous systems, some moisture usually appears in the final product due to the condensation of atmospheric moisture within the cold containers.

PRESSURE FILLING. By the pressure method, the product concentrate is quantitatively placed in the aerosol container, the valve assembly is inserted and crimped into place, and the liquefied gas, under pressure, is metered into the valve stem from a pressure burette. The desired amount of propellant is allowed to enter the container under its own vapor pressure. When

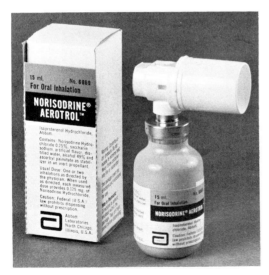

Fig. 9-3. *Example of a commercial package of a controlled-dose aerosol mist for oral inhalation. When the mouthpiece is placed in the mouth, the patient inhales through the mouthpiece, simultaneously pressing down on the spray head. The mist is automatically stopped when the dose has been administered. (Courtesy of Abbott Laboratories)*

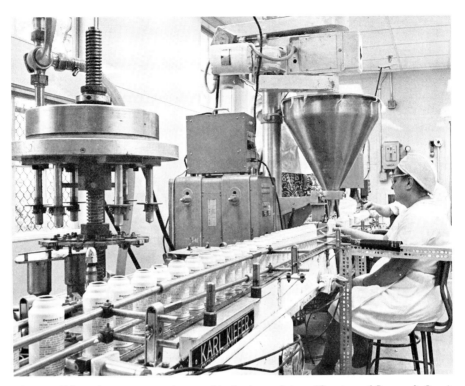

Fig. 9-4. *Filling the empty aerosol cans with the drug mixture. (Courtesy of Pennwalt Corp.)*

the pressure in the container equals that in the burette, the propellant stops flowing. Additional propellant may be added by increasing the pressure in the filling apparatus through the use of compressed air or nitrogen gas. The trapped air in the package may be ignored if it does not interfere with the quality or stability of the product, or it may be evacuated prior to filling or during filling, using special apparatus. After filling the container with sufficient propellant, the valve actuator is tested for proper function. This spray testing also rids the dip tube of pure propellant prior to consumer use.

Pressure filling is used for most pharmaceutical aerosols. It has the advantage over the cold filling method in that there is less danger of moisture contamination of the product, and also less propellant is lost in the process.

As mentioned earlier, compressed gases, rather than liquefied gases, may be employed as the propellant in aerosol systems. In these instances, a gas such as nitrogen, carbon dioxide, or nitrous oxide is transferred from large steel cylinders of the compressed gas into the aerosol containers. Prior to filling, the product concentrate is quantitatively placed in the container,

the valve assembly is crimped into place, and the air is evacuated from the container by a vacuum pump. The compressed gas is then passed into the container through a pressure reducing valve attached to the gas cylinder; when the pressure within the aerosol container is equal to the predetermined and regulated delivery pressure, the gas flow stops, and the aerosol valve is restored to the closed position. For gases, like carbon dioxide and nitrous oxide, which are slightly soluble in the product concentrate, the container is manually or mechanically shaken during the filling operation to achieve the desired pressure in the headspace of the aerosol container.

Testing the Filled Containers

After filling by either the cold method or the pressure method, the aerosol container is generally immersed in a heated water bath until the contents reach a minimum of 130°F to test for leaks or weakness in the valve assembly or container. This test conforms to the Interstate Commerce Commission regulations governing aerosol products. For pharmaceutical aerosols

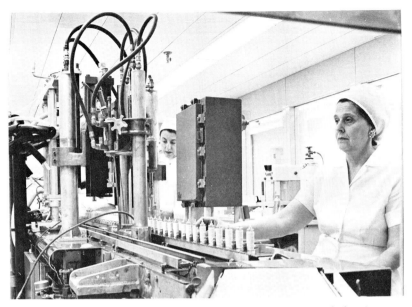

Fig. 9-5. *Pressure filling of aerosol containers. (Courtesy of Pennwalt Corp.)*

having thermolabile contents, the I.C.C. requires the successful testing of at least one completed container out of each product lot of 500 or less.

Filled aerosol containers are also tested for the proper function of the valve. The *valve discharge rate* is determined by discharging a portion of the contents of a previously weighed aerosol during a given period of time, and calculating, by the difference in weight, the grams of contents discharged per unit of time. As is deemed desirable, aerosols also may be tested for their spray patterns, for particle size distribution of the spray, and for accuracy and reproducibility of dosage when using metered valves.[1]

Packaging, Labeling, and Storage

A unique aspect of pharmaceutical aerosols compared to other dosage forms is that the aerosol is actually packaged as part of the manufacturing process. With most other dosage forms, the product is completely manufactured and then placed in the appropriate container.

Medicinal aerosols that are to be dispensed

only upon prescription usually may be labeled by the manufacturer with plastic peel-away labels or easily removed paper labels so that the pharmacist may easily replace the manufacturer's label with his label containing the directions for use specified by the prescribing practitioner. Most other types of aerosols have the manufacturer's label printed directly on the container or on firmly affixed paper. In all instances, aerosols should contain the following warning information as recommended by the USP XIX:

Warning: Avoid inhaling. Keep away from eyes or other mucous membranes.
(Note: warning not required for inhalation aerosols and those to be used on mucous membranes respectively)

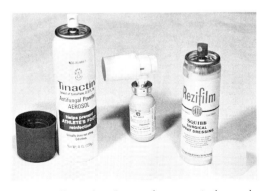

Fig. 9-6. *Examples of some pharmaceutical aerosols.*

[1] These and other tests are described in detail by J. J. Sciarra in *The Theory and Practice of Industrial Pharmacy*, 2nd Ed., by L. Lachman, H. A. Lieberman, and J. L. Kanig, Philadelphia, Lea & Febiger, 1976, pp. 291–294.

Warning: Contents under pressure. Do not puncture or incinerate container. Do not expose to heat or store at temperatures above 120°F. Keep out of reach of children.

For aerosols containing propellants of halocarbon or hydrocarbon:

Warning: Use only as directed; intentional misuse by deliberately concentrating and inhaling the contents can be harmful or fatal.

Aerosols should be maintained with the protective caps in place to prevent accidental activation of the valve assembly or its contamination by dust and other foreign materials.

Official Aerosols

The official aerosols are presented in Table 9-2.

Inhalations

Inhalations are drugs or solutions of drugs administered by the nasal or oral respiratory route. The drugs may be administered for their local action on the bronchial tree or for their systemic effects through absorption from the lungs. Certain gases, as oxygen and ether, are administered by inhalation as are finely powdered drug substances and solutions of drugs administered as fine mists.

Table 9-2. OFFICIAL AEROSOLS

Official Aerosol	Some Representative Commercial Products[a]	Category and Comments
Betamethasone Valerate Aerosol, NF	Valisone Aerosol (Schering)	Glucocorticoid; Sprayed topically to affected area. Used for management of inflammation of acute contact dermatitis. Aerosol contains 0.15% equivalent of betamethasone.
Dexamethasone Aerosol, NF	Decadron Topical (Merck Sharp & Dohme)	Glucocorticoid; sprayed topically on affected area. Dexamethasone is present in a lotion base
Isoproterenol Sulfate Aerosol, NF	Medihaler-Iso (Riker)	Adrenergic (bronchodilator). Isoproterenol sulfate is present as a suspension of microfine particles. The monograph contains a particle size requirement to assure that the great majority of particles are less than 5 microns in diameter. The commercial product is so metered that it delivers 75 mcg of isoproterenol sulfate per inhalation sequence. One or two such inhalations (2 to 5 minutes apart) constitutes the usual dose in treating dyspnea due to asthma, bronchitis, or emphysema.
Lidocaine Aerosol, USP	. . .	Topical anesthetic (dental)
Povidone-Iodine Aerosol, NF	Betadine (Purdue Frederick)	Local anti-infective; sprayed on affected area topically. The povidone-iodine is present as a 5% solution, equivalent to 0.5% of available iodine
Thimerosal Aerosol, NF	Merthiolate (Lilly)	Local anti-infective; sprayed on affected area topically. Thimerosal is present as a 0.1% solution containing stabilizers and usually colorants to delineate the area of application. Merthiolate is incompatible with iodine, strong acids, and heavy metal salts, and these should be avoided in its manufacture, storage, and use.
Trypsin Crystallized for Aerosol, NF	Granulex (Hickam)	Proteolytic; for debridement of eschar and other necrotic tissue.
Triamcinolone Acetonide, NF	Kenalog Spray (Squibb)	Anti-inflammatory; applied topically to the affected area from one to three times daily. Triamcinolone is present in solution (66 mcg/g).

[a]Products listed are examples and do not necessarily represent a complete listing.

As noted previously in Table 9-2, a number of drug substances are administered through pressure packaged *inhalation aerosols,* as the type shown in Figure 9-3. In order for the inhaled drug substance or solution to reach the bronchial tree, the inhaled particles must be just a few microns in size.

A unique form of powder administration that has recently been developed involves the inhalation of a micronized powder directly into the lungs using a special breath-activated device (Fig. 9-7). The drug present in the inhaled powder is cromolyn sodium, an agent used in the management of patients with severe perennial asthma. The drug is supplied to the patient in hard gelatin capsules as a powder mixture with the inert substance lactose. The particles of lactose are designed to be larger (30 to 60 μ) than the particles of cromolyn sodium powder (1 to 10 μ) and upon inhalation the cromolyn sodium passes deeply into the respiratory tract, whereas the lactose particles are retained in the upper airways (Fig. 9-8). The powder in the capsule is prepared for inhalation by placing it in the special inhaler device depicted in Figure 9-7. When ready for medication the patient makes two perforations in the capsule by a piercing mechanism present in the inhaler-device. When the mouth is placed on the mouthpiece and air inhaled, the turbo-vibratory action of the propeller causes the powdered drug to be dispensed into the inspired air

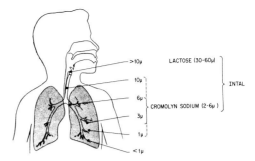

Fig. 9-8. *Relationship of INTAL (cromolyn sodium, Fisons) particle size to airway penetration. (Courtesy of Fisons Corporation.)*

through the perforations in the capsule wall.[1]

A widely used instrument capable of producing fine particles for inhalation therapy is the *nebulizer.* This apparatus, shown in Figure 9-9, contains an atomizing unit within a curved, glass, bulb-like chamber. A rubber bulb at the end of the apparatus is depressed and the medicated solution is drawn up a narrow glass tube and broken into fine particles by the passing airstream. The fine particles produced range between 0.5 and 5 microns. The larger, heavier droplets of the mist do not exit the apparatus but fall back into the reservoir of

[1]"Intal: Cromolyn Sodium a Monograph," Fisons Corporation, Bedford, Mass., 1973.

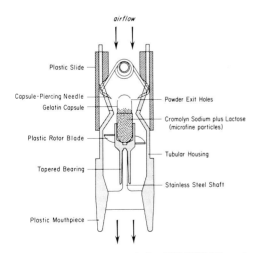

Fig. 9-7. *Cross section of the SPINHALER turbo inhaler, used in the administration of INTAL (cromolyn sodium, Fisons). (Courtesy of Fisons Corporation.)*

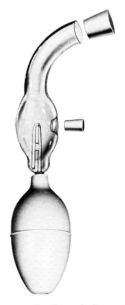

Fig. 9-9. *An example of a nebulizer used in inhalation therapy. See text for description of operation. (Courtesy of The DeVilbiss Co.)*

medicated liquid. The lighter particles do escape with the airstream and are inhaled by the patient who operates the nebulizer with the exit orifice in his mouth, inhaling as he depresses the rubber bulb.

The common household *vaporizer,* as the one depicted in Figure 9-10, produces a fine mist of steam which may be used to humidify a room. When a volatile medication is added to the water in the chamber or to a special medication cup present in some models, the medication volatilizes and is also inhaled by the patient. Humidifiers, as shown in Figure 9-11, are employed to provide a cool mist to the air in a room. Moisture in the air is important to prevent mucous membranes of the nose and throat from becoming dry and irritated. Vaporizers and humidifiers are commonly used in the adjunct treatment of colds, coughs, and chest congestion.

Official Inhalations

Epinephrine Inhalation, USP

A 1% aqueous solution of epinephrine in purified water is prepared with the aid of hydrochloric acid to form the water-soluble salt. The inhalation is employed orally to relieve bronchial asthma attacks. It is effective by virtue of its ability to shrink the congested bronchial mucosa and relax the bronchial musculature.

The inhalation is best stored in small, well-filled, tight, light-resistant containers and must not be used if the solution is brown or contains a precipitate.

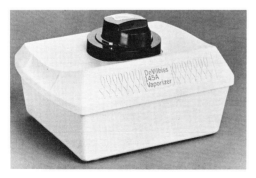

Fig. 9-10. *An example of a commercially available vaporizer. (Courtesy of The DeVilbiss Co.)*

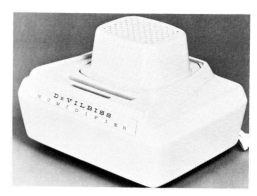

Fig. 9-11. *An example of a commercially available humidifier. (Courtesy of The DeVilbiss Co.)*

Isoproterenol Hydrochloride Inhalation, USP

This is a solution of isoproterenol hydrochloride, a sympathomimetic agent, in purified water rendered isotonic by the addition of the appropriate amount of sodium chloride. The solution is employed by oral inhalation for the relief of bronchial spasm in asthma, emphysema, and chronic bronchitis. The inhalation is usually packaged in an apparatus that permits the dosage regulation. The usual amount of drug administered is about 0.125 to 0.25 mg.

Because isoproterenol solutions darken on exposure to air and light, they must be preserved in small, well-filled, tight containers, protected from light. The inhalations must not be used if discolored brown or if a precipitate is present. The corresponding commercial product is Isuprel Mistometer (Winthrop).

Inhalants

Inhalants are drugs or combinations of drugs that by virtue of their high vapor pressure can be carried by an air current into the nasal passage where they exert their effect. The device in which the drug or drugs is contained and from which they are administered is termed an *inhaler.*

Official Inhalants

There are three official inhalants, described as follows.

Amyl Nitrite Inhalant, NF

Amyl nitrite is a clear, yellowish, volatile liquid which acts as a vasodilator when inhaled. The drug is prepared in sealed glass vials which are covered with a protective gauze cloth. Upon use, the glass vial is broken in the fingertips and the cloth soaks up the liquid which is then inhaled. The vials generally contain 0.3 ml of the drug substance. The effects of the drug are rapid and are used in the treatment of anginal pain.

Propylhexedrine Inhalant, NF

Propylhexedrine is a liquid adrenergic (vasoconstrictor) agent that volatilizes slowly at room temperature. This quality enables it to be effectively used as an inhalant. The official inhalant consists of cylindrical rolls of suitable fibrous material impregnated with propylhexedrine, usually aromatized to mask its amine-like odor, and contained in a suitable inhaler. The vapor of the drug is inhaled into the nostrils when needed to relieve nasal congestion due to colds and hay fever. It may also be employed to relieve ear block and the pressure pain in air travelers.

Each plastic tube of the commercial product contains 250 mg of propylhexedrine with aromatics. The containers should be tightly closed after each opening to prevent loss of the drug vapors. The counterpart commercial product is Benzedrex Inhaler (Smith Kline & French).

Tuaminoheptane Inhalant

Tuaminoheptane is a vasoconstrictor, used, as propylhexedrine, in the relief of nasal congestion. The commercial product is Tuamine Inhaler (Lilly). Each inhaler contains approximately 325 mg of tuaminoheptane.

Sprays

Sprays may be defined as aqueous or oleaginous solutions in the form of coarse droplets or as finely divided solids to be applied topically, most usually to the nasal-pharyngeal tract or to the skin. Many commercially available sprays are used intranasally to relieve nasal congestion and inflammation and to combat infection and contain antihistamines, sympathomimetic agents, and antibiotic substances. Other sprays are employed against sunburn and heat burn and contain local anesthetics, antiseptics, skin protectants, and antipruritics. Throat sprays containing antiseptics, deodorants, and flavorants may be effectively employed to relieve conditions such as halitosis, sore throat, or laryngitis. Other sprays may be employed to treat athlete's foot and other fungal infections. Numerous other medicinal and cosmetic uses of sprays are commonly available in pharmacies.

To achieve the breaking up of a solution into small particles so that it may be effectively sprayed or to facilitate the spraying of a powder, several mechanical devices have been developed and are commonly employed. The plastic spray bottle, which is gently squeezed to issue a spray of its contents, is familiar to most persons. It is commonly used for nasal decongestant sprays as well as cosmetically, especially for body deodorant products. Pharmacists are familiar with medicinal "atomizers," which are employed for the issuance of a medicated solution to the patient in the form of fine droplets (Fig. 9-12). One type of atomizer operates by the squeezing of a rubber bulb at the end of the apparatus, which causes a flow of air partially to enter the glass reservoir in which the solution is held and partially to exit from the opposite end of the system. The air forced into the reservoir causes the liquid to rise in a small dip tube, which is maintained below the level of the liquid, forcing the solution up and into the stream of air exiting the system. The air and the solution are forced through a jet opening and the liquid is broken up into a spray, the droplets being carried by the airstream. In other similar apparatuses, the stream of air caused by the depression of the bulb does not enter the reservoir of solution, but passes swiftly over it, creating a pressure change that causes a sucking up of the

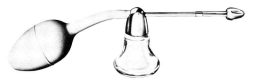

Fig. 9-12. *A common type of atomizer for the administration of a spray of liquid medication. The model shown has an adjustable tip for directing the spray upward or downward to reach otherwise inaccessible areas of the throat. (Courtesy of The DeVilbiss Co.)*

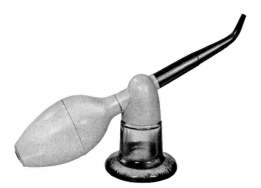

Fig. 9-13. *A general purpose insufflator, used in the application of powdered substances to the nose, throat, ear, tooth sockets, or to body surfaces. (Courtesy of The DeVilbiss Co.)*

liquid into the dip tube and into the airstream in which it exits the system. In instances in which powdered substances are employed rather than solutions, a *powder blower* or a powder *insufflator* may be employed to produce a powder spray. Such an apparatus is similar to the atomizer for liquids; the squeezing of the rubber bulb causes a turbulence within the reservoir of powder, forcing some up the dip tube and out of the tip of the apparatus by the exiting airstream (Fig. 9-13).

Official Sprays

Presently there are no official sprays; however, a number of official solutions, particularly the nasal solutions, are commercially packaged in plastic spray-bottles for use as sprays. Among the official solutions commercially packaged as nasal sprays are:

Naphazoline Hydrochloride Nasal Solution, USP [Privine Hydrochloride Nasal Spray (Ciba)]

Oxymetrazoline Hydrochloride Nasal Solution, USP [Afrin Nasal Spray (Schering)]

Phenylephrine Hydrochloride Nasal Solution, USP [Neo-Synephrine Hydrochloride Nasal Spray (Winthrop)]

Tetrahydrazoline Hydrochloride Nasal Solution, USP [Tyzine Nasal Solution (Pfizer)]

Each of these solutions is an adrenergic nasal solution employed for the vasoconstriction and decongestion of the nasal passages. The solutions will be discussed more fully in Chapter 12.

Selected Reading

Blaug, S. M., and Karig, A. W.: Oral Inhalation Aerosols. Amer. J. Hosp. Pharm., 24:603, 1967.

Contractor, A. M., Shangraw, R. F., and Richman, M. D.: Aerosol Metering Valves. Drug Cosmet. Industr., 95:36, 1964.

Goddard, R. F.: Inhalation Therapy for Infants and Children. Mod. Med., 38:90, 1970.

Harris, R. C.: Filling Pharmaceutical Aerosols. Drug Cosmet. Industr., 103:46, 1968.

Hartley, T. M.: The Big Switch to Propellant Blends. Drug Cosmet. Industr., 91:707, 1962.

Parisse, A. J.: Problems in Developing Inhalation Aerosols. Drug Cosmet. Industr., 105:40, 1969.

Parker, D. N.: Quality Assurance of Aerosol Pharmaceuticals. Drug Cosmet. Industr., 105:54, 1969.

Sciarra, J. J.: Pharmaceutical Aerosols. In *The Theory and Practice of Industrial Pharmacy*, 2nd Ed., L. Lachman, H. A. Lieberman, and J. L. Kanig, eds., Philadelphia, Lea & Febiger, 1976, pp. 270–295.

Sciarra, J. J.: Pharmaceutical and Cosmetic Aerosols, *J. Pharm. Sci.*, 63:1815–1837, 1974.

Yakubic, J.: Formulation of Aerosols. Drug Cosmet. Industr., 95:36, 1964.

Chapter 10

Ointments, Creams, Lotions, and Other Dermatological Preparations

THIS CHAPTER includes dosage forms and official preparations which are intended to be applied to the skin. Ointments, creams, lotions, topical solutions and tinctures represent the most frequently used dosage forms dermatologically; however, other preparations as pastes, liniments, powders, aerosols are also commonly used.

Preparations are applied to the skin either for their physical effects, that is, for their ability to act as skin protectants, lubricants, emollients, drying agents, etc., or for the specific effect of the medicinal agent(s) which may be present. Preparations sold over-the-counter without the requirement of a prescription frequently contain mixtures of medicinal substances and are used in the treatment of such conditions as minor skin infections, itching, burns, diaper rash, insect stings and bites, athlete's foot, corns, calluses, warts, dandruff, acne, psoriasis, and eczema. Skin applications which require a prescription generally contain a single medicinal agent intended to counter a specific diag-

nosed condition. Examples of the official ointments and creams are presented in Table 10-1.

Although it is generally desirable in treating skin diseases for the drug in the medicated application to penetrate past the surface and into the skin, it is not generally the intent that the medication enter the general circulation. However, once past the skin, a drug substance finds itself in proximity to blood capillaries feeding the subcutaneous tissues, and absorption into the general circulation is not unlikely. In fact, such absorption commonly results after topical application of certain preparations as evidenced by detectable blood levels of the drug and the urinary excretion of the drug or its metabolic products. Fortunately, most of the materials employed for topical use are sufficiently nontoxic in the amounts absorbed so that the effects of absorption are generally unrecognized by the patient.

Percutaneous Absorption

The absorption of substances from outside the skin to positions beneath the skin, including entrance into the blood stream, is referred to as *percutaneous absorption.* In general, the percutaneous absorption of a medicinal substance present in a dermatological preparation such as an ointment, cream, or paste depends not only upon the physical and chemical properties of the medicinal substance but also upon its behavior when placed in the pharmaceutical vehicle and upon the condition of the skin. It is well known that although a pharmaceutical vehicle may not penetrate the skin to any great extent nor actually carry the medicinal substance through the skin, the vehicle does influence the rate and degree of penetration of a medicinal agent, and the degree and rate vary with different drugs and with different vehicles. Each individual drug substance in each individual vehicle must therefore be examined to ascertain the rate and degree of drug release from the vehicle and the extent of percutaneous absorption after application in order to assess the therapeutic efficacy of the particular drug-vehicle combination.

The Skin

Upon the surface of the skin is a film of emulsified material composed of a complex mixture of sebum, sweat, and desquamating

Table 10-1. EXAMPLES OF OFFICIAL DERMATOLOGICAL OINTMENTS
AND CREAMS BY THERAPEUTIC CATEGORY

Preparation	Corresponding Commercial Product	Percentage of Active Ingredient*	Comments
Adrenocortical Steroids			
Betamethasone Valerate Cream, and Betamethasone Valerate Ointment, NF	Valisone Cream & Ointment (Schering)	0.1% (ointment) and 0.01% and 0.1% (cream)	
Dexamethasone Sodium Phosphate Cream, USP	Decadron Cream (Merck Sharp & Dohme)	0.1%	
Fluocinolone Acetonide Cream and Fluocinolone Acetonide Ointment, USP	Synalar Cream & Ointment (Syntex)	0.025 and 0.01% (cream) and 0.025% (ointment)	These preparations are indicated for the relief of the inflammatory manifestations
Flurandrenolide Ointment, USP	Cordran Ointment (Lilly)	0.025% and 0.05%	of corticosteroid responsive dermatoses. They are usu-
Hydrocortisone Acetate Ointment, USP	Cortef Acetate Ointment (Upjohn)	1% and 2.5%	ally applied to affected skin areas once to three times a day.
Hydrocortisone Cream and Hydrocortisone Ointment, USP	Cortril Ointment (Pfizer); Eldecort Cream (Elder)	1% (ointment) 0.5, 1.0, and 1.5% (cream)	
Triamcinolone Acetonide Cream and Triamcinolone Acetonide Ointment, USP	Aristocort Ointment (Lederle); Aristocort Cream (Lederle)	0.1% and 0.5% (ointment) and 0.1%, 0.025%, and 0.5% (cream)	
Antibacterial/Anti-infective			
Bacitracin Ointment, USP	Baciguent Ointment (Upjohn)	500 units/g	
Erythromycin Ointment, USP	Ilotycin Ointment (Dista)	1%	These antibiotic preparations are used in the treatment
Gentamicin Sulfate Cream and Gentamicin Sulfate Ointment, USP	Garamycin Cream and Ointment (Schering)	0.17%	of skin infections due to susceptible organisms amenable to local treatment.
Neomycin Sulfate Ointment, USP	Myciguent Ointment (Upjohn)	0.5%	
Neomycin Sulfate, Polymyxin B Sulfate, and Bacitracin Zinc Ointment, NF	Neo-Polycin Ointment (Dow)	Polymyxin B Sulfate, 8000 units/g; Neomycin Sulfate, 0.43%; Zinc Bacitracin, 400 units/g	
Ichthammol Ointment, NF	. . .	1%	See text for discussion.
Iodochlorhydroxyquin Cream and Iodochlorhydroxyquin Ointment NF	Vioform Cream and Ointment (Ciba)	3%	Used for eczema, dermatoses, impetigo, seborrheic dermatitis, and other conditions.
Methylbenzethonium Chloride Ointment	Diaparene Ointment (Breon)	0.1%	For diaper rash, prickly heat, chafing, etc.
Nitrofurazone Cream and Nitrofurazone Ointment, NF	Furacin (Eaton)	0.2%	Antibacterial agent indicated for adjunctive therapy in burn patients or skin-graft patients.
Antieczematic/Antipsoriatics			
Anthralin Ointment, USP	Anthra-Derm (Dermik)	0.25, 0.5, and 1.0%	Anthralin inhibits enzyme metabolism. Used in treating psoriasis.

Table 10-1. EXAMPLES OF OFFICIAL DERMATOLOGICAL OINTMENTS
AND CREAMS BY THERAPEUTIC CATEGORY (*Cont.*)

Preparation	Corresponding Commercial Product	Percentage of Active Ingredient*	Comments
Antieczematic/Antipsoriatics (cont.)			
Coal Tar Ointment, USP	. . .	1%	Used for its antipruritic, antieczematous and keratoplastic action in treating psoriasis and other chronic skin disorders. See text for additional discussion.
Antifungals			
Benzoic and Salicylic Acid Ointment, USP	. . .	6% benzoic acid and 3% salicylic acid	General antifungal preparations and skin keratolytic.
Nystatin Ointment, USP	Mycostatin Ointment (Squibb)	100,000 units/g	An antifungal antibiotic for cutaneous and mucocutaneous mycotic infections.
Compound Resorcinol Ointment, NF	. . .	6% resorcinol	Local antifungal and keratolytic. See text for additional discussion.
Compound Undecylenic Acid Ointment, USP	Desenex Ointment (Pharmacraft)	5% undecylenic acid and 20% zinc undecylenate	Used mainly for athlete's foot and ringworm.
Tolnaftate Cream, USP	Tinactin Cream (Schering)	1%	For topical treatment of tinea pedis, tinea cruris, tinea corporis and tinea manuum.
Antineoplastic			
Fluorouracil Cream, USP	Efudex Cream (Roche)	5%	For treatment of multiple actinic or solar keratoses.
Anesthetics (Local)			
Benzocaine Ointment, NF	Americaine Ointment (Arnar-Stone)	20%	
Cyclomethycaine Sulfate Cream and Cyclomethycaine Sulfate Ointment, NF	Surfacaine Cream and Ointment (Lilly)	0.5% (cream) and 1% (ointment)	Applied to skin to relieve pain and itching of sunburn, insect bites, etc.
Dibucaine Cream and Ointment NF	Nupercainal Cream and Ointment (Ciba)	0.5% (cream) and 1% (ointment)	
Tetracaine Ointment, NF and Tetracaine HCl Cream, NF	Pontocaine Cream and Ointment (Winthrop)	0.5% (ointment) and 1% (cream)	
Astringent/Protectant			
Zinc Oxide Ointment, USP	. . .	20%	See text for additional discussion
Depigmenting Agents			
Hydroquinone Ointment, USP	Eldopaque Ointment (Elder)	2% and 4%	Used in the temporary bleaching of hyperpigmented skin blemished due to freckles, old age spots, and cholasma.
Monobenzone Ointment, NF	Benoquin Ointment (Elder)	20%	

Table 10-1. EXAMPLES OF OFFICIAL DERMATOLOGICAL OINTMENTS
AND CREAMS BY THERAPEUTIC CATEGORY (*Cont.*)

Preparation	Corresponding Commercial Product	Percentage of Active Ingredient*	Comments
Scabicides			
Sulfur Ointment, USP	. . .	10%	Used in the treatment of ringworms, scabies, and pediculosis. See text for additional discussion.
Gamma Benzene Hexachloride Cream, USP	Kwell Cream (Reed and Carnrick)	1%	Used in the treatment of scabies and infestations with head lice and crab lice.
Crotamiton Cream, NF	Eurax Cream (Geigy)	10%	For eradication of scabies and symptomatic treatment of pruritus.
Sunscreening Agent			
Dioxybenzone and Oxybenzone Cream, USP	Solbar Cream (Person & Covey)	3% each of dioxybenzone and oxybenzone	Protects the skin against burning effects of the sun's ultraviolet rays.

* Unless otherwise indicated, the active constituent referred to is that agent named in the preparation's official title.

horny layer, the latter from the layer of dead epidermal cells, termed the "horny layer" or the "stratum corneum," and situated directly beneath the emulsified film. Beneath the horny layer in order is a "barrier layer," the living epidermis or the stratum germinativum, and the dermis or true skin.

Blood capillaries and nerve fibers rise from the subcutaneous fat tissue into the dermis and up to the epidermis. Sweat glands present in the subcutaneous tissue yield their products by way of sweat ducts which find their way to the surface of the skin. Sebaceous (oil) glands and hair follicles originating in the dermis and subcutaneous layers also find their way to the surface and are revealed as ducts and hairs respectively.

Penetration of the Skin by Drugs

Drugs could possibly penetrate intact skin after topical application through the walls of the hair follicles, through the sweat glands or the sebaceous glands, or between the cells of the horny layer. Naturally, broken or abraded skin is easily entered by applied substances, but such penetration does not really constitute true percutaneous absorption. In fact, the application of medicinal substances to skin areas devoid of their normal barrier may lead to very

rapid drug entrance into the blood stream, an event that is usually not welcomed in topical therapy.

If the skin is intact, the main route for the penetration of drug is generally through the epidermal layers, rather than through the hair follicles or the gland ducts, since the surface area of the latter is rather minute compared to the area of skin containing neither of these anatomical elements. The film covering the horny layer is not generally continuous and presents no real resistance to penetration. Since the composition of the film varies with the proportion of sebum and sweat produced and the degree of their removal through washing and sweat evaporation, the film is not a true barrier to drug transfer, since it has no definite composition, thickness, or continuity.

The horny layer of the skin, about 20 to 40 microns thick, is composed chiefly of keratin, a protein substance, and lipids. It is considered to act as a sponge, being capable of holding or absorbing water with both lipid- and water-soluble substances entering it. The barrier layer is only about 10 microns in thickness and is thought to prevent the penetration of molecules having molecular weights of greater than about 200 or 300. The resistance to penetration is considered to be due not to the smallness of the pores of the barrier layer, but rather to the molecular interactions between penetrating

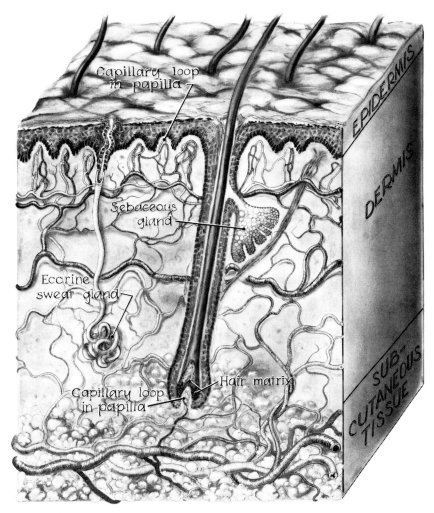

Fig. 10-1. *Stratified organization of the skin. (Pillsbury, D. M.: A Manual of Dermatology. Courtesy of W. B. Saunders Co., 1971.)*

substances and the pore contents. Molecules that do penetrate this barrier layer are either bound to the living epidermis or make their way to the lymphatic or blood vessels and are carried away for detoxication and excretion.

Factors Affecting Percutaneous Absorption

Among the factors playing a part in the percutaneous absorption of drugs are the nature of the drug itself, the nature of the vehicle, the condition of the skin, and the presence of moisture. There are many conflicting reports concerning the influence of each of these factors on the percutaneous absorption of specific drugs,

and general statements applicable to all possible combinations of drug, vehicle, and skin condition are difficult to draw. However, the consensus of the majority of the findings may be summarized as follows:[1]

1. The primary requirement for topical therapy is that the drug incorporated in a vehicle reach the skin surface at an adequate rate and in sufficient concentration.
2. Drug concentration is an important factor. Generally, the amount of drug percuta-

[1] Adapted largely from Barr, M.: Percutaneous Absorption. *J. Pharm. Sci.*, 51:395–409, 1962, and Idson, B.: Percutaneous Absorption., *J. Pharm. Sci.*, 64:901–924, 1975.

neously absorbed per unit of surface area per time interval increases as the concentration of the drug substance in the vehicle is increased.

3. More drug is absorbed through percutaneous absorption when the drug substance is applied to a larger surface area.

4. The drug substance should be attracted by the membranes of the skin to a greater extent than the drug molecule is attracted to the vehicle in which it is presented for percutaneous absorption in order for the drug to have the tendency to leave the vehicle in favor of the skin. On the other hand, the drug must not have such a great affinity for the tissues that it remains tightly bound and fails to penetrate as deeply as is required of it. For instance, a local anesthetic substance must penetrate to the nerve fibers to be effective.

5. In general, the greater the solubility of a drug in oil, the greater its percutaneous absorption. However, some degree of solubility of the drug substance in both oil and water is thought to be essential for effective percutaneous absorption. In essence, the aqueous solubility of a drug determines the concentration presented to the absorption site and the partition coefficient strongly influences the rate of transport across the absorption site.

6. Drug absorption appears to be best from vehicles that easily cover the skin surface, mix readily with the sebum, and bring the drug into contact with the tissue cells for absorption.

7. It is generally believed that the vehicle itself is incapable of promoting the absorption of "nonabsorbable" drugs distributed in it but that it may have the capability of modifying the absorption patterns of drugs that are "absorbable" without the presence of the vehicle.

8. The absorption of "absorbable" drugs is better from animal and vegetable oils than from mineral oils because the former types penetrate the skin more readily. Also, organic solvents such as ether, acetone, and benzene can enhance the absorption of a drug dissolved in them through their penetrability.

9. Vehicles that increase the amount of moisture imbibed by the skin generally favorably affect the percutaneous absorption of drugs.

Oleaginous vehicles act as moisture barriers through which the sweat from the skin cannot pass, and the skin therefore remains occluded, generally resulting in an increased hydration of the skin beneath the vehicle. Vehicles of the water-in-oil emulsion type are probably next in effectiveness to oleaginous vehicles in enhancing the hydration of the skin. Vehicles containing humectants like glycerin to keep the ointment moist and from drying out have a tendency to draw moisture from the skin when conditions of low humidity prevail and actually can reduce the moisture content of the skin.

10. The hydration of the skin is one of the most important factors in percutaneous absorption. The hydration of the stratum corneum appears to increase the rate of passage of all substances that penetrate the skin. Increased absorption is probably due to the softening of the tissue and the consequent "sponging" effect with an increase in the size of the pores, allowing a greater flow of substances, large and small, through them.

11. Hydration of the skin is influenced not only by the type of vehicle (e.g., oleaginous) but also by the absence or presence of a bandage (and the type) over the medicated application. In general, bandaging a nonocclusive application such as a water-miscible vehicle, will enhance the moisturizing effect of the skin through the inhibition of the evaporation of the sweat and thereby enhance absorption. An occlusive bandage is more effective in this regard than a loosely woven, nonocclusive one.

12. In general, the amount of rubbing in or inunction of the topical application will have a bearing on the amount of drug absorbed; the longer the period of inunction, the greater the absorption.

13. Percutaneous absorption appears to be greater when the drug is applied to skin with a thin horny layer than with one that is thick. Thus, the site of application may have a bearing on the degree of drug absorption, with the absorption from such sites as the palms of the hands and soles of the feet which have thick layers of horny layer being comparatively slow.

14. Generally, the longer the period of time the medicated application is permitted to remain in contact with the skin, the greater

will be the absorption. However, changes in the hydration of the skin during the application period or the saturation of the skin with the drug could preclude significant additional absorption with increasing time.

In conclusion, it should be pointed out that the above findings have been summarized from a great deal of data obtained from tests on human and animal skin which is generally in the normal state. Under the disease or injury conditions usually prevailing when topical preparations are used, the skin may be sufficiently abnormal to nullify many of the postulates stated above. Quite clearly, skin that has been abraded, cut, or broken will permit drugs, and for that matter other foreign substances, to gain direct access to the subcutaneous tissues.

Ointments

Ointments (*unguents*) are semisolid preparations intended for external application. Those intended for application to the eye are specially prepared and are termed *ophthalmic ointments*. They will be taken up in the next chapter. Ointments may be medicated or nonmedicated, the latter type being commonly referred to as *ointment bases* and used as such for their emollient or lubricating effect or used as vehicles in the preparation of medicated ointments.

Ointment Bases

The USP and the NF classify ointment bases into four general groups: (1) hydrocarbon bases, (2) absorption bases, (3) water-removable bases, and (4) water-soluble bases. Official examples are listed after the discussion of each group.

Official Hydrocarbon Bases

Hydrocarbon bases (oleaginous bases) are water-free, and aqueous preparations may only be incorporated into them in small amounts and then with difficulty. Hydrocarbon bases are used chiefly for their emollient effect. They are retained on the skin for prolonged periods, do not permit the escape of moisture from the skin to the atmosphere, and are difficult to wash off. As such they act as occlusive dressings. They do not change noticeably upon aging.

Petrolatum, NF

Petrolatum, NF, is a mixture of semisolid hydrocarbons obtained from petroleum. Petrolatum is an unctuous mass, varying in color from yellowish to light amber. It melts between 38° and 60°.

Synonyms: Yellow Petrolatum; Petroleum Jelly
Commercial Product: Vaseline (Chesebrough)

White Petrolatum, USP

White Petrolatum, USP is petrolatum that has been decolorized. It differs only in this respect to petrolatum and is used for the same purpose.

Synonym: White Petroleum Jelly
Commercial Product: White Vaseline (Chesebrough)

Yellow Ointment, NF

Each 100 g of Yellow Ointment, NF, contains 5 g of yellow wax and 95 g of petrolatum. Yellow Wax, NF, is the purified wax obtained from the honeycomb of the bee (*Apis mellifera*).

Synonym: Simple Ointment

White Ointment, USP

White Ointment, USP, contains 5% of white wax (bleached, purified beeswax) and 95% white petrolatum.

Paraffin, NF

Paraffin, NF, is a purified mixture of solid hydrocarbons obtained from petroleum. It is a colorless or white, more or less translucent mass that may be used to harden or stiffen oleaginous semisolid ointment bases.

Mineral Oil, USP

Mineral Oil, USP, is a mixture of liquid hydrocarbons obtained from petroleum. It is useful in the levigating of substances insoluble in it in the preparation of ointments in oleaginous bases.

Synonym: Liquid Petrolatum

Official Absorption Bases

Absorption bases may be of two types: (1) those that permit the incorporation of aqueous solutions, resulting in the formation of water-in-oil emulsions (e.g. *Hydrophilic Petrolatum* and *Anhydrous Lanolin*) and (2) those that are already water-in-oil emulsions (*emulsion bases*) that permit the incorporation of small, additional quantities of aqueous solutions (e.g. *Lanolin* and *Cold Cream*). These bases are useful as emollients although they do not provide the degree of occlusion afforded by the oleaginous bases. Like the oleaginous bases, absorption bases are not easily removed from the skin with water washing. They are also useful pharmaceutically in incorporating aqueous solutions into oleaginous bases. For example, an aqueous solution may be first absorbed into the absorption base, and then this mixture may be easily incorporated into the oleaginous base. In doing this, an equivalent amount of oleaginous base in the formula is replaced by the absorption base.

Hydrophilic Petrolatum, USP

Hydrophilic Petrolatum, USP, is composed of cholesterol, stearyl alcohol, white wax, and white petrolatum. It has the ability to absorb water, with the formation of a water-in-oil emulsion.

Anhydrous Lanolin, USP

Anhydrous lanolin may contain no more than 0.25% of water. Anhydrous lanolin is insoluble in water but mixes without separation with about twice its weight of water. The incorporation of water results in the formation of a water-in-oil emulsion.

Synonym: Refined Wool Fat

Lanolin, USP

Lanolin, USP, is a semisolid, fatlike substance obtained from the wool of sheep (*Ovis aries*). It is a water-in-oil emulsion that contains between 25 to 30% water. Additional water may be incorporated into lanolin by mixing.

Synonym: Hydrous Wool Fat

Cold Cream, USP

Cold Cream, USP, is a semisolid, white, water-in-oil emulsion prepared with spermaceti (a waxy substance obtained from the head of the sperm whale *Physeter macrocephalus*), white wax, mineral oil, sodium borate, and purified water. The sodium borate combines with the free fatty acids present in the waxes to form sodium soaps that act as the emulsifiers. Cold cream is employed as an emollient and ointment base.

Official Water-removable Base

Water-removable bases are oil-in-water emulsions that are capable of being washed from skin or clothing with water. For this reason, they are frequently referred to as "water-washable" ointment bases. These bases, which resemble creams in their appearance, may be diluted with water or with aqueous solutions. From a therapeutic viewpoint, they have the ability to absorb serous discharges in dermatologic conditions. Certain medicinal agents may be better absorbed by the skin when present in a base of this type than in other types of bases.

Hydrophilic Ointment, USP

Hydrophilic Ointment, USP, as the title indicates, is "water-loving." It contains sodium lauryl sulfate as the emulsifying agent, with stearyl alcohol and white petrolatum representing the oleaginous phase of the emulsion and propylene glycol and water representing the aqueous phase. Methylparaben and propylparaben are used to preserve the ointment against microbial growth. The ointment is employed as a water-removable vehicle for medicinal substances.

Official Water-soluble Base

Unlike water-removable bases, which contain both water soluble and water insoluble components, water-soluble bases contain only water-soluble components. Like water-removable bases, however, water-soluble bases are water washable. Water-soluble bases are commonly referred to as "greaseless" because of the absence of any oleaginous materials. Because they soften greatly with the addition of water, aqueous solutions are not effectively incorporated into these bases. Rather, they are better used for the incorporation of nonaqueous or solid substances.

Polyethylene Glycol Ointment, USP

The official formula for this base calls for the combining of 400 g of polyethylene glycol 4000 (a solid) and 600 g of polyethylene glycol 400 (a liquid) to prepare 1000 g of base. However, if a firmer ointment is required, the formula may be altered to permit up to equal parts of the two ingredients. If 6 to 25% of an aqueous solution is to be incorporated into the base, the USP permits the substitution of 50 g of the polyethylene glycol 4000 with an equal amount of stearyl alcohol to render the final product more firm.

Polyethylene glycols 400 and 4000 are polymers of ethylene oxide and water represented by the formula $HOCH_2(CH_2OCH_2)_nCH_2OH$ in which the average "n" varies from 8.2 to 9.1 for polyethylene glycol 400 and from 68 to 84 for polyethylene glycol 4000. The chain length may be varied to achieve polymers having desired physical (liquid, semisolid, or solid) form.

Selection of the Appropriate Base

The selection of the base to use in the formulation of an ointment depends upon the careful assessment of a number of factors, including (a) the desired release rate of the particular drug substance from the ointment base, (b) the desirability for enhancement by the base of the percutaneous absorption of the drug, (c) the advisability of occlusion of moisture from the skin by the base, (d) the short-term and long-term stability of the drug in the ointment base, and (e) the influence, if any, of the drug on the consistency or other features of the ointment base. All of these factors, and others, must be weighed one against the other to find the most suitable base. It should be understood that no ointment base is ideal nor possesses all of the desired attributes. For instance, for a drug that hydrolyzes rapidly, a hydrocarbon base would provide the greatest stability, even though from a therapeutic standpoint another base might be preferred. The idea is to find the base that provides the majority of what are considered to be the most essential attributes and to compromise when necessary.

In preparing ointments the official compendia permit the alteration of the proportions of substances constituting the base to maintain suitable consistency under different climatic conditions, provided the proportions of the active ingredients are not varied.

Preparation of Ointments

Both on a large and a small scale, ointments are prepared by two general methods: (1) incorporation and (2) fusion. The method for a particular preparation depends primarily upon the nature of the ingredients.

Incorporation

In the incorporation method, the components of the ointment are mixed together by various means until a uniform preparation has been attained. On a small scale, as in the extemporaneous compounding of prescriptions, the pharmacist may mix the components of an ointment in a mortar with a pestle, or he may employ a

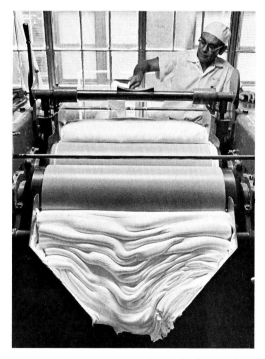

Fig. 10-2. *Day ointment roller mill. Standards of fineness and smoothness require that no grains of material be visible under a ten-power microscope after passage through this machine. (Courtesy of Eli Lilly and Company)*

spatula and an ointment slab (a large glass or porcelain plate) to rub the ingredients together. Some glass ointment slabs are of ground glass to permit greater friction in the rubbing process. Some pharmacists utilize nonabsorbent parchment papers that are large enough to cover the working surface and have the advantage of being disposable, eliminating much of the time-consuming chore of cleaning the ointment slab.

INCORPORATION OF SOLIDS. In preparing an ointment by spatulation, the pharmacist generally works the ointment with a stainless steel spatula with a long, broad blade and periodically removes the accumulation of ointment on the larger spatula with a smaller spatula. If the components of an ointment are reactive with the metal of the spatula (as for example, mercuric salts, iodine, and tannins), hard rubber spatulas are commonly used. The ointment is prepared by thoroughly rubbing and working the components together on the hard surface with the spatula until the product is smooth and uniform. Generally speaking, the ointment base is placed on one side of the working surface, and the powdered components, previously reduced to fine powders and thoroughly blended in a mortar, if there are more than one, are placed on the other. Then a portion of the powder is mixed with a portion of the base until uniform, and the process is repeated until all portions of the powder and base are combined. The portions of prepared ointment are then combined and thoroughly blended by continuous movement of the spatula over and through the combined portions of ointment.

When only a small portion of powder is to be added, it may be added in its entirety to a small portion of ointment base. After the two have been thoroughly mixed, another portion of base is added to this mixture, the process being repeated as in the "geometric method" of diluting until all of the ointment base has been incorporated.

Frequently it is desirable to reduce further the particle size of any solid material before incorporation into the ointment base so that the final product will not be gritty. This may be done by *levigating* the powder by mixing it in a vehicle in which it is insoluble to make a smooth dispersion of the material. Most commonly the solid substance is mixed with mineral oil or with a portion of the ointment base, using an amount of levigating agent about equal to the material to be levigated, and a mortar and pestle to accomplish the reduction of particle size as well as the dispersion of the substance. After levigation, the dispersion is incorporated with the remainder of the base by spatulation or by using the mortar and pestle.

Solid materials soluble in a common solvent that will affect neither the stability of the drug nor the efficacy of the product may first be dissolved in that solvent, and then the solution may be added to the appropriate ointment base by spatulation or by mixing in a mortar and pestle. Generally, the mortar and pestle is preferred when large volumes of any liquid are to be added to an ointment, as the liquid is more captive in the mortar and yields to more efficient incorporation.

INCORPORATION OF LIQUIDS. Liquid substances or solutions of drugs, as described above, are added to an ointment only after due consideration of the ointment's nature. For instance, an aqueous solution or preparation would be added with difficulty to an oleaginous ointment, except in very small amounts. However, water-absorbable or hydrophilic ointment bases would be quite suitable for the absorption and incorporation of the aqueous solution. Frequently when adding an aqueous preparation to a base that is hydrophobic in character, the pharmacist replaces a portion of the base with a hydrophilic base, incorporates the solution in the latter, and then mixes the product with the original base. It should be understood, however, that all bases, even if hydrophilic, have their limits of capacity; additional amounts of water render them too soft or semiliquid. Ointments must be semisolid, and sometimes pharmacists may find it appropriate to reduce the water content of a solution or utilize another dosage form of comparable merit in the preparation of the ointment. For instance, if a large amount of an alcoholic solution, such as a tincture, is to be added to an ointment base, the calculated equivalent of the fluidextract or the pilular extract of the same drug substance may be better incorporated.

Alcoholic solutions of small volume usually may be added quite well to oleaginous vehicles or emulsion bases. However, because the alcohol may evaporate and result in deposits of gritty solute on standing, it is usually best to evaporate the alcohol from the preparation (assuming the drug is heat stable) prior to incorporation into the base.

Other liquid material, for instance, natural balsams, are incorporated into ointment bases with difficulty. It is customary to mix a balsam such as Peru balsam with an equal portion of castor oil before incorporating it into the base. This procedure reduces the surface tension of the balsam and provides for the even distribution of the balsam throughout the vehicle.

On a large scale, mechanical ointment roller mills force coarsely formed ointments through moving stainless steel rollers, resulting in the formation of products that are smooth and uniform in composition and texture. Prior to passage through the mills, the ointment may be coarsely prepared in powerful ointment and paste mixers. Small ointment mills are available for the production of small batches of product, and pharmacies that routinely prepare medicated applications find these small mills useful additions to their equipment.

Fusion

By the fusion method, all or some of the components of an ointment are combined by being melted together and cooled with constant stirring until congealed. Those components not melted are generally added to the congealing mixture as it is being cooled and stirred. Naturally, heat-labile substances and any volatile components are added last when the temperature of the mixture is low enough not to cause decomposition or volatilization of the components. Many substances are added to the congealing mixture in solution, others are added as insoluble powders generally levigated with a portion of the base. On a small scale, the fusion process may be conducted in a porcelain dish or glass beaker; on a large scale, it is generally carried out in large steam-jacketed kettles. Once congealed, the ointment may be passed through an ointment mill (in large-scale manufacture) or rubbed with a spatula or in a mortar (in small-scale preparation) to ensure a uniform texture.

Many medicated ointments and ointment bases containing such components as beeswax, paraffin, stearyl alcohol, and high molecular weight polyethylene glycols, which do not lend themselves well to mixture by incorporation, are prepared by fusion. In preparing an ointment with these types of materials by fusion, it is generally found that the melting points of the individual components are quite varied; therefore, the temperatures required to achieve fusion may also vary from formula to formula. In a given formula, if the item having the highest melting point is melted first and the other components are added to this hot liquid, all of the components will be subjected to this high temperature, irrespective of their own individual melting points, and generally a temperature higher than necessary will have to be employed to achieve fusion. Either by melting the component having the lowest melting point first and adding the components of higher melting point in order of their individual melting points or by melting all of the components together very slowly, a lower temperature is usually sufficient to achieve fusion. This is apparently due to the solvent action exerted by the first melted component on the other components, and if the process is allowed to proceed by using only slowly rising temperatures, the fusion process does not generally require the high temperature normally required to melt the individual component having the highest melting point.

In the preparation of ointments having an emulsion type of formula—for example, cold cream—the general method of manufacture involves a melting process as well as an emulsification process. Usually, the water-immiscible components such as the oil and waxes are melted together on a steam bath to about 70° to 75°C. Meantime, an aqueous solution of all of the heat-stable, water-soluble components is being prepared in the amount of purified water specified in the formula and heated to the same temperature as the oleaginous components. Then the aqueous solution is slowly added, with constant stirring (usually with a mechanical stirrer), to the melted oleaginous mixture, the temperature is maintained for 5 to 10 minutes to prevent crystallization of waxes, and then the mixture is slowly cooled with the stirring continued until the mixture is congealed. If the aqueous solution were not the same temperature as the oleaginous melt, there would be solidification of some of the waxes upon the addition of the colder aqueous solution to the melted mixture.

Preservation of Ointments

Semisolid pharmaceutical preparations, as ointments, frequently require the addition of chemical antimicrobial preservatives to the formulation to inhibit the growth of contaminating microorganisms. These preservatives include p-hydroxybenzoates, phenols, benzoic acid, sorbic acid, quaternary ammonium compounds, mercurials and other compounds. Semisolid preparations utilizing bases which contain or hold water support microbial growth to a greater extent than those which have little moisture, and thus constitute the greater problem of preservation.

Semisolid preparations must also be protected through proper packaging and storage from the destructive influences of air, light, moisture, and heat, and the possible chemical interactions between the preparation and the container.

Packaging and Storage of Ointments

Ointments are usually packaged either in jars or in tubes. The jars may be made of glass, uncolored, colored green, amber, or blue, or opaque and porcelain-white. Plastic jars are also in use to a limited extent. Opaque and colored-glass containers are useful for ointments containing drugs that are light-sensitive. The tubes are made of tin or of plastic, some of them copackaged with special tips when the ointment is to be used for rectal, ophthalmic, vaginal, aural or nasal application. Tubes of ointments for ophthalmic use are most commonly packaged in small, tin, collapsible tubes holding about $\frac{1}{8}$ oz (about 3.5 g) of ointment. Tubes of ointments for topical use are more frequently of 5 g to 30 g size. Jars for ointments may vary in size from as little as a half ounce to a pound or more.

Ointment jars may be filled on a small scale by the pharmacist by packing the weighed amount of ointment into the jar by means of a flexible spatula and forcing the ointment down and along the sides of the jar to avoid the entrapment of air. In packing an ointment jar, the idea is to attain a level surface of ointment high enough to be near the top of the jar, but not so high as to touch the lid when it is placed on the jar. Some pharmacists like to finish the top of the ointment so that it has a gloss. This may be done by slightly melting a portion of the base by placing the filled jar under a heat-lamp for a few seconds. Through the adept use of the spatula, other pharmacists prefer to place a "curl" in the center of the surface of the ointment.

Ointments prepared by fusion may be poured directly into the ointment jars for congealing within the jar. These ointments normally assume a finished look. In the large-scale manufacture of ointments, pressure fillers force a specified amount of an ointment into a jar.

Tubes may be filled by pressure fillers from the open back end (opposite end from the cap end) of the tube, which is then closed and sealed. Ointments prepared by fusion may be poured directly into the tubes. On a small scale, as in the extemporaneous filling of an ointment tube by the community pharmacist, the tube may be filled in the following manner.

1. The prepared ointment is rolled into a cylinder shape in a piece of parchment paper, the cylinder being of a slightly lesser diameter than the tube to be filled but with the paper longer than the cylinder.
2. With the cap of the tube off to permit the escape of air, the cylinder of ointment with the paper is inserted into the open, bottom-end of the tube.
3. The piece of paper covering the ointment is grasped in one hand; the other hand forces a heavy spatula down on the extreme end of the tube, collapsing it and retaining the ointment while the paper is slowly pulled from the tube. About $\frac{1}{2}$ inch of the bottom of the tube is then flattened with the spatula.
4. About two $\frac{1}{8}$ inch folds are made from the flattened bottom end of the tube, and a sealing clip is placed over the folds to secure their closure. The clip may be applied with a hand plier or with a hand- or foot-operated "crimper" machine.

Industrially, automatic tube-filling, closing, and crimper machines are employed for the large-scale production of tube-filled ointments.

Tube-filled ointments predominate over jar-filled ointments primarily because they are more convenient for the patient, with less handling and mess resulting. Also, ointments in tubes are less exposed to air and to potential contaminants and are therefore likely to be more stable and to remain efficacious for longer periods of time than ointments packaged in jars.

Most ointments must be stored at temperatures below 30° to prevent the softening and even the liquefying of the base.

Examples of the official dermatologic ointments are presented in Table 10-1. The majority

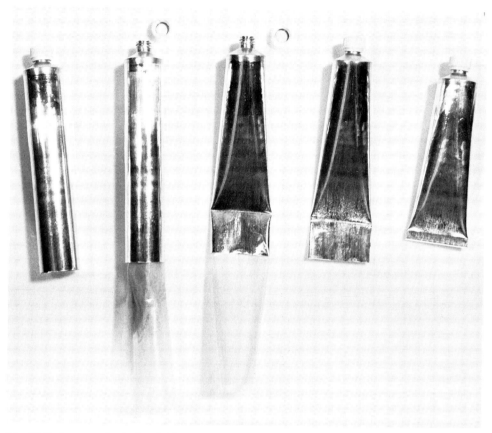

Fig. 10-3. *Sequence in the hand filling of ointment tubes.*

of these ointments are available commercially to the pharmacist and he usually dispenses the pre-manufactured product. Occasionally the pharmacist is called upon to fortify or reduce the strength of one of these commercial preparations, to add additional medicinal components to an existing ointment, or to combine two or more commercial ointments in compounding a prescription. In adding medicinal or pharmaceutical substances to a commercial preparation, the pharmacist should be certain that the material he adds is compatible with the existing preparation and does not adversely affect the required stability of the product.

In fortifying an ointment by the incorporation of additional active constituent, the pharmacist's source of the drug usually is pure powdered drug substance, or powder from the corresponding commercial tablet or capsule. In diluting the strength of active constituent in an ointment, the pharmacist mixes it with the appropriately calculated amount of an ointment base similar in physical features to that of the original ointment. The strength of an ointment may also be altered by combining it with other ointments of the same drug of greater or lesser strength.

Official ointments that are commonly used by the pharmacist from their commercial suppliers or which are protected by patents are not generally represented in the official compendia by specific formulations. Presently, the official compendia present pharmaceutical formulas for the following nonmedicated ointment bases: Cold Cream, Hydrophilic Ointment, Polyethylene Glycol Ointment, White Ointment, and Yellow Ointment. The composition of these ointment bases has been previously discussed. Of the medicated ointments, official formulas exist for the following: Coal Tar Ointment, Ichthammol Ointment, Compound Resorcinol Ointment, Sulfur Ointment and Zinc Oxide Ointment. These ointments are discussed briefly as follows:

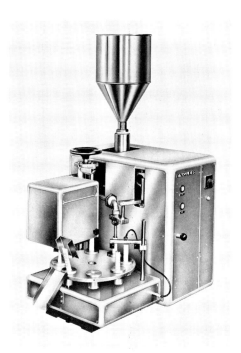

Fig. 10-4. *Example of a small-scale fully automatic filling and crimping machine for collapsible metal tubes. The capacity of the machine is up to 60 units per minute. (Courtesy of Chemical and Pharmaceutical Industry Co.)*

Coal Tar Ointment, USP

Coal Tar Ointment, USP, contains 1% of coal tar in a base of zinc oxide paste. A small amount of polysorbate 80, a nonionic surfactant, is employed in the preparation of the ointment and serves a dual purpose. It is mixed with the coal tar prior to incorporation with the base to increase the dispersion of the coal tar in the paste and to enhance the removal of the ointment from the skin during washing. The ointment is employed as an antieczematic.

Ichthammol Ointment, NF

Ichthammol is a reddish-brown to brownish-black, viscous liquid that is obtained by the destructive distillation of certain bituminous schists, sulfonating the distillate, and neutralizing the product with ammonia. Ichthammol is a local antibacterial and irritant. The ointment is prepared by mixing 10% each of ichthammol and anhydrous lanolin together and then mixing the product with petrolatum.

Compound Resorcinol Ointment, NF

Compound Resorcinol Ointment, NF, is a multicomponent ointment having resorcinol, bismuth subnitrate, zinc oxide, and juniper tar as the active ingredients. The resorcinol is dis-

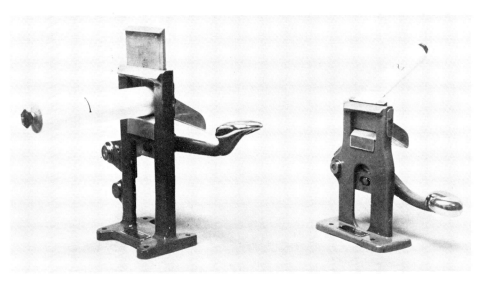

Fig. 10-5. *Hand-operated tube-closing apparatus. Model at left can close tubes up to about $1\frac{3}{4}$ inch diameter at an hourly rate of about 300 tubes. Model at right is for smaller tubes up to 1 inch in diameter. It can be operated at an hourly production of about 400 tubes. (Courtesy of Chemical and Pharmaceutical Industry Co., Inc.)*

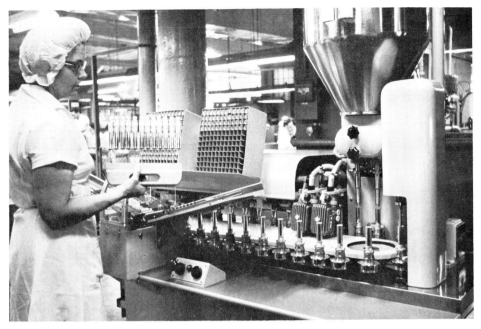

Fig. 10-6. *Arenco tube-filling machine automatically fills 125 tubes a minute with proper amount, tightens cap, orients each tube by electric eye so that label faces forward, then closes and crimps the end. (Courtesy of Eli Lilly and Company)*

solved in glycerin before incorporating into the ointment base to effect a smooth preparation. The ointment is categorized by the NF as an antifungal and keratolytic.

Sulfur Ointment, USP

Sulfur Ointment, USP, contains 10% of precipitated sulfur in white ointment and is prepared with mineral oil as the levigating agent for the sulfur. Precipitated sulfur is employed rather than sublimed sulfur (also official) because the former is of finer particle size and results in a smoother ointment with a greater reactive surface. The ointment is used in the treatment of ringworm, scabies, and pediculosis. The USP categorizes sulfur as a scabicide.

Zinc Oxide Ointment, USP

In the preparation of Zinc Oxide Ointment, USP, 20% of zinc oxide is levigated with mineral oil, and the mixture is incorporated into white ointment. The ointment is employed topically as an astringent and protective in various skin conditions.

Creams

Creams are defined by the USP and the NF simply as "semisolid emulsions of either the oil-in-water or the water-in-oil type." Creams are usually employed as emollients or as medicated applications to the skin.

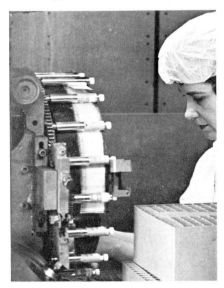

Fig. 10-7. *Industrial scale tube labeling machinery. (Courtesy of Eli Lilly and Company.)*

The term cream is widely used in the pharmaceutical and cosmetic industry, and many of the commercial products referred to as creams may not actually conform to the above definition. Many products that are creamy in appearance but do not have an emulsion-type base are commonly called creams.

So-called "vanishing creams" are generally oil-in-water emulsions containing large percentages of water and stearic acid. After application of the cream, the water evaporates leaving behind a thin residue film of the stearic acid.

Many patients and physicians prefer creams to ointments. For one thing, they are generally easier to spread, and, in the case of creams of the oil-in-water emulsion-type, easier to remove than many ointments. Pharmaceutical manufacturers frequently market their topical preparations in both cream and ointment bases to satisfy the preference of the patient and physician.

Creams are packaged and preserved in the same manner as discussed previously for ointments.

Official Creams

Examples of some of the official creams for use on the skin are presented in Table 10-1. Creams utilized by other means, as intravaginally, are presented in a later chapter. As is the case for ointments, the official compendia do not provide formulations for most creams since they generally are produced by large manufacturers using various formulative components. In fact, the only official cream having a formula given in the compendia is Cold Cream, USP. The components of this cream have been previously mentioned during the discussion of absorption bases.

Pastes

Pastes, like ointments, are intended for external application to the skin. They differ from ointments primarily in that they generally contain a larger percentage of solid material and as a consequence are thicker and stiffer than ointments. Because of their large percentage of solids, pastes are generally more absorptive and less greasy than ointments prepared with the same components.

Pastes are prepared similarly to ointments. However, when a levigating agent is to be used to render the powdered component smooth and more easily incorporable into the ointment base, the agent is sometimes a portion of the base, rather than a liquid like mineral oil that would soften the paste.

Because of the stiffness and absorptive qualities of pastes, they remain in place after application with little tendency to soften and flow and are therefore effectively employed to absorb serous secretions from the site of application. Pastes are therefore preferred over ointments for acute lesions that have a tendency toward crusting, vesiculation, or oozing. However, because of their stiffness and impenetrability, pastes are not generally suited for application to hairy parts of the body. When other medicaments are added to a paste, they are absorbed less readily than from ointments and therefore exert a more topical activity.

Official Pastes

There are only three official pastes: Triamcinolone Acetonide Dental Paste, USP, an anti-inflammatory preparation applied topically to the oral mucous membranes, Zinc Oxide Paste, USP, and Zinc Oxide Paste with Salicylic Acid, NF. The latter two pastes are intended for topical application to the skin and are described below.

Zinc Oxide Paste, USP

Zinc Oxide Paste, USP, is prepared by levigating and then mixing 25% each of zinc oxide and starch with white petrolatum. The product is very firm and difficult to manipulate with a spatula. It is capable of absorbing moisture to a much greater extent than zinc oxide ointment and is employed as an astringent and protective. The paste also frequently serves as a vehicle for other medicinal substances.

Synonym: Lassar's Plain Zinc Paste

Zinc Oxide Paste with Salicylic Acid, NF

Zinc Oxide Paste with Salicylic Acid, NF, is a 2% preparation of salicylic acid in zinc oxide paste. To avoid preparation of a gritty product, the salicylic acid must be reduced to a fine powder before incorporating it into the ointment. This paste is used for the same purpose as the plain zinc oxide paste. The presence of salicylic acid is thought to increase the penetrability of the paste.

Synonym: Lassar's Paste

Lotions

Lotions are liquid preparations intended for external application to the skin. Most lotions contain finely powdered substances that are insoluble in the dispersion medium and are suspended through the use of suspending agents and dispersing agents. Other lotions have as the dispersed phase liquid substances that are immiscible with the vehicle and are usually dispersed by means of emulsifying agents or other suitable stabilizers. One official lotion, Monobenzone Lotion, NF, is actually a solution of the drug in a vehicle of isopropyl alcohol and propylene glycol. Most commonly the vehicles of lotions are aqueous. Depending upon the nature of the ingredients, lotions may be prepared in the same manner as suspensions, emulsions, or solutions.

Lotions are intended to be applied to the skin for the protective or therapeutic value of their constituents. Their fluidity permits rapid and uniform application over a wide surface area. Lotions are intended to dry on the skin soon after application, leaving a thin coat of their medicinal components on the skin's surface.

Since the dispersed phase of lotions tends to separate from the vehicle upon standing, they should be shaken vigorously before each use to redistribute any separated matter. Containers of lotions should be labeled to instruct the patient to shake thoroughly before use and also to use externally only.

Official Lotions

The official lotions are presented in Table 10-2. Those lotions of particular pharmaceutical interest and those having formulas official in the USP and NF are discussed in greater detail below.

Benzyl Benzoate Lotion, USP

About 25% by volume of benzyl benzoate, a clear, colorless, oily liquid that is insoluble in water, is present in the benzyl benzoate lotion in the emulsified state. The emulsifying agent is an organic soap, triethanolamine oleate, formed during the preparation of the lotion by the combining of the two liquids, oleic acid and triethanolamine:

$$(HOCH_2CH_2)_3N + C_{17}H_{33}COOH \rightarrow$$

triethanolamine   oleic acid

$$(HOCH_2CH_2)_3NH\!-\!OOC(C_{17}H_{33})$$

triethanolamine oleate

In preparing the lotion, triethanolamine and oleic acid are mixed, then benzyl benzoate and water are added, and the mixture is shaken vigorously in an oversize vessel to ensure thorough agitation. Sufficient additional water is then added to the emulsion to make the required volume. The lotion is employed topically in the treatment of scabies and as a pediculicide. For scabies, it is applied to cleansed and still damp skin of the entire body, except the face.

The lotion is generally allowed to remain on the skin for about 24 hours, after which it is thoroughly washed off, and the patient is dressed in clean clothing. Adults may require 120 to 180 ml for a thorough application; a child, proportionately less, depending upon his size. The lotion is nonstaining and is water-washable.

Calamine Lotion, USP

Calamine Lotion, USP, contains 8 per cent each of zinc oxide and calamine, the latter composed primarily of zinc oxide with a small amount of ferric oxide, which gives calamine its characteristic pink color. In the preparation of the lotion, the two powders are levigated with a small portion of glycerin, the mixture being gradually diluted with a combination of bentonite magma and calcium hydroxide solution and the product made to volume with additional calcium hydroxide solution.

The bentonite magma is not totally effective in suspending the zinc oxide and calamine and on standing the powders do settle. The USP permits the increase in the amount of bentonite magma called for in the formula for the purpose of preparing a more viscous lotion if desired. Calamine is categorized as a protectant and is useful in relieving the itching and pain of sunburn, insect bites, and other minor skin irritations. The pink color helps disguise the presence of the lotion on the skin. Calamine lotion must be thoroughly shaken before use.

Table 10-2. OFFICIAL LOTIONS

Official Lotion	Corresponding Commercial Product	Percentage Strength of Active Constituent in Official or Commercial Lotion	Category and Comments
Benzoyl Peroxide Lotion, USP	Benoxyl Lotion (Stiefel)	5 and 10% benzoyl peroxide	Keratolytic. Applied to the skin once a day initially then two to four times a day thereafter. Lotion should be kept away from heat and contact with eyes and mucous membranes avoided.
Benzyl Benzoate Lotion, NF	. . .	25% benzyl benzoate	Scabicide. See text for additional discussion.
Betamethasone Valerate Lotion, NF	Valisone Lotion (Schering)	0.1% betamethasone	Glucocorticoid employed as an anti-inflammatory agent.
Calamine Lotion, USP	. . .	8% each of calamine and zinc oxide	Topical protectant. See text for additional discussion.
Phenolated Calamine Lotion, USP	. . .	1% liquefied phenol in calamine lotion	Topical protectant. See text for additional discussion.
Dimethisoquin HCl Lotion, NF	Quotane Lotion (Smith Kline & French)	0.5% dimethisoquin HCl	Local anesthetic. Used to relieve pain, itching, and burning of the skin.
Flurandrenolide Lotion, USP	Cordran Lotion (Dista)	0.05% flurandrenolide	Adrenocortical steroid. Anti-inflammatory agent.
Gamma Benzene HCl Lotion, USP	Kwell Lotion (Reed & Carnrick)	1% gamma benzene HCl	Pediculicide; scabicide. Applied topically to the skin once or twice a week. Contact with eyes or mucous membranes should be avoided.
Hexachlorophene Detergent Lotion, USP	pHisoHex (Winthrop)	3% hexachlorophene	Topical anti-infective; detergent.
Hydrocortisone Lotion, USP	Cort-Dome Lotion (Dome); Hydrocortone Topical Lotion (Merck Sharp & Dohme)	0.125 to 1.0% hydrocortisone	Adrenocortical steroid. Topical anti-inflammatory agent.
Methylbenzethonium Chloride Lotion, NF	Diaparene Lotion (Breon)	0.067% methylbenzethonium chloride	Local anti-infective. Used in diaper rash, prickly heat, chafing, etc.
Monobenzone Lotion, NF	Benoquin Lotion (Elder)	5% monobenzone	Depigmenting agent. Used in depigmenting freckles and other instances of hyperpigmention.
Selenium Sulfide Lotion, USP	Selsun and Selsun Blue (Abbott)	1% (Selsun Blue) and 2.5% (Selsun) of selenium sulfide	Anti-fungal; antiseborrheic. Used principally in the treatment of dandruff and seborrheic dermatitis. Contact with the eyes should be avoided.
White Lotion, NF	. . .	4% each of zinc sulfate and sulfurated potash	Local astringent and protectant. See text for additional discussion.

Phenolated Calamine Lotion, USP

Phenolated calamine lotion contains 1% of liquefied phenol in calamine lotion. Since phenol has anesthetic as well as antiseptic activity, it enhances the antipruritic action of the lotion. Like the plain calamine lotion, it must be shaken thoroughly before use. To maintain the phenol concentration, the container must be tightly closed.

White Lotion, NF

White lotion is prepared by dissolving separately 4% each of zinc sulfate and sulfurated potash in purified water, filtering each solution, and adding the solution of the sulfurated potash to the solution of the zinc sulfate slowly with constant stirring. A reaction takes place between the zinc sulfate and the sulfurated potash (the latter being a mixture composed primarily of potassium polysulfides and potassium thiosulfate) and may be represented in part by the following equation:

$$ZnSO_4 + K_2S \rightarrow K_2SO_4 + ZnS$$

The addition of the sulfurated potash solution to that of the zinc sulfate is necessary, rather than the reverse, in order to obtain a finely divided precipitate. The slow addition and constant mixing also contribute to the fineness of the precipitate. Despite these steps, the precipitate cakes on standing and cannot be uniformly redistributed. For this reason, the lotion must be freshly prepared to ensure uniformity and it must be shaken thoroughly to provide an even application to the skin.

The lotion is employed in the treatment of acne and other skin conditions responsive to the antiseptic activity of sulfur.

Synonyms: Lotio Alba; Sulfurated Lotion.

Topical Solutions and Tinctures

The official solutions and tinctures intended for application to the skin are presented in Tables 10-3 and 10-4. As shown in these tables, the majority of these preparations are used as anti-infective agents.

Generally, the topical solutions employ an aqueous vehicle, whereas the topical tinctures characteristically employ an alcoholic vehicle.

As required, co-solvents or adjuncts to enhance stability or the solubility of the solute are employed.

Topical solutions are prepared in the same general manner as the oral solutions previously discussed in Chapter 4, except of course the sweeteners and flavorants are not required. Most topical solutions and tinctures are prepared by simple solution of the solutes in the solvent. However, certain solutions are prepared by chemical reaction and these in particular are discussed later in this section. Of the official tinctures for topical use, one, Compound Benzoin Tincture, USP, is prepared by maceration of the natural components in the solvent, the others are prepared by simple solution.

Because of the nature of the active constituents or the solvents, many of the topical solutions and tinctures are self-preserved. Those that are not may contain suitable preservatives. Topical solutions and tinctures should be packaged in containers that make them convenient to use. Those that are used in small volume, as the anti-infectives, are usually packaged in glass bottles having an applicator tip as a part of the cap assembly, or in plastic squeeze bottles which deliver the medication dropwise. Many of the anti-infective solutions and tinctures contain a dye to delineate the area of application to the skin. In contrast to aqueous solutions, when the alcoholic tinctures are applied to abraded or broken skin, they cause a stinging sensation.

All medication intended for external use should be clearly labeled "FOR EXTERNAL USE ONLY" and maintained out of the reach of youngsters.

Official Topical Solutions

In addition to their listing in Table 10-3, the following official topical solutions are discussed below because of their particular pharmaceutic interest.

Aluminum Acetate Solution, USP

Each 100 ml of aluminum acetate solution yields between 1.20 g and 1.45 g of aluminum oxide and between 4.24 g and 5.12 g of acetic acid, corresponding to between 4.8 and 5.8 g of aluminum acetate. The requirement for the amount of acetic acid differentiates this solution from Aluminum Subacetate Solution, USP. In the later solution the ratio of aluminum oxide to

Table 10-3. OFFICIAL SOLUTIONS APPLIED TOPICALLY TO THE SKIN

Solution	Corresponding Commercial Product	Percent Active Constituent in Official or Commercial Solution*	Vehicle	Category and Comments
Aluminum Acetate Solution, USP	· · ·	5%	aqueous	Astringent. See text for additional discussion.
Aluminum Subacetate Solution, USP	· · ·	Approximately 2.45% aluminum oxide and 5.8% acetic acid	aqueous	Astringent. See text for additional discussion.
Benzethonium Chloride Solution, NF	Phemerol Solution (Parke Davis)	0.13 and 3%	aqueous	Local anti-infective. A quaternary ammonium compound used topically on the skin as well as on mucous membranes as those of the nose in dilute solution (e.g., 1:5000).
Calcium Hydroxide Solution, USP (Lime Water)	· · ·	0.14%	aqueous	Astringent. See text for additional discussion.
Cetylpyridinium Chloride Solution, NF	Ceepryn Chloride Aqueous Solution (Merrell)	0.05% (1:2000)	aqueous	Local anti-infective. Used topically to the skin (1:100 to 1:1000), to mucous membranes (1:2000 to 1:10,000), and to minor lacerations (1:1000)
Coal Tar Solution, USP (Liquor Carbonis Detergens; LCD)	· · ·	20%	alcoholic	Antieczematic; antipsoriatic. See text for additional discussion.
Fluocinolone Acetonide Topical Solution, USP	Synalar Solution (Syntex)	0.01%	propylene glycol	Adrenocortical steroid (topical anti-inflammatory)
Fluorouracil Topical Solution, USP	Efudex Topical Solution (Roche)	2 and 5%	propylene glycol	Antineoplastic (actinic keratoses).
Gentian Violet Solution, USP	· · ·	1%	hydro-alcoholic	Topical anti-infective. See text for additional discussion.
Hydrogen Peroxide Solution, USP	· · ·	3%	aqueous	Topical anti-infective. See text for additional discussion.
Iodine Solution, USP	· · ·	2%	aqueous	Topical anti-infective. See text for additional discussion.
Sulfurated Lime Solution, NF (Vleminckx's Solution)	· · ·	16.5% lime and 25% sublimed sulfur	aqueous	Scabicide. See text for additional discussion.
Nitrofurazone Solution, NF	Furacin Solution (Eaton)	0.2%	polyethylene glycols and water	Local anti-infective.
Nitromersol Solution, NF	Metaphen Solution (Abbott)	0.2%	aqueous	Local anti-infective. See text for additional discussion.

Table 10-3. OFFICIAL SOLUTIONS APPLIED TOPICALLY TO THE SKIN (*Cont.*)

Solution	Corresponding Commercial Product	Percent Active Constituent in Official or Commercial Solution*	Vehicle	Category and Comments
Podophyllum Resin Topical Solution, USP	· · ·	25%	alcoholic	Caustic. Used topically to treat papillomas; applied one to five times a day. The medication is extremely caustic to the skin and mucous membranes and care must be exercised in its use. It should be labeled "POISON" upon dispensing.
Povidone-Iodine Solution, USP	Betadine Solution (Purdue Frederick)	7.5 and 10%	aqueous	Topical anti-infective. See text for additional discussion.
Diluted Sodium Hypochlorite Solution, NF (Modified Dakin's Solution)	· · ·	0.475%	aqueous	Local anti-infective. See text for additional discussion.
Thimerosal Solution, NF	Merthiolate Solution (Lilly)	0.1%	alcohol-acetone	Local anti-infective. See text for additional discussion.
Tolnaftate Solution, USP	Tinactin Solution (Schering)	1%	polyethylene glycol	Topical anti-fungal.

* Unless otherwise indicated, the active constituent referred to is that agent named in the preparation's official title.

acetic acid is 1:2.35, whereas in aluminum acetate solution the ratio is 1:3.52. Aluminum subacetate solution is the stronger solution and is used in the preparation of the aluminum acetate solution.

The chemical aluminum acetate is very unstable and is difficult to obtain in pure form, and for this reason the solution is prepared by chemical reaction. Glacial acetic acid is added to aluminum subacetate solution, and sufficient water added to the prescribed volume. A reaction occurs between the acetic acid and basic aluminum acetate:

$$(CH_3COO)_2AlOH + CH_3COOH \rightarrow$$
$$(CH_3COO)_3Al + H_2O$$

The solution is filtered if necessary. Only clear aluminum acetate solution must be dispensed.

Aluminum acetate solution has the tendency to lose acetic acid on standing and deposit a basic form of aluminum acetate. This decomposition is hastened upon exposure to air. The USP permits the use of 0.6% of boric acid in the solution as a stabilizing agent. The pH of the solution should be maintained between pH 3.6 and 4.4. Because of its instability when exposed to air, the solution should be stored in tight containers. If the solution becomes turbid, it should be discarded.

The solution is colorless and has a faint acetous odor and a sweetish, astringent taste. It is widely applied topically as an astringent wash or wet dressing after dilution with 10 to 40 parts of water. It is frequently used as an ingredient in various types of dermatological preparations, as lotions, creams, and pastes.

Synonym: Burow's Solution.

Aluminum Subacetate Solution, USP

Aluminum subacetate solution yields from each 100 ml, between 2.30 g and 2.60 g of aluminum oxide and between 5.43 g and 6.13 g of acetic acid. It may be stabilized by the addition of not more than 0.9% of boric acid. The solution is a clear, colorless or faintly yellow liquid

Table 10-4. OFFICIAL TINCTURES APPLIED TOPICALLY TO THE SKIN

Tincture	Corresponding Commercial Product	Percent Active Constituent in Commercial or Official Tincture*	Vehicle	Category and Comments
Benzethonium Chloride Tincture, NF	Phemerol Tincture (Parke Davis)	0.2%	alcohol-acetone	Local anti-infective.
Green Soap Tincture, NF	. . .	65%	alcohol	Detergent. Also contains 2% lavender oil as perfume.
Iodine Tincture, USP	. . .	2%	alcohol-water	Topical anti-infective. See text for additional discussion.
Compound Benzoin Tincture, USP	. . .	10% benzoin; 2% aloe; 8% storax; 4% tolu balsam	alcohol	Topical protectant. Prepared by maceration of the ingredients in alcohol. See text for additional discussion.
Nitromersol Tincture, NF	Metaphen Tincture (Abbott)	0.5%	alcohol-acetone-water	Topical anti-infective.
Thimerosal Tincture, NF	Merthiolate Tincture (Lilly)	0.1%	ethylene diamine-mono-ethanolamine alcohol-acetone-water	Topical anti-infective. See text for additional discussion.

*Unless otherwise indicated, the active constituent referred to is that agent named in the preparation's official title.

having an acetous odor. It gradually becomes turbid on standing through separation of a more basic salt.

The solution may be prepared by the official method or by another method that results in a solution meeting the official requirements for strength, quality, and purity. In the official method, precipitated calcium carbonate is added in portions with constant stirring to a previously filtered solution of aluminum sulfate. Then acetic acid is slowly added, and the mixture is allowed to react during a period of 24 hours. The mixture is then filtered, and water is passed through the filter to make the required volume of solution. The reaction that takes place is as follows:

$$Al_2(SO_4)_3 \cdot 18H_2O + 3CaCO_3 + 4CH_3COOH \rightarrow$$
$$2(CH_3COO)_2AlOH + 3CaSO_4 + 3CO_2 + 19H_2O$$

The amount of acetic acid employed is insufficient to form the normal acetate, and the basic, or subacetate, results. The calcium carbonate is present to remove the sulfate radical from the solution by the formation of insoluble calcium sulfate, which is removed by filtration.

The solution, diluted first with 20 to 40 parts of water, is used externally as an astringent wash and wet dressing.

Calcium Hydroxide Solution, USP

Calcium hydroxide solution, commonly referred to as lime water, must contain not less than 140 mg of $Ca(OH)_2$ in each 100 ml of solution. Calcium hydroxide is less soluble in hot than in cold water, and, in the preparation of this solution cool purified water is employed as the solvent. The solution is intended to be saturated with solute, and to ensure saturation, an excess of calcium hydroxide, 300 mg for each 100 ml of solution to be prepared, is agitated with the purified water vigorously and repeatedly during a period of 1 hour. After this time, the excess calcium hydroxide is allowed to settle and remain at the bottom of the container. This permits the solution to remain saturated should a portion of the dissolved solute at the solution's surface react with the carbon dioxide of the air to form insoluble calcium carbonate:

$$Ca(OH)_2 + CO_2 \rightarrow CaCO_3 + H_2O$$

The calcium carbonate settles to the bottom of the container and by appearance is indistinguishable from the remaining excess of calcium hydroxide. The calcium hydroxide reserve dissolves as calcium is removed from solution in the form of the carbonate and in this way continually maintains the saturation of the solution. After the solution stands for an appreciable length of time, the undissolved material in the bottom of the container is composed of varying proportions of calcium hydroxide and calcium carbonate. Because of the uncertainty of the residue's composition the USP directs that additional quantities of calcium hydroxide solution may not be prepared by adding more purified water to the solution.

The solution should be stored in well-filled, tightly stoppered containers to deter the absorption of carbon dioxide and should be kept in a cool place to maintain an adequate concentration of dissolved solute. Only the clear supernatant liquid is dispensed. This is best accomplished by the use of a siphoning apparatus assembled so as to avoid the entrainment of the residue in the siphoning tubes.

The solution is officially categorized as an astringent. For this purpose it is generally employed in combination with other ingredients in dermatological solutions and lotions to be applied topically. The solution is also employed internally as an antacid, but its calcium hydroxide content is so low that large amounts of the solution (ranging from 15 to 120 ml) are required for this purpose. However, because of its mild antacid character, the solution has proven popular as an antacid for infants, sometimes being added to the feeding formulas.

Synonyms: Lime Water; Liquor Calcis

Coal Tar Solution, USP

Coal tar solution is an alcoholic solution containing 20% of coal tar and 5% of polysorbate 80. It is prepared by mixing the coal tar with two and a half times its weight of washed sand, adding the polysorbate 80 and most of the alcohol, and then macerating the mixture for 7 days in a closed vessel with frequent agitation followed by filtration and adjustment to the proper volume with alcohol. The final alcoholic content is between 81 and 86% ethyl alcohol.

Coal tar (pix carbonis) is a nearly black, viscous liquid having a characteristic naphthalene-like odor and a sharp, burning taste. It is the tar obtained as a by-product during the destructive distillation of bituminous coal. It is slightly soluble in water and partially soluble in most organic solvents, including alcohol. In the preparation of the official solution, the coal tar is mixed with the sand in order to distribute it mechanically and create a large surface area of tar exposed to the solvent action of the alcohol. During the period of maceration, or soaking, the alcohol-soluble components of the tar dissolve, leaving the undissolved portion clinging to the sand. Filtration removes the sand and the insoluble tar components from the solution. The container in which the solution was prepared should be rinsed with alcohol, and the washings should be passed through the filter paper in the adjustment of the final volume of the solution.

In the extemporaneous compounding of prescriptions and in the therapeutic application of this preparation on to the skin, the solution is frequently mixed with aqueous preparations or simply diluted with water. Since coal tar is only slightly soluble in water, in instances such as this it would separate from the solution were it not for the presence of the polysorbate 80 in the preparation. This agent, commercially available as Tween 80 (Atlas) and as other brand name products, is an oily liquid that is a nonionic surfactant. It is quite effective in dispersing the water-insoluble components of coal tar upon its admixture with an aqueous preparation.

Coal tar is categorized in the USP as a local antieczematic. The solution is used in the external treatment of a wide variety of chronic skin conditions after dilution with about 9 volumes of water, or in combination with other agents in various lotions, ointments, or solutions.

Synonyms: Liquor Carbonis Detergens: Liquor Picis Carbonis; LCD

Gentian Violet Solution, USP

This is a hydroalcoholic solution containing about 1% of gentian violet and about 10% of alcohol. Gentian violet, also known as methylrosaniline chloride, crystal violet, and methyl violet, is a medicinal dye composed largely of hexamethylpararosaniline chloride usually admixed with penta- and tetramethyl pararosaniline chlorides. Gentian violet is a dark green powder or glistening pieces having a metallic luster and is soluble in both alcohol and water. In the preparation of the official solution, gentian violet is dissolved in the hydroalcoholic solvent by agitation. The resulting liquid is purple and has a slight odor of alcohol.

The solution is used topically as a local anti-infective and is particularly effective against gram-positive bacteria and certain parasitic fungi.

Hydrogen Peroxide Solution, USP

Hydrogen peroxide solution contains between 2.5 and 3.5% (w/v) of hydrogen peroxide, H_2O_2. Suitable preservatives, totaling not more than 0.05%, may be added.

The USP does not specify a method for the preparation of the solution, largely because it may be prepared satisfactorily by one of several methods. One of these involves the action of either phosphoric acid or sulfuric acid on barium peroxide:

$$BaO_2 + H_2SO_4 \rightarrow BaSO_4 + H_2O_2$$

Another method involves the electrolytic oxidation of a cold solution of concentrated sulfuric acid to form persulfuric acid, which when hydrolyzed liberates hydrogen peroxide:

$$2H_2SO_4 \rightarrow H_2S_2O_8 + H_2$$
$$H_2S_2O_8 + 2H_2O \rightarrow H_2O_2 + 2H_2SO_4$$

A solution prepared by this method usually contains about 30% of hydrogen peroxide and is capable of liberating 100 times its volume of oxygen. A solution of this strength is commonly referred to as "100 volume peroxide." The official solution, which contains about 3% hydrogen peroxide and liberates 10 times its volume of oxygen, may be prepared from the concentrated solution by dilution.

The official solution is a clear, colorless liquid that may be odorless or may have the odor of ozone. It usually deteriorates upon long standing with the formation of oxygen and water. Preservative agents, as acetanilid, which have been found to retard the solution's decomposition are usually added in the amount stated above. Decomposition is enhanced by light and by heat, and for this reason the USP specifies that the solution should be preserved in tight, light-resistant containers, preferably at a temperature not exceeding 35° (95°F). The solution is also decomposed by practically all organic matter and other reducing agents and reacts with oxidizing agents to liberate oxygen and water; metals, alkalies, and other agents can catalyze its decomposition.

Hydrogen peroxide solution is categorized as a local anti-infective for use topically on the skin and mucous membranes. Its germicidal activity is based on the release of nascent oxygen on contact with the tissues. However, because of the short duration of this release, the chief value of the preparation in the reduction of infection is probably its ability to cleanse wounds by mechanical action through the effervescence and frothing caused by the release of oxygen.

Synonym: "Peroxide"

Iodine Solution, NF

Iodine solution contains about 2% of iodine and about 2.4% of sodium iodide in purified water. The solution is prepared by dissolving together the iodine and sodium iodide in a small portion of the required water and diluting the solution to the necessary volume with additional purified water. Sodium iodide is soluble in water to the extent of 1 g in 0.6 ml of water and dissolves rapidly, forming a concentrated solution. The iodine is soluble in water only to the extent of 1 g in about 3000 ml of water. When the two agents are added to the small portion of water, the sodium iodide forms a concentrated solution which has a solvent effect on the iodine due to the formation of a soluble polyiodide:

$$NaI + I_2 \rightarrow NaI_3$$

The solution is reddish brown and has the odor of iodine. It is best stored in tight, light-resistant containers and preferably at a temperature not above 35° (95°F.)

This solution contains the same concentration of iodine and sodium iodide as does Iodine Tincture, USP. However, the tincture is prepared with diluted alcohol as the solvent and is irritating upon application to cut tissue. For this reason, many persons prefer to use the aqueous solution. Both preparations are used topically as antiseptics.

Sulfurated Lime Solution, NF

Sulfurated lime solution is a clear, orange liquid with a slight odor of hydrogen sulfide. It is prepared by boiling lime (calcium oxide) and sublimed sulfur in water for about 1 hour, during which time the volume of the mixture is maintained by the periodic addition of water. After the solution is cooled, it is filtered and made to volume with water passed through the filter. The active constituents of the product are mainly calcium pentasulfide and calcium thiosulfate although some calcium disulfide may also be present:

$$CaO + H_2O \rightarrow Ca(OH)_2$$
$$3Ca(OH)_2 + 12S \rightarrow 2CaS_5 + CaS_2O_3 + 3H_2O$$

The NF recommends the storage of this solution in completely filled, tight containers to reduce the possibility of the absorption of carbon dioxide from the air with the consequent formation of insoluble calcium carbonate and free sulfur.

The solution is alkaline and is incompatible with mineral acids, which decompose the solution with the liberation of hydrogen sulfide and sulfur:

$$2CaS_5 + 4HCl \rightarrow 2CaCl_2 + 2H_2S + 4S_2$$

Sulfurated lime solution, diluted with 9 volumes of water, is used topically as a scabicide. It is also found in combination with other agents in various dermatological formulations.

Synonyms: Vleminckx's Solution; Vleminckx's Lotion

Nitromersol Solution, NF

Nitromersol, a local antibacterial agent used only in the form of the sodium salt, is among the best of the organic mercurial antiseptics. It is relatively nonirritating when applied to the skin or to mucous membranes. The official solution contains 0.2% of nitromersol dissolved in purified water through the action of sodium hydroxide and monohydrated sodium carbonate. Nitromersol itself is insoluble in water and practically insoluble in alcohol but dissolves in solutions of alkalies through the opening of the anhydride ring and the formation of the water-soluble salt:

The solution is prepared by dissolving the nitromersol in an aqueous solution of the alkalies and gradually adding purified water to the required volume. The NF cautions that dilutions of nitromersol solution should be prepared as needed, since they tend to precipitate upon standing. The solution is generally used in strengths of 1:500 to 1:10,000 as an antiseptic. It may also be used to sterilize surgical instruments. The solution is affected by light and must be stored in a light-resistant container.

Commercial Product: Metaphen Solution (Abbott)

Povidone-Iodine Solution, NF

The agent povidone-iodine is a chemical complex of iodine with polyvinylpyrrolidone, the latter agent being a polymer having an average molecular weight of about 40,000. The povidone-iodine complex contains approximately 10% of available iodine and slowly releases it when applied to the skin. The official povidone-iodine solution has no required strength; however the commercially available solutions contain 5, 7.5, 10, and 30% of povidone-iodine which is equivalent to 0.5, 0.75, 1, and 3% of available iodine. Although povidone-iodine is water soluble, the NF permits the presence of a small amount of alcohol in the solution.

The preparation is employed topically as a nonirritating antiseptic solution with its effectiveness directly attributable to the presence and the release of iodine from the complex.

Commercial Product: Betadine Solution (Purdue Frederick)

Diluted Sodium Hypochlorite Solution, NF

This solution is defined by the NF as a solution of chlorine compounds of sodium containing in each 100 ml not less than 450 mg and not more than 500 mg of NaClO. The solution is colorless or slightly yellow having a slight odor suggestive of chlorine.

The solution is prepared by diluting sodium hypochlorite solution with purified water. A solution of sodium bicarbonate is carefully added to the sodium hypochlorite solution, only partially diluted with purified water, in order to reduce its alkalinity. When a sample of the diluted solution no longer causes a red color to form on the addition of phenolphthalein, the sodium bicarbonate is no longer added, and the solution is adjusted to the proper sodium hypochlorite concentration by further dilution with purified water. It is necessary to reduce the alkalinity of the solution, since it is intended for use on open wounds, and alkalies are both irritant and caustic when brought into contact with raw tissue. The alkalinity of the solution is reduced by the lowering of the hydroxyl ion concentration to form carbonate ions and water:

$$OH^- + HCO_3^- \rightarrow CO_3^= + H_2O$$

or

$$NaOH + NaHCO_3 \rightarrow Na_2CO_3 + H_2O$$

It is important that the strength of this solution be accurately adjusted, for if too strong, the solution would be irritating to the tissues; if too weak, it would be an ineffective antibacterial. If the diluted preparation is to be used after standing a few days, it is recommended that its strength be redetermined.

Diluted sodium hypochlorite solution is employed in full strength and should be freshly prepared. The solution, which is used in the irrigation of suppurating wounds, exerts a germicidal action and dissolves necrotic tissue, thereby assisting in the cleansing of the wound.

Synonyms: Modified Dakin's Solution; Surgical Chlorinated Soda Solution; Carrel-Dakin Solution

Thimerosal Solution, NF

Thimerosal is a water-soluble, organic, mercurial, antibacterial agent used topically for its bacteriostatic and mild fungistatic properties. It is used mainly to disinfect skin surfaces and as an application to wounds and abrasions. In certain instances it has been applied to the eye, nose, throat, and urethra in dilutions of 1:5000. It is also used as a preservative for various pharmaceutical preparations, including many vaccines and other biological products.

Thimerosal Solution, NF, contains 0.1% thimerosal. Also present are ethylenediamine solution and sodium borate to maintain the alkalinity (usually pH 9.8 to 10.3) required for the solution's stability. Monoethanolamine is used as an additional stabilizer. The NF permits the addition of certified coloring agents to the preparation. The solution is affected by light and must be maintained in light-resistant con-

tainers. Also, the NF cautions that the solution must be manufactured and stored in glass or in suitably resistant metal containers.

Commercial Product: Merthiolate Solution (Lilly)

Official Topical Tinctures

The official tinctures for topical application to the skin are presented in Table 10-4. Those of particular pharmaceutic interest are discussed briefly below.

Iodine Tincture, USP

Iodine tincture is prepared by dissolving 2% of iodine crystals and 2.4% of sodium iodide in an amount of alcohol equal to half the volume of tincture to be prepared and then diluting the solution to volume with sufficient purified water. The sodium iodide reacts with the iodine to form sodium triiodide:

$$I_2 + NaI \rightleftharpoons NaI_3$$

This reaction prevents the formation of ethyl iodide from the interaction between iodine and the alcohol, which would result in the loss of the antibacterial activity of the tincture. An added benefit of the triiodide form of iodine is its water solubility which is important should the tincture, which contains between 44 and 50% alcohol, be diluted with water during use.

The tincture is a popular local anti-infective agent applied topically to the skin in general household first-aid procedures. The reddish-brown color, which produces a stain on the skin, is useful in delineating the application over the affected skin area.

The tincture should be stored in tight containers to prevent loss of alcohol.

Compound Benzoin Tincture, USP

Compound benzoin tincture is prepared by the maceration in alcohol of 10% of benzoin and lesser amounts of aloe, storax, and tolu balsam totaling about 24% of starting material. The drug mixture is best macerated in a wide-mouthed container, since it is difficult to introduce storax, a semi-liquid, sticky material into a narrow-mouthed container. Generally, it is advisable to weigh the storax in the container in which it will be macerated to avoid possible loss through a transfer of the material from one container to another.

The tincture is categorized as a protectant. It is used to protect and toughen skin in the treatment of bedsores, ulcers, cracked nipples, and fissures of the lips and anus. It is also commonly used as an inhalant in bronchitis and other respiratory conditions, one teaspoonful commonly being added to a pint of boiling water. The volatile components of the tincture travel with the steam vapor and are inhaled by the patient. Because of the incompatibility of the alcoholic tincture and water, mixture of the two produces a milky product with some separation of resinous material. Alcohol or acetone may be used as necessary to remove the residue from the vaporizer after use.

Compound benzoin tincture is best stored in tight, light-resistant containers. Exposure to direct sunlight or to excessive heat should be avoided.

The tincture originated in the 15th or 16th century and through the years probably has acquired more synonyms than any other official preparation. A few of these are indicated below.

Synonyms: Friar's Balsam; Turlington's Drops; Persian Balsam; Swedish Balsam; Jerusalem Balsam; Wade's Drops; Turlington's Balsam of Life.

Thimerosal Tincture, NF

The same general remarks made during the discussion of Thimerosal Solution, NF (page 326) apply to Thimerosal Tincture, NF, except that sodium chloride and sodium borate are absent from the tincture and the vehicle of the tincture is composed of water, acetone, and about 50% alcohol. A number of metals, notably copper, cause the decomposition of the tincture, and for this reason the monograph cautions: "manufacture and store Thimerosal Tincture in glass or suitably resistant containers." The tincture is normally packaged in glass containers with closures free of interfering metals. Monoethanolamine and ethylenediamine are used as stabilizers in the official solution and tincture and are thought to be effective because of their chelating action on traces of metallic impurities that may be present at the time of preparation or may later gain access to the preparation.

The commercial preparation is colored orange red and has a greenish fluorescence. The red stain it leaves on the skin defines the area of application. The preparation is a commonly used household antiseptic for application topically on the skin in abrasions and cuts and also in the preoperative preparation of patients for surgery.

Commercial Product: Merthiolate Tincture (Lilly)

Liniments

Liniments are alcoholic or oleaginous solutions or emulsions of various medicinal substances intended for external application to the skin, generally with rubbing. Liniments with an alcoholic or hydroalcoholic vehicle are useful in instances in which rubefacient, counterirritant, or penetrating action is desired; oleaginous liniments are employed primarily when massage is desired. By their nature, oleaginous liniments are less irritating to the skin than alcoholic liniments. Liniments are not generally applied to skin areas that are broken or bruised because excessive irritation might result. The vehicle for a liniment should therefore be selected on the basis of the type of action desired (rubefacient, counterirritant, or just massage) and also on the solubility of the desired components in the various solvents. For oleaginous liniments, the solvent may be a fixed oil such as almond oil, peanut oil, sesame oil, or cottonseed oil or a volatile substance such as wintergreen oil or turpentine, or it may be a combination of fixed and volatile oils.

All liniments should bear a label indicating that they are suitable only for external use and must never be taken internally. Liniments that are emulsions or that contain insoluble matter must be shaken thoroughly before use to ensure an even distribution of the dispersed phase, and for these preparations a "Shake Well" label is indicated. Liniments should be stored in tight containers.

Depending upon their individual ingredients, liniments are prepared in the same manner as solutions, emulsions, or suspensions, as the case may warrant.

There are presently no official liniments.

Collodions

Collodions are liquid preparations composed of pyroxylin dissolved in a solvent mixture usually composed of alcohol and ether with or without added medicinal substances. Pyroxylin (soluble gun cotton, collodion cotton) is obtained by the action of a mixture of nitric and sulfuric acids on cotton and consists chiefly of cellulose tetranitrate. It has the appearance of raw cotton when dry but is harsh to the touch. It is frequently available commercially moistened with about 30% alcohol or other similar solvent.

One part of pyroxylin is slowly but completely soluble in 25 parts of a mixture of 3 volumes of ether and 1 volume of alcohol. It is also soluble in acetone and glacial acetic acid. Pyroxylin is precipitated from solution in these solvents upon the addition of water. Pyroxylin, like collodions, is exceedingly flammable and must be stored away from flame in well-closed containers, protected from light.

Collodions are intended for external use. When applied to the skin with a fine camel's hair brush or glass applicator, the solvent rapidly evaporates, leaving a film residue of pyroxylin. This provides a protective coating to the skin, and when the collodion is medicated, it leaves a thin layer of that medication firmly placed against the skin. Naturally, collodions must be applied to dry tissues to effect adhesion to the skin's surface. The products must be clearly labeled "For External Use Only" or with words of similar effect.

Official Collodions

Collodion, USP

Collodion is a clear or slightly opalescent, viscous liquid prepared by dissolving pyroxylin (4% w/v) in a 3:1 mixture of ether and alcohol. The resulting solution is highly volatile and flammable and should be preserved in tight containers at a temperature not exceeding 30° remote from fire.

The product is capable of forming a protective film on application to the skin and the volatilization of the solvent. The film is useful in holding the edges of an incised wound together. However, its presence on the skin is uncomfortable due to its inflexible nature. The following product, which is flexible, has greater appeal when a nonpliable film is not required.

Flexible Collodion, USP

Flexible collodion is prepared by adding 2% of camphor and 3% of castor oil to collodion. The castor oil renders the product flexible, permitting its comfortable use over skin areas that are normally moved, such as fingers and toes. The camphor makes the product waterproof. Physicians frequently apply the coating over bandages or stitched incisions to make them waterproof and to protect them from external stress.

Salicylic Acid Collodion, USP

Salicylic acid collodion is a 10% solution of salicylic acid in flexible collodion. It is used for its keratolytic effects, especially in the removal of corns from the toes.

Synonym: Corn Solvent.

Glycerites

Glycerites are solutions or mixtures of medicinal or pharmaceutical substances in glycerin. Generally a minimum of 50% of glycerin is present in glycerites. Owing to the high concentration of glycerin and the presence of large amounts of dissolved or undissolved solids, glycerites are generally quite viscous with some of them reaching a jelly-like consistency.

Glycerin has a wide range of solvent power and is capable of dissolving a number of substances that may be insoluble or unstable in other solvents. Because glycerin possesses preservative capabilities, glycerites are considered to be stable preparations and are not usually as prone to microbial contamination as are aqueous preparations. Since glycerin is miscible with both water and alcohol, glycerites generally may be diluted with these solvents or with aqueous or alcoholic solutions as required.

Glycerites are not nearly as popular today as they once were probably due to increased methods of stabilizing and preserving aqueous solutions, an increased capability to create and utilize new salt forms of drugs having specifically desired chemical and physical features, the application of newly developed solubilizing agents, and also the expense of glycerin as a sole solvent. However, it should be remembered that glycerin is still today a valuable co-solvent in many liquid pharmaceutical preparations, adding permanency to the preparations in which it is used.

Presently there are no official glycerites. The two glycerites most recently official were starch glycerite, used topically as an emollient, and tannic acid glycerite, applied as an astringent.

Glycerogelatins

Glycerogelatins may be described as plastic masses intended for topical application and containing gelatin, glycerin, and water, in addition to any added medicinal substance. In dermatologic practice, such medicinal substances as zinc oxide, salicylic acid, resorcinol, and other appropriate agents may be added. Glycerogelatins are melted prior to application, cooled to only slightly above body temperature, and applied to the affected area with a fine brush. After application, the glycerogelatin hardens, is usually covered with a bandage, and is allowed to remain in place for periods up to 6 weeks and longer as is necessary.

Unless otherwise specified, glycerogelatins contain 10% of the medicinal substance prepared according to the formula:

Medicinal Substance	100 g
Gelatin	150 g
Glycerin	400 g
Purified Water	350 g
To make about	1000 g

In preparing a glycerogelatin, the gelatin is first softened in the purified water, being stirred when added, then allowed to stand for about 10 minutes after which time the mixture is heated on a steam bath until the gelatin is dissolved. The medicinal substance is mixed first with the glycerin (either dissolving in it or being dispersed by it) and then with the gelatin solution, the glycerogelatin being stirred until it congeals.

The only official glycerogelatin is Zinc Gelatin, USP.

Zinc Gelatin, USP

Zinc Gelatin, USP, is a firm, plastic mass containing 10% zinc oxide in a glycerogelatin base. It is used mainly for the treatment of varicose ulcers because of its ability to form a pressure bandage known as a "gelatin boot." The mass is softened on a water bath before being applied to the skin with a soft brush. This coating is then covered with a bandage and allowed to remain in place for up to 6 weeks, depending upon the degree of serous discharge from the lesion.

Synonym: Zinc Gelatin Boot.

Plasters

Plasters are solid or semisolid adhesive masses spread upon a suitable backing material and intended for external application to a part of the body to provide prolonged contact at that site. Among the backing materials used are paper, cotton, felt, linen, muslin, silk, moleskin, or plastic. The plasters are adhesive at body temperature and may be used to provide protection or mechanical support (nonmedicated plasters) or to provide localized or systemic effects (medicated plasters). The backings onto which the masses are placed are cut into different shapes appropriate to the contour and the extent of the body surface to be covered. Commonly used are back plasters, chest plasters, breast plasters, kidney plasters, and corn plasters. Common adhesive tape was formerly official under the title "Adhesive Plaster," the use of this material being well known.

Today, most plasters are prepared industrially, with few being prepared in the pharmacy. The adhesive material in many of the commercially available plasters consists of either a rubber base or a synthetic resin material.

There is presently only one official plaster, this being Salicylic Acid Plaster, USP.

Salicylic Acid Plaster, USP

Salicylic Acid Plaster, USP, is a uniform mixture of salicylic acid in a suitable base spread on a backing material and is intended to be placed on areas requiring the removal of horny layers of skin. The preparation is employed typically as corn plasters for the toes. The horny layers of skin are removed by virtue of the keratolytic action of salicylic acid. Although the USP does not specify the proportion of salicylic acid present in the base, the usual concentration is between 10 and 40% salicylic acid.

Powders for Application to the Skin

Nonmedicated and medicated powders are frequently applied to the skin. The use of plain talcum powder is common as a topical dusting powder to prevent skin irritation and chafing. Medicated powders are often employed to combat such conditions as diaper rash and athlete's foot.

Powders for topical use are prepared in the same manner as has been described previously in Chapter 6. Powders for use on the skin are generally packaged in paper, metal, or plastic containers having a sifter-type cap. Some commercial powders are also packaged in plastic squeeze bottles and in aerosol containers.

Two medicated powders which may be applied to the skin are presently official. Compound Iodochlorhydroxyquin Powder, NF contains 25% of iodochlorhydroxyquin, with zinc stearate and lactic acid also present in a vehicle of lactose, may be dusted on the skin as a local anti-infective agent. Methylbenzethonium Chloride Powder, NF, is commercially available as a 0.055% powder used as an anti-infective, primarily in diaper rash.

Topical Aerosols

Aerosol packages for topical use on the skin are prepared in the same manner as discussed in Chapter 9. Official aerosols used topically include the anti-infective agents, povidone-iodine and thimerosal, the adrenocortical steroids, betamethasone valerate, dexamethasone, and triamcinolone acetonide, and the local anesthetic dibucaine hydrochloride. These preparations have been presented in Table 9-2 in the previous chapter.

The use of topical aerosols provides to the patient a means of applying the drug in a convenient manner. The preparation may be applied to the desired surface area without the use of the fingertips, thus making the procedure less messy than with most other types of topical preparations. Among the disadvantages to the use of topical aerosols are the difficulty in applying the medication to a small area and the greater expense associated with the aerosol package.

Cataplasms

Cataplasms or poultices are viscous preparations intended for warm, external application to a body surface for the purpose of reducing inflammation and/or allaying pain. In addition to other agents, they characteristically contain the absorbent kaolin and the hygroscopic material glycerin, and because of these components, cataplasms were thought to be effective in drawing infectious material from the tissues. Presently, there are no official cataplasms.

Cerates

Cerates are soft, unctuous preparations made by fusion from hydrocarbon (oleaginous) bases and containing wax (cera) as a stiffening agent. They are intended to be spread on cloth and applied to the skin, historically to relieve inflammation. There are no cerates that are presently official.

Tapes and Gauzes

The USP contains monographs setting the standards for a number of topical dressings, including the following:

Adhesive Tape, USP—defined as "fabric or film evenly coated on one side with a pressure sensitive adhesive mixture." Standards are set for sterility of those tapes which are labeled to be sterile, as well as for the dimensions, tensile strength, and adhesive strength of the sterile and nonsterile tapes.

Flurandrenolide Tape, USP—this is adhesive-type tape having flurandrenolide impregnated in the adhesive material in the amount of 4 µg per sq cm. The tape is applied as an anti-inflammatory adrenocortical steroid once or twice daily.

Absorbent Gauze, USP—this is cotton in the form of a plain woven cloth. Official standards are set for thread count, length, width, weight, absorbency as well as sterility for absorbent gauze that has been rendered sterile.

Gauze Bandage, USP—this is one continuous piece of absorbent gauze, tightly rolled in various widths and lengths and substantially free from loose threads and ravelings. Standards are set for width, length, weight, absorbency, thread count, as well as for sterility for those products labeled to be sterile.

Adhesive Bandage, USP—this is a compress of four layers of absorbent or other suitable material, affixed to a film of fabric coated with a pressure-sensitive adhesive substance. Adhesive bandage is sterile and is protected by a suitable removable covering.

Petrolatum Gauze, USP—this is absorbent gauze saturated with white petrolatum. This gauze is sterile. It is prepared by adding molten, sterile, white petrolatum to dry, sterile absorbent gauze, previously cut to size, in the ratio of 60 g of petrolatum to each 20 g of gauze. Standards are set for packaging, labeling, and sterility.

Zinc Gelatin Impregnated Gauze, USP—this is absorbent gauze impregnated with zinc gelatin. The gauze is used as a topical protectant.

Miscellaneous Official Preparations for Topical Application to the Skin

Rubbing Alcohol, NF

Rubbing Alcohol, NF, contains about 70% of ethyl alcohol by volume, the remainder consisting of water, denaturants with or without color additives and perfume oils, and stabilizers. In each 100 ml it must contain not less than 355 mg of sucrose octa-acetate, a bitter substance that discourages its accidental or abusive oral ingestion. The denaturants employed in rubbing alcohol are according to the Internal Revenue Service, U.S. Treasury Department, Formula 23-H, which is composed of 8 parts by volume of acetone, 1.5 parts by volume of methyl isobutyl ketone, and 100 parts by volume of ethyl alcohol. The use of this denaturant mixture makes the separation of ethyl alcohol from the denaturants a virtually impossible task with ordinary distillation apparatus. This discourages the illegal removal and use as a beverage of the alcoholic content of rubbing alcohol.

The product is volatile and flammable and should be stored in tight containers remote from fire. It is employed as a rubefacient externally and as a soothing rub for bedridden patients, a germicide for instruments, and a skin cleanser prior to injection.

Synonym: Alcohol Rubbing Compound.

Isopropyl Rubbing Alcohol, NF

Isopropyl Rubbing Alcohol, NF, is about 70% by volume of isopropyl alcohol, the remainder consisting of water with or without color additives, stabilizers, and perfume oils. It is used externally as a rubefacient and soothing rub. This preparation and a commercially available 91% isopropyl alcohol solution are commonly employed by diabetic patients in preparing needles and syringes for hypodermic injections of insulin and for disinfecting the skin. The preparation is said not to interfere with the potency of the insulin protein, small amounts being compatible with most insulin preparations.

Hexachlorophene Liquid Soap, USP

Hexachlorophene Liquid Soap, USP, is a 0.24% solution, by weight, of hexachlorophene, a local anti-infective agent effective mainly against gram-positive microorganisms, in a 10 to 13% solution of a potassium soap. The USP permits the preparation of a more concentrated hexachlorophene liquid soap, provided it meets the requirements for the official product when diluted according to the labeling directions. The activity of the hexachlorophene may be affected by the simultaneous presence of large amounts of certain nonionic detergents, and the USP warns that such substances in amounts greater than 8% on a total weight basis may decrease the bacteriostatic activity of the preparation. The liquid soap, which is a clear, amber-colored liquid with a slight, characteristic odor, is employed topically to the skin as a local anti-infective and detergent. The preparation is best stored in well-closed, light-resistant containers.

Commercial Product: pHisoHex (Winthrop).

Liquefied Phenol, USP

Liquefied phenol is phenol maintained in a liquid condition by the presence of 10% of water. In its preparation, phenol crystals are melted with heat, and 1 ml of water is added for each 9 g of melted phenol. When the mixture cools, the liquid state is maintained. The USP requires that the preparation contain not less than 89% of phenol. Liquefied phenol is miscible with alcohol, ether, and glycerin, and a mixture of equal parts of glycerin and liquefied phenol is miscible with water. Phenol crystals are only soluble in water to the extent of 1 g of phenol in about 15 ml of water.

In compounding, the pharmacist finds it convenient to use the appropriate amount of liquefied phenol rather than phenol crystals when he is to add a small amount of phenol to an aqueous preparation. On the other hand, phenol crystals are preferred when phenol is to be added to a fixed oil, mineral oil, or to an ointment base such as petrolatum, since the water present in the liquefied phenol would not be miscible with these substances.

Liquefied phenol is categorized as a caustic and local antipruritic. It is applied locally, only after dilution to 0.1 to 2% of phenol. It is frequently added to calamine lotion by the pharmacist to increase its antipruritic action.

Because phenol gradually darkens from its colorless to light pink color upon exposure to air and light, liquefied phenol is best stored in tight, light-resistant containers.

Selected Reading

Barr, M.: Percutaneous Absorption. *J. Pharm. Sci.,* *51*:395–409, 1962.

Idson, B.: Percutaneous Absorption. *J. Pharm. Sci.,* *64*:901–924, 1975.

Chapter 11

Ophthalmic Preparations

DRUGS ARE commonly applied to the eye for the localized effect of the medication on the surface of the eye or on its interior. Most frequently aqueous solutions are employed; however, nonaqueous solutions, suspensions, and ophthalmic ointments are also commonly used. Recently, ophthalmic inserts, impregnated with drug, have been developed to provide for the continuous release of medication. These inserts are of particular usefulness for those drugs requiring frequent daytime and nighttime administration.

Since the capacity of the eye to retain liquid and ointment preparations is limited, they are generally administered in small volume. Liquid preparations are most frequently administered by drops and ointments by the application of a thin ribbon of ointment to the lid margin. Larger volumes of liquid preparations may be used to flush or wash the eye.

The effective "dose" of medication administered ophthalmically may be varied by the strength of medication administered, the volume administered, the retention time of the medication in contact with the surface of the eye, the frequency of administration, the pathologic condition of the eye and the pharmaceutic or formulative factors of the preparation used. It is important to recognize that although the local administration of medications to the eye is the main route of administration employed by the ophthalmologist in the treatment of diseases of the eye, other routes as oral and parenteral may also be used. The use of systemic antibiotic therapy to combat an intraocular infection is an example of this type of therapy.

Ophthalmic Solutions

By official definition, ophthalmic solutions are sterile solutions that are compounded and packaged for instillation into the eye. In addition to sterility, their preparation requires the careful consideration of such other pharmaceutical factors as the isotonicity value, the need for buffering agents, viscosity, the need for and the selection of antimicrobial agents, and proper packaging.

Sterility and Preservation

All ophthalmic solutions should be sterile when dispensed, and whenever possible, a suitable preservative should be added to ensure sterility during the course of use. However, ophthalmic solutions intended to be used during surgery or in the traumatized eye generally do not contain preservative agents, since these are irritating to the tissues within the eye; therefore it becomes imperative that solutions that may gain access to the interior of the eye be rendered and maintained sterile throughout their course of use. They should be packaged in single-dose containers, and any unused solution should be discarded.

Although it is preferable that ophthalmic solutions be sterilized by autoclaving in the final container, the method employed, as always, is dependent upon the nature of the particular preparation. Certain drugs that are thermostabile in acid media may become thermolabile when buffered near the physiological pH range (about 7.4). If the higher pH is desired for the product, the unbuffered solution of the drug may first be autoclaved, and the buffering agents added aseptically later. With the exception of basic salts of weak acids such as sodium fluorescein or sodium sulfacetamide, solutions of most of the common ophthalmic drugs, prepared in a boric acid vehicle, can be safely sterilized at 121° for 15 minutes as previously discussed in Chapter 8.

If necessary, a bacterial filter may be used to avoid the use of heat. Although bacterial filters work with a high degree of efficiency, they are not as trusted sterilizers as is the autoclave. The advantage of filtration, as was pointed out earlier, is the retention of all particulate matter, the removal of which is of prime importance in the manufacture and use of ophthalmic solutions. Figures 11-1 and 11-2 show filtration equipment which may be employed in the extemporaneous filtration of ophthalmic solutions.

Ophthalmic solutions to be used on eyes with intact corneal membranes may be packaged in multiple-dose containers. Even though sterile when dispensed, each of these solutions should contain a rapidly effective, topically nonirritating antibacterial agent or a mixture of such agents to prevent the growth of, or to destroy, microorganisms accidentally introduced into the solution when the container is opened during use. Suitable preservatives and their approximate concentrations for this purpose include (a) benzalkonium chloride, 0.01% (1:10,000); (b) chlorobutanol, 0.5%; (c) phenylmercuric nitrate, 0.002% (1:50,000); (d) p-chloro-m-cresol, 0.05% (1:2000); and (e) phenylethyl alcohol, 0.5%. Each of these has certain limitations with respect to stability, chemical compatibility with other formulative ingredients, and antibacterial activity. For example, chlorobutanol hydrolyzes and decomposes at autoclaving temperatures. Further, the hydrolysis of chlorobutanol may take place under moderate heat or slowly at room temperature with the formation of hydrochloric acid which not only may render the solution susceptible to microorganism growth but may change the pH of an unbuffered solution and affect the stability or the physiologic activity of the active ingredient. Benzalkonium chloride is one of the most reliable ophthalmic solution preservatives, since it has a broad antimicrobial spectrum of activity, but the pharmacist must be aware of its incompatibility with anionic drugs, salicylates, and nitrates, and for solutions containing any of these substances an alternative preservative, as phenylmercuric nitrate or phenylmercuric acetate, must be employed.

In concentrations tolerated by the tissues of the eye, all of the aforementioned preservative agents are ineffective against some strains of *Pseudomonas aeruginosa*, an organism that can invade an abraded cornea and cause ulceration and blindness. It has been found that a preservative mixture of benzalkonium chloride (1:10,000) and 1000 USP Units of polymyxin B sulfate, the latter in each ml of solution, is effective against most resistant strains of *Pseudomonas* and is nonirritating to the eye. In some ophthalmic preparations a mixture of benzalkonium chloride (1:10,000) and disodium ethylenediaminetetraacetate, 0.01 to 0.1%, is

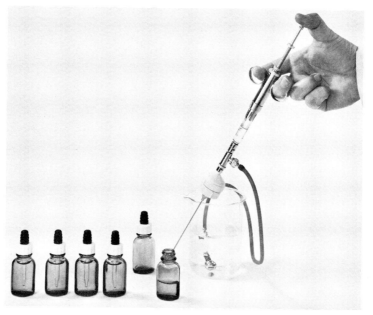

Fig. 11-1. *Sterilization by filtration. The preparation of a sterile solution by passage through a syringe affixed with a microbial filter. (Courtesy of Millipore Corporation.)*

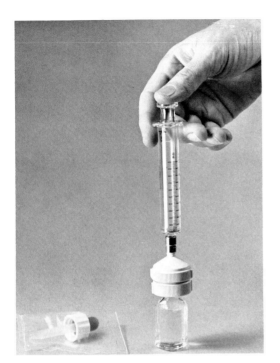

Fig. 11-2. *The preparation of a sterile ophthalmic solution by filtration. (Courtesy of Millipore Corporation.)*

employed for the same purpose. The latter agent is a chelating agent for metals, having the ability to render the resistant strains of *Pseudomonas aeruginosa* more sensitive to the benzalkonium chloride.

Isotonicity Value

If a solution is placed within or behind a membrane that is permeable only to solvent molecules and not to solute molecules (a *semipermeable membrane*) a phenomenon called *osmosis* occurs as the molecules of solvent traverse the membrane. If the solution-filled membrane is placed in a solution of a higher solute concentration than its own, the solvent, which has free passage in either direction, passes into the more concentrated solution. It does this until an equilibrium is established on both sides of the membrane and an equal concentration of solute exists on the two sides. The pressure responsible for this movement is termed *osmotic pressure*.

The concentration of a solution with respect to osmotic pressure is concerned with the number of "particles" of solute in solution. That is, if the solute is a nonelectrolyte (as sucrose), the concentration of the solution will depend solely on the number of molecules present. However, if the solute is an electrolyte (as sodium chloride), the number of particles that it contributes to the solution will depend not only upon the concentration of the molecules present, but also on their degree of ionization. A chemical that is highly ionized will contribute a greater number of particles to the solution than will the same amount of a poorly ionized substance. The effect is that a solution with a greater number of particles, whether they be molecules or ions, has a greater osmotic pressure than does a solution having fewer particles.

Body fluids, including blood and lacrimal fluid, have an osmotic pressure corresponding to that of a 0.9% solution of sodium chloride. Thus, a sodium chloride solution of this concentration is said to be *isosmotic*, or having an equal osmotic pressure, with physiologic fluids. The term *isotonic*, meaning equal tone, is commonly used interchangeably with isosmotic although the former term must be used with reference to some body fluid, and isosmotic really is a physical chemical term which compares the osmotic pressure of two liquids, one of which may or may not be a physiologic fluid. Solutions with a lower osmotic pressure than body fluids or a 0.9% sodium chloride solution are commonly referred to as *hypotonic*, whereas solutions having a greater osmotic pressure are termed *hypertonic*.

Theoretically, a hypertonic solution added to the body's system will have a tendency to draw water from the body tissues toward the solution in an effort to dilute and establish a concentration equilibrium. In the blood stream, a hypertonic injection could cause the *crenation* (shrinking) of blood cells; in the eye, the solution could cause the drawing of water toward the site of the topical application. Conversely, a hypotonic solution might induce the hemolysis of red blood cells, or the passage of water from the site of an ophthalmic application through the tissues of the eye.

In practice, the isotonicity limits of an ophthalmic solution in terms of sodium chloride, or its osmotic equivalent, may range from 0.6 to 2.0% without marked discomfort to the eye. As indicated, sodium chloride does not have to be used to establish the solution's osmotic pressure. Boric acid in a concentration of 1.9% produces the same osmotic pressure as does 0.9% sodium chloride. All of the ophthalmic solution's solutes, including the active ingredients, contribute to the osmotic pressure of the solution.

Various methods for the calculation of isotonic solutions may be found in textbooks of pharmaceutical calculations and physical pharmacy. However, as a convenience, the USP presents precalculated amounts of some common ophthalmic drugs which may be used to prepare isotonic solutions. These drugs and the related values are presented in Table 11-1. The data shown are utilized in the following manner. One gram of each of the drugs listed, when added to purified water, will prepare the corresponding volume of an isotonic solution. For instance, 1 g of atropine sulfate will prepare 14.3 ml of isotonic solution. This solution may then be diluted with an isotonic vehicle to maintain the isotonicity while changing the strength of the active constituent in the solution to any desired level. For instance, if a 1% isotonic solution of atropine sulfate is desired, the 14.3 ml of isotonic solution containing 1 g of atropine sulfate would be diluted to 100 ml with an isotonic vehicle (1 g atropine sulfate in 100 ml = a 1% w/v solution). By utilizing sterile drug, sterile purified water, a sterile isotonic vehicle, and aseptic techniques, a sterile product may be prepared. In addition to being sterile and isotonic, the diluting vehicles generally used are also buffered and contain suitable preservative to maintain the stability and sterility of the product.

Buffering

Buffers may be used in an ophthalmic solution for one or all of the following reasons: (1) to reduce discomfort to the patient, (2) to ensure drug stability, and (3) to control the therapeutic activity of the drug substance.

Normal tears, having a pH of about 7.4, possess some buffer capacity. The introduction of a medicated solution into the eye stimulates the flow of tears, which attempt to neutralize any excess hydrogen or hydroxyl ions introduced with the solution. Most drugs used ophthalmically, such as alkaloidal salts, are weakly acidic and have only weak buffer capacity. Normally, the buffering action of the tears is capable of neutralizing the ophthalmic solution and is thereby able to prevent marked discomfort. However, a few drugs—notably pilocarpine hydrochloride and epinephrine bitartrate

Table 11-1. ISOTONIC SOLUTIONS PREPARED FROM COMMON OPHTHALMIC DRUGS[1]

Drug (1.0 g)	Volume of Isotonic Solution Yielded (ml)
Atropine Sulfate	14.3
Chlorobutanol (hydrous)	26.7
Cocaine Hydrochloride	17.7
Colistimethate Sodium	16.7
Ephedrine Sulfate	25.7
Epinephrine Bitartrate	20.0
Eucatropine Hydrochloride	20.0
Fluorescein Sodium	34.3
Homatropine Hydrobromide	19.0
Neomycin Sulfate	12.3
Penicillin G Potassium	20.0
Phenylephrine Hydrochloride	35.7
Physostigmine Salicylate	17.7
Physostigmine Sulfate	14.3
Pilocarpine Hydrochloride	26.7
Pilocarpine Nitrate	25.7
Polymyxin B Sulfate	10.0
Procaine Hydrochloride	23.3
Proparacaine Hydrochloride	16.7
Scopolamine Hydrobromide	13.3
Silver Nitrate	36.7
Sodium Bicarbonate	72.3
Sodium Biphosphate	44.3
Sodium Borate	46.7
Sodium Phosphate (dibasic, heptahydrate)	32.3
Streptomycin Sulfate	7.7
Sulfacetamide Sodium	25.7
Sulfadiazine Sodium	26.7
Tetracaine Hydrochloride	20.0
Tetracycline Hydrochloride	15.7
Zinc Sulfate	16.7

[1] From USP XIX, p. 702.

—are quite acid and overtax the buffer capacity of the lacrimal fluid. For maximum comfort, an ophthalmic solution should have the same pH as the lacrimal fluid. However, this is not pharmaceutically possible, since at pH 7.4, many drugs are insoluble in water. Alkaloidal salts, for instance, are likely to precipitate as the free alkaloidal base at pH 7.4.

Most drugs, including many used in ophthalmic solutions, are most active therapeutically at pH levels which favor the undissociated molecule. However, the pH that permits greatest activity may also be the pH at which the drug is least stable. For this reason, a compromise pH is generally selected for a solution and maintained by buffers to permit the greatest activity while maintaining stability. The buffer system of an ophthalmic solution contributes to stability in another way by preventing an increase in the pH of the solution due to the normal leaching by the solution of alkali from the glass container.

Both the USP and the NF provide formulas for the preparation of buffer vehicles suitable for use for specific drugs.

Viscosity and Thickening Agents

Viscosity is a property of liquids that is closely related to the resistance to flow. The reciprocal of viscosity is *fluidity*. Viscosity is defined in terms of the force required to move one plane surface past another under specified conditions when the space between is filled by the liquid in question. More simply, it can be considered as a relative property with water as the reference material and all viscosities expressed in terms of the viscosity of pure water at 20°. The viscosity of water is given as one centipoise (actually 1.0087 centipoise). A liquid material ten times as viscous as water at the same temperature has a viscosity of 10 centipoises. The centipoise, abbreviated cp. (*cps.* plural), is a more convenient term than the basic unit, the poise; one poise is equal to 100 centipoises.

Specifying the temperature is important because viscosity changes with temperature; generally, the viscosity of a liquid decreases with increasing temperature. The determination of viscosity in terms of poise or centipoise results in the calculation of *absolute* viscosity. It is sometimes more convenient to use the kinematic scale in which the units of viscosity are *stokes* and *centistokes* (1 stoke equals 100 centistokes). The kinematic viscosity is obtained from the absolute viscosity by dividing the latter by the density of the liquid at the same temperature:

$$\text{kinematic viscosity} = \frac{\text{absolute viscosity}}{\text{density}}$$

Using water as the standard, examples of some viscosities at 20° are:

Ethyl alcohol—   1.19 cps
Olive oil   — 100   cps
Glycerin   — 400   cps
Castor oil   —1000   cps

Viscosity can be determined by any method that will measure the resistance to shear offered by the liquid. For ordinary liquids, it is customary to determine the time required for a given sample of the liquid to flow at a regulated temperature through a small vertical capillary tube and to compare this time with that required to perform the same task by the reference liquid. Many capillary tube viscosimeters have been devised, and nearly all are modifications of the Ostwald type. With an apparatus such as this, the viscosity of a liquid may be determined by the following equation:

$$\frac{\eta_1}{\eta_2} = \frac{\rho_1 t_1}{\rho_2 t_2}$$

where η_1 is the unknown viscosity of the liquid, η_2 is the viscosity of the standard, ρ_1 and ρ_2 are the respective densities of the liquids, and t_1 and t_2 are the respective flow times in seconds.

In the preparation of ophthalmic solutions, a suitable grade of methylcellulose or other thickening agent is frequently added to increase the viscosity and thereby aid in holding the drug in contact with the tissues so as to enhance the therapeutic effectiveness. Generally, methylcellulose of the 4000 cps viscosity type is used in concentrations of from 0.25 to 1% in ophthalmic solutions. Occasionally a 1% solution of methylcellulose without medication is used as a tear replacement.

Packaging

Ophthalmic solutions should be packaged so that they are easily administered and their sterility maintained. Most ophthalmic solutions, being administered by drop, are packaged in glass or plastic containers with a dropper service. Some plastic packages contain a fixed, built-in dropper which releases the medication when held in the inverted position. The patient must exercise care in protecting the ophthalmic solution from contamination. Obviously the ophthalmic solution packaged with the fixed dropper is less likely to acquire airborne contaminants than the screw-type bottle which must be opened and the dropper removed when using. However, each type is subject to contamination during use, brought about by the touching of the tip of the dropper to the tissues or to airborne contaminants. The prescribed amount of ophthalmic solution should be dropped quickly, but completely, into the eye without

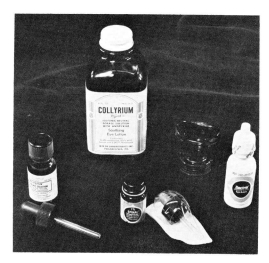

Fig. 11-3. *Typical commercial packages of ophthalmic solutions showing an ophthalmic wash solution with accompanying eye cup, dropper service bottles, and a plastic container with built-in dropper device.*

touching the dropper to the eye or surrounding tissue. Any ophthalmic solution that contains particulate matter or appears the least bit cloudy should be discarded.

Ophthalmic solutions used as eye washes are generally copackaged with an eye cup which should be cleaned and dried thoroughly after and prior to each use.

In selecting the packaging material for an ophthalmic solution, it must be determined that the container does not interfere with the stability or efficacy of the preparation. As pointed out previously in this text, plastic materials have been shown to interact with preservative agents rendering them unavailable for this function and to allow the sorption of certain medicinal agents; thus, particular precautions should be exercised when using plastic containers.

Official Ophthalmic Solutions

The major types of drugs used ophthalmically are as follows:

Miotics: Miotics are used primarily in the therapy of glaucoma but have been utilized in other conditions as accommodative esotropia, convergent strabismus, and for the local treatment of myasthenia gravis. Many miotics may be absorbed systemically after installation into the eye and may produce undesirable effects in some patients. Miotics reduce intraocular pressure associated with glaucoma. Among the miotics are physostigmine, pilocarpine, neostigmine, methacholine, carbachol, and isoflurophate.

Mydriatics and Cycloplegics: Mydriatics allow examination of the fundus through the dilation of the pupil. The stronger mydriatics having a long duration of action are called *cycloplegics.* Among the mydriatics and cycloplegics are atropine, hyoscyamine, scopolamine, homatropine, cyclopentolate, methentheline, naphazoline, cocaine, and tropicamide.

Local Anesthetics: Local anesthetics allow for the relief of pain preoperatively, postoperatively, following trauma, and during ophthalmic examination. Among the local anesthetics used ophthalmically are tetracaine, benoxinate, butacaine, piperocaine, and proparacaine.

Anti-inflammatory Agents: These agents combat inflammation of the eye. Most prominent among those employed topically are the steroids as prednisolone and dexamethasone salts.

Local Antiseptics: Local antiseptics are employed topically to reduce microbial presence on the eye. Among the agents so employed are certain organic mercury compounds as thimerosal and ammoniated mercury (the latter agent used primarily as an ophthalmic ointment), and silver nitrate.

Anti-infective Agents: Anti-infective agents are used specifically to combat infection of the eye. They are frequently employed both systemically and locally for their effect. Among those applied topically to the eye are chloramphenicol, sulfacetamide sodium, and neomycin. For viral infections, preparations of idoxuridine are employed.

Astringents: These agents are generally used in the treatment of conjunctivitis. Most preparations for this purpose utilize zinc compounds, particularly zinc sulfate, as the astringent.

Topical Protectants: These solutions are employed as artificial tears or as a contact lens fluid. Examples of agents used in these solutions are methylcellulose and hydroxypropyl methylcellulose.

Examples of some of the official ophthalmic solutions are presented in Table 11-2. There are several drugs utilized as ophthalmic solutions but because of their instability in solution, they are made available to the pharmacist by the

Table 11-2. EXAMPLES OF SOME OFFICIAL OPHTHALMIC SOLUTIONS BY CATEGORY

Ophthalmic Solution	Corresponding Commercial Product	Concentration of Active Ingredient*	Comments
Adrenergic			
Epinephrine Bitartrate Ophthalmic Solution, USP	Epitrate Ophthalmic Solution (Ayerst)	2%	Used in management of chronic simple (open angle) glaucoma.
Hydroxyamphetamine HBr Ophthalmic Solution, NF	Paredrine Ophthalmic Solution (Smith Kline & French)	1%	Produces pupillary dilatation which lasts a few hours.
Naphazoline HCl Ophthalmic Solution, USP	Privine HCl Ophthalmic Solution (Ciba)	0.1%	Used as a topical ocular vasoconstrictor.
Phenylephrine HCl Ophthalmic Solution, USP	Neo-Synephrine HCl Ophthalmic Solution (Winthrop)	2.5 and 10%	Used as a vasoconstrictor and mydriatic
Anesthetic			
Proparacaine HCl Ophthalmic Solution, NF	Ophthaine Ophthalmic Solution (Squibb)	0.5%	Rapid acting local anesthetic.
Tetracaine HCl Ophthalmic Solution, USP	Pontocaine Ophthalmic Solution (Winthrop)	0.5%	Rapid acting local anesthetic.
Antibacterial			
Chloramphenicol Ophthalmic Solution, USP	Chloramphenicol Ophthalmic Solution (Parke Davis)	0.5%	Used for superficial infections of the eye due to susceptible microorganisms.
Silver Nitrate Ophthalmic Solution, USP	. . .	1%	See text for discussion.
Sulfacetamide Sodium Ophthalmic Solution, USP	Sodium Sulamyd Ophthalmic Solution (Schering)	10 and 30%	See text for discussion.
Anticholinergic			
Atropine Sulfate Ophthalmic Solution, USP	Isopto Atropine Ophthalmic Solution (Alcon)	0.125 to 4%	
Homatropine HBr Ophthalmic Solution, USP	Isopto Homatropine Ophthalmic Solution (Alcon)	2 and 5%	Used to produce mydriasis and cycloplegia.
Scopolamine HBr Ophthalmic Solution, USP	Isopto Hyoscine Ophthalmic Solution (Alcon)	0.25%	
Tropicamide Ophthalmic Solution, USP	Mydriacyl Ophthalmic Solution (Alcon)	0.5 and 1%	
Antiviral			
Idoxuridine Ophthalmic Solution, USP	Dendrid Ophthalmic Solution (Alcon); Stoxil Ophthalmic Solution (Smith, Kline & French)	0.1%	Indicated in the treatment of herpes simplex keratitis.
Astringent			
Zinc Sulfate Ophthalmic Solution, USP	Op-Thal-Zin Ophthalmic Solution (Alcon)	0.25%	Used for angular conjunctivitis and acute catarrhal conjunctivitis (pink eye) caused by pneumococcus or Koch-Weeks bacillus as well as nonspecific infections of the eye. See text for additional discussion.

Table 11-2. Examples of Some Official Ophthalmic Solutions by Category (*Cont.*)

Ophthalmic Solution	Corresponding Commercial Product	Concentration of Active Ingredient*	Comments
Anti-inflammatory			
Dexamethasone Sodium Phosphate Ophthalmic Solution, USP	Decadron Phosphate Ophthalmic Solution Merck Sharp & Dohme)	0.1%	Combats inflammation due to mechanical, chemical, or immunologic causes.
Prednisolone Sodium Phosphate Ophthalmic Solution, USP	Metreton Ophthalmic Solution (Schering)	0.55%	
Cholinergic			
Carbachol Ophthalmic Solution, USP	Isopto Carbachol Ophthalmic Solution (Alcon)	0.75 to 3%	Reduces intraocular pressure in open-angle or narrow-angle glaucoma.
Isoflurophate Ophthalmic Solution, USP	Floropryl Ophthalmic Solution (Merck Sharp & Dohme)	0.1%	Long acting anticholinesterase miotic used in treating glaucoma. Commercial product in a solution in peanut oil. See text for additional discussion.
Pilocarpine HCl Ophthalmic Solution, USP	Isopto Carpine Ophthalmic Solution (Alcon)	0.25 to 10%	Used as a miotic in treating glaucoma, especially open-angle glaucoma. Also used to neutralize mydriasis following ophthalmoscopy or surgery.
Physostigmine Salicylate Ophthalmic Solution, USP	Isopto Eserine Ophthalmic Solution (Alcon)	0.25 and 0.5%	Short-acting anticholinesterase miotic used in reducing intraocular tension in glaucoma.
Protectant			
Methylcellulose Ophthalmic Solution, USP	Isopto Tears Ophthalmic Solution (Alcon)	0.5%	Preserved solutions used as artificial tears in the treatment of dry eyes and also as contact lens solutions.

*The active ingredient referred to is that agent named in the preparation's official title; the percent concentration is that amount generally present in the corresponding commercial product.

manufacturer in dry-form for constitution to solution-form prior to dispensing. Included among these are the following official preparations: Chloramphenicol for Ophthalmic Solution, USP, Chymotrypsin for Ophthalmic Solution, USP, and Tetracycline Hydrochloride for Ophthalmic Solution, NF.

The following ophthalmic solutions are discussed separately because of their special pharmaceutic or therapeutic interest.

Dexamethasone Sodium Phosphate Ophthalmic Solution, USP

The commercially available product contains 0.1% of dexamethasone sodium phosphate.

Dexamethasone is an adrenocorticoid steroid

that is practically insoluble in water; dexamethasone sodium phosphate has the same activity as the parent compound but is soluble in water to the extent of 1 g in 2 ml of water. This aspect is important not only from the pharmaceutical standpoint of preparing an aqueous solution, but also in the availability of the drug to the tissues at the site of its application.

The solution is used against a host of conditions of the eye, including conjunctivitis of various etiologies, keratitis, corneal injuries, lid allergies, and many and varied inflammatory conditions. Generally, therapy with dexamethasone is initiated with a regimen of 1 or 2 drops of solution into the conjunctival sac every hour during the day, and every 2 hours during the night until a favorable response is observed, after which time the dosage is reduced to 1 drop every 4 hours, and later yet, 1 drop three or four times a day.

Commercial Product: Decadron Phosphate Ophthalmic Solution (Merck Sharp & Dohme)

Isoflurophate Ophthalmic Solution, USP

Isoflurophate Ophthalmic Solution, USP, is a sterile solution of isopropyl phosphoro-fluoridate, $[(CH_3)_2CHO]_2P(F)O$, in a suitable vegetable oil. The official preparation contains about 0.1% of active ingredient. The label on the solution must bear an expiration date of not greater than 2 years after the date of manufacture.

Isoflurophate is not water soluble, but even if it were, water would not be used as the solvent, since the drug is hydrolyzed in the presence of moisture with resultant loss of potency and formation of the very irritating substance, hydrofluoric acid. For this reason, the nonaqueous solution must be handled carefully to prevent the absorption of moisture. The container of the solution must be sealed tightly at all times. The commercial solution contains anhydrous peanut oil as the solvent, and the manufacturer strongly urges that the solution not be diluted extemporaneously because of the chance of introducing moisture into the solution. Dangerous systemic absorption of isoflurophate is possible if the solution is accidentally placed on the skin or mucous membranes. Should this occur, the affected area must be immediately washed with voluminous amounts of water.

This solution is employed solely by application to the conjunctival sac for the treatment of certain types of glaucoma and strabismus. For the treatment of glaucoma 1 to 3 drops of the solution are carefully instilled in the affected eye every 8 to 72 hours, the frequency to be determined by the physician.

Commercial Product: Floropryl Solution (Merck Sharp & Dohme)

Silver Nitrate Ophthalmic Solution, USP

Silver Nitrate Ophthalmic Solution, USP, is a 1% aqueous solution of silver nitrate. The solution may be buffered by the addition of sodium acetate to a pH between 4.5 and 6.0. Although this solution is not required to be sterile, it is discussed in this section because of its use as an ophthalmic solution.

The USP requires that this clear, colorless solution be stored protected from light in inert, collapsible capsules or in other suitable single dose containers. In this form, the solution is packaged in units containing about 5 drops of a 1% solution.

Although many antibiotic preparations would serve the same purpose and perhaps with greater safety, many state laws still require the instillation of a few drops of silver nitrate ophthalmic solution into the conjunctival sac of the newborn infant for the prevention of *ophthalmia neonatorum*, a gonococcal infection of the eyes transmitted to the baby by his infected mother. In practice, a few drops of the solution are placed in the infant's eyes and rinsed out immediately with isotonic sodium chloride solution.

Sulfacetamide Sodium Ophthalmic Solution, USP

Sulfacetamide Sodium Ophthalmic Solution, USP, is a sterile solution containing up to 30% of sodium sulfacetamide, a sulfonamide drug, and suitable buffers, stabilizers, and preservatives selected by the manufacturer.

This solution is unusual because of the rather high concentration of active ingredient present. Ophthalmic solutions generally contain much smaller proportions of the therapeutic agent. The high concentration is permitted by the high water-solubility (1 g in 2.5 ml) of sodium sulfacetamide in alkaline media. The commercial preparations utilize phosphate buffers to maintain the pH at about 7.4. Sodium thiosulfate is employed as a stabilizer to prevent the darkening of the solution. The solution should be stored in light-resistant containers to minimize the chance of discoloration. One commercial preparation utilizes a combination of parabens as the antimicrobial preservative, and another uses chlorobutanol.

The solution is employed for its antibacterial properties when applied topically to the eye. It is effective against a number of different microorganisms commonly found in eye infections.

Commercial Products: Sodium Sulamyd Ophthalmic Solution (10 to 30%) (Schering); Isopto Cetamide Ophthalmic Solution (15%) (Alcon)

Zinc Sulfate Ophthalmic Solution, USP

Zinc Sulfate Ophthalmic Solution, USP, is a sterile solution of zinc sulfate in water, rendered sterile by the addition of suitable salts. The pH of the solution is between 5.8 and 6.2. The solution is usually available as a 0.25% solution.

This solution is frequently compounded by the pharmacist in his community practice, and he is often confronted by signs of the solution's instability. When boric acid is employed to make the solution isotonic to tears, zinc borate occasionally precipitates from solution. Cloudiness of a zinc sulfate solution may also be due to the partial hydrolysis of the zinc sulfate to a basic form. These solutions should be discarded, and only clear solutions should be dispensed.

The commercial preparation indicated below contains 0.25% of zinc sulfate, 1:10,000 of benzalkonium chloride, and barbital and sodium barbital as buffering agents. When taken internally, the latter agents have sedative effects; however, in the ophthalmic solution their physiologic effects are negligible.

Zinc sulfate solutions are employed in the eye for the temporary relief of discomfort and congestion occurring with minor irritations due to wind, dust, and glare. The USP categorizes the solution as an ophthalmic astringent. It is instilled into the conjunctiva three or four times a day.

Commercial Product: Op-Thal-Zin Ophthalmic Solution (Alcon)

Ophthalmic Suspensions

Ophthalmic suspensions are employed to a much lesser extent than are ophthalmic solutions. At the present time, there are only three official ophthalmic suspensions:

Hydrocortisone Acetate Ophthalmic Suspension, USP—an aqueous suspension of hydrocortisone acetate, a water-insoluble adrenocortical steroid, used topically as an anti-inflammatory agent. The suspension is generally of 0.5 to 2.5% in strength. [Corresponding Commercial Product: Hydro-Cortone Acetate Ophthalmic Suspension (Merck Sharp & Dohme)]
Medrysone Ophthalmic Suspension, USP—an aqueous suspension of medrysone, a sparingly water-soluble adrenocortical steroid, used topically for its anti-inflammatory action. The suspension is generally 1% in strength. [Corresponding Commercial Product: HMS Liquifilm (Allergan)]
Tetracycline Hydrochloride Ophthalmic Suspension, USP—a suspension of tetracycline HCl in oil. Used topically as an antibacterial preparation. [Corresponding Commercial Product: Achromycin Ophthalmic Oil Suspension (Lederle)]

Ophthalmic suspensions may be prepared when the medicinal agent is insoluble in the desired vehicle or unstable in solution-form. Ophthalmic suspensions may also be desired to provide a slower release of the drug from the vehicle and thus a more sustained effect.

Ophthalmic suspensions must possess the same characteristic of sterility as ophthalmic solutions, with proper consideration given also to preservation, isotonicity, buffering, viscosity and packaging. Additionally, ophthalmic suspensions must contain particles of such chemical characteristics and small dimensions that they are non-irritating to the eyes. The ophthalmic suspension must also be of such a quality that the suspended particles do not agglomerate into larger ones upon storage. The suspension must be shaken prior to use and the particles distributed uniformly throughout the vehicle. Ophthalmic suspensions are packaged in the same types of dropper containers as are the ophthalmic solutions.

Ophthalmic Ointments

Ophthalmic ointments, in contrast to the dermatological ointments discussed in the previous chapter, must be sterile. They are either manufactured from sterilized ingredients and under rigid aseptic conditions, or they are sterilized following manufacture. Ophthalmic ointments must meet the sterility tests as indicated in the official compendia.

The ointment base selected for an ophthalmic ointment must be non-irritating to the eye and must permit the diffusion of the medicinal substance throughout the secretions bathing the eye. Ointment bases utilized for ophthalmics have a melting or softening point close to body temperature. In most instances, mixtures of petrolatum and liquid petrolatum (mineral oil) are utilized as the ointment base. Sometimes a water miscible agent as lanolin is added. This permits water and water-soluble drugs to be retained within the delivery system.

The medicinal agent is added to the ointment base either as a solution or as a finely micronized powder. The drug is then intimately mixed with the base, usually by milling.

After preparation the ophthalmic ointments are filled into previously sterilized tin or plastic ophthalmic ointment tubes. These tubes are typically small, holding approximately 3.5 g of ointment, and fitted with narrow gauge tips which permit the expulsion of narrow bands of ointment (Fig. 11-4). This is convenient for placement of the ointment onto the margin of the eyelid, the usual site of application.

The primary advantage of an ophthalmic ointment over an ophthalmic solution is the increased ocular contact time of the drug. Studies have shown that the ocular contact time is

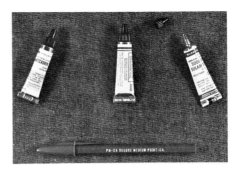

Fig. 11-4. *Examples of ophthalmic ointment products. Ball-point pen demonstrates the size of the ointment tubes. Each ointment tube contains $\frac{1}{8}$ oz (3.5 g) of ointment.*

Table 11-3. OFFICIAL OPHTHALMIC OINTMENTS

Ophthalmic Ointment	Corresponding Commercial Product	Concentration of Active Ingredient*	Category
Bacitracin Ophthalmic Ointment, USP	Baciguent Ophthalmic Ointment (Upjohn)	500 Units/g	Antibacterial
Chloramphenicol Ophthalmic Ointment, USP	Chloromycetin Ophthalmic Ointment (Parke Davis)	1%	Antibacterial
Chlortetracycline HCl Ophthalmic Ointment, NF	Aureomycin Ophthalmic Ointment (Lederle)	1%	Antibacterial
Dexamethasone Sodium Phosphate Ophthalmic Ointment, USP	Decadron Phosphate Ophthalmic Ointment (Merck Sharp & Dohme)	0.05%	Anti-inflammatory adrenocortical steroid
Erythromycin Ophthalmic Ointment, USP	Ilotycin Ophthalmic Ointment (Dista)	0.5%	Antibacterial
Gentamicin Sulfate Ophthalmic Ointment, USP	Garamycin Ophthalmic Ointment (Schering)	0.3%	Antibacterial
Hydrocortisone Acetate Ophthalmic Ointment, USP	Hydro-Cortone Acetate Ophthalmic Ointment (Merck Sharp & Dohme)	0.5 and 1.5%	Anti-inflammatory adrenocortical steroid
Idoxuridine Ophthalmic Ointment, USP	Stoxil Ophthalmic Ointment (Smith Kline & French)	0.5%	Antiviral
Isoflurophate Ophthalmic Ointment, USP	Floropryl Ophthalmic Ointment (Merck Sharp & Dohme)	0.025%	Cholinergic
Neomycin Sulfate Ophthalmic Ointment, USP	Myciguent Ophthalmic Ointment (Upjohn)	0.35%	Antibacterial
Sulfacetamide Sodium Ophthalmic Ointment, USP	Sodium Sulamyd Ophthalmic Ointment (Schering)	10 and 30%	Antibacterial
Sulfisoxazole Diolamine Ophthalmic Ointment, NF	Gantrisin Ophthalmic Ointment (Roche)	4%	Antibacterial
Tetracaine Ophthalmic Ointment, NF	Pontocaine Ophthalmic Ointment (Winthrop)	0.5%	Anesthetic

*The active ingredient referred to is that agent named in the preparation's official title; the percent concentration is that amount generally present in the corresponding commercial product.

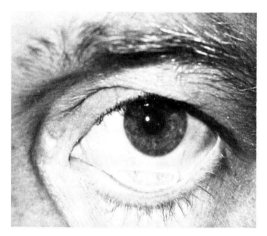

Fig. 11-5. *An OCUSERT ocular delivery system.* (*Courtesy of Alza Pharmaceuticals.*)

two to four times greater when ointments are used than when a saline solution is used.[1] One disadvantage to ophthalmic ointment use is the blurred vision which occurs as the ointment base melts and is spread across the lens.

Official Ophthalmic Ointments

The official ophthalmic ointments are presented in Table 11-3.

Ophthalmic Inserts

A recent development in the delivery of medication to the eyes has been that of ophthalmic inserts. One such device, the OCUSERT system (Alza Pharmaceuticals) is shown in Figure 11-5. The insert unit is designed to provide for the release of medication at predetermined and predictable rates permitting the elimination of frequent dosing by the patient, ensuring nighttime medication, and providing a better means of patient compliance.

The insert shown in Figure 11-5 is elliptical with dimensions of 13.4 by 5.7 mm and 0.3 mm

[1] Fraunfelder, F. T., and C. Hanna: Drug Delivery Systems, *Survey of Ophthalmology,* 18:292–298, 1974.

in thickness. The insert is flexible and is a multi-layered structure consisting of a drug-containing core surrounded on each side by a layer of copolymer membranes through which the drug diffuses at a constant rate. The rate of drug diffusion is controlled by the polymer composition, the membrane thickness, and the solubility of the drug. The devices are sterile and do not contain preservatives.

One such insert containing pilocarpine has been found to be effective and of great benefit in glaucoma therapy.[1] After placement in the conjunctival sac, the inserts are designed to release medication at the desired rates over a 7-day period at which time they are removed and replaced with new ones. Other drugs such as adrenocortical steroids have been utilized in the system with similar effectiveness.[2]

Soft contact lenses, composed of various polymeric materials, have also been used as drug delivery systems with success.[3] Readers interested in the use, composition, and care of both conventional hard contact lenses and the soft contact lenses may wish to refer to the papers noted below in footnote 4.

Selected Reading

Brown, M. R. W. and Norton, D. A.: The Preservation of Ophthalmic Preparations. *Journal of the Society of Cosmetic Chemists,* 16:369–387, 1965.

Fraunfelder, F. T. and Hanna, D.: Ophthalmic Drug Delivery Systems. *Survey of Ophthalmology,* 18:292–297, 1974.

[1] Worthen, D. M., Zimmerman, T. J., and Wind, C. A.: An Evaluation of the Pilocarpine Ocusert. *Investigative Ophthalmology,* 13:296–299, 1974.

[2] Dohlman, C. H., Pavan-Langston, D., and Rose, J.: A New Ocular Insert Device for Continuous Constant-Rate Delivery of Medication to the Eye. *Annals of Ophthalmology,* 4:823–832, 1972.

[3] Fraunfelder, F. T. and Hanna, C.: Ophthalmic Drug Delivery Systems. *Survey of Ophthalmology,* 18:292–297, 1974.

[4] Koetting, R. A.: Contact Lens Update. *Journal of the American Pharmaceutical Association,* NS15:575–577, 1975; *also,* Krezanoski, J. Z. and Lowry, J. B.: New Hydrophilic Contact Lenses and Their Pharmaceutical Accessories, *ibid,* NS15:578–580, 1975.

Chapter 12

Ear, Nose, and Topical Oral Preparations

P REPARATIONS USED topically in the ear, nose, and oral cavity include many of the types of pharmaceutical dosage forms previously discussed, as solutions, suspensions, and ointments. The purpose of this chapter is to identify more closely the types of dosage forms used with the sites of application and to define the purpose of any special formulative components.

Ear Preparations

Ear preparations are sometimes referred to as *otic* or *aural* preparations. Solutions are most frequently used in the ear, with suspensions and ointments also finding some application. Ear preparations are usually placed in the ear canal by drops or in small amounts for the removal of excessive cerumen (ear wax) or for the treatment of ear infections, inflammation, or pain. Since the outer ear is a skin-covered structure and susceptible to the same dermatologic conditions as other parts of the body's surface, skin conditions which arise are treated using the variety of topical dermatological preparations previously discussed in Chapter 10.

Cerumen-Removing Preparations

Cerumen is a combination of the secretions of the sweat and sebaceous glands of the exter-

nal auditory canal. The secretions, if allowed to dry, form a sticky semisolid which holds shed epithelial cells, fallen hair, dust and other foreign bodies that make their way into the ear canal. Excessive accumulation of cerumen in the ear may cause itching, pain, impaired hearing and is a deterrent to otologic examination. If not removed periodically, the cerumen may become impacted and its removal made more difficult and painful.

Through the years, light mineral oil, vegetable oils, and hydrogen peroxide have been commonly used agents to soften impacted cerumen for its removal. Recently, solutions of synthetic surfactants have been developed for their *cerumenolytic* activity in the removal of ear wax. One of these agents, triethanolamine polypeptide oleate-condensate, commercially formulated in propylene glycol, is used to emulsify the cerumen thereby facilitating its removal. Another commercial product utilizes carbamide peroxide in anhydrous glycerin. On contact with the cerumen, the carbamide peroxide releases oxygen which disrupts the integrity of the impacted wax, allowing its easy removal.

In removing cerumen, the procedure usually involves placing the otic solution in the ear canal with the patient's head tilted at a 45° angle, inserting a cotton plug to retain the medication in the ear for 15 to 30 minutes, followed by gentle flushing of the ear canal with lukewarm water using a soft rubber ear syringe.

Anti-infective, Anti-inflammatory and Analgesic Ear Preparations

Drugs used topically in the ear for their anti-infective activity include such agents as chloramphenicol, colistin sulfate, neomycin, polymyxin B sulfate, and nystatin, the latter agent used to combat fungal infections. These agents are generally formulated into ear drops (solutions or suspensions) in a vehicle of anhydrous glycerin or propylene glycol. These viscous vehicles permit maximum contact time between the medication and the tissues of the ear. In addition, their hygroscopicity causes them to draw moisture from the tissues thereby reducing inflammation and diminishing the moisture available for the life process of the microorganisms present. To assist in relieving the pain which frequently accompanies ear infections, a number of anti-infective otic preparations also contain analgesic agents as antipyrine and local anesthetics as lidocaine, dibucaine, and benzocaine.

Topical treatment of ear infections is frequently considered adjunctive, with concomitant systemic treatment with orally administered antibiotics also undertaken.

Liquid ear preparations of the anti-inflammatory agents hydrocortisone and dexamethasone sodium phosphate are prescribed for their effects against the swelling and inflammation which frequently accompany allergic and irritative manifestations of the ear as well as for the inflammation and pruritus which sometimes follow treatment of ear infections. In the latter instance, some physicians prefer the use of corticosteroids in ointment form, packaged in ophthalmic tubes. These packages allow the placement of small amounts of ointment in the ear canal with a minimum of waste. Many of the commercially available products used in this manner are labeled "eye-ear" to indicate their dual use.

Solutions of hydrogen peroxide, alcohol rubbing compound, and acetic acid (5%) in ethyl alcohol (85%) are frequently employed as ear rinses to prevent infection or irritation following such activities as swimming.

Pain in the ear frequently accompanies ear infection or inflamed or swollen ear tissue. Topical analgesic agents generally are employed together with internally administered analgesics, as aspirin, and other agents, as anti-infectives, to combat the cause of the problem.

Topical analgesics for the ear are usually solutions and frequently contain the analgesic antipyrine and the local anesthetic benzocaine in a vehicle of propylene glycol or anhydrous glycerin. Again, these hygroscopic vehicles reduce the swelling of tissues (and thus some pain) and the growth of microorganisms by drawing moisture from the swollen tissues into the vehicle. These preparations are commonly employed to relieve the symptoms of acute otitis media.

Although most of the drugs discussed in this section are officially recognized, there are presently no official ear drop formulations.

As determined on an individual-product basis, some liquid otic preparations require preservation against microbial growth. When preservation is required, such agents as chlorobutanol (0.5%), thimerosal (0.01%), and combinations of the parabens are commonly used.

Antioxidants, as sodium bisulfite, and other stabilizers are also included in otic formulations, as required.

Ear preparations are usually packaged in small (5 to 15 ml) glass or plastic containers with a dropper.

Nasal Preparations

The vast majority of preparations intended for intranasal use contain adrenergic agents and are employed for their decongestant activity on the nasal mucosa. Most of these preparations are in solution-form, and are administered as nose drops or sprays; however, a few are available as nasal jellies. The official products for intranasal use are presented in Table 12-1. Some nonofficial products including nasal jellies containing ephedrine sulfate and sticks of silver nitrate are commercially available for use in treating epistaxis (nose bleeds).

Nasal Decongestant Solutions

Most nasal decongestant solutions, as those presented in Table 12-1, are aqueous preparations, rendered isotonic to nasal fluids (approximately equivalent to 0.9% sodium chloride), buffered to maintain drug stability while approximating the normal pH range of the nasal fluids (pH 5.5 to 6.5), and stabilized and preserved as required. The antimicrobial preservatives used are the same as those used in preserving ophthalmic solutions. The concentration of adrenergic agent in the majority of nasal decongestant solutions is quite low, ranging from about 0.05 to 1.0%. Certain commercial solutions which are available for both pediatric and adult use, are generally available in two strengths, the pediatric strength being approximately one-half of the adult strength.

Nasal decongestant solutions are employed in the treatment of rhinitis of the common cold and for vasomotor and allergic rhinitis including hay fever, and for sinusitis. Their frequent use or their use for prolonged periods may lead to chronic edema of the nasal mucosa, aggravating the symptom that they are intended to relieve. Thus, they are best used for short periods of time with the patients advised not to exceed the recommended dosage and frequency of use.

Most of the adrenergic drugs used in nasal decongestant solutions are synthetic compounds similar in chemical structure, pharmacologic

Table 12-1. OFFICIAL NASAL SOLUTIONS AND NASAL INHALANTS

Official Preparation	Corresponding Commercial Product	Concentration of Active Constituent*	Category and Comments
Ephedrine Sulfate Nasal Solution, USP	Gluco-Fedrin Nasal Solution (Parke Davis)	1 and 3%	Nasal adrenergic.
Epinephrine Nasal Solution, USP	Adrenalin Chloride Solution (Parke Davis)	0.1%	Nasal adrenergic. See text for additional discussion.
Naphazoline HCl Nasal Solution, USP	Privine HCl Nasal Solution (Ciba)	0.05 and 0.1%	Nasal adrenergic.
Oxymetazole HCl Nasal Solution, USP	Afrin Nasal Solution (Schering)	0.05%	Nasal adrenergic.
Phenylephrine HCl Nasal Solution, USP	Neo-Synephrine HCl Nose Drops (Winthrop)	0.125 to 1.0%	Nasal adrenergic.
Tetrahydrozoline HCl Nasal Solution, USP	Tyzine Nasal Solution (Pfizer)	0.05 and 0.1%	Nasal adrenergic.
Amyl Nitrite Inhalant, NF	Amyl Nitrite Inhalant Capsules (Burroughs Wellcome)	0.3 ml per capsule	Vasodilator. Cloth covered glass capsule is broken and vapor inhaled in treatment of angina pectoris attack.
Propylhexedrine Inhalant, NF	Benzedrex Inhaler (Smith Kline & French)	250 mg per inhaler	Nasal adrenergic. See text for additional discussion.
Tuaminoheptane Inhalant, NF	Tuamine Inhaler (Lilly)	325 mg per inhaler	Nasal adrenergic. See text for additional discussion.

*The active constituent referred to is that agent named in the preparation's official title; the percent concentration is that amount generally present in the corresponding commercial product.

activity, and side effects to the parent compound, naturally occurring epinephrine. Epinephrine as a pure chemical substance was first isolated from suprarenal gland in 1901 and was called both *Suprarenin* and *Adrenalin*. Synthetic epinephrine was prepared just a few years later, and today either the natural form or the synthetic may be used in the preparation of the official solution.

Epinephrine is extremely sensitive to oxidizing agents and is decomposed by the slightest trace of iron, other metals, and alkalies. Thus in the preparation of epinephrine solutions, purified water is employed. Epinephrine solution is packaged in well-filled amber bottles to assist in its preservation; however, even with this precaution, the solution gradually decomposes on standing and changes in color. The USP directs that the solution must not be used if it is brown or contains a precipitate. The commercial product, Adrenalin Chloride Solution, contains about 0.15% of sodium bisulfite as an antioxidant, 0.5% of chlorobutanol as an antimicrobial preservative, and 0.1% of epinephrine hydrochloride in sodium chloride solution. The side

effects to the use of epinephrine solution and other such adrenergic solutions intranasally reflect the pharmacologic activity of the drug category and include an increase in blood pressure, headache, weakness and tremors. The drugs are used with caution in children under 6, in patients with coronary artery disease, hypertension and in other conditions in which the effects of the drugs are potentially harmful.

Most solutions for nasal use are packaged in dropper bottles or in plastic spray bottles, usually containing 15 to 30 ml of medication. The products should be determined to be stable in the containers used and the packages tightly closed during periods of nonuse. The patient should be advised that should the solution become discolored or contain precipitated matter, it should be discarded.

Decongestant Inhalers

As indicated in Table 12-1, there are two officially recognized nasal decongestants official in the form of inhalants. These two preparations are Propylhexedrine Inhalant and

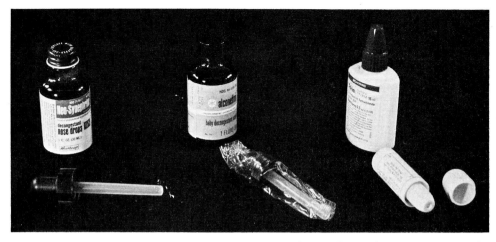

Fig. 12-1. *Examples of commercial packaging of nasal solutions, showing drop and spray containers, and nasal inhaler.*

Tuaminoheptane Inhalant, both official in the NF.

The drugs propylhexedrine and tuaminoheptane are liquids which volatilize slowly at room temperature. This quality enables them to be effective as inhalants. The inhalers in which they are held contain cylindrical rolls of fibrous material impregnated with the volatile drug substance. The medications which have amine-like odors are usually masked with added aromatic agents. The inhaler is placed in the nostril and vapor inhaled to relieve nasal decongestion. As with the other nasal adrenergic agents, excessive or too frequent use can result in nasal edema and increased rather than decreased congestion.

The inhalers are effective so long as the volatile drug remains present. To insure that the drug does not escape during periods of nonuse, the caps on the inhalers should be tightly closed.

Topical Oral Preparations

A variety of medicinal substances are employed topically in the oral cavity for a number of purposes and in a wide range of dosage forms. Among the official drugs and preparations included in this group are the following:

Camphorated Parachlorophenol, USP—Dental anti-infective. A eutectic liquid composed of 65% camphor and 35% parachlorophenol, used in dentistry for the sterilization of deep root canals.

Carbamide Peroxide Solution, NF—Dental anti-infective. Acts as a chemomechanical cleansing and debriding agent through the release of bubbling oxygen. The commercial product (Gly-Oxide, International Pharmaceutical) contains 10% carbamide in flavored anhydrous glycerin.

Cetylpyridinium Chloride Solution, NF and Cetylpyridinium Chloride Lozenges, NF—Local anti-infective. Commercial counterparts (Cepacol Mouthwash/Gargle and Cepacol Lozenges, Merrell-National) contain 1:2000 w/v and 1:1500 w/v of cetylpyridinium chloride respectively. Used primarily as a freshening mouth cleanser. Lozenges have benzyl alcohol present to act as a local anesthetic in soothing throat irritations.

Erythrosine Sodium Solution, USP and Erythrosine Sodium Tablets, USP—Diagnostic aid (dental disclosing agent). Solution applied topically to the teeth to reveal plaque left by inadequate brushing. Tablets chewed for the same purpose and are not to be swallowed.

Eugenol, USP—Dental analgesic. Applied topically to dental cavities and dental protectives. Eugenol is a pale yellow liquid having an aromatic odor of clove and a spicy taste.

Gutta Percha, USP—Dental restoration agent. Dried, purified latex from natural sources, insoluble in water, and used as needed for temporary dental restoration and permanent root canals.

Lidocaine Aerosol, NF—Topical dental anesthetic. Applied through metered spray in the amounts of 10 mg per spray; 20 mg per quadrant of gingiva and oral mucosa is usually employed.

Nystatin Oral Suspension, USP—Antifungal. May be employed for oral fungal infections by retaining in the mouth as long as possible before swallowing.

Pumice, NF—Dental abrasive. Pumice is a water-insoluble, gritty, grayish powder of volcanic origin containing silicates of aluminum, potassium, and sodium. It is used in small amounts and at infrequent intervals to clean the teeth.

Sodium Fluoride Solution, USP, and Sodium Fluoride Tablets, USP—Dental caries prophylactic. Solution applied to the teeth or, when drinking water does not contain adequate fluoride, a dilute solution may be swallowed. Tablets containing 1.1 or 2.2 mg of sodium fluoride are chewed or swallowed as required.

Sodium Fluoride and Orthophosphoric Acid Gel, NF, and Sodium Fluoride and Orthophosphoric Acid Solution, NF—Dental caries prophylactic. Gel and solution applied to the teeth; each contains 1.23% of fluoride ion and 1% of phosphoric acid.

Triamcinolone Acetonide Dental Paste USP—Topical anti-inflammatory agent. Applied to the oral mucous membranes as a 0.1% paste.

Zinc Chloride, USP—Dentin desensitizer. Applied topically to the teeth as a 10% solution.

Zinc-Eugenol Cement, USP—Topical dental protectant. Applied to the cleaned carious lesion as a temporary protectant. Cement made freshly before use by mixing a powder of zinc acetate, zinc stearate, zinc oxide and rosin, with a liquid containing eugenol and cottonseed oil.

In addition to the above-named official drugs and preparations, a host of nonofficial products for oral use are commercially available. Some of these products are medicated, as teething lotions and toothache drops, whereas others are used for hygienic purposes, as dentifrices, denture products, and many of the mouthwashes. Among the variety of products is a like variety of physical forms, as solutions, emulsions, ointments, pastes, aerosols, etc., with the manufacture of each following the same general procedures as has been previously outlined in this text. One type of dosage form for oral use, the lozenge, has not been previously described.

Lozenges

Lozenges, also called troches, are disk-shaped solid dosage forms containing a medicinal substance and generally flavoring and sweetening agents, intended to be slowly dissolved in the oral cavity for localized effects. Commercially, lozenges may be made by compression, using a tablet machine and large, flat punches. The tablet machines are operated at high compression to produce troches that are harder than ordinary tablets so that they slowly dissolve or disintegrate in the mouth. The use of adhesives such as mucilages or natural gums, added to effect the adhesion of the powders used, also contributes to the hardness of the resulting lozenges.

Medicinal substances that are heat stable may be prepared into hard, sugar candy lozenges by candy-making machines that process a warm, highly concentrated, flavored syrup as the base. These lozenges dissolve slowly, and because of their high sugar content are especially soothing to the throat. Most of the commercially available cough drops are of a hard candy base.

Chapter 13

Suppositories and Other Rectal, Vaginal, and Urethral Preparations

Suppositories

SUPPOSITORIES ARE solid dosage forms intended for insertion into body orifices where they melt, soften, or dissolve and exert localized or systemic effects.[1] Suppositories are commonly employed rectally and vaginally, occasionally urethrally, and rarely aurally and nasally. They have various shapes and weights. The shape and size of a suppository must be such that it is capable of being easily inserted into the intended body orifice without causing undue distension, and, once inserted, it must be retained for the appropriate period of time. Rectal suppositories are generally inserted with the fingers, but certain vaginal suppositories, particularly the vaginal "inserts" or vaginal tablets prepared by compression, may be in-

[1] According to Anschel and Lieberman, the Latin word *suppositorium* was first applied to this form of medication in the seventeenth century, with the word being derived from the verb *supponere*, meaning to "substitute for," and probably referred to the substitution of enemas with laxative suppositories. Reference: Anschel, J., and Lieberman, H. A.: Drug Cosmetic Ind., 97:341, 1965.

serted high in the vaginal tract with the aid of a special insertion appliance.

Generally speaking, rectal suppositories are usually about 32 mm (1½ inches) in length, are cylindrical, and have one or both ends tapered. Some rectal suppositories are shaped like a bullet, a torpedo, or the little finger. Depending upon the density of the base and the medicaments present in the suppository, the weight of rectal suppositories may vary. The USP and the NF state that adult rectal suppositories weigh about 2 g when cocoa butter (theobroma oil), the most common vehicle, is employed as the suppository base. Rectal suppositories for use by infants and children are about half the weight and size of the adult suppositories and assume a more pencil-like shape. Vaginal suppositories, also called *pessaries*, are usually globular, oviform, or cone-shaped. According to the official compendia they weigh about 5 g when cocoa butter is the base. Again, depending upon the base and the individual manufacturer's product, the weights of vaginal suppositories may vary widely. Urethral suppositories, also called *bougies*, are slender, pencil-shaped suppositories intended for insertion into the male or female urethra. Male urethral suppositories may be 3 to 6 mm in diameter and approximately 140 mm in length, although this may vary. When cocoa butter is employed as the base, these suppositories weigh about 4 g. Female urethral suppositories are about half the length and weight of the male urethral suppository, being about 70 mm in length and weighing about 2 g when of cocoa butter. Nasal suppositories and aural suppositories, also called *ear cones*, are each pencil-shaped suppositories similar in shape to urethral suppositories but shorter in length, generally being about 32 mm long. Aural suppositories have been generally prepared with a cocoa butter base and nasal suppositories, with a glycerinated gelatin base. As indicated earlier, nasal and aural suppositories are rarely encountered today.

Local Action

Once inserted, the suppository base melts, softens, or dissolves, distributing the medicaments it carries to the tissues of the region. These medicaments may be intended for retention within the cavity for localized drug effects, or they may be intended to be absorbed for the exertion of systemic effects. Rectal suppositories intended for localized action are most frequently employed to relieve constipation or the pain, irritation, itching, and inflammation associated with hemorrhoids or other anorectal conditions. Antihemorrhoidal suppositories frequently contain a number of components, including local anesthetics, vasoconstrictors, astringents, analgesics, soothing emollients, and protective agents. A popular laxative suppository is glycerin suppositories, which promote laxation by the local irritation of the mucous membranes, probably by the dehydrating effect of the glycerin on those membranes. Vaginal suppositories intended for localized effects are mainly employed as antiseptics in feminine hygiene and as specific agents to combat an invading pathogen. Most commonly, the drugs employed are trichomonacides to combat vaginitis caused by *Trichomonas vaginalis*, *Candida* (*Monilia*) *albicans*, and other microorganisms. Urethral suppositories may be used as antibacterials and as a local anesthetic preparative to urethral examination.

Systemic Action

For systemic effects, the mucous membranes of the rectum and vagina permit the absorption of many soluble drugs. Although the rectum is utilized quite frequently as the site for the systemic absorption of drugs, the vagina is not. However, this does not preclude the possibility of drug absorption from the vagina after the administration of a drug intended mainly for localized action.

Among the advantages over oral therapy of the rectal route of administration for achieving systemic effects are these: (a) drugs destroyed or inactivated by the pH or enzymatic activity of the stomach or intestines need not be exposed to these destructive environments; (b) drugs irritating to the stomach may be given without causing such irritation; (c) drugs destroyed by portal circulation bypass the liver after rectal absorption (drugs enter the portal circulation after oral administration and absorption); (d) the route is convenient for administration of drugs to adult or pediatric patients who may be unable or unwilling to swallow medication; and (e) it is an effective route in the treatment of patients with vomiting episodes.

Drugs administered rectally in the form of suppositories for their systemic effects include

(a) aminophylline and theophylline given to relieve asthma; (b) prochlorperazine and chlorpromazine for the relief of nausea and vomiting and as a tranquilizer; (c) chloral hydrate, as a sedative and hypnotic; (d) oxymorphone HCl for narcotic analgesia; (e) belladonna and opium, for analgesia and antispasmodic effects; (f) ergotamine tartrate, for the relief of migraine syndrome and (g) aspirin for its analgesic and antipyretic activity. Many others could be added to this group.

Some Factors of Drug Absorption from Rectal Suppositories

The dose of a drug administered rectally may be greater than or less than the dose of the same drug given orally, depending upon such factors as the constitution of the patient, the physicochemical nature of the drug and its ability to traverse the physiologic barriers to absorption, and the nature of the suppository vehicle and its capacity to release the drug and make it available for absorption.

The factors affecting the rectal absorption of a drug administered in the form of a suppository may be divided into two main groups: (1) physiologic factors, and (2) physicochemical factors of the drug and the base.[1]

Physiologic Factors

Included in the physiologic factors are such considerations as the colonic contents, circulation route, and the pH and lack of buffering capacity of the rectal fluids.

COLONIC CONTENT. When systemic effects are desired from the administration of a medicated suppository, greater absorption may be expected from a rectum that is void than from one that is distended with fecal matter. A drug will obviously have greater opportunity to make contact with the absorbing surface of the rectum and colon in the absence of fecal matter. Therefore, when deemed desirable, an evacuant enema may be administered and allowed to act before the administration of a suppository of a drug to

[1] Adapted in part from Anschel, J., and Lieberman, H. A.: Suppositories. Drug Cosmetic Ind., 97:341, 1965.

be absorbed. Other conditions such as diarrhea, colonic obstruction due to tumorous growths, and tissue dehydration can all influence the rate and degree of drug absorption from the rectal site.

CIRCULATION ROUTE. As pointed out in Chapter 3, drugs absorbed rectally, unlike those absorbed after oral administration, bypass the portal circulation, thereby enabling drugs otherwise destroyed in the liver to exert systemic effects. The lower hemorrhoidal veins surrounding the colon receive the absorbed drug and initiate its circulation throughout the body, bypassing the liver. Lymphatic circulation also assists in the absorption of rectally administered drugs.

pH AND LACK OF BUFFERING CAPACITY OF THE RECTAL FLUIDS. The rectal fluids are essentially neutral in pH and have no effective buffer capacity, the form in which the drug is administered will not generally be chemically changed by the rectal environment.

The suppository base employed has a marked influence on the release of active constituents incorporated into it. While cocoa butter melts rapidly at body temperature, because of its immiscibility with body fluids, it fails to readily release fat-soluble drugs. For systemic drug action, it is preferable to incorporate the ionized rather than the unionized form of a drug in order to maximize bioavailability. Although unionized drugs partition out of water-miscible bases such as glycerinated gelatin and polyethylene glycol more readily, the bases themselves tend to dissolve slowly and thus retard the release of the drug.

Physicochemical Factors of the Drug and Suppository Base

Physicochemical factors include such properties as the relative solubility of the drug in lipid and in water and the particle size of a dispersed drug. Physicochemical factors of the base include its ability to melt, soften, or dissolve at body temperature, its ability to release the drug substance, and its hydrophilic or hydrophobic character.

LIPID-WATER SOLUBILITY. The lipid-water partition coefficient of a drug (discussed in Chapter

3) is an important consideration in the selection of the suppository base and in anticipating drug release from that base. A lipophilic drug that is distributed in a fatty suppository base in low concentration has less of a tendency to escape to the surrounding aqueous fluids than would a hydrophilic substance present in a fatty base to an extent approaching its saturation. Water-soluble bases—for example, polyethylene glycols—which dissolve in the anorectal fluids, release for absorption both water-soluble and oil-soluble drugs. Naturally, the more drug a base contains, the more drug will be available for potential absorption. However, if the concentration of a drug in the intestinal lumen is above a particular amount, which varies with the drug, the rate of absorption is not changed by a further increase in the concentration of the drug.

PARTICLE SIZE. For drugs present in the suppository in the undissolved state, the size of the particle will influence the amount released and dissolved for absorption. As indicated many times previously, the smaller the particle size, the more readily the dissolution of the particle and the greater the chance for rapid absorption. A recent study has shown that aspirin, prepared in cocoa butter-based suppositories, dissolved in the rectal canal faster, and was absorbed and excreted more readily when present in small particle size than when present in larger particle size.[1]

NATURE OF THE BASE. As indicated earlier, the base must be capable of melting, softening, or dissolving to release its drug components for absorption. If the base interacts with the drug inhibiting its release, drug absorption will be impaired or even prevented. Also, if the base is irritating to the mucous membranes of the rectum, it may initiate a colonic response and prompt a bowel movement, negating the prospect of thorough drug release and absorption.

In a recent study of the bioavailability of aspirin from five brands of commercial suppositories, it was shown that the absorption rates varied widely, and that even with the best product only about 40% of the dose was absorbed when the retention time in the bowel was lim-

[1] Parrott, E. L.: Influence of Particle Size on Rectal Absorption of Aspirin. *Journal of Pharmaceutical Sciences, 64*:878–880, 1975.

ited to 2 hours. Thus, the absorption rates were considered exceedingly low, especially when compared to orally administered aspirin, and of dubious dependability.[1]

Because of the possibility of chemical and/or physical interactions between the medicinal agent and the suppository base, which could affect the stability and/or bioavailability of the drug, the absence of any drug interaction between the two agents should be ascertained prior to formulation or use.

Suppository Bases

Analogous to the ointment bases, suppository bases play an important role in the release of the medication they hold and therefore in the availablility of the drug for absorption for systemic effects or for localized effects. Of course, one of the first requisites for a suppository base is that it remains solid at room temperature but softens, melts, or dissolves readily at body temperature so that the drug it contains may be made fully available soon after insertion. Certain bases are more efficient in drug release than others. For instance, cocoa butter (theobroma oil) melts quickly at body temperature, but since the resulting oil is immiscible with the body fluids, fat-soluble drugs tend to remain in the oil and have little tendency to enter the aqueous physiologic fluids. For water-soluble drugs incorporated into cocoa butter, the reverse is generally true, and good release results. Fat-soluble drugs seem to be released more readily from bases of glycerinated gelatin or polyethylene glycol, both of which dissolve slowly in body fluids. When irritation or inflammation is to be relieved, as in the treatment of anorectal disorders, cocoa butter appears to be the superior base because of its emollient or soothing, spreading action.

Classification of Suppository Bases

For most purposes, it is convenient to classify suppository bases according to their physical characteristics into two main categories and a third miscellaneous group: (1) fatty or oleaginous bases, (2) water-soluble or water-miscible bases, and (3) miscellaneous bases, generally combinations of lipophilic and hydrophilic substances.

FATTY OR OLEAGINOUS BASES. Fatty bases are undoubtedly the most frequently employed suppository bases, principally because cocoa butter is a member of this group of substances. When the base is not specified, cocoa butter is generally employed in the preparation of suppositories. Among the other fatty or oleaginous materials used in suppository bases are many hydrogenated fatty acids of vegetable oils such as palm kernel oil and cottonseed oil. Also, fat-based compounds containing compounds of glycerin with the higher molecular weight fatty acids, such as palmitic and stearic acids, may be found in fatty suppository bases. Such compounds as glyceryl monostearate and glyceryl monopalmitate are examples of this type of agent. The suppository bases in many commercial products employ various and varied combinations of these types of materials to achieve a base possessing the desired hardness under conditions of shipment and storage and the desired quality of submitting to the temperature of the body to release their medicaments. In some instances, suppository bases are prepared with the fatty materials emulsified or with an emulsifying agent present to prompt emulsification when the suppository makes contact with the aqueous body fluids. These types of bases are arbitrarily placed in the third, or "miscellaneous," group of suppository bases.

Cocoa Butter, USP, is defined as the fat obtained from the roasted seed of *Theobroma cacao*. At room temperature it is a yellowish, white solid having a faint, agreeable chocolate-like odor. Chemically, it is a triglyceride (combination of glycerin and one or different fatty acids) primarily of oleopalmitostearin and oleodistearin.[1] Since cocoa butter melts between 30 to 36°, it is an ideal suppository base, melting just below body temperature and yet maintaining its solidity at usual room temperatures. However, because of its triglyceride content, cocoa butter exhibits marked *polymorphism*, or the property of existing in several different crystalline forms. Because of this, when cocoa butter is hastily or carelessly melted at a temperature greatly exceeding the minimum re-

[1]Gibaldi, M. and Grundhofer, B.: Bioavailability of Aspirin from Commercial Suppositories. *Journal of Pharmaceutical Sciences*, 64:1064–1066, 1975.

[1]Oleopalmitostearin has a molecule each of oleic, palmitic, and stearic acids esterified with the glycerin, and oleodistearin has one molecule of oleic acid and two of stearic acid esterified with glycerin.

quired temperature and then quickly chilled, the result is a metastable crystalline form (α crystals) with a melting point much lower than the original cocoa butter. In fact, the melting point may be so low that the cocoa butter will not solidify at room temperature. However, since the crystalline form represents a metastable condition, there is a slow transition to the more stable β form of crystals having the greater stability and the higher melting point. This transition may require several days. Consequently if suppositories that have been prepared by melting cocoa butter for the base do not harden soon after molding, they will be useless to the patient and a loss of time, materials, and prestige to the pharmacist. Cocoa butter must be slowly and evenly melted, preferably over a water bath of warm water, to avoid the formation of the unstable crystalline form and ensure the retention in the liquid of the more stable β crystals that will constitute nuclei upon which the congealing may occur during chilling of the liquid.

It should be mentioned here that such substances as phenol and chloral hydrate have a tendency to lower the melting point of cocoa butter when incorporated with it. If the melting point is lowered to such an extent that it is not feasible to prepare a solid suppository using cocoa butter alone as the base, solidifying agents like spermaceti (about 20%) or beeswax (about 4%) may be melted with the cocoa butter to compensate for the softening effect of the added substance. However, the additions of hardening agents must not be so excessive as to prevent the melting of the base after the suppository has been inserted into the body, nor must the waxy material interfere with the therapeutic agent in any way so as to alter the efficacy of the product.

WATER-SOLUBLE AND WATER-MISCIBLE BASES. The main members of this group are bases of glycerinated gelatin and bases of polyethylene glycols.

The USP gives the following directions for the preparation of glycerinated gelatin suppositories:

Weigh the medicinal substance into a tared container, add purified water to make a total of 10 g, and dissolve or mix, depending upon the solubility of the medicinal substance. Add 70 g of glycerin, and mix. To the mixture add 20 g of granular gelatin, mix carefully to avoid incorporating air, and heat on a steam bath until the gelatin is dissolved. Pour the melted mixture into molds, and allow to congeal.

A glycerinated gelatin base is most frequently used in the preparation of vaginal suppositories, where the prolonged localized action of the medicinal agent is usually desired. The glycerinated gelatin base is slower to soften and mix with the physiologic fluids than is cocoa butter and therefore provides a more prolonged release.

Because glycerinated gelatin-based suppositories have a tendency to absorb moisture due to the hygroscopic nature of glycerin, they must be protected from atmospheric moisture in order for them to maintain their shape and consistency. Due also to the hygroscopicity of the glycerin, the suppository may have a dehydrating effect and be irritating to the tissues upon insertion. The water present in the formula for the suppositories minimizes this action; however, if necessary, the suppositories may be moistened with water prior to their insertion to reduce the initial tendency of the base to draw water from the mucous membranes and irritate the tissues.

Urethral suppositories are also commonly prepared from a glycerinated gelatin base of a formula somewhat different from the one indicated above. For urethral suppositories, the gelatin constitutes about 60% of the weight of the formula, the glycerin about 20%, and the medicated aqueous portion about 20%. Urethral suppositories of glycerinated gelatin are much more easily inserted than suppositories with a cocoa butter base, owing to the brittleness of cocoa butter and its rapid softening at body temperature.

Polyethylene glycols are polymers of ethylene oxide and water, prepared to various chain lengths, molecular weights, and physical states. They are available in a number of molecular weight ranges, the more commonly used being polyethylene glycol 200, 400, 600, 1000, 1500, 1540, 4000, and 6000. The numerical designations refer to the average molecular weights of each of the polymers. Polyethylene glycols having average molecular weights of 200, 400, and 600 are clear, colorless liquids. Those having molecular weights of greater than 1000 are wax-like, white solids with the hardness increasing with an increase in the molecular weight. Various combinations of these polyethylene glycols may be combined by fusion, using two or more of the various types to achieve a suppository base of the desired consistency and characteristics.

Polyethylene glycol suppositories do not melt at body temperature but rather dissolve slowly in the body's fluids. Therefore, the base need not be formulated to melt at body temperature. Thus it is possible, and in fact routine, to prepare suppositories from polyethylene glycol mixtures having melting points considerably higher than that of body temperature. Not only does this property permit a slower release of the medication from the base once the suppository has been inserted, but it also permits the convenient storage of these suppositories without need of refrigeration and without danger of their softening excessively in warm weather. Their solid nature also permits them to be inserted slowly without the fear that they will melt in the fingertips (as cocoa butter suppositories sometimes do). Since they do not melt at body temperature, but mix with mucous secretions upon their dissolution, polyethylene glycol-based suppositories do not "leak" from the orifice as do many cocoa butter-based suppositories. If the polyethylene glycol suppositories do not contain at least 20% of water to avoid the irritation of the mucous membranes after insertion, they should be dipped in water just prior to use. This procedure prevents moisture being drawn from the tissues after insertion and the "stinging" sensation.

MISCELLANEOUS BASES. In the miscellaneous group of bases are included those which are mixtures of the oleaginous and water-soluble or water-miscible materials. These materials may be chemical or physical mixtures. Some are preformed emulsions, generally of the w/o type, or they may be capable of dispersing in aqueous fluids. One of these substances is polyoxyl 40 stearate, a surface-active agent that is employed in a number of commercial suppository bases. Polyoxyl 40 stearate is a mixture of the monostearate and distearate esters of mixed polyoxyethylene diols and the free glycols, the average polymer length being equivalent to about 40 oxyethylene units. The substance is a waxy, white to light tan solid that is water-soluble. Its melting point is generally between 39° and 45°. Other surface active agents useful in the preparation of suppository bases also fall into this broad grouping. Mixtures of many fatty bases (including cocoa butter) with emulsifying agents capable of forming w/o emulsions have been prepared. These bases have the ability to hold water or aqueous solutions and are sometimes referred to as "hydrophilic" suppository bases.

Suppositories employing a soap as a base are also included in this miscellaneous category. Glycerin Suppositories, USP, which have sodium stearate, a soap, as the base are included here.

Preparation of Suppositories

Suppositories are prepared by three methods: (1) *molding* from a melt, (2) *compression*, and (3) *hand rolling* and *shaping*. The method most frequently employed in the preparation of suppositories both on a small scale and on an industrial scale is molding.

Preparation by Molding

Basically, the steps in molding include (a) the melting of the base, (b) incorporating of any required medicaments, (c) pouring the melt into molds, (d) allowing the melt to cool and congeal into suppositories, and (e) removing the formed suppositories from the mold. Suppositories of cocoa butter, glycerinated gelatin, polyethylene glycol, and most other suppository bases are suitable for preparation by molding.

SUPPOSITORY MOLDS. Suppository molds are commercially available with the capability of producing individual or large numbers of suppositories of various shapes and sizes. Individual plastic suppository molds may be obtained to form a single suppository. Other molds, as those most commonly found in the community pharmacy, are capable of producing 6 or 12 suppositories in a single operation. Industrial molds produce hundreds of suppositories from a single molding.

Molds in common use today are made from stainless steel, aluminum, brass, or plastic. The molds, which separate into sections, generally longitudinally, are opened for cleaning before and after the preparation of a batch of suppositories, closed when the melt is poured, and opened again to remove the cold, molded suppositories. Care must be exercised in cleaning the molds, as any scratches on the molding sur-

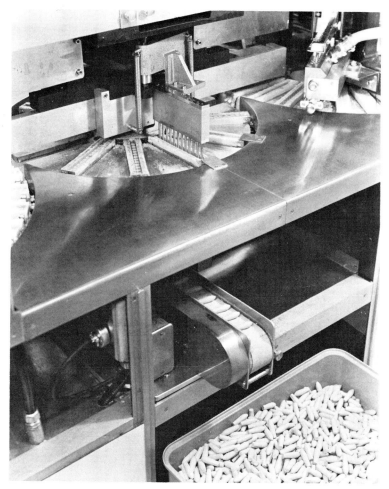

Fig. 13-1. *Highly automated large-scale production of molded suppositories. Molding operation (at the right) is followed by the removal of the suppositories from the molds, dropping them onto a conveyor belt and into a collection basket. (Courtesy of Wyeth Laboratories)*

faces will take away from the desired smoothness of the resulting suppositories. Plastic molds are especially prone to scratching.

Although satisfactory molds are commercially available for the preparation of suitable rectal, vaginal, and urethral suppositories, if necessary in the extemporaneous preparation of suppositories, temporary molds may be successfully formed by pressing heavy aluminum foil about an object having the shape of the desired suppository, then carefully removing the object, and filling the shaped foil with the melt. For instance, glass stirring rods, may be used to form molds for urethral suppositories, rounded eraser ends of cylindrical (not hexagonal) pencils or the ends of pens (even the writing end of many ball-point pens is suitable) may be used to

form molds for rectal suppositories, and any cone-shaped object may be used to form vaginal suppositories.

LUBRICATION OF THE MOLD. Depending upon the formulation, suppository molds may require lubrication before the melt is poured to facilitate the clean and easy removal of the molded suppositories. Lubrication is seldom necessary when the suppository base is cocoa butter or polyethylene glycol, as these materials contract sufficiently on cooling within the mold to separate from the inner surfaces and allow their easy removal. Lubrication is usually necessary when glycerinated gelatin suppositories are prepared. A thin coating of mineral oil or expressed almond oil applied with the finger to the mold-

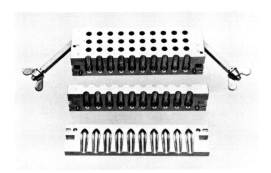

Fig. 13-2. *Partially opened suppository mold capable of producing 50 torpedo-shaped suppositories in a single molding. (Courtesy of Chemical and Pharmaceutical Industry Co., Inc.)*

ing surfaces usually suffices to provide the necessary lubrication. It should be stressed, however, that any materials which might cause irritation to the mucous membranes should not be employed as a mold lubricant.

CALIBRATION OF THE MOLD. Each individual mold is capable of holding a specific volume of material in each of its openings. If the material is cocoa butter, the weight of the resulting suppositories will differ from the weight of suppositories prepared in the same mold with a mixture of polyethylene glycols as the base because of the difference in the densities of the materials. Similarly, any added medicinal agent would further alter the densities of the bases, and the weights of the resulting suppositories would be different from those prepared with base material alone.

It is important that the pharmacist calibrate each of his suppository molds for the suppository bases that he generally employs (usually cocoa butter and a polyethylene glycol base) in order that he may prepare medicated suppositories each having the proper quantity of medicaments.

The first step in the calibration of a mold is to prepare molded suppositories from base material alone. After removal from the mold, the suppositories are weighed, and the total weight and the average weight of each suppository are recorded (for the particular base used). To determine the volume of the mold, the suppositories are then carefully melted in a calibrated beaker, and the volume of the melt is determined for the total number as well as for the average of one suppository.

DETERMINATION OF THE AMOUNT OF BASE REQUIRED. In his prescriptions for medicated suppositories to be prepared extemporaneously by the pharmacist, the prescribing physician generally indicates the amount of a medicinal substance that he desires in each suppository, but he leaves the amount of base to the discretion of the pharmacist. Generally, in filling such prescriptions, the pharmacist calculates the amounts of materials needed for the preparation of one or two more suppositories than the number prescribed to compensate for the inevitable loss of some material and to ensure having enough material to prepare the last required suppository.

In determining the amount of base to be incorporated with the medicaments, the pharmacist must be certain that the required amount of drug is provided in each suppository. Since the volume of the mold is known (from the determined volume of the melted suppositories formed from the base), the volume of the drug substances subtracted from the total volume of the mold will give the volume of base required. In instances in which the added amounts of medicaments are slight, they may be considered to be negligible, and no deduction from the total volume of base may be deemed necessary. However, if considerable quantities of substances are to be incorporated into the suppository, the volumes of these materials are important and should be used to calculate the amount of base actually required to fill the mold completely. The total volumes of these materials are subtracted from the volume of the mold, and the appropriate amount of base is added. Since the suppository bases are solids at room temperature, the volume of base determined may be converted to weight from the density of the material. For example, if 12 ml of cocoa butter are required to fill a suppository mold and if the medicaments in the formula have a collective volume of 2.8 ml, then 9.2 ml of the cocoa butter will be required. By multiplying 9.2 ml times the density of cocoa butter, 0.86 g/ml, it may be calculated that 7.9 g of cocoa butter will be required. After adjusting for the preparation of an extra suppository or two, the calculated amount is weighed.

Another method for the determination of the amount of base in the preparation of medicated suppositories requires the following steps: (a) weigh the active ingredient for the preparation of a single suppository; (b) dissolve it or mix it (depending upon its solubility in the base) with a portion of melted base insufficient to fill one cavity of the mold, and add the mixture to a cavity; (c) add additional melted base to the cavity to completely fill it; (d) allow the suppository to congeal and harden; and (e) remove the suppository from the mold and weigh it. The weight of the active ingredients present, subtracted from the weight of the suppository yields the weight of the amount of base used. This amount of base multiplied by the number of suppositories to be prepared in the mold is the total amount of base required.

A third method involves the placing of all of the required medicaments for the preparation of the total number of suppositories (including one extra) in a calibrated beaker. To this is added a portion of the melted base and the drug substances incorporated. Then sufficient additional melted base is added until the volume of mixture is reached that is required for the preparation of the necessary suppositories, based on the original calibration of the volume of the mold.

PREPARING AND POURING THE MELT. Using the least possible heat, the weighed suppository base material is melted, generally over a water bath, since a great deal of heat is not usually required. A porcelain casserole, which is a dish having a pouring lip and a handle, is perhaps the best utensil to use, since it later permits the convenient pouring of the melt into the cavities of the mold. Medicinal substances are usually incorporated into a portion of the melted base by mixing on a glass or porcelain tile with a spatula. After incorporation, this material is added with stirring to the remaining base which has been allowed to cool almost to its congealing point. Any volatile materials or heat labile substances should be incorporated at this point with thorough stirring.

It is generally best to chill the mold in the refrigerator before pouring the melt. Then, the melt is added carefully and continuously in the filling of each cavity in the mold. If any undissolved materials in the mixture are of greater density than the base so that they have a tendency to settle, constant stirring, even during pouring, is required, else the last filled cavity will contain a disproportionate share of the undissolved materials. The solid materials remain suspended if the pouring is performed just above the congealing point and not when the base is too fluid. The chilled mold encourages prompt congealing and discourages any settling

of the materials within the mold's cavities. If the melt is not near the congealing point when poured, the solids may settle within each cavity of the mold to reside at the tips of the suppositories, with the result that the suppositories may be broken when removed from the mold. In filling each suppository cavity, the pouring must be continuous to prevent *layering*, which may lead to a product easily broken on handling. To ensure a completely filled mold upon congealing, the melt is poured excessively over each opening, actually rising above the level of the mold. The excessive material may actually form a continuous ribbon along the top of the mold above the cavities. This use of extra suppository material prevents the formation of recessed dips in the ends of the suppositories and justifies the preparation of extra suppository melt. When solidified, the excess material is evenly scraped off of the top of the mold with a spatula. The mold is usually placed in the freezer section of the refrigerator to hasten the hardening of the suppositories.

When the suppositories are hard, the mold is removed from the freezer, and slight pressure is exerted with the thumb on the ends of each suppository to loosen it in the mold. Then the sections of the mold are separated, and the suppositories are dislodged with the pressure being exerted principally on their ends and only if needed on the tips. Generally, little, if any, pressure is required, and the suppositories simply fall out of the mold when it is opened.

Preparation by Compression

Suppositories may be prepared by forcing the mixed mass of the suppository base and the medicaments into special molds using suppository-making machines. In preparation for compression into the molds, the suppository base and the other formulative ingredients are combined by thorough mixing, the friction of the process causing the base to soften into a paste-like consistency. On a small scale, a mortar and pestle may be used. If the mortar is heated in warm water before use and then dried, the softening of the base and the mixing process is greatly facilitated. On a large scale, a similar process may be used, employing mechanically operated kneading mixers and a warmed mixing vessel.

The process of compression is especially suited for the making of suppositories containing medicinal substances that are heat labile

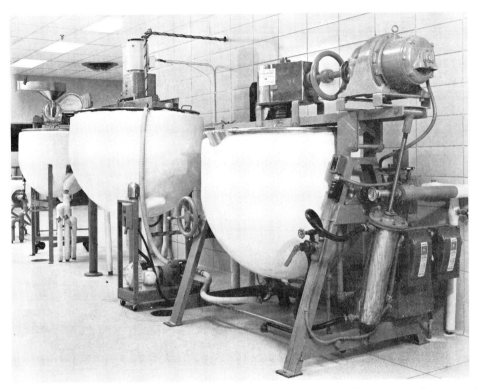

Fig. 13-3. *Large heated tanks for the preparation of the melt in the commercial production of suppositories by molding.* (*Courtesy of Wyeth Laboratories*)

and for suppositories containing a great deal of substances insoluble in the base. In contrast to the molding method, there is no likelihood of insoluble matter settling during the preparation of suppositories by compression. The disadvantage to the process is that the special suppository machine is required and there is some limitation as to shapes of suppositories that can be made from the available molds.

In preparing suppositories with the compression machine, the suppository mass is placed into a cylinder which is then closed, and pressure is applied from one end, mechanically, or by turning a wheel, and the mass is forced out of the other end into the suppository mold or die. When the die is filled with the mass, a movable end plate at the back of the die is removed and when additional pressure is applied to the mass in the cylinder, the formed suppositories are ejected. The end plate is returned, and the process is repeated until all of the suppository mass has been used. Various sizes and shapes of dies are available. It is possible to prepare suppositories of uniform circumference by extrusion through a perforated plate and cutting the extruded mass to the desired length.

Preparation by Hand Rolling and Shaping

With the ready availability of suppository molds of accommodating shapes and sizes, there seems little requirement for today's pharmacist to shape suppositories by hand. However, since hand rolling and shaping is a historic part of the art of the pharmacist and the possibility exists that he may be called upon, for instance, to adjust the size of a commercially prepared adult rectal suppository to the size and weight appropriate for a child, it seems within the realm of both historic importance and practicality that the method at least be briefly outlined.

Although the process requires no special equipment, it does demand patience and a certain degree of manual dexterity. Generally, hand-prepared suppositories are limited to those utilizing cocoa butter as the base. A plastic-like mass is formed from the base of grated cocoa butter and the other formulative ingredients by severe trituration in a mortar. During the process of mixing, a spatula is employed to scrape the material from the pestle and the upper part of the mortar to the working surface of the mortar. Once the mass has been prepared, it is quickly formed into a ball in the palms of the hands, which have been previously cooled in ice water, and a broad-bladed spatula or a flat board is used to roll it into a cylinder on a pill tile. The diameter of the cylinder must be that of the thickest part of the suppository to be shaped. When the rolling process has been completed, the cylinder is cut with a spatula or razor blade into the appropriate number of sections, each one representing a suppository. Then, each piece is shaped with the fingertips, sometimes with a glassine powder paper between the fingers and the suppository to prevent excessive warmth against the suppository and undue softening. One end or both ends of the suppositories may be shaped as desired. In the preparation of vaginal suppositories, the diameter of the original cylinder would generally be greater than when rectal suppositories are prepared. As mentioned earlier, urethral suppositories made from a cocoa butter base are generally inadequate due to the insertion problem caused by the brittleness of the cocoa butter. However, if prepared, sections the size of rectal suppositories are generally first cut, and these individual sections of mass are further rolled to the rod shape of a urethral suppository.

Many pharmacists find that they must periodically soak their hands in ice water during the hand shaping of suppositories to prevent the excessive melting of the base. Rather than hand shaping, some pharmacists prefer to force the sections of the cut cylinder into the cavities of a suppository mold, emulating the compression method for the preparation of suppositories. This method might be preferred over molding with a melt by pharmacists having a suppository mold because of the heat instability of the medicament or the large percentage of insoluble solids in the formula. When compressing a mass in a suppository mold, it is usually necessary to lubricate the mold with a dusting powder such as starch to prevent sticking. Homemade plungers may be used to force or pack the mass into the cavities of the mold.

Packaging and Storage

Glycerin suppositories and glycerinated gelatin suppositories are generally packaged in tightly closed glass containers to prevent a moisture change in the content of the suppositories. Suppositories prepared from a cocoa butter base are usually individually wrapped or otherwise separated in compartmentalized boxes to prevent contact and adhesion. Suppositories containing light-sensitive drugs are generally individually wrapped in an opaque material such as a metallic foil. In fact, most commercially available suppositories are individually wrapped in either foil or a plastic material. Some are packaged in a continuous strip with suppositories being separated by tearing along perforations placed between suppositories. Suppositories are also commonly packaged in slide boxes or in plastic boxes.

Since suppositories are adversely affected by heat, it is necessary to maintain them in a cool place. Suppositories having cocoa butter as the base must be stored below 30°, preferably in a refrigerator. Glycerinated gelatin suppositories are best stored at temperatures below 35°. Suppositories made from a base of polyethylene glycol may be stored at usual room temperatures without the requirement of refrigeration.

Suppositories stored in environments of high humidity may absorb moisture and tend to become spongy, whereas suppositories stored in places of extreme dryness may lose moisture and become brittle.

Official Rectal Suppositories

The official rectal suppositories are presented in Table 13-1. As noted earlier, drugs as aspirin, and oxymorphone HCl, given for pain, ergotamine tartrate for treating migraine headaches, theophylline as a smooth muscle relaxant in

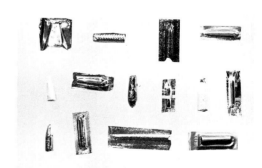

Fig. 13-4. *Some commercially available suppositories wrapped in paper, foil, and plastic.*

Table 13-1. OFFICIAL RECTAL SUPPOSITORIES

Suppository	Corresponding Commercial Product	Active Constituent per Suppository	Type of Effect	Category and Comments
Aminophylline Suppositories, USP	various	125, 250 and 500 mg	Systemic	Smooth muscle relaxant, bronchodilator; useful in treating asthmatics
Aspirin Suppositories, USP	various	65, 130, 162, 195, 325, 650, and 975 mg, and 1.3 g	Systemic	Analgesic and antipyretic. See text for additional discussion.
Bisacodyl Suppositories, USP	Dulcolax Suppositories (Boehringer-Ingelheim)	10 mg	Local	Cathartic. See text for additional discussion.
Chlorpromazine Suppositories, USP	Thorazine Suppositories (Smith Kline & French)	25 and 100 mg	Systemic	Anti-emetic; tranquilizer.
Cyclomethycaine Sulfate Suppositories, NF	Surfacaine Suppositories (Lilly)	10 mg	Local	Local anesthetic. See text for additional discussion.
Dibucaine Suppositories, NF	Nupercainal Suppositories (Madison)	2.5 mg	Local	Local anesthetic. See text for additional discussion.
Ergotamine Tartrate and Caffeine Suppositories, NF	Cafergot Suppositories (Sandoz)	2 mg ergotamine tartrate and 100 mg caffeine	Systemic	Antiadrenergic; central
Glycerin Suppositories, USP	various	about 1.8 g	Local	Cathartic
Oxymorphone HCl Suppositories, NF	Numorphan Suppositories (Endo)	10 mg	Systemic	Narcotic analgesic
Prochlorperazine Suppositories, USP	Compazine Suppositories (Smith Kline & French)	2.5, 5, and 25 mg	Systemic	Anti-emetic
Theophylline Olamine Suppositories, NF	Monotheamin Suppositories (Lilly)	500 mg	Systemic	Smooth muscle relaxant.

treating asthma, and chlorpromazine and prochlorperazine, which act as antiemetics and tranquilizers are intended to be absorbed into the general circulation to provide systemic drug effects. The rectal route of administration is especially useful in instances in which the patient is unwilling or unable to take medication orally.

Several of the official rectal suppositories are intended to provide local action within the perianal area. These include the local anesthetic agents cyclomethycaine sulfate and dibucaine, and the cathartics bisacodyl and glycerin. Local anesthetic suppositories are commonly employed to relieve *pruritus ani* of various causes, and the pain sometimes associated with hemorrhoids. Many of the commercial hemorrhoidal suppositories contain a number of medicinal agents including astringents, protectives, anesthetics, lubricants, and others, intended to relieve the discomfort of the condition. Cathartic suppositories are contact-type agents which act directly on the colonic mucosa to produce normal peristalsis. Since the contact action is restricted to the colon, the motility of the small intestine is not appreciably affected. Cathartic suppositories are more rapid-acting than orally administered medication. Suppositories of bisacodyl are usually effective in 15 minutes to an hour, and glycerin suppositories usually within a few minutes following insertion.

Some commercially prepared suppositories are available for both adult and pediatric use. The difference is in the shape and drug content.

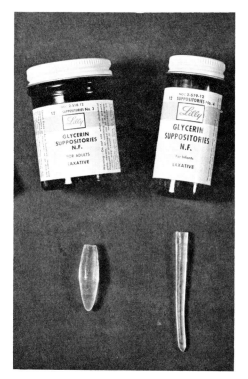

Fig. 13-5. *Glycerin suppositories intended for adult and pediatric patients (Courtesy of Eli Lilly and Company).*

Pediatric suppositories are more narrow and pencil-shaped than the typical bullet-shaped adult suppository. Glycerin suppositories are commonly available in each type. In terms of varying drug content, a good example is aspirin

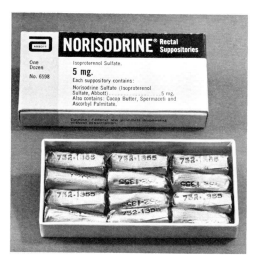

Fig. 13-6. *Example of commercial packaging of rectal suppositories. (Courtesy of Abbott Laboratories)*

suppositories which are commercially available containing 65, 130, 162, 195, 325, 650, and 975 mg, and 1.3 g each of aspirin.

Upon dispensing suppositories the pharmacist should instruct the patient as to the proper method and frequency of insertion for the most efficacious effects. Most suppositories are dispensed in paper, foil, or plastic wrappings, and the patient must be instructed to remove the wrapping thoroughly before insertion.

The only official medicated suppository for which a formula is given in the USP or NF is Glycerin Suppositories, USP. The formula is as follows:

Glycerin	91 g
Sodium Stearate	9 g
Purified Water	5 g
To make about	100 g

In the preparation of this suppository, the glycerin is heated in a suitable container to about 120°. Then the sodium stearate is dissolved with stirring in the hot glycerin, the purified water added and the mixture immediately poured into the suppository mold. It is recommended that if the mold is of metal, that it also be heated prior to the addition of the glycerin mixture. After cooling to solidification, the suppositories are removed. From the above formula, about fifty adult suppositories may be prepared.

Glycerin, a hygroscopic material, contributes to the laxative effect of the suppository by drawing water from the intestine and also from its irritant action on the mucous lining. The sodium stearate, a soap, is the solidifying agent in the suppository and may also contribute to the laxative action. Because of the hygroscopic nature of glycerin, the suppositories attract moisture and should be maintained in tight containers, preferably at temperatures below 25°.

Official Vaginal Suppositories

The official vaginal suppositories are presented in Table 13-2. These preparations as well as the various commercial products are employed principally for two purposes: (1) to combat infections occurring in the female genitourinary area, and (2) to restore the vaginal mucosa to its normal state. In combating vaginal infections, the usual pathogenic organisms involved

Table 13-2. OFFICIAL VAGINAL SUPPOSITORIES

Suppository	Corresponding Commercial Product	Active Constituent per Suppository	Category and Comments
Candidicin Suppositories, NF	Candeptin Vagelettes (Schmid)	3 mg	Antifungal; commercial product contains drug dispersed in petrolatum and prepared into vaginal capsules; used in treatment of *Candida albicans* and other *Candida* infections.
Diethylstilbestrol Suppositories, USP	various	0.1, 0.5 and 1 mg	Estrogen; indicated for the treatment of postmenopausal and senile vulvovaginitis, atrophic vaginitis, and pruritus vulvae.
Iodochlorhydroxyquin Suppositories, NF	Vioform Inserts (Ciba)	250 mg	Anti-infective used in the treatment of Trichomonas vaginalis vaginitis. Commercial product is actually a tableted insert rather than a suppository.
Metronidazole Suppositories, USP	Flagyl Vaginal Inserts (Searle)	500 mg	Antitrichomonal; possesses trichomonacidal activity; commercial product is a tableted insert.

are *Trichomonas vaginalis, Candida (Monilia) albicans* or other species, and *Hemophilus vaginalis*. Among the anti-infective agents found in commercial vaginal preparations are: candidicin and nifuroxime (antifungals), 9-aminoacridine, nitrofurazone, and sulfanilamide (antibacterials), and furazolidone and metronidazole (antitrichomonals). Estrogenic substances as estrone, dienestrol, and diethylstilbestrol are found in vaginal preparations to restore the vaginal mucosa to its normal state.

In the preparation of vaginal suppositories, the most commonly used base consists of combinations of the various molecular weight polyethylene glycols. To this base is frequently added surfactants and preservative agents, commonly the parabens. Many of the vaginal suppositories and other types of vaginal dosage forms are buffered to an acid pH, usually around pH 4.5 which resembles that of the normal vagina. This acidity discourages pathogenic organisms and at the same time provides a favorable environment for eventual recolonization by the acid-producing bacilli normally found in the vagina.

The polyethylene glycol-based vaginal suppositories are water-miscible and are generally sufficiently firm for the patient to handle and insert without great difficulty. However, to make the task even easier, many manufacturers provide plastic insertion devices with their products which are used to hold the suppository or vaginal tablet during insertion for proper placement within the vagina (Fig. 13-7).

Urethral Suppositories

At the present time there are no official urethral suppositories; in fact, few are in use today.

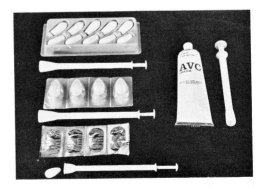

Fig. 13-7. *Dosage forms used intravaginally, including suppositories (top and middle), vaginal tablets packaged in foil (bottom), vaginal cream, and corresponding insert devices.*

One commercial urethral insert [Furacin Urethral Inserts (Eaton)] contains nitrofurazone, an anti-infective agent, and diperodon HCl, a local anesthetic, in a water dispersible base of glyceryl monolaurate and polyoxyethylene (4) sorbitan monostearate. The product is recommended for urethritis and for topical anesthesia and prophylaxis of infection preceding and following urethral instrumentation examination. The insert is usually held in place for 10 minutes following insertion in the male patient to permit melting and the coating of the entire urethra. It is sometimes necessary in warm weather to hold the wrapped insert under cold water prior to its use to prevent softening and to enable insertion. These suppositories which may be utilized in both male and female patients are about 50 mm in length and weigh about 1.3 g.

Other Dosage Forms Used Rectally, Vaginally, and Urethrally

Tablets and Capsules

Vaginal tablets are more widely used nowadays than are vaginal suppositories. The tablets are easier to manufacture, they are more stable, and less messy to handle in use. Vaginal tablets, frequently referred to as *vaginal inserts*, are usually ovoid in shape and are accompanied in their packaging with a plastic inserter, a device for easy placement of the tablet within the vagina. Vaginal tablets contain the same types of anti-infective and hormonal substances as the vaginal suppositories. They are prepared by tablet compression, and are commonly formulated to contain lactose as the base or filler, a disintegrating agent, as starch, a dispersing agent, as polyvinylpyrrolidine, and a tablet lubricant, as magnesium stearate. The tablets are intended to disintegrate within the vagina releasing their medication.

Some vaginal inserts are capsules of gelatin containing medication to be released intravaginally. Capsules may also be used rectally, especially in pediatrics to administer medication to children unwilling or unable to tolerate the drug orally. Their insertion into the rectum is facilitated by first lightly wetting the capsule with water. Drugs are absorbed from the rectum, but frequently at unpredictable rates and in varying amounts as has been previously noted in this chapter. Drugs which do not dissolve rapidly and which are irritating to mucous membranes should not be placed in direct contact with such membranes.

Ointments, Creams, and Aerosol Foams

Rectal and vaginal ointments and vaginal creams are in common use. Rectal ointments are used primarily to allay local conditions as pruritus ani and to relieve the pain and discomfort associated with hemorrhoids. The drugs present are generally the same as previously discussed for rectal suppositories, including local anesthetics, analgesics, protectives, and anti-inflammatory agents. To facilitate the insertion of ointment into the rectum, each rectal ointment tube is accompanied with a special rectal insertion and delivery tip. This tip replaces the ordinary ointment cap prior to use (Fig. 13-8). After placement of the rectal tip on the ointment tube, the tip is slowly and carefully inserted into the anus. The ointment tube is depressed to release the medication through the rectal tip and into the anal canal. After use, the tip should be removed from the ointment tube and replaced with the original cap. The rectal tip should be thoroughly cleaned following each use.

Vaginal ointments and creams are typically

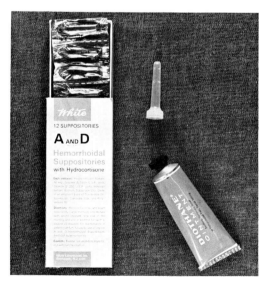

Fig. 13-8. *Typical commercial packaging of rectal suppositories and rectal ointment with rectal applicator tip.*

available containing anti-infective agents, estrogenic hormonal substances, and contraceptive agents. The anti-infective and hormonal substances used are the same as have previously been discussed for vaginal suppositories. The contraceptive creams contain spermacidal agents as nonylphenoxy polyethylene ethanol and octoxynol and are used alone or in combination with a cervical diaphragm to prevent conception. When used with a diaphragm, the cream is placed on the diaphragm surface in contact with the cervix and around the edges of the diaphragm. When used alone, the cream is first squeezed into the special inserter-applicator tube provided. This applicator is then inserted well into the vagina, the plunger of the applicator depressed and the cream deposited. The contraceptive creams are utilized just prior to intercourse.

Aerosol foams are commercially available containing estrogenic substances and contraceptive agents. The foams are used intravaginally in the same manner as that employed for creams. The aerosol package contains an inserter device which is filled with foam and the contents placed in the vagina through activation of the plunger. The foams are generally oil-in-water emulsions, resembling light creams. They are water-miscible and non-greasy.

There are some commercial preparations of rectal foams available which utilize rectal inserters for the presentation of the foam to the anal canal. One such product, Proctofoam-HC (Reed & Carnrick), contains hydrocortisone acetate and promoxine hydrochloride and is used in relieving inflammatory anorectal disorders.

Jellies and Gels

Jellies are a class of gels in which the structural coherent matrix contains a high proportion of liquid, usually water. Pharmaceutical jellies are usually formed by adding a thickening agent as tragacanth or carboxymethyl cellulose to an aqueous solution of a drug substance. The resultant product is usually clear and of a uniform semisolid consistency.

There are three official jellies, Lidocaine Hydrochloride Jelly, USP, Cyclomethycaine Sulfate Jelly, NF and Pramoxine Hydrochloride Jelly, NF. Each is a topical local anesthetic. Jellies of lidocaine hydrochloride and cyclomethycaine sulfate are usually used in the prevention and control of pain in examination procedures in-

volving male and female urethra, and in the topical treatment of painful urethritis. Pramoxine hydrochloride jelly finds its greatest application in allaying rectal pain and for topical application to itching and irritated skin.

There are a number of commercially available contraceptive jellies and gels containing the same types of spermatocidal agents and used intravaginally in the same manner as previously discussed for contraceptive creams. Also, a number of antiseptic and nonmedicated lubricant jellies are available, primarily for use by physicians in their rectal and vaginal examination procedures.

Jellies are subject to bacterial contamination and growth and thus most are preserved with antimicrobial preservatives. The tubes of jellies should be tightly closed when not in use, as they have a tendency to lose water to the air and dry out.

Powders

Powders are used to prepare solutions for vaginal *douche*, that is, for the irrigative cleansing of the vagina. The powders themselves may be prepared and packaged in bulk or as unit packages. A unit package is designed to contain the appropriate amount of powder to prepare the specified volume of douche solution. The bulk powders are utilized by the teaspoonful or tablespoonful amounts in the preparation of the desired solution. The user simply adds the prescribed amount of powder to the appropriate volume of warm water and stirs until dissolved. Among the components of douche powders are the following:

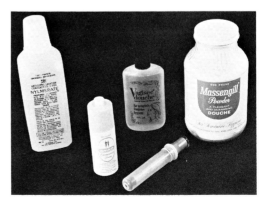

Fig. 13-9. *Products for vaginal use, including solution concentrates, powder, and aerosol foam with insert device.*

a. Boric acid or sodium borate.
b. Astringents, as potassium alum, ammonium alum, zinc sulfate.
c. Antimicrobials, as oxyquinoline sulfate, povidone-iodine.
d. Quaternary ammonium compounds, as benzethonium chloride.
e. Detergents, as sodium lauryl sulfate.
f. Oxidizing agents, as sodium perborate.
g. Salts, as sodium citrate, sodium chloride.
h. Aromatics, as menthol, thymol, eucalyptol, methyl salicylate, phenol.

Douche powders are generally employed for their hygienic effects. A few douche powders, containing specific therapeutic anti-infective agents as those mentioned previously in the discussion of vaginal suppositories, are employed against Monilial and Trichomonal infections.

Solutions

Vaginal douche solutions may be prepared from powders as indicated above or from liquid solutions or liquid concentrates. In using liquid concentrates, the patient is instructed to add the prescribed amount of concentrate (usually a teaspoonful or bottle-capful) with a certain amount of warm water (frequently a quart). The resultant solution then contains the appropriate amount of chemical agents in proper strength. The agents present are similar to the ones described above for douche powders.

Rectal enemas are employed to cleanse the bowel. Commercially, many enemas are available in disposable plastic squeeze bottles containing a premeasured amount of enema solution. The agents present are solutions of sodium phosphate and sodium biphosphate, glycerin and dioctyl potassium sulfosuccinate, and light mineral oil.

As mentioned previously in Chapter 8, there are a number of sterile irrigation solutions that are employed in urological procedures and treatment.

Suspensions

Barium Sulfate for Suspension, USP, previously discussed in Chapter 5, may be employed orally or rectally for the diagnostic visualization of the gastrointestinal tract.

Selected Reading

Anschel, J., and Lieberman, H. A.: Suppositories: Part I. Bases, *Drug Cosmetic Ind.*, 97:341, 1965; Part II. Formulation Problems, *ibid.*, 97:507, 1965.

Gibaldi, M. and Grundhofer, B.: Bioavailability of Aspirin from Commercial Suppositories. *Journal of Pharmaceutical Sciences*, 64:1064–1066, 1975.

Lowenthal, W., and Borzelleca, J. F.: Drug Absorption from the Rectum I. Suppository Bases: A Preliminary Report. *J. Pharm. Sci.*, 54:1790–1794, 1965.

Parrott, E. L.: Influence of Particle Size on Rectal Absorption of Aspirin. *Journal of Pharmaceutical Sciences*, 64:878–880, 1975.

Chapter 14

Miscellaneous Preparations: Aromatic Waters, Diluted Acids, Spirits, and Radiopharmaceuticals

Aromatic Waters

AROMATIC WATERS may be defined as clear, aqueous solutions saturated (unless otherwise specified) with volatile oils or other aromatic or volatile substances. The currently official aromatic waters contain the volatile substances of orange flower oil, peppermint oil, and rose oil. In previous compendia, aromatic waters of other oils such as anise oil, spearmint oil, and wintergreen oil and of pure chemicals such as camphor and chloroform were also official. Naturally, the odors and tastes of aromatic waters are of the volatile substances from which they are prepared. Aromatic waters having foreign or empyreumatic (smokelike) odors, which result from contamination or product deterioration, must be discarded.

Most of the aromatic substances in the prep-aration of aromatic waters have very low solubilities in water, and even though a water may be saturated, its concentration of aromatic material is still rather small. Aromatic waters are used for perfuming, and to a lesser extent, flavoring other pharmaceutical preparations. Water-soluble drugs intended for oral administration may be dissolved in an appropriate aromatic water, as that of peppermint water, with the taste of the drug being masked by the pleasant-tasting vehicle. Aromatic waters as rose water that are not generally taken internally are intended to serve as perfuming agents in various external pharmaceutical preparations. Certain aromatic waters have found widespread use in a specific manner. For instance, camphor water is frequently the vehicle in ophthalmic solutions, owing to its ability to contribute a refreshing, stimulating effect to the preparation. Hamamelis water, known popularly as witch hazel, is commonly employed as a rub and as a perfume and astringent in various cosmetic preparations, particularly in aftershave lotions.

Preparation of Aromatic Waters

Aromatic waters may be prepared by any of the three general methods outlined in the *United States Pharmacopeia*. They are (a) distillation method, (b) solution method, and (c) alternative solution method.

Distillation Method

The distillation method involves the placing of the contused or coarsely ground odoriferous portion of the plant or drug from which the aromatic water is to be prepared in a suitable still with sufficient purified water. Most of the volume of water is then distilled, carefully avoiding the development of empyreumatic odors through the scorching or charring of the plant or drug materials. The excess oils collected with the distillate generally rise to the top of the aqueous product and are removed. The remaining aqueous solution, saturated with volatile material, frequently requires clarification by filtration.

Because it involves special apparatus and is time-consuming, the distillation process is not generally employed in instances when a product of equal merit may be prepared by the simpler solution method. However, there are instances when the distillation method must be used due to the unavailability or the high cost of suitable volatile oils from certain plant materials. Certain aromatic waters such as those of rose petals, orange flowers, and hamamelis leaves and twigs are prepared by the more complex method of distillation. Whenever it is thought that the distillate obtained is not a saturated solution of the volatile principles of a plant or drug substance, the process of distillation may be repeated, returning the first distillate to a fresh portion of plant or drug and the distillation process repeated. This procedure may be repeated several times in the preparation of a saturated aromatic water. Such multiple distillations are frequently indicated on the labels of commercially prepared products, especially with witch hazel, by the usage of one X for each distillation. Therefore a package bearing four X's, for instance, indicates that the preparation was subjected to four separate distillations and is an attestation of the quality of the product. The process of redistillation is frequently referred to as *cohobation*.

Of the presently official waters, Orange Flower Water, NF and Stronger Rose Water, NF are prepared by distillation. Peppermint Water, NF may be prepared by either of the official methods.

Solution Method

The aromatic constituents of most plants can be separated from the plant part in which they are contained by steam distillation. These aromatic constituents are generally separated as a volatile oil (also called essential oils), which is a complex blend of organic substances that are extremely difficult to isolate and identify. Thus, the exact composition of most volatile oils is largely undetermined except for a few of their major and assayable components. The composition of a volatile oil from a single plant species may vary, depending upon such factors as the plant's habitat, the various environmental conditions it encountered during its growth, the age of the plant, the season of year at harvest, the storage conditions of the harvested plant. Since the precise chemical composition of a volatile oil cannot be unerringly predicted, neither can it be made an unyielding requirement of the official compendia, nor can its exact solubility

be unequivocably stated.[1] For this reason, aromatic waters prepared by solution generally utilize a large excess of solute to insure the water's saturation, and the pharmacist does not depend upon solubility information of the oil to calculate the required amount to prepare a saturated solution. The general formula to permit such an excess of aromatic substance is presented in the USP as:

The volatile oil, or other specified
    volatile substance........................2 ml or 2 g
Purified water,
    a sufficient quantity, to make..............1000 ml

By this formula, an aromatic water is prepared by intermittently shaking 2 ml (if a liquid) or 2 g (if a solid) of the volatile substance with 1000 ml of purified water in a suitable container for a period of 15 minutes. If the aromatic substance is a solid, it is comminuted prior to the addition of the water in order that a large surface area of material be made available for more rapid dissolution. If the aromatic substance is a liquid, the repeated agitation causes minute oil droplets to separate from the larger oil droplets, thereby exposing an increased surface area to the water for the dissolution process. After the period of agitation, the mixture is set aside for a period of 12 hours or longer to permit the excess oil droplets to coalesce into large globules of oil, and the solid substance (if used) to settle. During this period of standing, the aromatic substances continue to dissolve and are afforded ample opportunity to saturate the solution. Without further agitation, the mixture is passed through a wetted filter paper, and as the USP directs, purified water is passed through the filter, if needed, to bring the volume of the filtrate up to the prescribed amount (1000 ml in the above formula). Since the volume of water required to bring the product up to the desired volume is generally quite small and since the addition of water may render the solution unsaturated, the final dilution step is

---

[1] Although the exact composition and solubility of volatile oils cannot be unerringly stated in advance, the official compendia have established requirements that generally state the minimum permitted amounts of some known and easily determined main components. For example, the USP monographic statement for peppermint oil states that the oil "yields not less than 5% of esters, calculated as menthyl acetate ($C_{12}H_{22}O_2$), and not less than 50% of total menthol ($C_{10}H_{20}O$), free and as esters."

frequently disregarded. The filter paper is moistened with purified water before filtering to provide a physical barrier to the passage of the excess oil in the mixture onto the filter paper and into the filtrate. The moistened filter also prevents the absorption into the paper of the dissolved aromatics in the aqueous solution. Even with these precautions, aromatic waters prepared by simple solution are not always crystal clear because of the passage of minute particles through the filter paper. These particles are difficult to remove, even upon repeated filtration.

The preparation of aromatic waters by solution has the advantage over the distillation method in that the solution method does not require special equipment or the expenditure of a great deal of time on the part of the operator. However, when an aromatic water must be prepared extemporaneously for immediate use, it is necessary to employ a more rapid method of preparation than the two methods already described. For reasons of expediency with respect to both time and the clarity of the resulting product, the compendia permit the use of an "Alternative Solution Method" in the preparation of aromatic waters.

Alternative Solution Method

By this method, the volatile oil (2 ml) or suitably comminuted aromatic solid (2 g) is thoroughly incorporated with 15 g of talc or with a sufficient quantity of purified siliceous earth or pulped filter paper.[1] To this mixture is added 1000 ml of purified water, and the resulting slurry is thoroughly agitated several times during a period of 10 minutes. The mixture is then filtered, returning the first portions

of the filtrate to the filter, if necessary, to obtain a clear product.

DISTRIBUTING AGENTS. The talc, or other inert material, serves both as a filter aid to help render the product more clear and as a distributing agent for the aromatic substance. In the latter capacity it serves to accelerate the rate of solution by permitting the aromatic substance to be adsorbed and spread over its entire surface, thereby increasing the surface area of the aromatic substance exposed to the solvent action of the water. It is for this reason that a saturated solution of the aromatic substance can be effected in as short a period as the prescribed 10 minutes.

At one time it was thought that any apparently insoluble material was suitable for use as a distributing agent in the preparation of aromatic waters, and magnesium carbonate and calcium phosphate were among the agents recommended. However, it was later learned that each of these two agents dissolved slightly in the water being prepared, imparting to it an alkaline character. Because of the effects of the alkaline material on the volatile substance, the alkaline waters that resulted frequently developed a faintly yellowish tint upon standing. More importantly, however, the alkaline waters were responsible for a number of incompatibilities, including the precipitation of alkaloids from solution. The calcium ions, present to a small extent in waters prepared with calcium phosphate (or other slightly soluble calcium salts) as the distributing agent, had the undesired ability to form insoluble calcium salts with many anions. It is now generally recognized that an effective distributing agent must possess the following characteristics:

(a) It must be insoluble in water.
(b) It must not react chemically with the aromatic solute.
(c) It must be sufficiently coarse to be easily filtered from the mixture, leaving a sparkling clear filtrate. Occasionally the filtering agent selected for use in the preparation of an aromatic water is found to be too finely ground to be retained by the filter paper employed, and the result is sedimentation in the filtrate and a waste of time and materials. This can be avoided through the proper selection of the particle size of the filtering agent and the pore size of the filter.

---

[1] Talc is a native, hydrous magnesium silicate, sometimes containing a small proportion of aluminum silicate. It is found in commerce as a very fine white or grayish white crystalline powder which is insoluble in water. It is used in medicine as a dusting powder, and in pharmacy as a filtering medium.

Purified siliceous earth is a form of silica (SiO_2) consisting of the frustules and fragments of diatoms, purified by boiling with diluted hydrochloric acid, washing, and calcining. It is an amorphous, very fine, white, light gray or pale buff powder that is insoluble in water. It is used pharmaceutically as a filtering medium. Purified siliceous earth may also be referred to as: purified infusorial earth, purified kieselguhr, and terra silicea purificata.

Storage of Aromatic Waters

Once prepared by any of the recommended methods, aromatic waters are best stored in airtight, light-resistant containers maintained at room temperature. Aromatic waters are not considered to be permanently stable preparations; they deteriorate with time and are prone to contamination by mold. In general, aromatic waters tend to lose their aromatic fragrance several months after preparation and should be discarded upon notice of any change in odor or appearance. Some of the changes are due to the oxidative decomposition of the aromatic substances. Since atmospheric oxygen dissolved in water plays a role in this decomposition and since light and trace metals have the ability to catalyze oxidation reactions, aromatic waters should be maintained as free from these materials as possible. Maintenance of aromatic waters in tightly closed containers is doubly important, since the aromatic substances are volatile and are easily lost to the atmosphere upon prolonged exposure. This volatilization is hastened at elevated temperatures, and for this reason aromatic waters should be maintained at room temperature and never heated when employed as a solvent. Storage at low temperatures may cause the separation from solution of some of the aromatic materials, since their solubilities in water are generally decreased with decreasing temperatures. The clarity of the product can generally be restored by allowing the preparation to reach room temperature. To avoid light, aromatic waters are generally stored in a dark place or in an opaque or dark colored-glass container.

Since aromatic waters are not long lasting, they are generally prepared in small volumes in the pharmacy. The use of recently boiled purified water instead of unboiled water in the preparation of aromatic waters is beneficial, since it reduces the possibility of mold growth in the resultant preparation. Outside of this precaution, no other means of preserving the solution should be undertaken.

In prescription compounding with aromatic waters, the most frequently encountered incompatibility is the "salting out" of the volatile principles from the water upon the addition of large amounts of soluble salts. In using aromatic waters as vehicles, it is entirely permissible to replace a portion of the aromatic water with purified water in order to maintain a clear product.

Official Waters Prepared by Distillation

Orange Flower Water, NF

Orange flower water is a saturated solution of the odoriferous principles of the flowers of *Citrus aurantium*, prepared by distilling the fresh flowers with water and separating the excess volatile oil from the clear water portion of the distillate. The product possesses the pleasant odor and taste of orange blossoms and is employed as a vehicle, flavor, and perfume.

Stronger Rose Water, NF

Stronger Rose Water, NF, (Aqua Rosae Fortier) is prepared by distilling the fresh flowers of *Rosa centifolia* according to the general procedure. The NF prescribes that when rose water is required, it may be prepared by diluting stronger rose water with an equal volume of purified water. Rose water (Aqua Rosae) was formerly official for use as a perfuming agent in rose water ointment; however the present formula for the latter preparation, now official in the NF, calls for stronger rose water in half the volume of that formerly required of the diluted water.

Official Waters Prepared by Distillation or Solution

Peppermint Water, USP

Peppermint Water, USP, (Aqua Menthae Piperitae) is perhaps the most popular of all of the waters. It is prepared from the oil of leaves and flowering tops of *Mentha piperita*, either by solution of the oil or by distillation of the plant parts. However, since the oil is readily available at a reasonable price, the simpler solution method is generally used in the preparation of the water. The oil, which is composed of approximately 50% of menthol, imparts a refreshing taste and fragrance to the water. Peppermint water is employed pharmaceutically as a flavored vehicle and medicinally as a carminative at an unofficial dose of about 15 ml.

Diluted Acids

The official diluted acids are aqueous solutions prepared by diluting the corresponding

Table 14-1. SOME FORMERLY OFFICIAL
AROMATIC WATERS

Title and Synonyms	Comments
Camphor Water, NF XI	Prepared by solution after powdering the camphor by dissolving it in a small portion of solvent such as ether, alcohol, or chloroform and gently stirring the solution in a mortar until the solvent completely evaporates. The water is employed as a vehicle in ophthalmic preparations.
Chloroform Water, NF XI	Prepared by solution with an excess of chloroform (which is heavier than water) being permitted to remain at the bottom of the solution to maintain the solution's saturation of this volatile agent. The water must be carefully dispensed by decantation, making certain that the undissolved chloroform remains behind. Chloroform decomposes to the poisonous substance phosgene through oxidation, and thus the water must be protected from the catalyst to that reaction, light. The water is used as a vehicle and has mild analgesic qualities.
Hamamelis Water, NF XI (Witch Hazel; Distilled Witch Hazel Extract)	Contains about 15% alcohol as a preservative and is used externally as an astringent.

concentrated acids with purified water. The strength of a diluted acid is generally expressed on a per cent weight-to-volume (% w/v) basis, that is, the weight in grams of solute per 100 ml of solution, whereas the strength of a concentrated acid is generally expressed in terms of per cent weight-to-weight (% w/w), which indicates the number of grams of solute per 100 g of solution. In order to prepare a diluted acid from a concentrated one, it is first necessary to calculate the amount of solute required in the diluted product. Then, the amount of concentrated acid

required to supply the needed amount of solute can be determined.

To illustrate, Hydrochloric Acid, USP, the concentrated acid, contains not less than 35 g and not more than 38 g of solute (absolute HCl) per 100 g of acid and therefore is considered to be, on the average, 36.5% w/w in strength. Diluted Hydrochloric Acid, USP, is required to contain between 9.5 and 10.5 g of solute per 100 ml of solution and is therefore considered to be approximately 10% w/v in strength. If, for example, one wished to prepare 100 ml of the diluted acid from the concentrated acid, he would require 10 g of solute. The amount of concentrated hydrochloric acid required to supply this amount of solute may be calculated by the following proportion:

$$\frac{36.5 \text{ g (solute)}}{100 \text{ g (conc. acid)}} = \frac{10 \text{ g (solute)}}{x \text{ (g conc. acid)}}$$

solving for x:

$$36.5x = 1000 \text{ g}$$
$$x = 27.39 \text{ g (conc. acid)}$$

Thus, 27.39 g of concentrated acid are required to supply 10 g of solute needed for the preparation of 100 ml of the diluted acid. Although the required amount of concentrated acid may be accurately weighed, it is a cumbersome task, and as a rule pharmacists prefer to measure liquids volumetrically. Therefore, in the preparation of diluted acids, the calculations are generally carried one step further to determine the *volume* of concentrated acid that corresponds with the calculated weight. Since this additional step requires the use of the concentrated acid's specific gravity, a brief review of specific gravity seems appropriate.

By definition, specific gravity is a ratio, expressed decimally, of the weight of a substance to the weight of an equal volume of a standard, both substances having the same temperature or the temperature of each being known. Water is used as the standard for liquids and solids; hydrogen or air, for gases. In pharmacy, specific gravity calculations mainly involve liquids and solids, and water is an excellent choice for a standard, since it is readily available and easily purified.

At 4°C, the density of water is 1 g per cubic centimeter (cc). Since the USP states that 1 ml may be considered the equivalent of 1 cc, in pharmacy, water is assumed to weigh 1 g per ml. By the following equation, used to calculate specific gravity, a substance having a density the same as water would have a specific gravity of 1.0:

$$\text{sp gr} = \frac{\text{weight of a substance}}{\text{weight of an equal volume of water}}$$

In solving this equation, the same units of weight must be used in each part of the ratio. These units cancel out, and the ratio is expressed decimally.

Specific gravity indicates the relative weight of a substance compared to an equal volume of water. For example, if 10 ml of a liquid weigh 20 g, an equal volume of water would weigh 10 g, and the ratio in the equation would be 20 g/10 g yielding a specific gravity of 2.0. This would indicate that the liquid is twice as heavy as water in equal volume. By the same token, a liquid having a specific gravity of 0.5 would be half as heavy as water; a liquid with a specific gravity of 0.8 would be eight-tenths as heavy as water, etc.

If both the volume of a liquid and its specific gravity are known, its weight may be calculated. For instance, if concentrated hydrochloric acid has a specific gravity of 1.17, it is that number times as heavy as water, and 100 ml of the acid would weigh 1.17 times as much as 100 ml of water. Since 100 ml of water weigh 100 g, 100 ml of the acid would weigh 1.17 times that or 117 g.

If one knows the weight of a liquid and its specific gravity, the volume of the liquid may be determined. For example, a liquid that is twice as heavy as water would have a specific gravity of 2.0 and would occupy half the volume that an equal weight of water would occupy. If one had 100 g of this liquid and substituted in the above equation as indicated below, the volume of the liquid could be arrived at:

$$2.0 = \frac{100 \text{ g}}{\text{weight of an equal volume of water}}$$

$$\text{weight of an equal volume of water} = \frac{100 \text{ g}}{2.0} = 50 \text{ g}$$

Since 50 g is the weight of an equal volume of water, it follows that the water must measure 50 ml. Since the volume of the water is an "equal volume" to the other liquid, that liquid must also measure 50 ml.

The volume represented by 27.39 g of the concentrated hydrochloric acid may be similarly determined by dividing the specific gravity of

the concentrated acid into its weight and equating the answer of weight of an equal volume of water to the volume of the acid:

$$\frac{27.39 \text{ g}}{1.17} = 23.41 \text{ g, weight of equal volume of water.}$$

Thus, since 23.41 g of water measures 23.41 ml and since it is equal in volume to the concentrated acid, the latter also measures 23.41 ml and would be required to prepare 100 ml of the 10% w/v diluted acid.

Once the above is thoroughly understood, the following simplified formula can be used to calculate the amount of a concentrated acid required in the preparation of a specific volume of the corresponding diluted acid:

$$\frac{\begin{array}{c}\text{Percentage strength}\\\text{(w/v) of diluted acid}\end{array} \times \begin{array}{c}\text{Volume of diluted}\\\text{acid to be prepared}\end{array}}{\begin{array}{c}\text{Percentage strength (w/w)}\\\text{of concentrated acid}\end{array} \times \begin{array}{c}\text{Specific gravity of}\\\text{concentrated acid}\end{array}}$$

= Volume of concentrated acid to use.

Recalculating the preparation of 100 ml of diluted hydrochloric acid from the concentrated acid gives the following:

$$\frac{10 \times 100 \text{ ml}}{36.5 \times 1.17} = 23.41 \text{ ml of concentrated acid to use.}$$

All of the official diluted acids have a strength of 10% w/v, with the exception of Diluted Acetic Acid, NF, which is 6% w/v. The strengths of these acids are commensurate with the concentrations generally used for medicinal or pharmaceutical purposes. The concentrations of the corresponding concentrated acids vary widely from one acid to another, depending upon various properties of the solute such as solubility, stability, and ease of preparation. For instance, concentrated sulfuric acid is generally between 95 and 98% w/w, nitric acid between 69 and 71% w/w, and concentrated phosphoric acid between 85 and 88% w/w. As a result, the amounts of each concentrated acid required to prepare the corresponding diluted acid vary widely and must be calculated on an individual basis.

Official Diluted Acids

Diluted Acetic Acid, NF

Diluted Acetic Acid, NF, is an aqueous solution containing approximately 6% of CH_3COOH. It is prepared by diluting either

Acetic Acid, USP, approximately a 36.5% acid, or the more concentrated Glacial Acetic Acid, USP, which is not less than 99.4% in strength and which is itself diluted to prepare the Acetic Acid, USP. Glacial acetic acid is so named because of its solid glassy appearance when congealed, an event that occurs at various temperatures depending upon the concentration of the acid. For example, an acid of 99.4% strength will congeal at a temperature of 15.47°C, whereas acids of a lesser concentration will require colder temperatures to reach their congealing points. Diluted acetic acid is officially categorized as a pharmaceutical aid (solvent). Medicinally, acetic acid is bactericidal to many types of microorganisms and finds application in 1% solutions in surgical dressings, as an irrigating solution to the bladder in 0.25% concentration, and also as a spermatocidal in some proprietary contraceptive preparations. The concentrated acids are useful to the pharmaceutical chemist in the preparation of acetate salts and esters of numerous drugs.

Diluted Hydrochloric Acid, USP

Diluted Hydrochloric Acid, USP, is a 10% solution of HCl prepared by adding 234 ml of the concentrated acid (about 36.5% w/w) with a sufficient amount of purified water to make a liter of solution. The concentrated acid was first prepared commercially by distilling sea salt with sulfuric acid, and for this reason, it has become widely known as muriatic acid, a name derived from the Latin *murea* for salt and meaning the acid from salt. The diluted acid is used medicinally in the treatment of achlorhydria, a condition generally associated with pernicious anemia and characterized by failure of the gastric secretion to produce gastric acid. It is also used in the less severe hypochlorhydria. Diluted hydrochloric acid as a gastric acidifier has a dose of 5 ml, well diluted with water. Even after dilution, the product should be administered through a glass tube or drinking straw to prevent the solvent action of the acid upon the enamel of the teeth. It is usually taken during or after meals to aid the digestive process. Officially, the diluted acid is categorized as a pharmaceutic aid (acidifying agent).

Diluted Phosphoric Acid, NF

Diluted Phosphoric Acid, NF, is a 10% preparation of H_3PO_4 made by diluting the concentrated acid (about 85 to 88% w/w). The concentrated phosphoric acid is a rather heavy liquid with a specific gravity of 1.71 and a syrupy consistency, which is responsible for its synonym, "syrupy phosphoric acid." Both the diluted and the concentrated acids are mainly pharmaceutical necessities as chemical reagents and in the preparation of various phosphate salts. The diluted acid has been used medicinally as a gastric and urinary acidifier.

Other Diluted Acids

Two additional diluted acids, diluted nitric acid and diluted sulfuric acid, are listed in the "Reagents" section of the USP. Each of these diluted acids is a 10% acid prepared from the corresponding concentrated acids. Because of the spattering that occurs when water is added to sulfuric acid, the acid should be added to the purified water in the preparation of diluted sulfuric acid. Although the latter product finds its principal use as a chemical reagent, it was formerly employed medicinally for the same purpose as diluted hydrochloric acid, to augment the acid content of the stomach.

Spirits

Spirits, formerly called essences, may be defined as alcoholic or hydroalcoholic solutions of volatile substances. Generally, the alcoholic concentration of spirits is rather high, the range of alcoholic content among the currently official preparations being from a low of 62 to 68%, required for Aromatic Ammonia Spirit, NF, to a high of 79 to 85%, required for Peppermint Spirit, NF. Because of the greater solubility of aromatic or volatile substances in alcohol than in water, spirits generally contain a greater concentration of these materials than do the corresponding aromatic waters. When mixed with water or with an aqueous preparation, the volatile substances present in spirits generally separate from solution and form a milky preparation. During the preparation of spirits contact with water must be avoided, and all glassware and utensils must either be dry or final-rinsed with alcohol rather than with water. For instance, if a spirit is to be filtered, it is best to filter it through a dry filter paper or one moistened with a small portion of alcohol rather than through a paper moistened with water. Because spirits contain volatile solutes as well as a volatile solvent and because many volatile substances deteriorate in the presence of air and light, they should be stored in tightly closed, light-resistant containers.

Spirits are employed pharmaceutically as flavoring agents and medicinally for the therapeutic value of the aromatic solute. As flavoring agents they are used to impart the flavor of their solute to other pharmaceutical preparations, especially elixirs, which are not incompatible with the alcoholic solution. For medicinal purposes, spirits may be taken orally, applied externally, or used by inhalation, depending upon the particular preparation. In any case, they are employed for the therapeutic merit of their solute. When taken orally, they are generally mixed with a portion of water to reduce the pungency of the spirit.

Preparation of Spirits

In general, spirits are prepared by four methods: (1) simple solution of the volatile substance in the solvent by agitation, (2) solution with maceration, (3) chemical reaction, and (4) distillation.

SIMPLE SOLUTION. The majority of spirits are prepared by dissolving the solute in alcohol by agitation. Filtration is generally desirable to obtain a sparkling clear product.

SOLUTION WITH MACERATION. Spirits prepared from plant material may be prepared by macerating the vegetable material in a suitable solvent to remove an undesired constituent or to extract one which is desired. Generally in the preparation of spirits, the desired constituents are alcohol-soluble and the undesired ones, water-soluble.

CHEMICAL REACTION. Among the official spirits, only the preparation of Aromatic Ammonia Spirit, NF, involves a chemical reaction, and that is one which merely converts official ammonium carbonate to the true ammonium carbonate to increase its solubility. A formerly official spirit, ethyl nitrite spirit, was prepared by a method in which the solute ethyl nitrate was first prepared by the action of sodium nitrite on a mixture of alcohol and sulfuric acid in the cold.

DISTILLATION. No spirits currently official are prepared by distillation. However, two products

of historical significance, which were official in the NF XI, are prepared by distillation; they are Brandy (*Spiritus Vini Vitis*), prepared by the distillation of the fermented juice of sound ripe grapes, and Whisky (*Spiritus Frumenti*), prepared by the distillation of the fermented mash of wholly or partly malted cereal grains. Each of these preparations contains about 50% of alcohol, and both were officially categorized as central depressants.

Aromatic Ammonia Spirit, NF

Aromatic Ammonia Spirit, NF, is a hydroalcoholic solution of ammonia and ammonium carbonate, flavored and perfumed with lemon, lavender, and myristica oils. It is prepared by dissolving translucent pieces of official ammonium carbonate in strong ammonia solution and purified water by agitation. Following a 12-hour standing period, the aqueous solution is added to an alcoholic solution of the oils, and enough purified water is added to prepare the required volume. The hydroalcoholic mixture is set aside for 24 hours with intermittent agitation and is then filtered, using a covered filter.

Official ammonium carbonate is a mixture of ammonium bicarbonate (NH_4HCO_3), which is insoluble in alcohol, and ammonium carbamate (NH_2COONH_4), which is alcohol-soluble. Upon standing, the compound takes up moisture, and the carbamate portion releases ammonia, leaving a white powdery residue of ammonium bicarbonate on the surface of the compound:

$$NH_2COONH_4 + H_2O \rightarrow NH_4HCO_3 + NH_3$$

The liberation of ammonia renders the total compound less potent, and in order to obtain fully potent ammonium carbonate, the powdery ammonium bicarbonate must be scraped from the surface of the compound (generally with a spatula) until the translucent pieces of the original compound are exposed. The translucent pieces of material are then dissolved in strong ammonia solution, and a true ammonium carbonate is formed:

$$NH_4HCO_3 \cdot NH_2COONH_4 + NH_4OH \rightarrow 2(NH_4)_2CO_3$$
$$\text{or}$$
$$NH_4HCO_3 + NH_3 \rightarrow (NH_4)_2CO_3$$
$$\text{and}$$
$$NH_2COONH_4 + H_2O \rightarrow (NH_4)_2CO_3$$

The mixture is allowed to stand to insure the completion of the reaction and the potency of the spirit, which is required to be about 1.9%, by weight, of ammonia. After the alcoholic and aqueous solutions have been mixed, a second standing period is required to allow any unconverted bicarbonate to precipitate and to permit the hydroalcoholic mixture to become fully saturated with the oils.

The spirit has only a faint color when fresh but gradually acquires an amber color, probably due to the effect of the alkali on the oils. The spirit remains potent, even after a color change, so long as the concentration of ammonia is maintained. The spirit is best stored in tight, light-resistant containers, preferably at a temperature not exceeding 30°.

The spirit is used as a reflex stimulant in cases of fainting, by the inhalation of the ammonia vapor. It may be taken orally, well diluted with water, in an unofficial dose of 2 ml. When taken in this manner, it forms a milky preparation due to the liberation of some of the oils by the water.

Camphor Spirit, NF

Camphor Spirit, NF, contains about 10% of camphor dissolved in alcohol by agitation. The spirit is officially categorized as a "local irritant" and is employed topically in the treatment of cold sores and fever blisters and to relieve the itching of insect bites. Camphor spirit may be taken internally in an unofficial dose of 1 ml as a carminative and to combat diarrhea.

Compound Orange Spirit, NF

Compound Orange Spirit, NF, contains approximately 27.5% of combined oils of orange, coriander, lemon, and anise dissolved by simple solution in alcohol. The appealing flavor of the spirit is utilized in the preparation of other pharmaceutical products, particularly elixirs.

Peppermint Spirit, NF

Peppermint spirit is an alcoholic solution containing 10% peppermint oil and the green colorant, chlorophyll, extracted with alcohol from coarsely ground peppermint.

Peppermint, NF, consists of the dried leaf and flowering top of *Mentha piperita*. When fresh, peppermint contains about 2% of peppermint oil. However, the oil is lost when the peppermint is air-dried prior to packaging.

The peppermint therefore is used in the preparation of the spirit not for its oil content, but rather for the purpose of imparting a pleasant green color to the product. In extracting the green chlorophyll from the peppermint, the drug first must be macerated with water for about 1 hour to remove the brown water-soluble pigments. Then, the leaves are drained, expressed of water, and macerated in alcohol with frequent agitation for a period of about 6 hours. If the peppermint were only macerated with alcohol, all coloring material, brown and green, would be extracted, and the resulting spirit would not be as brilliantly colored as it is from green chlorophyll alone. Chlorophyll resists extraction by water but is easily soluble in the alcohol. After the peppermint is macerated in the alcohol, the mixture is filtered, and the peppermint oil dissolved in the green-colored alcoholic filtrate. The spirit is then made to volume with additional alcohol.

Peppermint spirit may be taken internally as a digestive aid in a dose of 1 ml. If it is mixed with water, the mixture is milky but retains its medicinal value.

Radiopharmaceuticals

A *radiopharmaceutical* is a chemical containing a radioactive isotope for use in humans for the purpose of diagnosis, mitigation, or treatment of a disease. It should be recalled from general chemistry that substances which have the same number of protons but have varying numbers of neutrons are called *isotopes*. Isotopes may be stable or unstable; those that are unstable are radioactive because their nuclei undergo a rearrangement while changing to a stable state, and energy is given off.

All of the atoms of an unstable isotope do not completely rearrange at the same instant. The time required for a radioisotope to decay to 50% of its original activity is termed its radioactive half-life. Isotopes vary widely in their half-life; carbon-14 has a radioactive half-life of some 5730 years, whereas that for sodium-24 is only 15 hours.

The activity of a radioactive material is expressed as the number of nuclear transformations per unit time. The fundamental unit of radioactivity is the *curie* (Ci), defined as 3.700×10^{10} nuclear transformations per second. The *millicurie* (mCi) and *microcurie* (μCi) are commonly used subunits:

1 millicurie = 10^{-3} curie
1 micorcurie = 10^{-6} curie

The three types of radiation most frequently emitted from radioactive nuclei are *alpha, beta,* and *gamma* radiations. Alpha particles which constitute alpha radiation consist of two protons and two neutrons, thus being identical with the helium nucleus. As an alpha particle loses energy, its velocity decreases. It then attracts electrons and becomes a helium atom. Most alpha particles are unable to pierce the outer layers of skin or penetrate a thin piece of paper. Beta particles may be either electrons with negative charge, *negatrons,* or positive electrons, *positrons.* These two particles, β^- and β^+ have a range of over 10 feet in air and up to about 1 mm in tissue. Nuclear medicine has been dependent mostly on radiopharmaceuticals that decay by gamma (γ) emission. Gamma rays are electromagnetic vibrations comparable with light but of much shorter wavelength. Because of their short wavelength and high energy, they are very penetrating.

The majority of radiopharmaceuticals are produced by the process of nuclear activation in a nuclear reactor. In such a reactor, stable atoms are bombarded with excess neutrons present in the reactor. The resulting neutron additions to the stable atoms produce unstable atoms and radioactive isotopes. The facilities for the production, use, and storage of radioactive pharmaceuticals are subject to licensing by the Nuclear Regulatory Commission, or in certain instances to appropriate state agencies. As for all pharmaceuticals, the Federal Food and Drug Administration enforces strict adherence to good manufacturing practice and proper labeling and use of the products. The Federal Department of Transportation regulates the conditions of shipment of the radiopharmaceuticals, as do state and local agencies.

Radioactive pharmaceuticals require highly specialized techniques in their preparation, handling, and use in order that correct results may be obtained from their use and hazards to personnel minimized. All operations must be conducted or supervised by personnel having expert training in the handling and use of radioactive materials.

Living cells may be damaged by all types of radiation. The degree being dependent upon the type of radiation and the length of exposure. Damaging exposure may occur externally as on the skin, or internally through ingestion, inhalation, or absorption or penetration through the tissues.

Different radioisotopes tend to concentrate in different tissues or organs. Their presence may be determined by scanning and their amounts in the tissues determined from their radiation emissions. Because of their ability to become attracted to certain tissues and organs, radioactive isotopes can perform diagnostic as well as therapeutic functions within those tissues and organs. In diagnostic work, a tracer dose is employed which is much smaller than the therapeutic dose of the same material and cellular damage is minimal. The therapeutic use of radioactive isotopes is based on their ability to destroy the cells for which they have an affinity.

Official Radiopharmaceuticals

The official radiopharmaceuticals are presented below. The category for each indicates the types of cells or tissues for which the isotope has an affinity.

Chlormerodrin Hg 197 Injection, USP—Diagnostic aid (renal scanning)

Chlormerodrin Hg 203 Injection, NF—Diagnostic aid (tumor localization)

Cyanocobalamin Co 57 Capsules, USP—Diagnostic aid (pernicious anemia)

Cyanocobalamin Co 57 Solution, USP—Diagnostic aid (pernicious anemia)

Cyanocobalamin Co 60 Capsules, NF—Diagnostic aid (pernicious anemia)

Cyanocobalamin Co 60 Solution, NF—Diagnostic aid (pernicious anemia)

Gold Au 198 Injection, NF—Antineoplastic; diagnostic aid (liver scanning)

Iodinated I 125 Serum Albumin, USP—Diagnostic aid (blood volume determination)

Iodinated I 131 Serum Albumin, USP—Diagnostic aid (blood volume determination)

Iodohippurate Sodium I 131 Injection, USP—Diagnostic aid (renal function)

Macroaggregated Iodinated I 131 Serum Albumin, NF—Diagnostic aid (pulmonary clearance)

Sodium Rose Bengal I 131 Injection, USP—Diagnostic aid (hepatobiliary function)

Sodium Chromate Cr 51 Injection, USP—Diagnostic aid (blood volume determination)

Sodium Iodide I 125 Solution, NF—Diagnostic aid (thyroid function)

Sodium Iodide I 131 Capsules, USP—Diagnostic aid (thyroid function); thyroid inhibitor

Sodium Iodide I 131 Solution, USP—Diagnostic aid (thyroid function); thyroid inhibitor

Sodium Pertechnetate Tc 99m Solution, USP—Diagnostic aid (brain scanning; thyroid scanning)

Sodium Phosphate P 32 Solution, USP—Antipolycythemic; diagnostic aid (ocular tumor localization)

Strontium Sr 85 Injection, USP—Diagnostic aid (bone scanning)

Technetium Tc 99m Aggregated Albumin, USP—Diagnostic aid (lung scanning)

Technetium Tc 99m Sulfur Colloid Injection, USP—Diagnostic aid (liver scanning)

Definitions of Official Drug Categories

Abrasive—an agent that rubs off an external layer, such as dental plaque. (Pumice NF)

Absorbent—a drug that takes up chemicals into the drug substance, useful in reducing the free availability of toxic chemicals. (Polycarbophil NF, gastrointestinal absorbent)

Acidifier, Systemic—a drug that lowers internal body pH, useful in restoring normal body pH (pH 7.4 for blood) in patients with systemic alkalosis. (Ammonium Chloride NF)

Acidifier, Urinary—a drug that lowers the pH of the renal filtrate and urine. (Methionine NF)

Adrenergic—a drug that activates organs innervated by the sympathetic branch of the autonomic nervous system; a sympathomimetic drug. (Epinephrine USP)

Adrenocortical Steroid, Anti-inflammatory—an adrenal cortex hormone or analog that regulates organic metabolism and inhibits inflammatory response; a glucocorticoid. (Hydrocortisone USP)

Adrenocortical Steroid, Salt-regulating—an adrenal cortex hormone or analog that regulates sodium/potassium electrolyte balance in the body; a mineralocorticoid. (Desoxycorticosterone Acetate USP)

Adsorbent—a drug that binds chemicals to the drug surface, useful in reducing the free availability of toxic chemicals. (Kaolin NF, gastrointestinal adsorbent)

Alcohol Deterrent—a drug that alters physiology so that unpleasant symptoms occur following ingestion of ethanol-containing beverages and products. (Disulfiram NF)

Alkalizer, Systemic—a drug that raises internal body pH, useful in restoring normal body pH (pH 7.4 for blood) in patients with systemic acidosis. (Sodium Bicarbonate USP)

Analgesic—a drug that selectively suppresses pain perception without inducing unconsciousness. (Morphine Sulfate USP, narcotic analgesic; Aspirin USP, nonnarcotic analgesic)

Androgen—a hormone that stimulates and maintains male reproductive function and sex characteristics. (Testosterone Propionate USP)

Anesthetic, General—a drug that eliminates pain perception by inducing unconsciousness. (Ether USP, inhalation anesthetic; Thiopental Sodium USP, intravenous anesthetic)

Anesthetic, Local—a drug that eliminates pain perception in a limited body area by local action on sensory nerves. (Procaine Hydrochloride USP)

Anesthetic, Topical—a local anesthetic (q.v.) that is effective by application to mucous membranes. (Tetracaine Hydrochloride USP)

Anorexic—a drug that suppresses appetite, usually by central stimulation of mood. (Phenmetrazine Hydrochloride NF)

Antacid—a drug that neutralizes excess gastric acid locally. (Aluminum Hydroxide Gel USP)

Anthelmintic—a drug that kills or inhibits pathogenic nematodes and cestodes; causative agents of intestinal worm infestations. (Piperazine Citrate USP)

Anti-adrenergic—a drug that prevents response to sympathetic nerve impulses and to adrenergic drugs (q.v.). (Propranolol Hydrochloride USP)

Anti-amebic—a drug that kills or inhibits the pathogenic protozoan *Entamoeba histolytica*, causative agent of intestinal and extraintestinal amebiasis. (Diiodohydroxyquin USP, intestinal anti-amebic; Emetine Hydrochloride USP, extraintestinal anti-amebic)

Anti-anemic—a drug that stimulates production of erythrocytes in normal number, size and hemoglobin content, useful in treating anemia or in antidoting overdosage of anemia-causing drugs. (Leucovorin Calcium USP)

Anti-anginal—a coronary vasodilator (q.v.) useful in preventing or treating attacks of angina pectoris. (Nitroglycerin Tablets USP)

Anti-arrhythmic—a cardiac depressant (q.v.), useful in suppressing cardiac rhythm irregularities. (Procainamide Hydrochloride USP)

Anti-arthritic—an anti-inflammatory drug (q.v.) useful in treating rheumatoid arthritis and other types of joint inflammation. (Oxyphenbutazone NF)

Antibacterial—a drug that kills or inhibits pathogenic bacteria, causative agents of many systemic, gastointestinal, and topical infections. (Penicillin G Potassium USP, systemic antibacterial; Nitrofurantoin USP, urinary antibacterial; Bacitracin USP, topical antibacterial)

Anticholesteremic—a drug that lowers plasma cholesterol level. (Dextrothyroxine Sodium NF)

Anticholinergic—a drug that prevents response to parasympathetic nerve impulses and to cholinergic drugs (q.v.). (Atropine Sulfate USP)

Anticoagulant, Systemic—a systemically acting drug that slows clotting of circulating blood. (Warfarin Sodium USP)

Anticoagulant, For Storage of Whole Blood—a drug that when added to collected blood prevents clotting. (Anticoagulant Citrate Dextrose Solution USP)

Anticonvulsant—An antiepileptic drug (q.v.), or a drug that arrests convulsions by inducing general anesthesia (*Phenytoin Sodium USP*, antiepileptic anticonvulsant; Thiopental Sodium USP, anesthetic anticonvulsant)

Antidepressant—a central acting drug that selectively induces mood elevation, useful in treating mental depression. (Amitriptyline Hydrochloride USP)

Antidiabetic—a drug that replaces insulin or stimulates secretion of insulin, useful in treating diabetes mellitus. (Insulin Zinc Suspension USP)

Antidote, General Purpose—a drug that prevents or minimizes the effects of an ingested poison (or drug overdose) by adsorption of the toxic material while in the gastrointestinal tract. (Activated Charcoal USP)

Antidote, Specific—a drug that terminates or minimizes the systemic effects of a poison (or drug overdose) by a mechanism of action that is specific for the particular poison. (Dimercaprol USP, specific antidote for arsenic, mercury and gold poisoning; Naloxone Hydrochloride USP, specific antidote for narcotic analgesic overdosage)

Anti-eczematic—a topical drug that aids in control of chronic exudative skin lesions. (Coal Tar USP)

Anti-emetic—a drug that prevents vomiting. (Prochlorperazine Maleate USP)

Anti-epileptic—an anticonvulsant drug (q.v.) that selectively suppresses epileptic seizures without inducing loss of consciousness. (Ethosuximide USP)

Antifilarial—a drug that kills or inhibits pathogenic filarial worms, causative agents of infections such as loaiasis. (Diethylcarbamazine Citrate USP)

Antiflatulent—a drug that reduces gastrointestinal gas. (Simethicone NF)

Antifungal, Systemic—a systemically active drug that kills or inhibits pathogenic fungi that cause systemic, gastrointestinal or topical infections. (Griseofulvin USP)

Antifungal, Topical—a topically active drug that kills or inhibits pathogenic fungi that cause topical infections. (Tolnaftate USP)

Antihemophilic—a drug that replaces the blood clotting factors absent in the hereditary disease hemophilia. (Antihemophilic Factor, Human USP)

Antihistaminic—a drug that prevents response to histamine, including histamine released by allergic reactions. (Chlorpheniramine Maleate USP)

Antihyperlipidemic—a drug that lowers plasma cholesterol and lipid levels. (Clofibrate USP)

Antihypertensive—a drug that lowers arterial blood pressure, especially the elevated diastolic pressure of hypertensive patients. (Guanethidine Sulfate USP)

Antihypocalcemic—a drug that elevates plasma calcium level, useful in treating plasma hypocalcemia, especially that associated with hypoparathyroidism. (Parathyroid Injection USP)

Antihypoglycemic—a drug that elevates plasma glucose level, useful in treating hypoglycemia, including that induced by overdosage with antidiabetic drugs. (Glucagon USP)

Anti-infective, Topical (or Local)—a drug that kills or inhibits a variety of pathogenic microorganisms, and is suitable for sterilizing the skin or wounds. (Hexachlorophene Liquid Soap USP)

Anti-inflammatory—a drug that inhibits the physiologic response to cell damage (inflammation). (Prednisolone USP, adrenocortical steroid; Oxyphenbutazone NF, nonsteroid)

Antileishmanial—a drug that kills or inhibits protozoa of the genus *Leishmania*, causative agents of infections such as kala-azar. (Hydroxystilbamidine Isethionate USP)

Antimalarial—a drug that kills or inhibits pathogenic protozoa that cause malaria. (Chloroquine Phosphate USP)

Antineoplastic—a drug that is selectively toxic to the rapidly multiplying cells of malignant tumors. (Busulfan USP)

Antiparkinsonian—a drug that reduces the neurologic disturbances and symptoms present in the disease parkinsonism (shaking palsy). (Levodopa USP)

Antiperistaltic—a drug that inhibits intestinal motility, useful in treating diarrhea. (Paregoric USP)

Antipolycythemic—a drug that reduces the number of erythrocytes, useful in treating patients with abnormally high erythrocyte count (polycythemia). (Sodium Phosphate P 32 Solution USP)

Antiprotozoal—a drug that kills or inhibits pathogenic protozoa, such as *Giardia lamblia*. (Quinacrine Hydrochloride USP, antiprotozoal for giardiasis)

Antipruritic—a drug that prevents or inhibits itching (pruritus). (Trimeprazine Tartrate USP, systemic antipruritic; Menthol USP, topical antipruritic)

Antipsoriatic—a drug that suppresses the lesions or otherwise alleviates the symptoms of the skin disease psoriasis. (Methotrexate USP, systemic antipsoriatic; Anthralin USP, topical antipsoriatic)

Antipsychotic—a potent tranquilizer (q.v.), useful in treating psychoses. (Acetophenazine Maleate NF)

Antipyretic—a drug that lowers body temperature in the presence of fever. (Acetaminophen USP)

Antirachitic—a drug with vitamin D activity, useful in preventing or treating vitamin D deficiency and its symptoms such as rickets. (Cholecalciferol USP)

Antirheumatic—a drug that alleviates inflammatory symptoms of arthritis and related rheumatic diseases. (Phenylbutazone USP)

Antirickettsial—a drug that kills or inhibits pathogenic microorganisms of the genus *Rickettsia*, causative agents of infectious diseases such as Rocky Mountain spotted fever. (Chloramphenicol USP)

Antischistosomal—a drug that kills or inhibits pathogenic flukes of the genus *Schistosoma*, causative agents of schistosomiasis. (Antimony Potassium Tartrate USP)

Antiscorbutic—a drug with vitamin C activity, useful in preventing or treating vitamin C deficiency and its symptoms such as scurvy. (Ascorbic Acid USP)

Antiseborrheic—a drug that aids in the control of seborrheic dermatitis (dandruff). (Selenium Sulfide USP)

Antitrichomonal—a drug that kills or inhibits pathogenic protozoa of the genus *Trichomonas*, causative agents of infections such as trichomonal vaginitis. (Metronidazole USP)

Antitussive—a drug that suppresses coughing. (Codeine Phosphate USP)

Antiviral, Ophthalmic—a topically acting drug that kills or inhibits viral infections of the eye. (Idoxuridine USP, ophthalmic antiviral for ocular herpes simplex infection)

Antiviral, Prophylactic—a drug useful in preventing (rather than treating) viral infections. (Amantadine Hydrochloride USP, prophylactic for A_2 (Asian) influenza)

Antixerophthalmic—a drug with vitamin A activity, useful in preventing or treating vitamin A deficiency and its symptoms such as xerophthalmia. (Vitamin A USP)

Astringent—a mild protein precipitant suitable for topical application to toughen and shrink tissues. (Aluminum Acetate Solution USP)

Astringent, Ophthalmic—an astringent (q.v.) suitable for use in the eye. (Zinc Sulfate USP)

Blood Neutralizer—a drug which when added to group 0 blood neutralizes the traces of anti-A and anti-B isoagglutinins present and makes the blood suitable for universal administration. (Blood Group Specific Substances A and B NF)

Blood Volume Supporter—an intravenous drug containing solutes that are retained in the vascular system to supplement osmotic activity of plasma and so to expand plasma volume. (Plasma Protein Fraction, Human USP)

Bronchodilator—a drug that expands bronchiolar airways, useful in treating asthma and related conditions. (Isoproterenol Hydrochloride USP, adrenergic bronchodilator; Oxitriphylline NF, smooth muscle relaxant bronchodilator)

Carbonic Anhydrase Inhibitor—a drug that inhibits the enzyme carbonic anhydrase, the therapeutic effects of which are diuresis and reduced formation of intraocular fluid. (Acetazolamide USP)

Cardiac Depressant, Antiarrhythmic—a drug that depresses myocardial function, useful in treating cardiac arrhythmias. (Procainamide Hydrochloride USP)

Cardiotonic—a drug that increases myocardial contractile force, useful in treating myocardial inadequacies such as congestive heart failure. (Digitoxin USP)

Cathartic—a drug that promotes defecation. (Aromatic Cascara Fluidextract USP, peristaltic stimulant; Milk of Magnesia USP, fecal fluid volume expander; Mineral Oil USP, fecal lubricant)

Caustic—a topical drug that destroys tissue on contact, useful in removing abnormal skin lesions. (Toughened Silver Nitrate USP)

Centrally Acting Drug—a drug that produces its therapeutic effect by action on the central nervous system, usually designated by type of therapeutic action (sedative, hypnotic, anticonvulsant, etc.).

Choleretic—a drug that increases secretion of bile by the liver. (Dehydrocholic Acid NF)

Cholinergic—a drug that activates organs innervated by the parasympathetic branch of the autonomic nervous system; a parasympathomimetic drug. (Neostigmine Bromide USP, systemic cholinergic; Pilocarpine Nitrate USP, ophthalmic cholinergic)

Coagulant, Clotting Factor—a blood derivative that replaces a deficient factor necessary for coagulation. (Fibrinogen USP)

Contraceptive, Oral—an orally effective drug that prevents conception. All currently available oral contraceptives are for use by females. (Norethindrone Acetate and Ethinyl Estradiol Tablets USP)

Dental Caries Prophylactic—a drug applied to the teeth to reduce the incidence of cavities. (Stannous Fluoride USP)

Dentin Desensitizer—a drug applied to the teeth to reduce the sensitivity of exposed subenamel material (dentin). (Zinc Chloride USP)

Depigmenting Agent—a topical drug that inhibits formation of skin pigment (melanin), useful in lightening localized areas of darkened skin. (Hydroquinone USP)

Detergent—an emulsifying agent used as a cleanser, as for the skin. (Hexachlorophene Liquid Soap USP, anti-infective detergent)

Diagnostic Aid—a drug used to determine the functional state of a body organ, or to determine the presence of disease, usually designated specifically by type of diagnostic test. (Betazole USP, gastric secretion indicator; Fluorescein Sodium USP, corneal trauma indicator)

Digestive Aid—a drug that promotes digestion, usually by supplementing a naturally occurring digestive enzyme. (Pancreatin NF)

Disinfectant—an agent that destroys microorganisms on contact and suitable for sterilizing inanimate objects. (Formaldehyde Solution USP)

Diuretic—a drug that promotes renal excretion of electrolytes and water, useful in treating generalized edema. (Furosemide USP)

Emetic—a drug that induces vomiting, useful in removing unabsorbed accidentally ingested poisons. (Ipecac USP)

Emollient—a topical drug, especially an oil or fat, used to soften the skin and make it more pliable. (Cold Cream USP)

Enzyme, Proteolytic—an enzyme that hydrolyzes proteins, useful in eye surgery to facilitate lens removal, useful topically to digest necrotic material, etc. (Chymotrypsin USP, ophthalmic and systemic use; Trypsin NF, topical and systemic use)

Estrogen—a hormone that stimulates and maintains female reproductive organs and sex characteristics, and functions in both the proliferative and secretory phases of the uterine cycle. (Ethinyl Estradiol USP)

Expectorant—a drug that increases respiratory tract secretion, lowering its viscosity and promoting its removal. (Potassium Iodide USP, Glyceryl Guaiacolate NF)

Fecal Softener—a drug that promotes defecation by softening the feces. (Dioctyl Calcium Sulfosuccinate NF)

Glucocorticoid—an anti-inflammatory adrenocortical steroid (q.v.), useful in suppressing the inflammatory process. (Betamethasone NF)

Gonad-stimulating Principle—a hormone or other drug that stimulates function of the ovaries or testes (gonads). (Chorionic Gonadotropin USP)

Hematopoietic—a vitamin that stimulates formation of blood cells, useful in treating vitamin deficiency anemia. (Cyanocobalamin USP)

Hematinic—a drug that promotes hemoglobin formation by supplying iron needed for incorporation. (Ferrous Sulfate USP)

Hemostatic, Local—a drug applied to a bleeding surface to promote the clotting process or to serve as a matrix for the clot. (Thrombin USP, clot promoter; Oxidized Cellulose USP, clot matrix)

Hemostatic, Systemic—a drug that inhibits systemic dissolution of clots (fibrinolysis), useful in treating hyperfibrinolysis. (Aminocaproic Acid NF)

Hormone, Adrenocorticotropic—the pituitary hormone that stimulates the adrenal cortex to produce glucocorticoids. (Corticotropin Injection USP)

Hormone, Posterior Pituitary, Antidiuretic—the pituitary hormone that promotes water reabsorption from the distal and collecting renal tubules, useful in treating antidiuretic hormone deficiency (diabetes insipidus). (Vasopressin Injection USP).

Hormone, Thyroid—the thyroid gland hormone that stimulates mature metabolic function and maintains normal basal metabolic rate. (Levothyroxine Sodium USP)

Hypnotic—a central nervous system depressant that, with suitable dosage, induces sleep. (Amobarbital Sodium USP)

Immunizing Agent, Active—an antigen that induces production of antibodies against a pathogenic microorganism, used to provide permanent but delayed protection against infection with the microorganism. (Tetanus Toxoid USP)

Immunizing Agent, Passive—a biological product containing antibodies against a pathologic microorganism, used to provide immediate but temporary protection against infection with the microorganism. (Tetanus Antitoxin USP)

Immunosuppressive—a drug that inhibits immune response to foreign materials, useful in suppressing rejection of homografts (organ transplants). (Azathioprine USP)

Ion-Exchange Resin—an ion-containing solid resin which, when perfused with an ion-containing solution, gives up its ions in exchange for those in solution. (Sodium Polystyrene Sulfonate USP, sodium-potassium exchanger)

Irritant, Local—a drug that reacts weakly and nonspecifically with biological tissue, used topically to induce a mild inflammatory response. (Camphor NF)

Keratolytic—a topical drug that softens the superficial keratin-containing layer of the skin and promotes its desquamation. (Salicylic Acid USP)

Leprostatic—a drug that kills or inhibits the pathogenic bacterium *Mycobacterium leprae,* causative agent of leprosy. (Dapsone USP)

Mineralocorticoid—a salt-regulating adrenocortical steroid (q.v.), useful in regulating sodium/potassium electrolyte balance. (Desoxycorticosterone Acetate Pellets NF)

Metal Complexing Agent—a drug that binds certain metals tightly, removing them from ionic solution, useful in treating poisoning with the metal. (Edetate Calcium Disodium USP, complexing agent for lead)

Mucolytic—a drug that hydrolyses mucoproteins, useful in reducing the viscosity of pulmonary mucous. (Acetylcysteine NF)

Narcotic—a drug that induces its pharmacologic action by reacting with central nervous system receptors that respond to morphine, or a drug legally classified as a narcotic with regard to prescribing regulations.

Oxytoxic—a drug that stimulates uterine motility, useful in obstetrics to initiate labor or to control postpartum hemorrhage. (Oxytocin USP)

Parasiticide—a drug that kills or inhibits invertebrate parasites, especially those that infest the skin or hair follicles. (Sublimed Sulfur NF)

Pediculicide—an insecticide suitable for eradicating louse infestations of humans (pediculosis). (Gamma Benzene Hexachloride USP)

Pigmenting Agent—a drug that promotes skin darkening by increasing melanin synthesis, used to promote repigmentation or to increase tolerance to solar exposure. (Trioxsalen USP, oral pigmenting agent; Methoxsalen USP, topical pigmenting agent)

Potentiator—an adjunctive drug that enhances the action of a primary drug, the total response being greater than the sum of the individual actions. (Hexafluorenium Bromide NF, potentiator for Succinylcholine)

Progestin—a hormone that stimulates the secretory phase of the uterine cycle. (Dydrogesterone NF)

Protectant—a topical drug that serves as a physical barrier to the environment. (Zinc Gelatin USP, skin protectant; Methylcellulose USP, ophthalmic protectant)

Proteolytic—an enzyme that hydrolyzes protein, useful in digesting necrotic and other proteinaceous material. (Trypsin Crystallized NF)

Prothrombogenic—a drug with vitamin K activity, useful in treating vitamin K deficiency (or overdosage with vitamin K antagonist) and associated symptoms such as hypoprothrombinemia. (Phytonadione USP)

Relaxant, Skeletal Muscle—a drug that inhibits contraction of voluntary muscles, usually by interfering with innervation. (Tubocurarine C1 USP)

Relaxant, Smooth Muscle—a drug that inhibits contraction of involuntary (visceral) muscles usually by action on their contractile elements. (Aminophylline USP)

Repellant, Arthropod—an agent applied to the skin or clothing to ward off insects and other members of the phylum *Arthropoda*. (Diethyltoluamide NF)

Rubefacient—a topical drug that induces mild irritation with erythema of the skin, sometimes used as a toughening agent. (Rubbing Alcohol NF)

Scabicide—an insecticide suitable for topical use on humans to eradicate the itch mite *Sarcoptes scabiei* (scabies). (Gamma Benzene Hexachloride USP)

Sclerosing Agent—an irritant drug suitable for injection into varicose veins to induce their fibrosis and obliteration. (Morrhuate Sodium Injection NF)

Sedative—a central nervous system depressant which, in suitable dosage, induces mild relaxation and reduces emotional tension. (Phenobarbital USP)

Specific—a drug peculiarly adpated to its indicated use, usually because of unique functional relationship between drug mechanism and pathologic condition. (Methysergide Maleate USP, specific analgesic for migraine)

Stimulant, Central—a drug that increases the general functional state of the central nervous system, sometimes used in convulsive therapy of mental disorders, or as antidote for barbiturate overdosage. (Flurothyl NF, convulsant)

Stimulant, Respiratory—a drug that selectively stimulates respiration, either by peripheral initiation of respiratory reflexes, or by selective central nervous system stimulation. (Carbon Dioxide USP, reflex respiratory stimulant; Ethamivan NF, central respiratory stimulant)

Sun Screening Agent—a skin protectant (q.v.) that absorbs light energy at the wavelengths that cause sunburn. (Aminobenzoic Acid USP)

Suppressant—a drug that inhibits the progress of a disease but does not cure it. (Colchicine USP, suppressant for gout)

Systemically Acting Drug—a drug administered for absorption into systemic circulation, from which the drug diffuses into all tissues including the site of therapeutic action.

Thyroid Inhibitor (or Suppressant)—a drug that reduces thyroid hormone production, either by inhibiting hormone synthesis or by destroying thyroid tissue. (Methimazole USP, thyroid hormone synthesis inhibitor)

Topically Acting Drug—a drug applied to the body surface for local therapeutic action without drug absorption into systemic circulation.

Tranquilizer—a psychotherapeutic drug that induces emotional repose without significant sedation. (Chlorpromazine USP)

Tuberculostatic—a drug that kills or inhibits the pathogenic bacterium *Mycobacterium tuberculosis*, causative agent of tuberculosis. (Isoniazid USP)

Uricosuric—a drug that promotes renal excretion of uric acid, useful in treating gout. (Probenecid USP)

Vasodilator, Coronary—a drug that widens blood vessels in the heart and improves coronary blood flow, useful in treating angina pectoris; an anti-anginal drug (q.v.). (Amyl Nitrite NF)

Vasodilator, Peripheral—a drug that widens peripheral blood vessels and improves blood flow to the extremities of the body. (Nylidrin NF)

Vasopressor—an adrenergic drug (q.v.) administered systemically to constrict arterioles and elevate arterial blood pressure. (Levarterenol Bitartrate USP)

Vitamin—an organic chemical essential in small amounts for normal body metabolism, used therapeutically to supplement the vitamin content of foods. (Niacinamide USP, enzyme co-factor)

Xanthine Oxidase Inhibitor—a drug that inhibits the enzyme xanthine oxidase, the therapeutic effect of which is inhibition of uric acid synthesis, useful in treating gout. (Allopurinol USP)

Nomograms for Calculating Body Surface Area

NOMOGRAMS FOR CALCULATING BODY SURFACE AREA*

Nomogram for Calculating the Body Surface Area of Children[1]

Nomogram for Calculating the Body Surface Area of Adults[1]

1) From the formula of DuBois and DuBois, Arch. intern. Med., 17, 863, 1916: $S = W^{0.425} \times H^{0.725} \times 71.84$, or log $S = 0.425$ log $W + 0.725$ log $H + 1.8564$, where S = body surface area in square centimeters, W = weight in kilograms, H = height in centimeters.

*From *Documenta Geigy Scientific Tables*, 6th ed., pp. 632–633. By permission of J. R. Geigy S.A.

Pharmaceutical Systems and Techniques of Measurement

the methods of applying these systems in pharmaceutical measurement.

Systems of Pharmaceutical Measurement

In pharmacy today, three systems of measurement have common application. They are the *metric system*, the *apothecary system*, and the *avoirdupois system*. The metric and apothecary systems include units of weight and volume measure with the metric system additionally having units of linear measure. The pharmacist utilizes these systems in his pharmaceutical measurements. The avoirdupois system is the common commercial system of weight used in the United States that is slowly being replaced by the metric system. The avoirdupois system is used by the pharmacist in his purchase of bulk chemicals and commercial packages from manufacturers.

The Metric System

The metric system is the most widely used system in pharmacy. It is the system used by the official compendia and in the labeling of most of the commercial pharmaceutical products. Most of the prescriptions and medication orders written today are in the metric system.

In the metric system, the *gram* is the main unit of weight, the *liter* the main unit of volume, and the *meter* the main unit of length. Subunits and multiples of these basic units are indicated by the following prefix notations:

nano—used to denote one billionth (10^{-9}) of the basic unit

micro—used to denote one millionth of the basic unit

milli—used to denote one thousandth of the basic unit

centi—used to denote one hundredth of the basic unit

deci—used to denote one tenth of the basic unit

deka—used to denote 10 times the basic unit

hekto—used to denote 100 times the basic unit

kilo—used to denote 1000 times the basic unit

myria—used to denote 10,000 times the basic unit

The "metric weight scale" on page 389 is intended to depict the relationship between the

The pharmacist's knowledge and application of accurate pharmaceutical measurement is essential to his practice of pharmacy. Whether practicing in the community or institutional pharmacy or in the large industrial pharmaceutical manufacturing firm, accuracy of measurement is a prime requisite in the preparation of medications.

Pharmaceuticals prepared industrially pass numerous inspections and assays during the course of their manufacture to ensure conformance to standards of quality and quantity. However, prescriptions and medication orders filled extemporaneously in the community and institutional pharmacy usually lack the advantage of such control by assay, and the pharmacist must be absolutely certain that his calculations and measurements are accurate. He should double check his work, and when possible he should have a colleague do the same. An error in the placement of a decimal point, for instance, represents an error of a *minimum* factor of ten, as an overdose or an underdose.

The student must have a working knowledge of the systems of pharmaceutical measurement as presented in this appendix, including factors of conversion between the systems used, and

METRIC WEIGHT SCALE

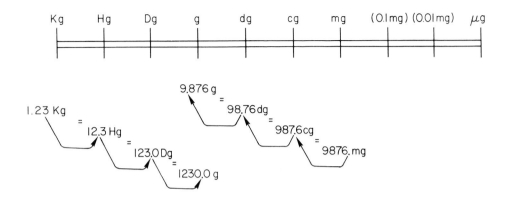

DECIMAL MOVEMENT

◉► TO CONVERT FROM LARGER TO SMALLER UNITS
◄◉ TO CONVERT FROM SMALLER TO LARGER UNITS

units of weight in the metric system and to provide an example of an easy method of converting from one unit to another. In the example, 1.23 kilograms (kg) are to be converted to grams (g). On the scale, the gram position is three decimal positions from the kilogram position. Thus, the decimal point is moved three places toward the right. In the other example, the conversion from milligrams (mg) to grams also requires the movement of the decimal point three places, but this time to the left. The same method may be used to convert metric units of volume or length.

Table of Metric Weight:

1 kilogram (Kg or kg)   = 1000.000 grams
1 hektogram (Hg or hg)   =   100.000 grams
1 dekagram (Dg or dg)   =   10.000 grams
1 gram (Gm, gm or g)   =   1.000 gram
1 decigram (dg)   =   0.100 gram
1 centigram (cg)   =   0.010 gram
1 milligram (mg)   =   0.001 gram
1 microgram (μg or mcg) = 0.000,001 gram
1 nanogram (ng)   = 0.000,000,001 gram

or

1 gram = 0.001 kilogram
          = 0.010 hektogram
          = 0.100 dekagram
          = 10 decigram
          = 100 centigram
          = 1000 milligram
          = 1,000,000 microgram
          = 1,000,000,000 nanograms

Table of Metric Volume:

1 kiloliter (Kl or kl)   = 1000.000 liters
1 hektoliter (Hl or hl) =   100.000 liters
1 dekaliter (Dl)   =   10.000 liters
1 liter (L or l)   =   1.000 liter
1 deciliter (dl)   =   0.100 liter
1 centiliter (cl)   =   0.010 liter
1 milliliter (ml)   =   0.001 liter
1 microliter (μl)   = 0.000,001 liter

or

1 liter = 0.001 kiloliter
         = 0.010 hektoliter
         = 0.100 dekaliter
         = 10 deciliters
         = 100 centiliters
         = 1000 milliliters
         = 1,000,000 microliters

Table of Metric Length:

1 kilometer (Km or km) = 1000.000 meters
1 hektometer (Hm)   =   100.000 meters
1 dekameter (Dm)   =   10.000 meters
1 meter (M or m)   =   1.000 meter
1 decimeter (dm)   =   0.100 meter
1 centimeter (cm)   =   0.010 meter
1 millimeter (mm)   =   0.001 meter
1 micrometer (μm)   = 0.000,001 meter
1 nanometer (nm)   = 0.000,000,001 meter

or

1 meter = 0.001 kilometer
       = 0.010 hektometer
       = 0.100 dekameter
       = 10 decimeters
       = 100 centimeters
       = 1000 millimeters
       = 1,000,000 micrometers
       = 1,000,000,000 nanometers

The Apothecary System

The apothecary system provides for the measurement of both weight and volume. The tables of the system are presented below.

TABLES OF APOTHECARY SYSTEM

Table of Apothecaries' Fluid Measure:

60 minims (♏)	= 1 fluidrachm (f℥ or ℥)*
8 fluidrachms (480 minims)	= 1 fluidounce (f℥ or ℥)*
16 fluidounces	= 1 pint (pt or 0)
2 pints (32 fluidounces)	= 1 quart (qt)
4 quarts (8 pints)	= 1 gallon (gal or C)

Table of Apothecaries' Measure of Weight:

20 grains (gr)	=1 scruple (℈)
3 scruples (60 grains)	=1 dram (℥)
8 dram (480 grains)	=1 ounce (℥)
12 ounces (5760 grains)	=1 pound (℔)

* When there is no doubt that the material referred to is a liquid, the *f* is usually omitted from this symbol. *Dram* is also spelled *drachm.*

The Avoirdupois System

The avoirdupois system is used in commerce generally in the supplying of drugs, chemicals, and other materials by weight. The pharmacist who purchases bulk or prepackaged amounts of chemicals, as sodium bicarbonate powder or epsom salts, purchases them in the avoirdupois system. When he resells them "over the counter" in their original packages, he likewise sells them in the avoirdupois system. The "grain" in each of the apothecary and avoirdupois systems are equivalent. The other units (ounce and pound) are of different weights. It should also be noted that the symbols for the ounce and pound are different in the two systems.

TABLE OF AVOIRDUPOIS MEASURE OF WEIGHT

437.5 grains (gr)	= 1 ounce (oz)
16 ounces (7000 grains)	= 1 pound (lb)

Intersystem Conversion

It is sometimes advantageous or convenient for the pharmacist to convert the weight, volume, or dimensions of length from one system to another. Depending upon the circumstances and requirements of accuracy, conversion equivalents of different exactness may be used. The following is a table of those equivalents commonly used in prescription practice. They are not the exact equivalents, but are over 99% accurate and suffice nicely for most pharmaceutical measurements. Exact equivalents may be found in the USP.

Conversion Equivalents of Weight

1 g	= 15.432 gr
1 Kg	= 2.2 Avoirdupois lb
1 gr	= 0.0648 g or 64.8 or 65 mg
1 ℥	= 31.1 g
1 oz (Avoir)	= 28.35 g
1 ℔ (Apoth)	= 373.2 g
1 lb (Avoir)	= 453.6 or 454 g

Conversion Equivalents of Volume

1 ml	= 16.23 minims
1 minim	= 0.06 ml
1 f℥	= 3.69 ml
1 f℥	= 29.57 ml
1 pt	= 473 ml
1 gal (U.S.)	= 3785 ml
1 gal (British Imperial)	= 4546 ml

Conversion Equivalents of Length

1 inch	= 2.54 cm
1 meter	= 39.37 inches

Approximate Dose Equivalents

Oftentimes in communicating medication information to one another, health professionals may utilize "approximate equivalents." For instance, in ordering commercially prepared tablets, a physician may indicate "60 mg tablets." The pharmacist may find the commercial tablets labeled to contain "65 mg" or "1 gr." According to the Food and Drug Administration, when such prepared dosage forms are prescribed in the metric system, the pharmacist may dispense the corresponding "approximate dose equivalent" in the apothecary system, and vice versa, for drugs prescribed in the apothecaries' system.

The approximate or prescribing equivalents are not intended for use by the pharmacist in his calculations involving the compounding of prescriptions or the manufacture of pharmaceutical products.

Among the approximate dose equivalents listed in the *United States Pharmacopeia* are the following:

Liquid Measure

1000 ml = 1 quart
500 ml = 1 pint
30 ml = 1 fluidounce
4 ml = 1 fluid dram
1 ml = 15 minims
0.06 ml = 1 minim

Weight

30 g   = 1 Apothecary ounce
1 g   = 15 grains
60 mg = 1 grain
30 mg = $\frac{1}{2}$ grain
15 mg = $\frac{1}{4}$ grain
1 mg = $\frac{1}{60}$ grain
0.6 gm = $\frac{1}{100}$ grain
0.4 mg = $\frac{1}{150}$ grain

Common Household Measure

Liquid and powdered medications which are not packaged in unit dose systems are usually measured at home by the patient with common household measuring devices as the teaspoon, tablespoon, and various cooking measure utensils. Although the household teaspoon may vary in volume capacity from approximately 3 to 8 ml, the American Standard Teaspoon has been established as having a volume of 4.93 ± 0.24 ml by the American Standards Association. For practical purposes, most pharmacy practitioners and pharmacy references utilize 5 ml as the capacity of the teaspoon. This is approximately equivalent to $1\frac{1}{3}$ fluid drams although physicians commonly utilize the dram symbol (ʒ) to indicate a teaspoonful in their prescription directions to be transcribed by the pharmacist to the patient. The tablespoon is considered to have a capacity of 15 ml, equivalent to three teaspoonfuls or approximately one-half fluid ounce.

Occasionally the pharmacist will dispense a special medicinal spoon which the patient may use in measuring this medication. These spoons are available in half-teaspoon, teaspoon, and tablespoon capacities. Some manufacturers provide specially designed devices to be used by the patient in measuring his medication. These include specially calibrated droppers, measuring wells or tubes, and calibrated bottle caps. In health care institutions, disposable measuring cups are commonly employed in administering liquid medication (Fig. A-1).

Weighing and The Prescription Balance

In weighing materials, the selection of the instrument to use is based on the amount of material involved and the accuracy desired. In the large scale manufacture of pharmaceuticals, large industrial *scales* of varying capacity and sensitivity are employed, and later, highly sensitive analytical balances are utilized in the quality control and analytical work.

In the hospital and community pharmacy, most weighings are made on the *prescription balance*. Two examples of these balances are shown in Figure A-2. Prescription balances are divided into two classes, *Class A* and *Class B* prescription balances, which meet the prescribed standards of the National Bureau of Standards. Every prescription department is required by law to have a Class A prescription balance, which is the more sensitive of the two. The sensitivity of a balance is usually represented by the term *sensitivity requirement* (SR) which is defined as the maximum change in load that will cause a specified change in the position of rest of the indicating element(s) of the balance.[1] A Class A balance has a SR of 6 mg with no load as well as with 10 g on each pan. This means that under the above conditions, the addition of 6 mg of weight to one pan of the balance will disturb the equilibrium and move

[1] The *sensitivity requirement* (SR) of a balance is determined in the following manner: (1) level the balance, (2) determine the rest point, (3) place a 6-mg weight on one of the empty pans, (4) the rest point is shifted *not less than* one division on the index plate. The entire operation is repeated with a 10-g weight placed in the center of each balance pan.

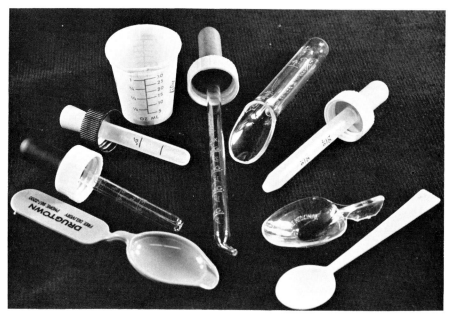

Fig. A-1. *Examples of medicinal spoons of various shapes and capacities, calibrated medicine droppers, an oral medication tube, and a disposable medication cup.*

the balance pointer one division marking on the scale.

The official compendia direct that to avoid errors in weighing of 5% or greater, which may be due to the limits of accuracy of the Class A prescription balance, one must weigh a minimum of 120 mg (approximately 2 grains) of any material in each weighing (5% of 120 mg being the 6 mg SR or error inherent with the balance). If a smaller weight of material is desired, it is directed that the pharmacist mix a larger, calculated weight of the ingredient (120 mg or over), dilute it with a known weight of an inert dry diluent (as lactose), mix the two uniformly,

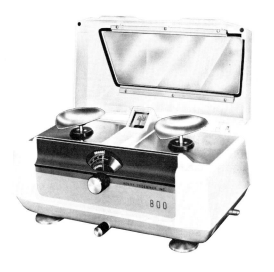

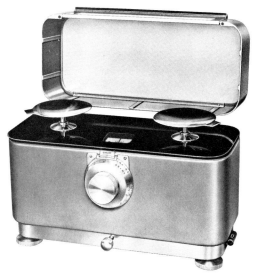

Fig. A-2. *Examples of commonly used Class A prescription balances. On left is the Troemner Model 800 Prescription Balance (Courtesy of Henry Troemner, Inc.); on right, the Model DRX2 Torsion balance (Courtesy of Torsion Balance Company).*

and weigh an aliquot portion of the mixture (again 120 mg or over) calculated to contain the desired amount of agent. The Class A balance which has a capacity of 120 g should be used for all weighings required in prescription compounding.

The Class B prescription balance has a SR of 30 mg and a 120 g capacity. It must not be used for weighing loads of less than 600 mg. Both the Class A and Class B balance must be distinctively marked as to its class on the balance itself. The Class B balance is only rarely found and used in pharmacies.

Weights

Pharmacies usually have two sets of weights for use, one metric set and one apothecary set. Some commercial sets contain both systems of weights in a single container. Prescription weights meet the National Bureau of Standards' specifications for analytical weights. Metric weights of 1 g and greater, and apothecaries' weights of 1 scruple and greater, are generally conical in shape with a narrow neck and head which allows them to be easily grasped and picked up with a small forceps. Most of these weights are made of polished brass, with some coated with nickel or chromium or other materials to resist corrosion. Fractional gram weights are made of aluminum and are generally square-shaped and flat with one raised end or corner for picking up with the forceps. Apothecaries' weights of one-half scruple are frequently coin-shaped brass and those of 5 grains and less are usually bent aluminum wires, with each straight side representing 1 grain of weight. The half-grain weight is usually a smaller gauge wire bent in half.

To prevent the deposit of moisture and oils from the fingertips being deposited on the weights, all weights should be transferred with the forceps provided in each weight set.

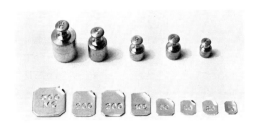

Fig. A-3. *Examples of some metric weights, showing their shape and markings.*

Care and Use of a Prescription Balance

First and foremost, the prescription balance should be located in a well-lighted location, placed on a firm level counter approximately waist-high to the operator. The area should be as free from dust as is possible and in an area that is draft-free. There should be no corrosive vapors present nor high humidity or vibration. When not in use, the balance should be clean and covered with the balance cover. Any agent spilled on the balance during use should be wiped off immediately with a soft brush or cloth. When not in use, the balance should always be maintained with the weights off and the beam in the fixed or locked (arrested) position.

Before weighing an article, the balance must be made level. This is accomplished with the leveling screws on the bottom of the balance, according to the instructional materials accompanying the balance. The balance should be level, front-to-back and side-to-side, as indicated by the leveling bubble of the balance.

In using a prescription balance, neither the weights nor the substance to be weighed should be placed on the balance while the beam is in the *un*arrested position and free to oscillate. Before weighing, powder papers of equal size should be placed on both pans of the balance and the equilibrium of the balance tested by releasing the arresting knob. If the balance is unbalanced due to differences in the weight of the powder papers, additional weight may be added to the "light pan" by adding small tearings of powder papers. When balanced, the balance is placed in the arrested position and the desired weight added to the right-hand pan. Then, an amount of substance, considered to be approximately the desired weight, is carefully placed on the left hand pan, with the assistance of a spatula. The beam should then be slowly released by means of the locking device in the front of the balance. If the substance is in excess, the beam is fixed again and a small portion of the substance removed with the spatula. The process is continued until the two pans balance, as indicated by central position of the balance pointer. If the amount of weight on the balance is initially too little, the reverse process is undertaken. The powder paper used on the left hand pan, intended to hold the substance to be weighed, is usually folded either diagonally or with the edges of the sides folded upwards to contain the material being weighed.

In transferring material by spatula, the material may be lightly tapped from the spatula when the correct amount to be measured is approached. Usually this is done by holding the spatula with a small amount of material on it in the right hand, and tapping the spatula with the forefinger. As material comes off the spatula, the left hand is working the balance arresting mechanism and the status of the weight observed alternately with the tappings of the spatula. Most balances have a "damping" mechanism which slows down the balance oscillations and permits more rapid determinations of the balance or imbalance positions of the pans.

Once the material has been weighed, the balance beam is again put in the fixed position and the paper holding the weighed substance carefully removed. If more than a single weighing is to be performed, the paper is usually marked with the name of the substance it holds. After the final weighing, all weights are removed with the forceps and the balance cleaned, closed, and the balance cover placed over the balance.

Most prescription balances contain built-in mechanisms whereby external weights are not required for weighings under 1 gram. Some balances utilize a rider, which may be shifted from the zero position toward the right side of the balance to add increments of weight marked on the scale in 10-mg units, up to 1 gram. Another type of balance uses a centrally located dial, calibrated in 10-mg units, to add weight up to 1 gram. Both types of devices add the weight internally to the right-hand pan. In each case, the pharmacist may use a combination of the internal weights and external weights in his weighings. For instance, if 1.2 g are to be weighed, the pharmacist can place a 1-g weight on the right hand pan and place the rider or adjust the dial to add 0.2 g additionally. Care must always be exercised to bring the rider or dial to zero between weighings to avoid the inadvertent weighing of rider- or dial-amounts on subsequent weighings.

Most weighings on the prescription balance involve the weighing of powders or semisolid materials, as ointments. However, liquids may also be weighed through the use of tared (weighed) vessels of appropriate size, by placing the liquid inside of the vessel. The pharmacist must always be certain that he has accounted for the weight of the vessel in calculating the amount of liquid weighed.

Materials should never be "downweighed;" that is, substances should never be placed on the pan with the balance in the unarrested position forcing the pan to drop suddenly and forcefully as the excess material is placed on it. The sudden slamming down of the pan can do serious damage to the balance, affecting its sensitivity and the accuracy of subsequent weighings.

The two most popular types of prescription balances are the compound lever balance and the torsion balance. The former type operates through the use of a series of knife edges held in delicate contact and suspension. The torsion type operates on the tension of taut wires, which when twisted through the addition of weight, tend to twist back to the original balance position. The compound lever principle is the basis for the Troemner balance and the torsion principle is applied in the Torsion Balance (Fig. A-2).

Measuring Volume

The common instruments for pharmaceutical measurement are presented in Figure A-4. Two types of graduates are used in pharmacy, those which are *conical* in shape and those which are *cylindrical*. Cylindrical graduates are generally calibrated in metric units, whereas conical graduates may be graduated in both the metric and apothecaries' units (dual scale) or with a single scale of either of the systems. Graduates of both shapes are available in a wide variety of capacities, ranging from 5 to 1000 ml or more. Most graduates in use are made of a good quality, heat-treated glass, although graduates of polypropylene are also available. In measuring small volumes of liquids, as less than 1.5 ml, the pharmacist should utilize a pipet as the one shown in Figure A-4. The bulb-like device shown with the pipet is a pipet filler, used for drawing acids or other toxic solutions into the pipet without the necessity of using the mouth. The device, without being removed from the pipet, also allows for the accurate delivery of the liquid.

In measuring volumes of liquids, the pharmacist should select the measuring device most appropriate to the volume of liquid to be measured and the degree of accuracy desired. It should be recognized that in measuring liquids, the more narrow the column of liquid, the more accurate is likely to be the measurement. Figure

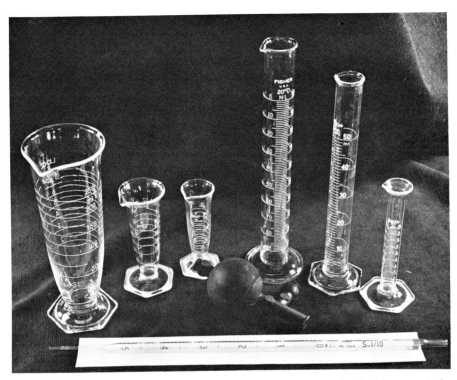

Fig. A-4. *Typical equipment for the pharmaceutical measurement of volume. On the left are conical graduates and on the right, cylindrical graduates. In the front is a pipet for the measurement of small volumes. Behind the pipet is a pipet filler, used instead of the mouth to draw acids and other dangerous liquids into the pipet.*

A-5 demonstrates this point. A reading error of the same dimension will produce a small volume-error when using a pipet, a greater volume-error when using a cylindrical graduate,

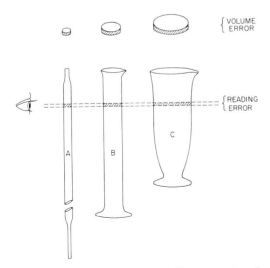

Fig. A-5. *Drawing showing the difference in the volume-error occurring with the same reading-error in measuring devices of different diameters.*

and the greatest volume-error when using a conical graduate. The greater the flair in the design of the conical graduate, the greater is the volume-error due to an error in reading.

In reading the level of liquid in a graduate, it is important to recognize the error which could result due to the error of parallax. Figure A-6 depicts this point. A liquid in a graduate tends to be drawn to the inner surface of the graduate and rises slightly against that surface and above its true meniscus. If one measured looking downward, it would appear as though the meniscus of the liquid is at this upper level, whereas it is slightly lower, at the actual level of the liquid within the center of the graduate. Thus, measurements of liquids in graduates should be taken with the eyesight level with the liquid in the graduate.

If a pharmacist was in error in his reading of a graduate, the *percentage of error* of his measurement would be affected by the volume of liquid that he was measuring. According to the *National Formulary*, an acceptable 10-ml graduate cylinder with an internal diameter of 1.18 cm contains 0.109 ml of liquid in each

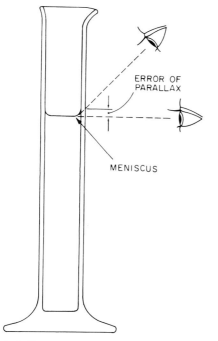

ERROR OF
PARALLAX

MENISCUS

Fig. A-6. *Drawing depicting the error in the reading of the meniscus of a liquid in a graduate cylinder when the reading is made from above the level of the liquid rather than at the same level.*

1 mm of column. A reading error of 1 mm in magnitude would cause a percentage error in the measurement of only 1.09% when 10 ml were being measured, 2.18% when 5 ml were being measured, 4.36% when 2.5 ml were being measured, and 7.26% when 1.5 ml were being measured. It is apparent that the greatest percentage error occurs when the smallest amount is being measured. Thus, the rule of thumb for measuring liquids in graduates is that a graduate should be used having a capacity *equal to or just exceeding* the volume to be measured.

According to Goldstein and Mattocks,[1] based

---

[1] Goldstein, S. W. and Mattocks, A. M.: How to Measure Accurately, *Journal of the American Pharmaceutical Association*, 12:421, 1951.

on a deviation of 1 mm from the mark and an allowable error of 2.5%, the smallest amounts that should be measured in the following size cylindrical graduates having the stated internal diameters are as follows:

Graduate Cylinder Size	Internal Diameter	Deviation in Actual Volume	Minimum Volume Measurable
5 ml	0.98 cm	0.075 ml	3.00 ml
10 ml	1.18 cm	0.109 ml	4.36 ml
25 ml	1.94 cm	0.296 ml	11.84 ml
50 ml	2.24 cm	0.394 ml	15.76 ml
100 ml	2.58 cm	0.522 ml	20.88 ml

For a 5% error, the minimum volumes measurable would be one-half of those stated. It is apparent that for accuracy, one should not select a graduate for use when the measurement involves utilization of only the bottom portion of the scale.

In using graduates, the pharmacist pours the liquid into the graduate slowly, observing the level as he proceeds. In measuring viscous liquids, adequate time must be allowed for the liquid to settle in the graduate, as some may run slowly down the innersides of the graduate. It is best to attempt to pour such liquids toward the center of the graduate, avoiding contact with the sides. In emptying the graduate of its measured contents, adequate drain time should be allowed.

When pouring liquids from bottles, it is considered good pharmaceutical technique to keep the label on the bottle facing upwards; this avoids the possibility of drops of liquid running down the label as the bottle is righted after use. Naturally, the bottle orifice should be wiped clean after each use.

Index

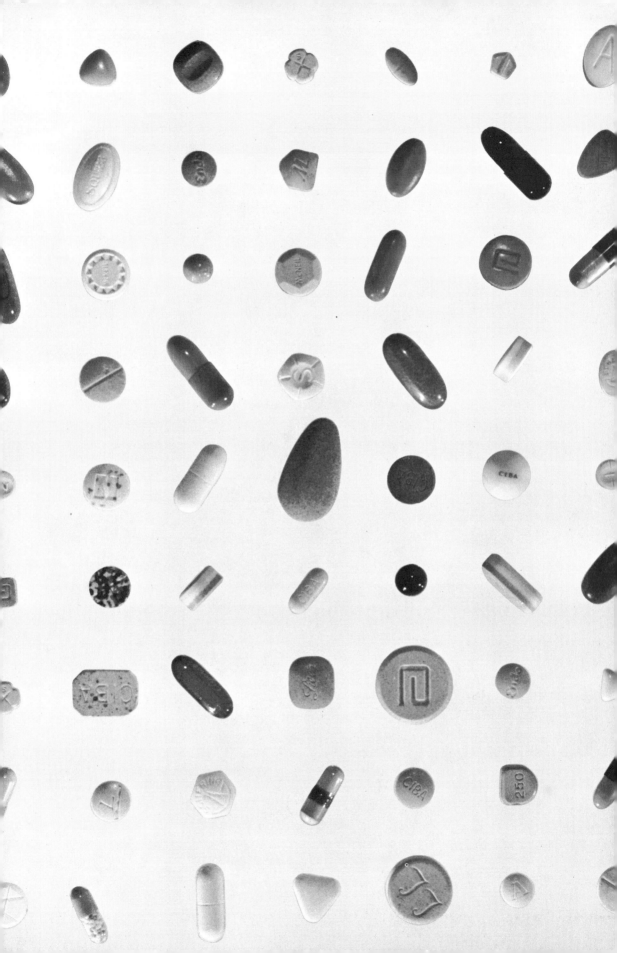